Bethesda Handbook of Clinical Hematology

Second Edition

Provided as an
educational service by
Genentech BioOncology

Genentech
BIO ONCOLOGY™

Translating science into life

Bethesda Handbook of Clinical Hematology

Second Edition

Editors

Griffin P. Rodgers, MD, MACP

Director, National Institute of Diabetes, Digestive, and Kidney Disorders
Chief, Molecular and Clinical Hematology Branch
National Heart, Lung, and Blood Institute
National Institutes of Health
Bethesda, Maryland

Neal S. Young, MD, MACP

Chief, Hematology Branch
National Heart, Lung, and Blood Institute
National Institutes of Health
Bethesda, Maryland

Wolters Kluwer | Lippincott Williams & Wilkins
Health
Philadelphia · Baltimore · New York · London
Buenos Aires · Hong Kong · Sydney · Tokyo

Acquisitions Editor: Jonathan Pine
Managing Editor: Joyce Murphy
Associate Production Manager: Kevin Johnson
Manufacturing Manager: Benjamin Rivera
Marketing Manager: Angela Panetta
Design Coordinator: Doug Smock
Production Service: Maryland Composition/ASI

530 Walnut Street
Philadelphia, PA 19106 USA
LWW.com

Printed in China

Library of Congress Cataloging-in-Publication Data

Bethesda handbook of clinical hematology / [edited by] Griffin P. Rodgers, Neal Young. — 2nd ed.
    p. ; cm.
  Includes bibliographical references and index.
  ISBN 978-0-7817-7583-0
  1. Blood—Diseases—Handbooks, manuals, etc. 2. Hematology—Handbooks, manuals, etc. I. Rodgers, Griffin P. II. Young, Neal S. III. Title: Handbook of clinical hematology.
  [DNLM: 1. Hematologic Diseases—Handbooks. WH 39 B562 2009]
  RC633.B49 2009
  616.1′5—dc22

                              2008052574

Care has been taken to confirm the accuracy of the information presented and to describe generally accepted practices. However, the authors, editors, and publisher are not responsible for errors or omissions or for any consequences from application of the information in this book and make no warranty, expressed or implied, with respect to the currency, completeness, or accuracy of the contents of the publication. Application of the information in a particular situation remains the professional responsibility of the practitioner.

The authors, editors, and publisher have exerted every effort to ensure that drug selection and dosage set forth in this text are in accordance with current recommendations and practice at the time of publication. However, in view of ongoing research, changes in government regulations, and the constant flow of information relating to drug therapy and drug reactions, the reader is urged to check the package insert for each drug for any change in indications and dosage and for added warnings and precautions. This is particularly important when the recommended agent is a new or infrequently employed drug.

Some drugs and medical devices presented in the publication have Food and Drug Administration (FDA) clearance for limited use in restricted research settings. It is the responsibility of the health care provider to ascertain the FDA status of each drug or device planned for use in their clinical practice.

To purchase additional copies of this book, call our customer service department at (800) 638-3030 or fax orders to (301) 223-2320. International customers should call (301) 223-2300.

Visit Lippincott Williams & Wilkins on the Internet: at LWW.com. Lippincott Williams & Wilkins customer service representatives are available from 8:30 am to 6 pm, EST.

RRS0902

To our wives, Sherry and Genoveffa

And, for our children, with love:
Chris and Gregory Rodgers
Andrea, Max, and Giorgio Young

Contents

CONTENTS

Preface

Life is short, the art long.

—*Hippocrates* c. 460–357 BC

The accessibility of blood and bone marrow has made hematology, historically, the engine of basic research in internal medicine. Hematology has thrived at the National Institutes of Health because of this close relationship with the research laboratory. Investigators from the various institutes in Bethesda have contributed to the knowledge of blood diseases from the study of individual patients with sometimes rare diseases, and to the development of clinical protocols for the rigorous assessment of diagnostic criteria or treatments, both established and novel. Our hematology fellowship programs have fostered a scientific approach to hematology, not only to assess outcomes but also to advance the experimental basis of our understanding of blood diseases and the application of laboratory insights to their treatment in practice. The collegial relationships among local institutions and individuals in the greater Washington area who share training and patients have greatly furthered these efforts.

Handbooks are intended to be highly accessible, both literally and figuratively. Our Handbook has been designed to be carried in the white coat pocket of the student, resident, and fellow on a hematology or oncology service, and in the briefcase of the internist, hospitalist, family practitioner, and pediatrician, whose practice includes patients with blood diseases. We have purposely combined authors who are recognized experts in their fields with senior fellows who have had current experience learning hematology and caring daily for hematology patients, and encouraged a thoughtful approach to the presentation of the core knowledge using tables, algorithms, meaningful figures, and bulleted text structures. The Handbook is organized according to disease categories and hematological problems of importance to the consulting and treating hematologist, and additional chapters are provided to acquaint the reader with familiar and new laboratory methodologies that underlie modern clinical approaches to diagnosis and treatment.

The appearance of a second edition of the BHOCH is a testimonial to our readers, who have supported our efforts with their kind comments and concrete purchases of the book, more remarkable in an age of internet-based medical information. The Handbook remains focused on providing the practitioner at every level of training practical, authoritative, and current guidance to the diagnosis and treatment of blood diseases and to consultative problems in hematology. All the chapters have been revised and updated. We look forward to your responses to our authors' efforts.

Griffin P. Rodgers, MD, MACP
Neal S. Young, MD, MACP

Disclaimer: This work was not performed as official NIH duties.

Contributors

Jame Abraham, MD, FACP   *Associate Professor of Medicine; Chief, Section of Hematology/Oncology; Medical Director, Mary Babb Randolph Cancer Center; West Virginia University, Morgantown, West Virginia*

Firoozeh Alvandi, MD   *Medical Officer, Food and Drug Administration/ Center for Drug Evaluation and Research, Fairfax, Virginia*

Barbara M. Alving, MD   *Professor of Medicine, Uniformed Services University of Health Sciences, Bethesda, Maryland*

Georg Aue, MD   *Hematology Branch, National Heart, Lung, and Blood Institute, National Institutes of Health, Bethesda, Maryland*

Kristin Baird, MD   *Staff Clinician, National Cancer Institute, National Institutes of Health, Bethesda, Maryland*

John A. Barrett, MD   *Chief, Stem Cell Allotransplantation Section, Hematology Branch, National Heart, Lung, and Blood Institute, National Institutes of Health, Bethesda, Maryland*

Minoo Battiwalla, MD   *Staff Physician, Department of Medicine, Roswell Park Cancer Institute, Buffalo, New York*

Charles D. Bolan, MD   *Professor of Medicine, Uniformed Services University; Staff Clinician, Hematology Branch; National Heart, Lung, and Blood Institute; National Institutes of Health; Bethesda, Maryland*

Richard W. Childs, MD   *Senior Clinical Investigator, Hematology Branch, National Heart, Lung, and Blood Institute, National Institutes of Health, Bethesda, Maryland*

Michael Craig, MD   *Assistant Professor of Medicine, West Virginia University, Morgantown, West Virginia*

Sandeep S. Dave, MD, MS   *Assistant Professor of Medical Oncology, Duke University Medical Center, Durham, North Carolina*

Cynthia E. Dunbar, MD   *Head, Molecular Hematopoiesis Section, Hematology Branch, National Heart, Lung, and Blood Institute, National Institutes of Health, Bethesda, Maryland*

Thomas A. Fleisher, MD   *Chief, Department of Laboratory Medicine, National Institutes of Health, Bethesda, Maryland*

Patrick F. Fogarty, MD   *Associate Clinical Professor of Medicine, Division of Hematology/Oncology, Department of Medicine, University of California, San Francisco, San Francisco, California*

Lukasz P. Gondek, MD, PhD   *Experimental Hematology and Hematopoiesis Section, Cleveland Clinic, Cleveland, Ohio*

Peiman Hematti, MD   *Assistant Professor of Hematology/Oncology, University of Wisconsin-Madison School of Medicine and Public Health, Madison, Wisconsin*

McDonald K. Horne, III, MD   *Senior Clinical Investigator, Department of Laboratory Medicine, W. G. Magnuson Clinical Center, National Institutes of Health, Bethesda, Maryland*

Matthew M. Hsieh, MD   *Staff Clinician, Chief Molecular and Clinical Hematology Branch, National Heart, Lung, and Blood Institute, National Institute of Diabetes and Digestive and Kidney Diseases, National Institutes of Health, Bethesda, Maryland*

Elaine S. Jaffe, MD   *Chief, Hematopathology Section, Laboratory of Pathology, Center for Cancer Research, National Cancer Institute, Bethesda, Maryland*

Craig M. Kessler, MD   *Professor of Pathology, Division of Hematology/ Oncology, Director, Clinical Coagulation Laboratory, Georgetown University Hospital, Washington, DC*

Harvey G. Klein, MD   *Chief, Transfusion of Medicine, Clinical Center, National Institutes of Health, Bethesda, Maryland*

Pallavi P. Kumar, MD   *Instructor in Medicine, Department of Internal Medicine, John Hopkins University, Baltimore, Maryland*

Roger Kurlander, MD   *Staff Clinician, Hematology Service, Clinical Pathology Department, Clinical Center, National Institutes of Health, Bethesda, Maryland*

Susan F. Leitman, MD   *Chief, Blood Services Section, Department of Transfusion Medicine, National Institutes of Health, Bethesda, Maryland*

Steven J. Lemery, MD   *Hematology Branch, National Heart, Lung, and Blood Institute, National Institutes of Health, Bethesda, Maryland*

Richard F. Little, MD, MPH   *Senior Investigator, Head, Hematologic and AIDS-related Cancers and Marrow Transplant Therapeutics Section, Clinical Investigations Branch, Divisions of Cancer Therapy and Diagnosis, National Cancer Institute, National Institutes of Health Clinical Research Center, Bethesda, Maryland*

Johnson M. Liu, MD *Associate Professor of Pediatrics, Albert Einstein College of Medicine; Schneider Children's Hospital, New York, New York*

Jaroslaw P. Maciejewski, MD, PhD *Professor of Medicine, Section Head, Center for Hematology and Oncology Molecular Therapeutics, Cleveland Clinic, Cleveland, Ohio*

Harry L. Malech, MD *Laboratory Chief and Senior Investigator, Laboratory of Host Defenses, National Institutes of Health, Bethesda, Maryland*

Vera Malkovska, MD *Director of Hematology, Washington Cancer Institute at the Washington Hospital Center, Washington, DC*

Jeffery L. Miller, MD *Tenured Investigator, Chief, Section on Molecular Genomics and Therapeutics, Molecular Medicine Branch, National Institutes of Health, Bethesda, Maryland*

Pierre Noel, MD *Chief, Hematology Services, Department of Laboratory Medicine, W. G. Magnuson Clinical Center, National Institutes of Health, Bethesda, Maryland*

Patricia A. Oneal, MD *Assistant Professor of Medicine, Howard University Hospital, Washington, DC*

Antonio M. Risitano, MD, PhD *Research Associate, Department of Hematology, Department of Biochemistry and Biotechnology, Federico II University of Naples, Naples, Italy*

Jamie A. Robyn, MD, PhD *Laboratory of Allergic Diseases, National Institute of Allergy and Infectious Diseases, National Institutes of Health, Bethesda, Maryland*

Griffin P. Rodgers, MD, MACP *Director, National Institute of Diabetes, Digestive, and Kidney Disorders; Chief, Molecular and Clinical Hematology Branch; National Heart, Lung, and Blood Institute; National Institutes of Health, Bethesda, Maryland*

Geraldine P. Schechter, MD *Chief, Hematology Section, Washington VA Medical Center; Professor of Medicine, George Washington University, Washington, DC*

Phillip Scheinberg, MD *Staff Clinician, Hematology Branch, National Heart, Lung, and Blood Institute, National Institutes of Health, Bethesda, Maryland*

Carmine Selleri, MD *Associate Professor of Medicine, Department of Hematology, Department of Biochemistry and Biotechnology, Federico II University of Naples, Naples, Italy*

Aarthi Shenoy, MD *Hematology Branch, National Heart, Lung, and Blood Institute, National Institutes of Health, Bethesda, Maryland*

Elaine M. Sloand, MD   *Senior Clinical Investigator, Department of Hematology, National Heart, Lung, and Blood Institute, National Institutes of Health, Bethesda, Maryland*

Scott R. Solomon, MD   *Blood and Marrow Transplant Group of Georgia, Atlanta, Georgia*

Ramaprasad Srinivasan, MD, PhD   *Staff Clinician, Urologic Oncology Branch, Center for Cancer Research, National Cancer Institute, Bethesda, Maryland*

Louis M. Staudt, MD, PhD   *Head, Molecular Biology of Lymphoid Malignancies Section; Deputy Branch Chief, Metabolism Branch; National Cancer Institute, Bethesda, Maryland*

Vijay S. Suhag, MD   *Attending Physician, Department of Hematology and Oncology, Sutter Auburn Faith Hospital, Auburn, California*

John F. Tisdale, MD   *Senior Investigator, Molecular and Clinical Hematology Branch, National Heart, Lung, and Blood Institute, National Institute of Diabetes and Digestive and Kidney Diseases, National Institutes of Health, Bethesda, Maryland*

Alan S. Wayne, MD   *Clinical Director, Pediatric Oncology Branch, National Cancer Institute; National Institutes of Health, Bethesda, Maryland*

Adrian Wiestner, MD, PhD   *Principal Investigator, Hematology Branch, National Heart, Lung, and Blood Institute, National Institutes of Health, Bethesda, Maryland*

Wyndham H. Wilson, MD, PhD   *Senior Investigator, Center for Cancer Research, National Cancer Institute, Bethesda, Maryland*

Agnes S. M. Yong, MD, PhD   *Senior Research Fellow, Hematology Branch, National Heart, Lung, and Blood Institute, National Institutes of Health, Bethesda, Maryland*

Neal S. Young, MD, MACP   *Chief, Hematology Branch, National Heart, Lung, and Blood Institute, National Institutes of Health, Bethesda, Maryland*

1

Iron Deficiency

McDonald K. Horne, III

Iron deficiency is the most common cause of anemia throughout the world. In the United States roughly 10% of women of childbearing age and young children are depleted of iron (1). Iron deficiency anemia is particularly common in elderly patients, who also have a high frequency of anemia resulting from inadequate utilization of iron stores (2).

ABSOLUTE VERSUS FUNCTIONAL IRON DEFICIENCY

Iron deficiency anemia is caused by:

- a lack of endogenous iron ("absolute" iron deficiency) or
- inadequate utilization of endogenous iron ("functional" iron deficiency).

IRON METABOLISM

Most iron in the body is contained in the hemoglobin of circulating red cells (Fig. 1.1). After senescent erythrocytes are phagocytosed in the reticuloendothelial system (RES), predominantly in the spleen, the majority of their iron is released into the plasma bound to transferrin and returns to supply the marrow (Fig. 1.1). Through this circuit, an average adult reutilizes about 20 mg of iron each day derived from about 20 mL of red cells reaching the end of their life span.

Each transferrin molecule can bind one or two iron atoms, but diferric transferrin is taken up by developing red cells more easily than monoferric transferrin and delivers twice as much iron per molecule (3). Therefore, the concentration of diferric transferrin is critical to the support of erythropoiesis. Basal (i.e., nonanemic, steady state) erythropoiesis requires a serum concentration of diferric transferrin that is achieved when the transferrin saturation is at least ~16% (4).

A relatively small amount of iron is normally lost from the body in epithelial cells sloughed from the skin and gastrointestinal (GI) tract and in red cells lost in menses and in a miniscule amount of normal GI bleeding (5). To balance this loss:

- *Adult males must absorb about 1 mg of iron each day from their diet, and menstruating females require about twice this much.*
- *During pregnancy and periods of rapid growth iron, balance must be positive to support increased production of hemoglobin and myoglobin.*
- *Negative iron balance results from increased loss of iron (nearly always due to bleeding), inadequate dietary intake, and increased utilization of iron (Table 1.1).*

When the need for iron exceeds the dietary intake, iron is mobilized from ferritin stored in the RES. At most 3–4 mg of iron can be absorbed from the diet each day, enough to produce 3 or 4 mL of red cells (5). In contrast, about 40–60 mg of iron can be transferred from ferritin to transferrin per day to produce 40–60 mL of red cells, but this is a maximum (6). No more can be produced unless supplemental (i.e., medicinal) iron is provided.

Dietary iron is present in ferric (Fe^{+3}) salts in meat and vegetables and in heme in meat (5). Heme iron is the most bioavailable because it is soluble at the alkaline pH of the duodenum, where it is

1

Earliest   <u>Causes of misleading results</u>

Reduced RES iron

     Marrow hemosiderin .... Inadequate sample, poor staining

     Serum ferritin .... Inflammation, liver disease

Reduced serum Fe,
     transferrin saturation   Inflammation
Elevated serum transferrin

Elevated serum transferrin receptor .... Erythroid hyperplasia (hemolysis,
                                         megaloblastosis)

Reduced red cell count, hemoglobin .... Inflammation

Elevated RDW
Reduced MCV   .... Inflammation, thalassemia, hemoglobin E,
                                       chronic lead poisoning, hereditary sideroblastic anemia
Latest

FIG. 1.2. Development of laboratory abnormalities during negative iron balance.

FUNCTIONAL IRON DEFICIENCY

Functional iron deficiency is characterized by *hypoferremia despite seemingly adequate or increased iron stores*. It is one of several pathophysiologic processes underlying the anemia that develops in patients with chronic infectious, inflammatory, or neoplastic diseases (14,15). Functional iron deficiency can also occur in patients recovering from absolute iron deficiency if the rate of supply of iron from their stores limits the rate of red cell production (6,16). This situation occurs, for example, when patients begin hemodialysis and start receiving erythropoietin. Although they may have iron stores at the time, their response to erythropoietin is blunted until they are given iron supplements to enhance the flow of iron to the developing red cells.

Characteristically anemia associated with functional iron deficiency is mild and asymptomatic (14,15). Although *usually normocytic, the MCV is often on the low end of normal and may be in the microcytic range. The serum iron concentration and transferrin saturation often suggest absolute iron deficiency, but the transferrin concentration is not elevated and may be low.* Furthermore, there is evidence of storage iron in the form of an *elevated serum ferritin*.

Patients with chronic illnesses, of course, can also have absolute iron deficiency, which can be particularly difficult to diagnose because of the effects of inflammation on the laboratory parameters of iron status. Chronic inflammation, for example, can suppress transferrin and elevate serum ferritin even in the true absence of storage iron (12,15).

The most reliable diagnostic parameter to identify absolute iron deficiency in patients with chronic inflammatory diseases is reported to be *the ratio of serum transferrin receptor concentration (mg/L) to the log of the serum ferritin concentration* (13,17).

TABLE 1.2. *Oral Iron Supplements (Over-the-Counter)*

		Elemental Fe (mg)	AWP of maximum dose per month*
Ferrous Sulfate			
Tablet	325 mg/tablet	65	$3.05
Elixir	220 mg/5 mL	44	$5.56
Ferrous Gluconate	320 mg/tablet	40	$6.49

*Average wholesale price for 3 doses/day (April 2007; Pharmacy Department, W.G. Magnuson Clinical Center, Bethesda, MD).

Because soluble transferrin receptor concentration and ferritin concentration change in opposite directions with iron absolute deficiency, the ratio of the two is especially sensitive to iron status and appears to distinguish patients with anemia of chronic inflammation from patients who have absolute iron deficiency with or without a chronic disease.

TREATMENT OF IRON-DEFICIENCY ANEMIA

Oral Iron Therapy

A daily supplement of ~200 mg of elemental iron taken fasting provides the marrow with enough iron to raise the blood hemoglobin concentration ~0.25 g/dL per day in an otherwise healthy individual (Table 1.2) (18).

Oral iron, however, causes nausea or constipation in some patients. Because these symptoms correlate with the amount of iron ingested, the dose should be lowered until tolerable, or the medication should be stopped altogether until the symptoms resolve and then restarted at a lower dose. Using an elixir of iron allows doses as low as 10–20 mg (1/4 to 1/2 teaspoon), and multivitamins often contain even smaller amounts. Low doses of iron can be therapeutic; the response is just slower (19). Patients should be prescribed stool softeners as needed. Often they can avoid nausea by taking their iron with food. This practice reduces iron absorption, but it usually does not make patients refractory to iron. Ascorbic acid is sometimes given with iron to improve its absorption, although it is doubtful that this enhances the response to the medicinal ferrous salts.

Slow-release formulations of iron are touted to cause fewer gastrointestinal side effects, but they also often contain less iron per dose and are considerably more expensive than the salts in Table 1.2. Furthermore, they may release their iron below the duodenum, too distal for significant absorption.

A variety of medications can reduce oral iron absorption (Table 1.3) and should not be taken within several hours of iron tablets. Conversely, oral iron supplements can hinder the absorption of other medications (Table 1.4).

TABLE 1.3. *Medications and Foods That Reduce Iron Absorption*

Antacids (alkaline liquids, H2-blockers, proton pump inhibitors)
Tetracyclines (especially doxycycline)

Pancreatic enzyme supplements
Biphosphonates

Cholestyramine
Calcium supplements

Tea
Dairy products
Phosphonates (vegetables)

TABLE 1.4. *Medications Malabsorbed*
Because of the Co-administration of Iron

Quinolone antibiotics	Thyroxine
Biphosphonates	Penicillamine
Cefdinir	Mycophenolate mofetil
Levodopa, carbidopa, methyldopa	Zinc or copper salts

Another way to replenish iron is by increasing lean meat intake. Because the heme of meat is so readily absorbed and without gastrointestinal side effects, it is an excellent source of iron. The presence of heme in the diet also increases the absorption of inorganic iron.

Iron supplements should obviously be taken until the anemia resolves, which usually only requires a few weeks. To accumulate storage iron, the supplements must be continued for several months because the rate of iron absorption becomes slower once the patient is no longer anemic (20). The serum ferritin can be followed to determine when iron stores are sufficient.

Intravenous Iron Therapy

Other than in patients on hemodialysis, negative iron balance is rarely so marked or so protracted that oral iron supplements are insufficient (Table 1.5). However, when patients cannot tolerate an adequate dose of oral iron, such as during pregnancy, or when they have severe and recurrent gastrointestinal or uterine hemorrhage, parenteral iron may be necessary.

Three formulations of parenteral iron are currently marketed in the United States: iron dextran (DexFerrum [American Regent Laboratories, Shirley, NY], INFeD [Watson Pharma, Corona, CA]), sodium ferric gluconate in sucrose (Ferrlecit [Watson Pharma, Corona, CA]), and iron sucrose (Venofer [American Regent Laboratories, Shirley, NY]) (21,22). Whereas the U.S. Food and Drug Administration (FDA) has approved iron dextran for replacement of iron whenever the parenteral route is preferred, the FDA's indications for the two newer preparations are limited to the treatment of absolute or functional iron deficiency associated with renal disease. However, the relative safety of these agents argues for their use in other settings as well. Iron dextran has been associated with serious adverse reactions in 2% to 3% of patients, including rare deaths. Although ferric gluconate has only been available in the United States since 1999 and iron sucrose since 2000, a longer experience in Europe has indicated that serious adverse reactions associated with these agents are rare. No deaths have been reported. Because of this safety record, test doses are not required for ferric gluconate or iron sucrose. Dosing regimens approved by the FDA for patients with renal disease are shown in Table 1.5. The only disadvantage to the newer agents is that the total amount of iron indicated must be given in divided doses every 2 or 3 days to avoid acute toxic effects from the iron.

TABLE 1.5. *Intravenous Iron Supplements*

	FDA-Approved Dosing for Renal Patients	AWP per Dose*
Ferric gluconate complex in sucrose (Ferrlecit™: 12.5 mg/mL Fe)	125 mg Fe in 10 mL over at least 10 minutes or same dose plus 90 mL 0.9% sodium chloride over 1 hour	$86
Iron sucrose (Venofer™: 20 mg/mL Fe)	100 mg Fe in 5 mL into hemodialysis line over 2–5 minutes or same dose plus 95 mL 0.9% sodium chloride over at least 15 minutes	$69

*Average wholesale price (April 2007; Pharmacy Department, W.G. Magnuson Clinical Center, Bethesda, MD).

RESPONSE TO IRON THERAPY

When iron therapy is given orally in full doses or parenterally to otherwise healthy individuals,

- within *3 or 4 days* peripheral blood *reticulocytes* increase, and
- within *the first week* the *hemoglobin* begins to rise.

A failure to observe a rise in hemoglobin after 1 to 2 weeks suggests several problems: an incorrect diagnosis of iron deficiency, continued bleeding (in which case reticulocytes will increase despite no improvement in the anemia), noncompliance with the therapy, and iron malabsorption.

A patient can be tested for iron malabsorption by measuring his serum iron concentration immediately before and 2 to 4 hours after taking his usual dose of iron in his usual fasting or nonfasting state (23). Although this test is not standardized and can yield misleading results if the post sample is not drawn at the optimal time, it can be helpful when the serum iron clearly rises into the normal range.

TREATING THE ANEMIA OF FUNCTIONAL IRON DEFICIENCY

The only truly satisfactory solution to functional iron deficiency is adequate treatment of its underlying cause. Although the anemia of functional iron deficiency is typically mild, treatment with iron supplements should be considered if transfusions are required to relieve symptoms. The aim is a hemoglobin level of 10–12 g/dL. Hemoglobin concentrations above this increase the risk of serious cardiovascular and thromboembolic events and mortality and are associated with increased tumor progression in patients with cancer (24,25).

Functional iron deficiency usually occurs together with other pathophysiologic mechanisms, such as erythropoietin deficiency or erythroid suppression by inflammatory cytokines (14). Therefore, iron alone may not correct the anemia, but if the erythroid marrow can be stimulated with pharmacologic doses of erythropoietin at the same time that the iron supply is being enhanced, red cell production may increase (26). In general, the iron supply is adequate for accelerated erythropoiesis if the transferrin saturation is >20% and the serum ferritin is >100 μg/L. Even with the combination of iron and erythropoietin, the hemoglobin may only rise about 0.5–1 g/dL per month.

Patients with functional iron deficiency are more likely to respond to *parenteral* iron than to oral supplements. Some of the iron delivered to macrophages by parenteral injections apparently escapes over the raised hepcidin "fence" surrounding the macrophages. Once this iron returns to the macrophages in the hemoglobin of a phagocytosed red cell, however, it can no longer escape. Although giving both erythropoietin and iron can eliminate the need for red cell transfusions, the effect of this combination on a patient's distribution of iron is the same as that of transfusions: more and more iron accumulates in inaccessible stores.

ADMINISTRATION OF ERYTHROPOIETIN

Indications for the administration of pharmacologic erythropoietin are limited to the treatment of anemia associated with chronic renal failure, human immunodeficiency virus (HIV) infection, and cancer chemotherapy, not the anemia related to cancer itself (Table 1.6). Erythropoietin should not be used before correctable causes of anemia have been excluded, such as bleeding. The FDA has recently stressed the importance of using the lowest dose of erythropoietin that will eliminate the need for transfusions (27). To protect against a potentially hazardous rise in hemoglobin, it is recommended that the hemoglobin concentration be checked twice weekly for 2 to 6 weeks after any increase in dose. Erythropoietin should be withheld if the hemoglobin exceeds 12 g/dL or rises more than 1 g/dL in any 2-week period.

Erythropoietin for injection is a recombinant form (epoetin alfa) that is marketed as two pharmacologically identical products, Epogen (Amgen, Thousand Oaks, CA) and Procrit (Ortho Biotech, Bridgewater, NJ) and formulated in vials of 2000, 3000, 4000, 10,000, 20,000, and 40,000 units. Darbepoietin alfa (Aranesp, Amgen) is the same protein that has been hyperglycosylated to make its circulatory half-life threefold longer than native erythropoietin. Darbopoietin alfa is formulated in vials

TABLE 1.6. *Erythropoietin Regimens for Iron Replete Patients**

	Initial Dose	
	Epoetin alpha	Darbepoetin alpha
Cancer chemotherapy[†]	40,000 units sc once weekly[2]	200 μg sc every 2 weeks[‡]
Anemia of chronic disease	150 units/kg sc 2–3 times per week	
HIV/zidovudine	100 units/kg sc 3 times per week	
(if serum Epo <500 U/L)		
Chronic hemodialysis	50–100 units/kg sc 2–3 times per week	0.45 μg/kg sc once weekly

Dose adjustment: If hemoglobin rises ≥1 g/dL per 2 weeks, reduce dose by 25%.
If hemoglobin rises <1 g/dL by 4 weeks, increase dose by 25% to 50%.

*Goal: maximum hemoglobin 10–12 g/dL.
[†]Practice Guidelines in Oncology, March 2007, National Comprehensive Cancer Network.
[‡]Average wholesale price ~$600 per week (March 2007; Pharmacy Department, W.G. Magnuson Clinical Center, Bethesda, MD).

of 25, 40, 60, 100, 150, 200, 300, and 400 micrograms. One microgram of darbopoietin alfa is approximately equivalent to 200 units of epoetin alfa. In comparable doses, the responses to darbopoietin and epoietin are very similar (28).

Subcutaneous administration of erythropoietin is preferable to intravenous because it requires about one third less drug (29). The prescribed dose should be rounded to the nearest vial size to avoid waste. Erythropoietin was first used to treat the anemia of chronic renal failure, which is largely caused by a deficiency of the hormone, and therefore was traditionally given at the time of hemodialysis two or three times per week. Although this schedule is often used in other settings, it may require otherwise unnecessary trips to a medical facility. Therefore, a quest for convenience drove the development of a weekly regimen of 40,000–60,000 units for cancer patients with chemotherapy-related anemia (30).

IRON DEFICIENCY IN PATIENTS WITH ADVANCED MALIGNANCY

Absolute iron deficiency is always a risk in patients with advanced malignancies and is likely to respond to oral iron regimens, although the response may be slower than in healthy individuals. Worsening anemia due to the effect of cytotoxic chemotherapy can often be controlled with erythropoietin without supplemental iron, but including parenteral iron appears to be beneficial (31). Oral iron in this setting is usually not effective. The hemoglobin target for erythropoietin treatment should be limited to 10–12 g/dL because there is evidence that higher levels increase the risk of tumor progression and death (26).

ANEMIA ASSOCIATED WITH CHRONIC INFLAMMATORY DISEASES

The anemia of rheumatoid arthritis has been reported to respond to parenteral iron alone, as well as to erythropoietin alone, with elevations of hemoglobin from ~11.5 to ~12.5 g/dL in both instances (32,33). Adding parenteral iron to erythropoietin when the ferritin is less than 50 μg/mL enhances the response, with hemoglobin reaching a median of 13.3 g/dL in one series (34). In inflammatory bowel disease, absolute iron deficiency is common, and the anemia typically responds to iron alone, although parenteral iron is usually required because of gastrointestinal intolerance. Including erythropoietin magnifies the response (35). In contrast, anemic patients with chronic infections, including HIV, should only receive iron if they have absolute iron deficiency because of concern that an increased iron supply will promote the invasion of microorganisms (36,37). Although the anemia of associated with chronic inflammation is usually treated with two or three erythropoietin injections per week, there is no reason to believe that once weekly injections of 40,000 units would not be just as effective.

Before launching treatment, however, the chronic nature of the disease should be considered. Unless the primary disease is controlled, treatment with iron and/or erythropoietin will likely be necessary indefinitely to maintain an elevated hemoglobin level. In the case of erythropoietin, this incurs enormous expense, and in the case of iron there is a risk of adverse events from iron overload. Unfortunately, any increase in red cell mass generated by treatment cannot be sustained if the treatment is discontinued.

REFERENCES

1. Looker AC, Dallman PR, Carroll MD, et al. Prevalence of iron deficiency in the United States. JAMA 1997;277:973–976.
2. Ania BJ, Suman VJ, Fairbanks VF, et al. Incidence of anemia in older people: an epidemiologic study in a well defined population. J Am Geriatr Soc 1997;45:825–831.
3. Huebers HA, Csiba E, Huebers E, et al. Competitive advantage of diferric transferrin in delivering iron to reticulocytes. Proc Natl Acad Sci 1983;80:300–304.
4. Bainton DF, Finch CA. The diagnosis of iron deficiency anemia. Am J Med 1964;37:62–70.
5. Bothwell TH, Baynes RD, MacFarlane BJ, et al. Nutritional iron requirements and food iron absorption. J Intern Med 1989;226:357–365.
6. Hillman RS, Henderson PA. Control of marrow production by the level of iron supply. J Clin Invest 1969;48:454–460.
7. Andrews NC. Understanding heme transport. N Engl J Med 2005;353:2508–2509.
8. McKie AT, Barrow D, Latunde-Dada GO, et al. An iron-regulated ferric reductase associated with absorption of dietary iron. Science 2001;291:1755–1759.
9. Atanasiu V, Manolescu B, Stoian I. Hepcidin – central regulator of iron metabolism. Europ J Haematol 2006;78:1–10.
10. Pak M, Lopez MA, Gabayan V, et al. Suppression of hepcidin during anemia requires erythropoietic activity. Blood 2006;108:3730–3735.
11. Nemeth E, Rivera S, Gabayan V, et al. IL-6 mediates hypoferremia of inflammation by inducing the synthesis of the iron regulatory hormone hepcidin. J Clin Invest 2004;113:1271–1276.
12. Lipschitz DA, Cook JD, Finch CA. A clinical evaluation of serum ferritin as an index of iron stores. N Engl J Med 1974;290:1212–1216.
13. Beguin Y. Soluble transferrin receptor for the evaluation of erythropoiesis and iron status. Clin Chim Acta 2003;329:9–22.
14. Weiss G, Goodnough LT. Anemia of chronic disease. N Engl J Med 2005;352:1011–1023.
15. Cash, JM, Sears, DA. The anemia of chronic disease: spectrum of associated diseases in a series of unselected hospitalized patients. Am J Med 1989;87:638–644.
16. Brugnara C, Chambers LA, Malynn E, et al. Red blood cell regeneration induced by subcutaneous recombinant erythropoietin: iron-deficient erythropoiesis in iron-replete subjects. Blood 1993;81:956–964.
17. Punnonen K, Irjala K, Rajamaki A. Serum transferrin receptor and its ratio to serum ferritin in the diagnosis of iron deficiency. Blood 1997;89:1052–1057.
18. Pritchard JA. Hemoglobin regeneration in severe iron-deficiency anemia. JAMA 1966;195:97–100.
19. Radtke H, Tegtmeier J, Rocker L, et al. Daily doses of 20 mg of elemental iron compensate for iron loss in regular blood donors: a randomized, double-blind, placebo-controlled study. Transfusion 2004;44:1427–1432.
20. Pritchard JA, Mason RA. Iron stores of normal adults and replenishment with oral iron therapy. JAMA 1964;190:119–123.
21. Danielson BG. Structure, chemistry, and pharmacokinetics of intravenous iron agents. J Am Soc Nephrol 2004;15:S93–S98.
22. Michael B, Fishbane S, Coyne DW, et al. Drug insight: safety of intravenous iron supplementation with sodium ferric gluconate complex. Nature Clin Pract 2006;2:92–100.
23. Crosby WH, O'Neil-Cutting MA. A small-dose iron tolerance test as an indicator of mild iron deficiency. JAMA 1984;251:1986–1987.

24. Singh AK, Szczech L, Tang KL, et al. Correction of anemia with epoetin alfa in chronic kidney disease. N Engl J Med 2006;355:2085–2098.
25. Procrit (epoetin alfa), WARNINGS: Erythopoiesis-stimulating agents [package insert]. Amgen, Inc., Thousand Oaks, CA.
26. Eschbach JW. Iron requirements in erythropoietin therapy. Best Pract Res Clin Haematol 2005;18:347–361.
27. Mitka M. FDA sounds alert on anemia drugs. JAMA 2007;297:1868–1869.
28. Glaspy J, Vadhan-Raj S, Patel R, et al. Randomized comparison of every-2-week darbepoetin alfa and weekly epoetin aflf for the treatment of chemotherapy-induced anemia: the 20030125 study group trial. J Clin Oncol 2006;24:2290–2297.
29. Kaufman JS, Reda DJ, Fye CL, et al. Subcutaneous compared with intravenous epoetin in patients receiving hemodialysis. N Engl J Med 1998;339:578–583.
30. Gabrilove JL, Cleeland CS, Livingston RB, et al. Clinical evaluation of once-weekly dosing of epoetin alfa in chemotherapy patients: improvements in hemoglobin and quality of life are similar to three-times-weekly dosing. J Clin Oncol 2001;19:2875–2882.
31. Henry DH, Dahl NV, Auerbach M, et al. Intravenous ferric gluconate significantly improves response to epoetin alfa versus oral iron or no iron in anemic patients with cancer receiving chemotherapy. Oncologist 2007;12:231–242.
32. Bentley DP, Williams P. Parenteral iron therapy in the anaemia of rheumatoid arthritis. Rheumatol Rehabil 1982;21:88–92.
33. Pincus T, Olsen NJ, Russell IJ, et al. Multicenter study of recombinant human erythropoietin in correction of anemia in rheumatoid arthritis. Am J Med 1990;89:161–168.
34. Nordstrom D, Lindroth Y, Marsal L, et al. Availability of iron and degree of inflammation modifies the response to recombinant human erythropoietin when treating anemia of chronic disease in patients with rheumatoid arthritis. Rheumatol Int 1997;17:67–73.
35. Gasche C, Lomer MCE, Cavill I, et al. Iron, anaemia, and inflammatory bowel disease. Gut 2004;53:1190–1197.
36. Henry DH, Beall GN, Benson CA, et al. Recombinant human erythropoietin in the treatment of anemia associated with human immunodeficiency virus (HIV) infection and zidovudine. Ann Intern Med 1992;117:739–748.
37. Gordeuk VR, Delanghe JR, Langlois MR, et al. Iron status and the outcome of HIV infection: an overview. J Clin Virol 2001;20:111–115.

2

Deficiencies of Vitamin B12 and Folate

McDonald K. Horne, III

Besides iron deficiency, shortages of vitamin B12 (cobalamin) and folate are the most common nutritional causes of anemia. The frequencies of these deficiencies are highly dependent upon the population under study. Because vitamin B12 deficiency usually develops as a consequence of insidious malabsorption that occurs over many years, it becomes more prevalent with advancing age. Because folate deficiency is largely a consequence of inadequate dietary folate, it is most prevalent in populations at risk for malnutrition.

VITAMIN REQUIREMENTS, SOURCES, STORES

To avoid clinically apparent ill effects, the daily adult requirement for vitamin B12 is 1–3 μg and for folic acid ~200 μg (Table 2.1) (1). However, recent information indicates that at least 6 μg/day of B12 is necessary to prevent biochemical changes secondary to a limiting supply of the vitamin (2). The daily requirement for folate has been more easily met since 1996, when the U.S. Food and Drug Administration mandated that all grains be fortified with the vitamin to reduce the risk of neural tube defects in developing fetuses (3).

Bacteria in the gut of herbivorous animals synthesize vitamin B12 and supply it to their hosts, who in turn supply it to humans in the form of meat. There is no vitamin B12 in plant products other than that attributable to bacterial contamination. Plants synthesize folic acid and provide it to man directly in fruits and vegetables and indirectly in meat from herbivores.

The human body normally stores 2 to 3 months' supply of folic acid, although marginally nourished patients, such as chronic alcoholics, may have stores that can be depleted much sooner (4). In contrast, body stores of vitamin B12 are normally sufficient for 5 to 10 years (Table 2.1).

METABOLIC ROLES OF FOLATE AND VITAMIN B12

The metabolic roles of folate and vitamin B12 are closely interrelated (Fig. 2.1). Folate derivatives are essential cofactors in thymidylate synthesis, which is a rate-limiting step in the synthesis of DNA. RNA synthesis, however, is not dependent upon folate. Therefore, deficiency of folate limits gene transcription but not RNA translation, retarding cell division but not cytoplasmic protein synthesis. This leads to *the typical cytonuclear dissociation of maturation characteristic of megaloblastic hematopoiesis.* Because cobalamin supports the recycling of folate, vitamin B12 deficiency causes megaloblastic changes by restricting the folate supply. This restriction can be at least partially overcome by increasing dietary folate, *allowing the hematopoietic effects of cobalamin deficiency to be ameliorated by high doses of folic acid.* In contrast, the hematopoietic effects of folate deficiency cannot be overcome by treatment with vitamin B12.

Cobalamin is also necessary in the pathway leading to the synthesis of S-adenosyl-methionine, which is the only donor of methyl groups for numerous reactions in the brain involving proteins, membrane phospholipids, and neurotransmitters (5). Presumably *this explains the frequent neuropsychiatric signs and symptoms* associated with vitamin B12 deficiency (6). Folate is not involved in these reactions and cannot reverse the neuropsychiatric deficits caused by vitamin B12 deficiency. However, methyl-tetrahydrofolic acid is the methyl donor for the synthesis of methionine, the precursor of

TABLE 2.1. *Vitamin B12 and Folic Acid: Biology and Dosing*

	Vitamin B12	Folic Acid
Source	Bacteria → Meat	Plants → Meat
Daily requirement	1–3 μg	~200 μg
Body store	2–5 mg	~20 mg
Time to deficiency	5–10 years	2–3 months
Dosing, oral	2 mg/d	1 mg/d
parenteral	1 mg/month	
**Cost of dose, oral*	$3.40/month	$2.34/month
parenteral	$1.80/month	

*Average wholesale price (April 2007; Pharmacy Department, W.G. Magnuson Clinical Center, Bethesda, MD.)

S-adenosyl-methionine. Therefore, *folate deficiency may restrict the synthesis of S-adenosyl-methionine and produce some neuropsychiatric effects as well* (7).

DEVELOPMENT OF VITAMIN B12 DEFICIENCY

Cobalamin deficiency is rarely caused by inadequate intake or increased utilization of the vitamin (Table 2.2). Although strict vegetarians become depleted of vitamin B12, vegetables often contain sufficient bacteria to provide a marginally adequate supply. A developing fetus shunts cobalamin from its mother, placing her at risk of deficiency, particularly if her baseline stores are low.

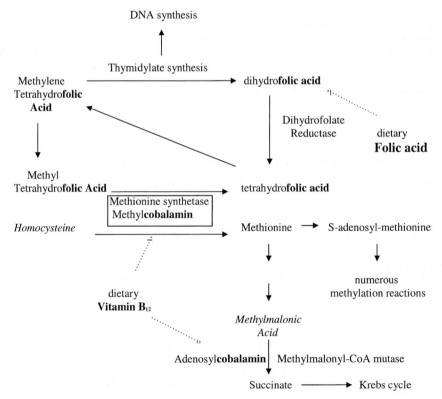

FIG. 2.1. Metabolic pathways involving folic acid and vitamin B12 (cobalamin).

TABLE 2.2. *Causes of Vitamin B12 Deficiency*

Gastrointestinal	Gastric atrophy: achlorhydria
	  achlorhydria + intrinsic factor deficiency
	Bariatric surgery
	Gastrectomy
	Gastric bypass
	Terminal ileal resection
	Extensive celiac disease
	Crohn's disease of the stomach
	Bacterial overgrowth in the small bowel
	  (achlorhydria, anatomical defects,
	  impaired motility)
	Zollinger-Ellison syndrome
	Pancreatic insufficiency
	HIV

Medications	Megadoses of vitamin C, metformin, proton pump inhibitors (?)
Increased utilization	Pregnancy
Toxin	Nitrous oxide
Dietary	Strict vegetarianism

Far more commonly, defects in any of three levels of the gastrointestinal tract can lead to vitamin B12 malabsorption: the fundus of the stomach, the pancreas, or the small bowel. Obviously surgical removal or bypass of any of these regions leads to B12 malabsorption (8). Otherwise, the etiology is inflammatory.

- *Stomach*: In the stomach, food (protein)-bound vitamin B12 must be freed by digestion with pepsin and bound to "R-proteins," which is a generic term for proteins that bind B12 (1). The parietal cells in the fundus secrete both the acid necessary for this digestion and intrinsic factor, the protein to which cobalamin is later transferred in the alkaline duodenum. Therefore, any process that damages the parietal cells can lead to vitamin B12 malabsorption and eventually deficiency. The most common cause is autoimmune atrophic gastritis, which increases in prevalence with age and is sometimes associated with other autoimmune diseases, such as thyroiditis. Helicobacter pylori, however, which typically causes antral gastritis, can occasionally also infect the fundus (9,10). Proton pump inhibitors induce chronic hypochlorhydria but rarely cause clinically significant B12 malabsorption. Parodoxically, the hypersecretion of acid in the Zollinger-Ellison syndrome leads to B12 malabsorption by acidifying the small bowel, which must remain alkaline for the transfer of B12 from the R-binders to intrinsic factor.
- *Pancreas*: Deficiency of pancreatic enzymes retards the digestion of R-binders in the small bowel and therefore the release of B12 to intrinsic factor. Although pancreatic insufficiency causes cobalamin malabsorption, it rarely is significant enough to become clinically apparent.
- *Small bowel*: Vitamin B12-intrinsic factor complexes are endocytosed by the mucosa of the terminal ileum. Inflammatory bowel disease or particularly extensive celiac or tropical sprue will interfere with this process (11). Bacterial overgrowth in the small bowel, especially common in the elderly, competes for B12 and makes it less available for absorption (12). Human immunodeficiency virus (HIV) infection is also sometimes also associated with B12 malabsorption.

DEVELOPMENT OF FOLIC ACID DEFICIENCY

A diet poor in fresh vegetables is a major cause of folic acid deficiency (Table 2.3). Cooked vegetables and meat are less satisfactory sources because cooking destroys much of the folate. (This is less of a problem for vitamin B12.) The other major causes are gastrointestinal diseases that affect the jejunum, where folic acid is absorbed, and conditions such as pregnancy that increase folate consumption. Ethanol abuse and several chronic medications (Table 2.3) lead to folate deficiency by interrupting folate metabolism or inhibiting its absorption.

TABLE 2.3. *Causes of Folic Acid Deficiency*

Diet	Lack of fresh vegetables
Gastrointestinal disease	Celiac disease (gluten-sensitive enteropathy)
	Dermatitis herpetiformis
	Tropical sprue
	Small bowel resection
	Crohn's disease
	Enterohepatic diversion
Medications	Cytotoxic agents: methotrexate
	Antibiotics: pyrimethamine, cycloserine, trimethoprim (?)
	Diuretics: triamterene
	Anticonvulsants: phenytoin, carbamazepine, phenobarbital, primidone
	Oral contraceptives (?)
Ethanol	
Increased utilization/loss	Pregnancy
	Chronic hemolysis
	Exfoliative dermatitis
	Chronic hemodialysis

PATIENT POPULATIONS AT RISK

Vitamin B12 deficiency due to lack of intrinsic factor ("pernicious anemia") is sometimes believed to be limited to elderly patients of European descent. In this population, the median age at presentation is almost 70 years.

Nevertheless, intrinsic factor deficiency may be almost as prevalent in African Americans and Latinos, who tend to present with vitamin B12 deficiency a decade earlier (13,14).

Older patients are actually more likely to become B12 deficient from achlorhydria or small bowel bacterial than lack of intrinsic factor (10,15).

Whereas cobalamin deficiency is generally found in older age groups, folic acid deficiency is likely to occur in any patient who has an inadequate diet or who has an increased need for the vitamin hemolysis (Table 2.3).

CLINICAL PRESENTATION

The clinical presentation of vitamin B12 and folic acid deficiency covers a wide range (Table 2.4). The investigation of any new neuropsychiatric changes should include an evaluation of folate and vitamin B12 status even in the absence of hematologic signs of a deficiency (6).

LABORATORY EVALUATION

Hematologic Abnormalities

Macrocytosis develops before anemia when either folic acid or vitamin B12 is limiting (Table 2.5) (4,16). With the advent of automated blood cell analyzers, isolated macrocytosis has become a typical presentation of deficiencies of either vitamin, although other causes of macrocytosis are more common (Table 2.6) (17). *An unexplained rise in mean cell volume (MCV) of 5 fL or more even within the normal range should also attract suspicion.* However, the macrocytosis may be masked if the patient is also iron deficient or has a thalassemic trait. At hemoglobin concentrations below ~10 g/dL, B12 or folate deficiency leads to elevations of serum lactate dehydrogenase, which can become quite high (4,16). This results from marked intramedullary death of developing red cells and a shortening of the circulating red cell life span but can mislead the clinician to suspect metastatic disease or a primary hemolytic anemia.

TABLE 2.4. *Clinical and Laboratory Presentations of Vitamin B12 or Folic Acid Deficiency*

Hematologic:
  Macrocytosis
  Anemia, usually macrocytic but normo- or microcytic if
    accompanied by iron deficiency or thalassemia
  Pancytopenia
Neuropsychiatric:
  Peripheral neuropathy (paresthesias, hyporeflexia)
  Spinal cord degeneration (weakness, hyperreflexia, reduced
    vibratory, and position sense)
  Memory loss, disorientation, depression
Gastrointestinal:
  Malabsorption (weight loss, diarrhea, abdominal pain), glossitis
Reproductive:
  Infertility, fetal loss

The earliest change in the peripheral blood caused by folate or vitamin B12 deficiency is hyper-segmentation of the neutrophils, which can be easily overlooked unless a blood smear is carefully examined. Finding even 5% of neutrophils with five lobes or just 1% with six lobes is highly suggestive of a deficiency, although this could also be seen with myelodysplasia. In advanced deficiencies pancytopenia can develop.

There is rarely if ever a need to perform a bone marrow examination in the evaluation of vitamin B12 and folic acid status. The megaloblastic changes in the marrow are identical in both deficiencies and are variable in intensity. A marrow examination cannot rule out myelodysplasia or even a smoldering leukemic process until cobalamin and folate deficiencies have been excluded first.

Serum Vitamin Concentrations

When vitamin B12 and folate deficiency is suspected, a common diagnostic starting point is measurement of the serum concentrations of the vitamins, which should be done after the patient has been fasting. The results, however, can be difficult to interpret (Table 2.7). *Serum folic acid* does not reliably reflect the body's supply of the vitamin, unless it is consistently below ~3 ng/mL, and even then

TABLE 2.5. *Progression of Laboratory Parameters*

Folic Acid Deficiency

	Normal	Negative Balance	Deplete Stores	Tissue Deficiency	Anemia
Serum folic acid (ng/mL)	5–20	<3	<3	<3	<3
RBC folic acid (ng/mL)	>200	>200	<200	<200	<200
Serum Hcy (μmol/L)	5–15	5–15	5–15	15–250	15–250
Hypersegmented neutrophils	0	0	0	+	++
MCV (fL)	80–5	80–95	80–95	90–110	100–130
Hemoglobin (g/dL)	12–15	12–15	12–15	12–15	<12

Vitamin B12 Deficiency

	Normal	Negative Balance	Deplete Stores	Tissue Deficiency	Anemia
Serum cobalamin (pg/mL)	200–900	150–500	100–300	50–250	50–250
Serum MMA (μmol/L)	<0.4	<0.4	<0.4	0.4–20	1–20
Hypersegmented neutrophils	0	0	0	+	++
MCV (fL)	80–95	80–95	80–95	90–110	100–130
Hemoglobin (g/dL)	12–15	12–15	12–15	12–15	<12

Hcy, homocysteine; MCV, mean cell volume; MMA, methylmalonic acid; RBC, red blood cell.

TABLE 2.6. *Causes of Macrocytosis with or without Anemia*

	Macrocytosis Alone	Macrocytic Anemia
Medications		
Cytotoxic chemotherapy (methotrexate, hydroxyurea cytosine arabinoside, azathioprine, others)	+	+
Anticonvulsants (phenytoin, carbamazepine primadone)	+	+
Antiretrovirals	+	+
Antibiotics (cotrimoxazole)	+	+
Liver disease	+	+
Alcoholism ± liver disease	+	+
Reticulocytosis	0	+
Folate deficiency	+	+
Vitamin B12 deficiency	+	+
Myelodysplasia	+	+
Hypothyroidism	+	+
>75 years old	+	+
Down's syndrome	+	0
Artifact (RBC agglutination)	+	0

RBC, red blood cell.

it does not distinguish between negative balance and actual tissue deficiency (18). Because *red cell folate* is packaged at the time the cell is made and remains in the cell throughout its 3- to 4-month life span, the measured mean value may fail to reflect relatively recent reductions in dietary folate. Furthermore, the reproducibility of assays for red cell folate is relatively poor so that borderline values can be misleading (18). To complicate matters further, red cell folate can be reduced by vitamin B12 deficiency and lead to an erroneous diagnosis (Table 2.7).

Interpreting *serum vitamin B12 levels* can also be problematic because serum B12 can actually be decreased in cases of folate deficiency (1). A more frequent problem, like that with folic acid, relates to uncertainties in the physiologic levels of the vitamin. The "normal range" of serum cobalamin typically extends down to 200 pg/mL, because healthy, nonanemic donors occasionally have B12 concentrations that are this low. However, patients who are truly deficient in vitamin B12 can have serum cobalamin levels as high as 300 pg/mL and maybe higher (18,19). The reason for this discrepancy is that the total cobalamin is measured, rather than just the vitamin B12 bound to transcobalamin, which is the metabolically available B12 but represents only ~20% of the total serum vitamin. Therefore, individuals who have relatively low concentrations of haptocorrin, which binds the other ~80% of the serum vitamin B12, can have alarmingly low B12 levels (<100 pg/mL) without any harmful effect

TABLE 2.7. *Laboratory Tests in Folic Acid and Vitamin B12 Deficiency*

	Folic Acid	Vitamin B12
Serum folic acid	↓→	→↑
Red cell folic acid	↓→	→↓
Serum vitamin B12	→↓	↓→
Methylmalonic acid	→	↑
Homocysteine	↑	↑
Lactate dehydrogenase	↑	↑
Haptoglobin	→↓	→↓

because they have adequate amounts of B12 bound to transcobalamin. Occasional healthy patients have been described with low haptocorrin levels (20). Haptocorrin can also be low in patients with multiple myeloma (21). Such patients will be easier to identify when tests become available to measure B12 specifically bound to transcobalamin rather than total serum B12 (22).

Serum Methylmalonic Acid and Homocysteine

Measurements of Serum methylmalonic (MMA) and homocysteine (Hcy), although they are more expensive than the vitamin assays, answer the question of vitamin deficiency more reliably (23). Although these metabolites can be elevated for other reasons (Table 2.8), if these causes are excluded, these metabolites become specific reflections of vitamin B12 and folate depletion at the tissue level (14,23). Usually MMA and Hcy both become elevated when B12 is the limiting factor, whereas only Hcy becomes elevated with folate is limiting. However, in 1% to 2% of cases of vitamin B12 deficiency only Hcy will be elevated, whereas in ~10% of cases of folate deficiency MMA will be high. Therefore, elevated Hcy alone does not always differentiate B12 and folate deficiency but makes folate deficiency more likely.

Although normal levels of MMA and Hcy were reported to exclude a metabolic effect from B12 deficiency, the negative predictive value of these assays has recently been questioned because of reports of patients with normal metabolites who clearly respond to vitamin B12 (14,24).

Therapeutic Trial

If the laboratory evaluation is impossible because resources are lacking or is inconclusive, a therapeutic trial can be diagnostic if a single vitamin is given at a time. Vitamin B12 should be given first because it will do nothing for folic acid deficiency, whereas replacement with folic acid will improve the anemia secondary to B12 deficiency but not the neuropathic changes. The response to treatment can be judged by following the reticulocyte count and hemoglobin (see below). A more expensive way is to remeasure Hcy or MMA levels 2 to 5 days after one or the other of the vitamins has been administered. The metabolites will fall only in response to replacement of the deficient vitamin (23).

DETERMINING THE CAUSE OF VITAMIN B12 OR FOLATE DEFICIENCY

The *etiology of folate deficiency* must always be determined because virtually all causes are either preventable or treatable. If the patient appears to have an adequate diet, a gastrointestinal evaluation is indicated to search for the underlying causes shown in Table 2.3.

In contrast, *if vitamin B12 is deficient* and the patient is not a vegan and there are no symptoms of gastrointestinal disease, an argument can be made to take the evaluation no further and simply to treat the individual with the vitamin.

If the patient and/or his or her physician feels compelled to confirm that the pathology lies in the stomach, however, a test for anti-intrinsic factor antibodies should be done (25). A positive test is diagnostic

TABLE 2.8. *Causes of Elevated Methylmalonic Acid and Homocysteine*

	Methylmalonic Acid	Homocysteine
Vitamin deficiencies		Folic acid deficiency
	Vitamin B12 deficiency	Vitamin B12 deficiency
		Vitamin B6 (pyridoxine) deficiency
Genetic traits		Homozygous thermolabile tetrahydrofolate reductase
Renal disease	Renal insufficiency	Renal insufficiency
Endocrine	Pregnancy	Hypothyroidism
Drugs		Niacin, L-dopa
Metabolic	Volume contraction	Volume contraction

of pernicious anemia and is found in half the cases. Antiparietal cell antibodies are more common but are also found in a small percentage of normal individuals. Demonstrating an elevation in serum gastrin also strongly supports the diagnosis of gastric atrophy (26).

If the patient is unusually young to have achlorhydria or pernicious anemia (e.g., <50 years old or younger if African American), a gastrointestinal evaluation is indicated (Table 2.2) (13). In the past, the Schilling test was used in an attempt to detect vitamin B12 malabsorption, but Schilling tests are no longer performed because of lack of a commercial source for radiolabeled cobalamin and the realization that this test also often gives misleading results. Because the incidence of many malignancies, especially gastric cancer, is slightly higher in patients with pernicious anemia than in age- and sex-matched controls, following the patient for any signs of gastrointestinal blood loss is wise, although more aggressive surveillance is not indicated (27).

TREATMENT/RESPONSE

There are two treatment goals: replacement of the deficient vitamin and correction of the cause of the deficiency. The first goal is always achievable; the second may not be. Treatment should always be given if the clinical presentation is suspicious, even if the laboratory data are confusing, because the laboratory data are not totally sensitive and the consequences of undertreating can be devastating (23,24).

In the past, vitamin B12 was always given intramuscularly in North America, although the oral route was used in Sweden (28). Recently, however, the effectiveness of oral B12 was demonstrated in two randomized, controlled clinical trials (29,30). This works even in patients with pernicious anemia because approximately 1% of any oral dose of vitamin B12 is absorbed by simple diffusion across the mucosa. So the recommended daily dose of 1–2 mg of vitamin B12 results in the absorption of ~10–20 μg, which is much more than the daily requirement. A caveat, however, is that 1-mg tablets of vitamin B12 are sometimes difficult to find in hospital pharmacies.

Intramuscular B12, of course, is perfectly acceptable if it is more practical for a patient, and this route would still be preferred by most physicians to treat a patient with neurologic symptoms. Daily injections of 50–100 μg should be given for a week, followed by weekly injections for a month, and then monthly injections of 1 mg. For most patients with vitamin B12 deficiency, *lifelong treatment is required* because the underlying cause is not reversible.

The usual dose of oral folic acid is 1 mg/d (Table 2.1). This is ample even during pregnancy or chronic hemolysis. If the deficiency is dietary, replacement with folic acid should continue until the diet has become adequate. A month of daily folic acid should be sufficient to replenish body stores. If the etiology of the deficiency is small bowel dysfunction, higher doses for longer periods of time may be necessary.

The response to correction of vitamin B12 or folate deficiency is the same:

- Mental changes and tongue soreness improve almost immediately after starting to replace the deficient vitamin (1).
- After 4 to 5 days, reticulocytosis appears and may elevate the MCV even further.
- Soon thereafter the hemoglobin concentration begins to rise.
- Neuropathic abnormalities, such as paresthesias, improve slowly, over several months, but may never disappear entirely if they have been longstanding.

If the hematologic response is blunted, additional etiologies for the anemia should be sought. It is not unusual for iron deficiency to accompany folate or vitamin B12 deficiency. An underlying anemia of chronic disease is always a possibility.

REFERENCES

1. Chanarin I. The Megaloblastic Anaemias, 3rd Ed. Oxford: Blackwell Scientific Publications;1990.
2. Bor MV, Lydeking-Olsen E, Moller J, et al. A daily intake of approximately 6 μg vitamin B-12 appears to saturate all the vitamin B-12-related variables in Danish postmenopausal women. Am J Clin Nutr 2006;83:52–58.

3. Jacques PF, Selhub J, Bostom AG, et al. The effect of folic acid fortification on plasma folate and total homocysteine concentrations. N Engl J Med 1999;340:1449–1454.
4. Lindenbaum J, Allen RH. Clinical spectrum and diagnosis of folate deficiency. In: Folate in Health and Disease. New York: Marcel Dekker;1995:43–74.
5. Reynolds EH, Carney MWP, Toone BK. Methylation and mood. Lancet 1984;2:196–198.
6. Lindenbaum J, Healton EB, Savage DG, et al. Neuropsychiatric disorders caused by cobalamin deficiency in the absence of anemia or macrocytosis. N Eng J Med 1988;318:1720–1728.
7. Shorvon SD, Carney MWP, Chanarin I, et al. The neuropsychiatry of megaloblastic anaemia. Br Med J 1980;281:1036–1038.
8. Skroubis G, Sakellaropoulos G, Pouggouras K, et al. Comparison of nutritional deficiencies after Roux-en-Y gastric bypass and after biliopancreatic diversion with Roux-en-Y gastric bypass. Obes Surg 2002;12:551–558.
9. Kaptan K, Beyan C, Ural AU, et al. Helicobacter pylori – is it a novel causative agent in vitamin B12 deficiency? Arch Intern Med 2000;160:1349–1353.
10. Hershko C, Ronson A, Souroujon M, et al. Variable hematologic presentation of autoimmune gastritis: age-related progression from iron deficiency to cobalamin depletion. Blood 2006;107: 1673–1679.
11. Dahele A, Ghosh S. Vitamin B12 deficiency in untreated celiac disease. Am J Gastroenterol 2001; 96:745–750.
12. Haboubi NY, Montgomery RD. Small-bowel bacterial overgrowth in elderly people: clinical significance and response to treatment. Age Aging 1992;21:13–19.
13. Carmel R, Johnson CS. Racial patterns in pernicious anemia. N Engl J Med 1978;298:647–650.
14. Savage DG, Lindenbaum J, Stabler SP, et al. Sensitivity of serum methylmalonic acid and total homocysteine determinations for diagnosing cobalamin and folate deficiencies. Am J Med 1994; 96:239–246.
15. Dharmarajan TS, Adiga GU, Norkus EP. Vitamin B12 deficiency, recognizing subtle symptoms in older patients. Geriatrics 2003;58:30–38.
16. Stabler SP, Allen RH, Savage DG, et al. Clinical spectrum and diagnosis of cobalamin deficiency. Blood 1990;76:871–881.
17. Savage DG, Ogundipe A, Allen RH, et al. Etiology and diagnostic evaluation of macrocytosis. Am J Med Sci 2000;319:343–352.
18. Klee GG. Cobalamin and folate evaluation: measurement of methylmalonic acid and homocysteine vs vitamin B12 and folate. Clin Chem 2000;46:1277–1283.
19. Tucker KL, Rich S, Rosenberg I, et al. Plasma vitamin B-12 concentrations relate to intake source in the Framingham Offspring Study. Am J Clin Nutr 2000;71:514–522.
20. Carmel R. A new case of deficiency of the R binder for cobalamin, with observations on minor cobalamin-binding proteins in serum and saliva. Blood 1982;59:152–156.
21. Hansen OP, Drivsholm A, Hippe E. Vitamin B12 metabolism in myelomatosis. Scand J Haematol 1977;18:395–402.
22. Ulleland M, Eilertsen I, Quadros EV, et al. Direct assay for cobalamin bound to transcobalamin (holo-transcobalamin) in serum. Clin Chem 2002;48:526–532.
23. Lindenbaum J, Savage DG, Stabler SP, et al. Diagnosis of cobalamin deficiency II: relative sensitivities of serum cobalamin, methylmalonic acid, and total homocysteine concentrations. Am J Hematol 1990;34:99–107.
24. Solomon LR. Cobalamin-responsive disorders in the ambulatory care setting: unreliability of cobalamin, methylmalonic acid, and homocysteine testing. Blood 2005;105:978–986.
25. Fairbanks VF, Lennon VA, Kokmen E, et al. Tests for pernicious anemia: serum intrinsic factor blocking antibody. Mayo Clin Proc 1983;58:203–204.
26. Lindgren A, Lindstedt G, Kilander AF. Advantages of serum pepsinogen A combined with gastrin or pepsinogen C as first-line analytes in the evaluation of suspected cobalamin deficiency: a study in patients previously not subjected to gastrointestinal surgery. J Intern Med 1998;244:341–349.
27. Schafer LW, Larson DE, Melton LJ, et al. Risk of development of gastric carcinoma in patients with pernicious anemia: a population-based study in Rochester, Minnesota. Mayo Clin Proc 1985; 60:444–448.

28. Hvas A-M, Nexo E. Diagnosis and treatment of vitamin B12 deficiency. An update. Haematologica 2006;91:1506–1512.
29. Kuzminski AM, Giacco EJD, Allen RH, et al. Effective treatment of cobalamin deficiency with oral cobalamin. Blood 1998;92:1191–1198.
30. Bolaman Z, Kadikoylu G, Yukselen V, et al. Oral versus intramuscular cobalamin treatment in megaloblastic anemia: a single-center, prospective, randomized, open-label study. Clin Therap 2003;25:3124–3134.

3

Hemolytic Anemia: General Overview with Special Consideration of Membrane and Enzyme Defects

Patricia A. Oneal, Geraldine P. Schechter, Griffin P. Rodgers, and Jeffery L. Miller

Many diseases share the clinical feature of red blood cell hemolysis. Hemoglobinopathies and immune-mediated hemolysis are the most common causes (see discussions in Chapters 4 and 24, respectively). Very rare inherited or acquired diseases may also directly or indirectly result in increased red cell destruction (1). Understanding the mechanisms that lead to hemolysis assists with the diagnosis, prognosis, and consideration of the most appropriate therapy. In this postgenomic era, correlations between genotype and phenotype are being pursued in cases of inherited hemolytic syndromes. Those genetic-based discoveries are also being translated into new clinical tools in anticipation of mechanism-specific therapies.

Hemolytic anemia is defined as decreased levels of erythrocytes in circulating blood (anemia) because of their accelerated destruction (hemolysis). All circulating erythrocytes are subject to physiologic stresses such as turbulence in blood flow, endothelial damage, and age-related catabolic changes. Normally, damaged red blood cells (RBC) are removed from the circulation by the reticuloendothelial system. In hemolytic syndromes, erythrocyte clearance by the reticuloendothelial system may be increased (extravascular hemolysis) or the cells may be lysed within the circulation (intravascular hemolysis). As a result, RBC survival is generally shortened to less than 100 days (normal is approximately 120 days). When sufficient numbers of erythrocytes are destroyed, oxygen delivery to tissues is impaired. Tissue hypoxia leads to increased release of erythropoietin, which signals the bone marrow to produce more red blood cells.

A hallmark of hemolytic anemia is an elevated number of immature erythrocytes (reticulocytes) in the peripheral blood. In low-level hemolysis, erythrocyte production may adequately compensate for blood cell destruction and minimize the anemia. Alternatively, patients with hemolysis and underlying defects in hematopoiesis may present with pronounced anemia without reticulocytosis. Hence, the evaluation of suspected hemolysis requires consideration of the hemolysis itself as well as the marrow's ability to compensate. The diagnostic strategy usually begins with a search for common causes of hemolysis and proceeds toward rare etiologies. The extent of diagnostic studies should be guided by the magnitude of hemolysis and the available therapeutic options. With the information contained here, practicing clinicians should be able to develop a clinical approach, differential diagnosis, and therapeutic plan for patients with suspected hemolysis.

ETIOLOGY AND DIFFERENTIAL DIAGNOSIS

Grouping the various causes of the disease generates a differential diagnosis for hemolysis. As shown in Figure 3.1, hemolysis results from pathology intrinsic or extrinsic to the erythrocytes. Intrinsic hemolysis may then be categorized further according to hemoglobin, membrane, or enzyme-based factors. Alternatively, the patient's immune status or infectious agents can lead to hemolysis in the absence of intrinsic defects. Other chemical or physical features of the erythrocyte environment also cause hemolysis. A more complete differential organized according to these categories is shown in Table 3.1 (2–5).

Low-level or chronic hemolysis should be suspected in all patients with unexplained anemia. A detailed history and physical examination should be the cornerstone of each patient's evaluation.

History
Onset/duration (hereditary versus acquired)
History of fatigue
History of jaundice
Abdominal pain/cholelithiasis (chronic hemolysis)
Medications (may exacerbate enzyme deficiencies)
Travel (consider infection)
History of recent or current infection
Vascular/cardiac surgery
Blood loss or sequestration (increases reticulocytes in the absence of hemolysis)
Discolored urine (intravascular hemolysis)
Complete family history (jaundice, gallbladder disease, splenectomy, hereditary anemia, or other inherited diseases)

Physical
Pallor
Increased temperature
Rapid pulse
Jaundice (chronic hemolysis)
Mechanical click from heart valves
Splenomegaly

The laboratory evaluation is performed to confirm the suspected diagnosis, provide insight regarding the underlying mechanism, and gauge a therapeutic response. The complete blood count (CBC) usually confirms the diagnosis of anemia. Reticulocytosis increases the mean cell volume (MCV) and red cell distribution width (RDW). A critical test in the evaluation of all patients with suspected hemolysis is the reticulocyte count. An increased number of reticulocytes are present in hemolysis unless erythropoiesis is suppressed. Stressed erythropoiesis associated with hemolysis also causes the release of large polychromatic reticulocytes with a decreased area of central pallor into the circulation, called shift cells (8). Reticulocytes are also identified by their RNA content, so automated detection of RNA in the cells provides an accurate alternative to manual inspection. Normal values for reticulocytes in newborn infants range from 2.5% to 6.5%, and then the percentage falls to less than 2% by the second week of life. In adults, reticulocytes comprise 0.5% to 1.5% of circulating erythrocytes in the absence of anemia, consistent with the normal turnover of 1% of normal red cell mass per day in adults. Percentages above the normal range are usually detected in the setting of hemolysis because of increased erythropoiesis. However, in the setting of anemia, an uncorrected reticulocyte percentage may also reflect the prolonged survival of stress reticulocytes and the lower total number of circulating RBC. Therefore, an absolute reticulocyte count more accurately measures the compensatory response than does the uncorrected reticulocyte percentage (9).

$$\text{Absolute reticulocyte count (ARC)} = \text{Reticulocyte percentage}/100 \times \text{RBC count}/\mu L$$

The normal ARC ranges between 25,000 and 75,000/μL. In patients with hemolysis, the ARC is usually elevated to levels greater than 100,000/mm^3. If hemolysis is acute, a rise in reticulocytes may be delayed.

While a bone marrow examination is generally not required to determine the etiology of uncomplicated hemolysis, the peripheral blood smear should never be overlooked. This simple test is rapid, inexpensive, and can provide important clues regarding the mechanism of hemolysis (Table 3.2).

ACUTE INTRAVASCULAR HEMOLYSIS

The clinical syndrome associated with acute intravascular hemolysis deserves special attention because of its potential catastrophic consequences. Its recognition can lead to rapid institution of specific therapies

TABLE 3.2. *Erythrocyte Morphologies and Associated Pathology*

Cell type	Intrinsic	Extrinsic
Acanthocyte	Glutathione peroxidase deficiency Hereditary choreoacanthocytosis Abetalipoproteinemia McLeod syndrome LCAT deficiency	Liver disease Asplenia
Basophilic stippling	Hemoglobinopathies Ineffective erythropoiesis	Lead poisoning 5′ nucleotidase deficiency
Elliptocyte	G6PD deficiency Hereditary elliptocytosis Protein band 4.1 Glycophorin C deficiency Pyropoikilocytosis	Malaria
Heinz bodies	G6PD deficiency Thalassmemias Unstable hemoglobins	Drug-induced oxidant injury
Parasites		Malaria (shown) Babesiosis Bartonellosis
Pyropoikilocytes	Hereditary pyropoikilocytosis α-Spectrin mutation	Burns
Schistocyte		Microangiopathic hemolytic anemia (see Table 3.1)
Sickle cell	Hemoglobin SS Hemoglobin SC Hemoglobin S beta-thalassemia	

(continued)

TABLE 3.2. *Erythrocyte Morphologies and Associated Pathology (continued)*

Cell type	Intrinsic	Extrinsic
Spherocyte	Hereditary spherocytosis Ankyrin/Spectrin deficiency Hemoglobin C disease Band 3 defects Protein 4.2 defects	Immune-mediated hemolysis Infections Chemical injuries
Stomatocyte	Hereditary stomatocytosis Rh null disease	Alcohol intoxication Liver disease
Target cell	Thalassemias Hemoglobin C disease Unstable hemoglobins	Liver disease

and prevent acute renal failure and death. Diagnosis and treatment of *Clostridium perfringens* sepsis or thrombotic thrombocytopenia purpura may be triggered by a hemolysis workup. The causes of intravascular hemolysis are almost exclusively extrinsic (Table 3.1).

Examination of several key laboratory values may also be used to assess the severity of intravascular hemolysis. Lactate dehydrogenase is released from hemolyzed red blood cells. Small amounts of hemoglobin released into the circulation are metabolized in the liver after binding and clearance by haptoglobin. With robust intravascular hemolysis, a rapid decrease of serum haptoglobin to undetectable levels occurs. Free hemoglobin not bound to haptoglobin can be oxidized to methemoglobin or bound to transport proteins such as hemopexin or albumin, which the liver will then remove from the circulation. Free hemoglobin at levels of 100 to 200 mg/dL can be detected by visual examination of plasma or serum. The capacity of renal tubular cells to reabsorb free hemoglobin is limited to producing hemoglobinuria. As renal tubular cells slough, iron staining can identify the tubular epithelium containing hemosiderin in the urine sediment. Cessation of hemolysis leads to a rapid recovery of the haptoglobin levels, but urine hemosiderin is detectable for longer periods (Fig. 3.3). Urine hemosiderin

FIG. 3.3. Indicators of acute intravascular hemolysis. With permission from Hillman RS, Finch CA. Red Cell Manual, 7th Ed. Philadelphia: F. A. Davis Co.;1996.

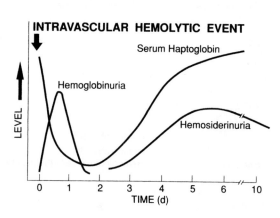

in the absence of urine hemoglobin provides clinical evidence for subacute or chronic intravascular hemolysis. Reduced levels of haptoglobin and increased levels of lactate dehydrogenase provide 96% specificity for predicting hemolytic anemia (10).

SPECIAL CONSIDERATION OF ENZYME AND MEMBRANE DEFECTS

Once the more obvious causes of hemolysis are ruled out, the clinician must consider those etiologies less frequently encountered in daily practice, including enzyme or membrane defects. The laboratory evaluation can be confusing because of the numerous etiologies and the diversity of tests available. Therefore, the extent of diagnostic testing is dictated by the magnitude of hemolysis and the impact of a specific diagnosis on therapy. Paroxysmal nocturnal hemoglobinuria is diagnosed by flow cytometry because of the associated absence of glycosylphosphatidylinositol-anchored proteins (e.g., CD59) on the plasma membranes of hematopoietic cells (see Chapter 6). General evaluation of the erythroid cytoskeleton abnormalities can usually be assessed by peripheral blood smear evaluation, and osmotic fragility assays may be helpful in subtle cases. In the case of enzymopathies, specific functional assays are available from reference laboratories. With the exception of G6PD, pyruvate kinase, and glucose phosphate isomerase, enzyme abnormalities are a rare cause of hemolysis.

ERYTHROID ENZYMOPATHIES

Enzyme deficiencies are most often associated with congenital nonspherocytic hemolytic anemia. Inheritances of G6PD and phosphoglycerate kinase deficiencies are chromosome X-linked; the other red cell enzyme abnormalities exhibit an autosomal recessive mode of inheritance. Based on their low incidence, laboratory evaluation of suspected enzymopathies requires assays performed at specialized or research laboratories (e.g., Mayo Medical Laboratories, Rochester, MN), which measure the functional properties of each enzyme. In the setting of acute hemolysis, however, the magnitude of the functional deficit may be underestimated because of the generally higher levels of enzyme activity in reticulocytes and other "young" erythrocytes. As the clinical application of information contained in the human genome improves, genetic testing may become more practical for these enzymopathies. The success of clinical genotyping in this regard will depend upon the number of mutations identified, as well as the strength of correlation between genotype and phenotype. A genome-based profile of the known hemolysis-related enzymes is available on the Internet (http://hembase.niddk.nih.gov/).

Enzyme deficiencies most commonly associated with hemolysis are linked to the prevention of oxidative damage or the generation of energy (ATP) in RBCs. Glutathione reduction (hexose monophosphate shunt) is necessary for the prevention of oxidative damage from hydrogen peroxide to cellular proteins including hemoglobin. Glycolysis (Embden-Meyerhof pathway) provides the sole source of energy to the red blood cells once they lose their mitochondria. Below is a brief synopsis of the enzymopathies associated with hemolysis (organized according to the involved metabolic pathway).

Enzymes Involved in Glutathione Metabolism

Glucose-6-phosphate dehydrogenase (G6PD) deficiency is the most common RBC enzyme disorder associated with hemolysis. As an X-linked disorder, it is far more common in males, but females do present with the disease because of mosaicism of the X chromosome as well as compound heterozygocity of inheritance. It has been estimated that this disorder affects 400 million of people throughout the world, with the highest frequencies occurring in populations from the Mediterranean region, Africa, and China (11). Approximately 10% to 15% of African American males are deficient in G6PD activity. Clinical classification is made according to the magnitude of the enzyme deficiency and the severity of hemolysis.

- Class I: Severe enzyme deficiency (less than 10% of normal enzyme activity). These rare patients present at birth and manifest chronic active hemolysis.
- Class II: Severe enzyme deficiency but with only intermittent hemolysis (Mediterranean and Asian populations).

- Class III: Moderate enzyme deficiency (10% to 60% of normal) with intermittent hemolysis usually associated with infection or drugs (African populations).
- Class IV: No enzyme deficiency or hemolysis.
- Class V: Increased enzyme activity.

Importantly, the severity of hemolysis among all classes of G6PD deficient patients depends on two major variables: G6PD protein and oxidative stress. G6PD deficiency is defined at the genetic level by mutations that cause either reduced synthesis of functional G6PD (quantitative defect) versus production of abnormal G6PD (qualitative defect). The World Health Organization (http://www.who.int/en/) has classified the known 400 G6PD variants. Patients with class I G6PD possess genetic mutations that are central to the production or function of the G6PD protein. These defects are so severe that erythrocytes cannot withstand the normal stresses encountered in the circulation. The neonatal hyperbilirubinemia in G6PD-deficient infants is caused by increased bilirubin production from erythrocyte breakdown and inadequate clearance by an immature liver. Neonates with the class I variant are at greatest risk of developing neonatal hyperbilirubinemia.

The second major factor in determining the level of hemolysis is the level of intracellular oxidative stress. G6PD acts to catalyze the conversion of glucose-6-phosphate to 6-phosphogluconate. That biochemical reaction is coupled to the production of NADPH and subsequent reduction of glutathione. Erythrocytes that are exposed to oxidants or oxidative stresses become depleted of reduced glutathione (GSH). Once GSH is depleted, oxidation of other red blood cell sulfhydryl-containing proteins (including hemoglobin) occurs. Oxidation of hemoglobin leads to the formation of sulfhemoglobin and hemoglobin precipitates called Heinz bodies. Heinz body inclusions are generated during acute, drug-induced hemolytic episodes. Patients with the most prevalent G6PD variants, class II and III, are generally asymptomatic in the steady state. They present episodically with acute hemolytic anemia because of oxidative stress from infections such as infections or certain drugs (Table 3.3). A complete list of drugs and chemicals associated G6PD deficiency is available on the Internet (http://www.uptodate.com or http://www.g6pd.org/favism/english/index.mv). Favism is a term used to describe hemolysis associated with the ingestion of fava beans, which contain pyrimidine aglycones (divicine and isouramil). Favism is most commonly associated with the G6PD Mediterranean variant.

Testing for suspected G6PD deficiency is performed by a simple fluorescence test that measures the production of NADPH. A more definitive diagnosis of G6PD deficiency requires familial genetic testing of the involved family. Genetic testing is expected to supplant enzyme electrophoretic mobility assays. Treatment of a G6PD-deficient individual depends on the degree of hemolysis. Potentially harmful drugs should always be avoided, and patients with infection should be carefully monitored for early

TABLE 3.3. *Drugs and Chemicals to Avoid
in Patients with Glucose-6-phosphate
Dehydrogenase Deficiency*

Dapsone
Methylene blue
Naphthalene
Nitrofurantoin
Phenzopyridine (Pyridium)
Phenylhydrazine
Primaquine
Sulfacetamide
Sulfamethoxazole (Bactrim, Septra)
Sulfanilamide
Sulfapyridine
Thiazosulfone
Toluidine blue
Trinitrotoluene
Quinolones

signs of increased hemolysis. Blood transfusion may be life saving during acute hemolytic episodes. While controversial, splenectomy may be considered in cases of G6PD deficiency presenting with severe hemolysis that do not respond to other measures (12).

γ-Glutamylcysteine synthetase is the rate-limiting enzyme in glutathione biosynthesis. Hemolytic anemia is associated with low activity of this enzyme and normal glutathione synthetase levels. These rare patients present with a history of lifelong anemia, intermittent jaundice, and spinocerebellar degeneration in adulthood (13).

Glutathione peroxidase (GSH-Px) is primarily responsible for the elimination of hydrogen peroxide from erythrocytes. Production of this protein is dependent on adequate nutritional levels of selenium (14). Moderate deficiencies in GSH-Px activity may result in the formation of Heinz bodies and nonspherocytic hemolytic anemia in infants. Like G6PD deficiency, oxidizing agents should be avoided in these patients.

Glutathione reductase is the enzyme that reduces oxidized GSH in the presence of flavin adenine dinucleotide. Reduction in glutathione reductase causes increased susceptibility to drug-induced hemolysis. Glutathione reductase activity increases with dietary supplementation of riboflavin, and a subset of these patients responds well to riboflavin dietary supplements. In some cases of glutathione reductase deficiency, the enzymatic activity cannot be restored by riboflavin supplementation because of a 2246 base pair deletion found in the gene encoding for glutathione reductase (15).

Glutathione synthetase deficiency is caused by autosomal recessive inheritance of mutations of the glutathione synthetase gene with subsequently low levels of glutathione in RBCs. The disease is marked by accumulation of the metabolite oxyproline in the urine (16). The patients present with the clinical triad of hemolysis, metabolic acidosis, and mental deterioration. Treatment includes vitamin C, vitamin E, bicarbonate, and avoidance of oxidative drugs.

Enzymes Involved in Glycolysis

Pyruvate kinase (PK) deficiency is the second most common enzymopathy associated with congenital nonspherocytic hemolytic anemia. Over 150 genetic mutations are associated with PK deficiency. Pyruvate kinase converts phosphoenolpyruvate to pyruvate, simultaneously generating adenosine triphosphate (ATP) from adenosine diphosphate (ADP). Pyruvate kinase activity decreases during RBC aging, as the enzyme is gradually denatured. The eventual result is failure of glycolysis as PK activity falls below a critical level. Because glycolysis is the sole source of ATP synthesis in the mature RBC, ATP depletion soon follows glycolytic failure.

Consistent with several other inherited causes of hemolysis, pyruvate kinase deficiency is postulated to provide some protection from malarial infection (17). Selection for variations of this gene may involve other factors as well, because pyruvate kinase deficiency is common among northern Europeans. Most patients are compound-heterozygotes for the two most common mutant forms of the enzyme. Approximately one third of the cases present with jaundice during the newborn period, and one third of those cases are severe enough to require transfusion. Death during the neonatal period may result from severe anemia. The anemia is less severe in individuals with milder forms of the enzymopathy, and the diagnosis may not be established until later in childhood. Unfortunately, poor correlation between PK activity and the severity of clinical hemolysis confounds the accuracy of prognosis (18). There is currently no reliable method to predict success of splenectomy for individual cases.

Glucose phosphate isomerase (GPI) deficiency is the third most common glycolytic enzyme associated with hemolytic anemia. GPI catalyzes the production of fructose-6-phosphate from glucose-6-phosphate. It is found in all ethnic groups, but is prevalent in individuals of European descent. Over two dozen genetic variants have been identified to date with considerable variability in disease severity. In severe cases, anemia and hyperbilirubinemia are evident at birth. In addition to chronic hemolysis and hyperbilirubinemia, acute hemolytic crises can occur with viral and bacterial infections (19).

Aldolase deficiency has been found to cause moderately severe lifelong hemolytic anemia, sometimes requiring transfusions during acute hemolytic crises. Aldolase catalyzes the conversion of fructose-1,6-diphosphate to dihydroxyacetone phosphate and glyceraldehyde-3-phosphate. Abnormal expression of the aldolase variant causes hemolysis and myopathy (20). Other congenital anomalies include short stature, mental retardation, delayed puberty, and a distinct facial appearance.

Hereditary pyropoikilocytosis is a severe type of HE resulting from a mutation in either protein 4.1 or α-spectrin. The usual presentation involves mild to moderate hemolytic anemia with evidences of poikilocytosis. The spectrin in these abnormal cells has an increased sensitivity to thermal denaturation, and the cells exhibit mechanical fragility. As a result, the red cell volume distribution is broad, and a striking number of fragmented cells and microspherocytes are observed on the peripheral smear (37).

TREATMENT OPTIONS FOR CONFIRMED HEMOLYSIS

Therapeutic strategies for hemolytic anemia are determined by the underlying cause of red cell destruction, the magnitude of the anemia, and cardiopulmonary status of the patient.

For extrinsic causes, the treatment plan usually becomes obvious at the time of diagnosis. Immune-mediated hemolysis may require immunoglobulin infusion, corticosteroids, or other immunosuppressive therapies. Transfusion therapy (packed RBCs) should be avoided unless absolutely necessary. However, RBC transfusion should not be withheld if a severely compromised cardiopulmonary status exists even when compatibility of the donor cells is incomplete. In those rare cases, the involved department of transfusion medicine should be asked to identify the most compatible product available, and the transfusion should be closely monitored. Infections are treated with antimicrobials. For thrombotic thrombocytopenic purpura, plasmapharesis is specifically indicated. Prevention of immune- or G6PD-mediated hemolysis involves discontinuation or avoidance of associated medications. Monitoring urine hemoglobin and hemosiderin levels can determine the response to intravascular hemolysis therapy.

Intrinsic causes of hemolysis are usually inherited. They are present during infancy or childhood and result in chronic hemolysis. In those cases, prognosis and treatment are complex, because the hemolytic picture may change over time. Despite the considerable advances in defining these genetic diseases at the molecular level, equally specific treatment regimens are lacking. The first question to ask is whether treatment is necessary. Chronic hemolysis may only require a yearly clinical evaluation with CBC, absolute reticulocyte count, and blood smear to determine if the patient is able to maintain adequate levels of erythropoiesis. Parvovirus infections in these patients may result in acute worsening of their anemia because of a sudden decrease in their erythropoiesis. Folic acid should be given to all patients with chronic hemolysis (1 mg per day) because this vitamin is consumed with the accelerated production of erythrocytes. Transfusion regimens should be tailored for individual patients, and iron overload should be anticipated. Even in the absence of transfusion, iron overload may result from ineffective erythropoiesis. The increased metabolism of heme also leads to a significant increase in pigmented gallstone formation.

Treatments such as splenectomy or bone marrow transplantation should be reserved for marked hemolysis producing life-threatening anemia. As stated above, patients with hereditary stomatocytosis syndromes should not be considered candidates for splenectomy (35). When severe hemolysis is because of other membrane defects, splenectomy may be beneficial and indicated. In children, splenectomy should be delayed until the age of 6 (if possible) because of the increased risk of sepsis. In general, splenectomy risks must be compared with those associated with lifelong transfusion. After a splenectomy is performed, special care must be taken to compensate for the loss of splenic function. The spleen is responsible for the clearance of encapsulated bacteria such as *Streptococcus pneumoniae, Haemophilus influenzae,* or *Neisseria meningitis.* The combined use of pneumococcal polysaccharide immunization and early empiric antibiotic therapy offer a high level of protection for postsplenectomy patients. It is estimated that sepsis is fatal in 40% to 50% of all splenectomized patients. Within that group, children with thalassemia and sickle cell syndromes have the highest risk of death (38). In all cases, patients must be informed that the asplenic state carries a significant risk of overwhelming and life-threatening infection.

CONCLUSION

A broad range of genetic and acquired diseases is manifested by hemolysis. The differential diagnosis is useful in developing diagnostic and therapeutic strategies and should be thought of in terms of intrinsic or extrinsic causes of erythrocyte damage. A careful search for the cause of hemolysis should be pursued because treatments are so different. When a common cause of hemolysis is not found, an underlying enzyme or membrane defect should be sought.

Clinical severity in all cases of hemolysis is determined by the rate of red cell destruction and the host's ability to compensate by producing fresh erythrocytes. Disease can vary from a subtle and clinically silent syndrome to hemolysis of sufficient intensity to dominate the clinical picture and even cause death if left untreated. Every therapeutic plan should be designed for both the severity of disease as well as the cause of hemolysis.

HELPFUL INTERNET SITES

http://www.ncbi.nlm.nih/omim
http://hembase.niddk.nih.gov/
http://www.g6pd.org/favism/english/index.mv
http://www.uptodate.com

REFERENCES

1. Lichtman MA, Beutler E, Kipps TJ, et al. Williams Hematology, 7th Ed. New York: Mcgraw-Hill Publishers; 2006.
2. Nathan DG, Orkin SH, Oski FA. Hematology of Infancy and Childhood, 6th Ed. Philadelphia: WB Saunders; 2003.
3. Hoffman, R, Benz EJ, Shattil, SJ, et al. Hematology: Basic Principles and Practice, 4th Ed. Philadelphia: Elsevier; 2005.
4. Beutler E, Luzzatto L. Hemolytic anemia. Semin Hematol 1999;36:38–47.
5. Dhaliwal G, Cornett PA, Tierney LM. Hemolytic anemia. Am Fam Physician 2004;69: 2599–2606.
6. Dacie JV. The Haemolytic Anaemias: Secondary or Symptomatic Haemolytic Anaemias, 3rd Ed. Vols. 1–5. New York: Churchill Livingstone; 1967.
7. Nowicki MJ, Poley JR. The hereditary hyperbilirubinaemias. Baillieres Clin Gastroenterol 1998; 12:355–367.
8. McArthur JR. Morphology Glossary. American Society of Hematology Education Book. 2000; 457–474.
9. Riley RS, Ben-Ezra JM, Tidwell A, et al. Reticulocyte analysis by flow cytometry and other techniques. Hematol Oncol Clin North Am 2002;16:373–420.
10. Marchand A, Galen RS, Van Lente F. The predicative value of serum haptoglobin in hemolytic disease. JAMA 1980;243:1909–1911.
11. Ronquist G, Theodorsson E. Inherited, non-spherocytic haemolysis due to deficiency of glucose-6-phosphate dehydrogenase. Scand J Clin Lab Invest 2007;67:105–111.
12. Hamilton JW, Jones FG, McMullin MF. Glucose-6-phosphate dehydrogenase Guadalajara—a case of chronic non-spherocytic haemolytic anaemia responding to splenectomy and the role of splenectomy in this disorder. Hematology 2004;4:307–309.
13. Ristoff E, Larsson A. Patients with genetic defects in the gamma-glutamyl cycle. Chem Biol Interact 1998;111–121.
14. Takahashi K, Newburger PE, Cohen HJ. Glutathione peroxidase protein. Absence in selenium deficiency states and correlation with enzymatic activity. J Clin Invest 1986;77:1402–1404.
15. Kamerbeek NM, vanZwieten R, deBoer M, et al. Molecular basis of glutathione reductase deficiency in human blood cells. Blood 2007;109:3560–3566.
16. Ristoff E, Larsson A. Inborn errors in the metabolism of glutathione. Orphanet J Rare Dis 2007; 2:16–24.
17. Williams TN. Human red blood cell polymorphisms and malaria. Curr Opin Microbiol 2006;9: 388–394.
18. Zanella A, Fermo E, Bianchi P, et al. Red cell pyruvate kinase deficiency: molecular and clinical aspects. Br J Haematol 2005;130:11–25.

19. Kugler W, Lakomek M. Glucose-6-phosphate isomerase deficiency. Baillieres Clin Haematol 2000;13:89–101.
20. Yao DC, Tolan DR, Murray MF, et al. Hemolytic anemia and severe rhabdomyolysis caused by compound heterozygous mutations of the gene for erythrocyte/muscle isozyme of aldolase, ALDOA. Blood 2004;103:2401–2403.
21. Jacobasch G, Rapoport SM. Hemolytic anemias due to erythrocyte enzyme deficiencies. Mol Aspects Med 1996;17:143–170.
22. Boulard-Heitzmann P, Boulard M, Tallineau C. Decreased red cell enolase in 40 year old woman with compensated haemolysis. Scand J Haemotol 1984;33:401–404.
23. Kanno H. Hexokinase: gene structure and mutations. Baillieres Clin Haematol 2000;13:83–88.
24. Sabina RL, Waldenström A, Ronquist G. The contribution of Ca^2†-calmodulin activation of human erythrocyte AMP deaminase (isoform E) to the erythrocyte metabolic dysregulation of familial phosphofructokinase deficiency. Haematologica 2006;91:652–655.
25. Beutler E. PGK deficiency. Br J Haematol 2007;136:3–11.
26. Oláh J, Orosz F, Keserü GM, et al. Triosephosphate isomerase deficiency: a neurodegenerative misfolding disease. Biochem Soc Trans 2002;30:30–38.
27. Zanella A, Bianchi P, Fermo E, et al. Hereditary pyrimidine 5'-nucleotidase deficiency: from genetics to clinical manifestations. Br J Haematol 2006;133:113–123.
28. Chottiner EG, Cloft, HJ, Tartaglia AP, et al. Elevated adenosine deaminase activity and hereditary hemolytic anemia: evidence for abnormal translational control of protein synthesis. J Clin Invest 1987;79:1001–1005.
29. Koizumi S. Human heme oxygenase-1 deficiency: A lesson on serendipity in the discovery of the novel disease. Pediatr Int 2007;49:125–132.
30. Hovingh GK, de Groot E, van der Steeg W et al. Inherited disorders of HDL metabolism and atherosclerosis. Curr Opin Lipidol 2005;16:139–145.
31. Nash R, Shojania AM. Hematological aspect of Rh deficiency: a case report and review of literature. Am J Hematol 1987;24:267–275.
32. Walker RH, Danek A, Uttner I, et al. McLeod phenotype without the McLeod syndrome. Transfusion 2007;47:299–305.
33. Bolton-Maggs PH, Stevens RF, Dodd NJ, et al. Guidelines for the diagnosis and management of hereditary spherocytosis. Br J Haematol 2004;126:455–474.
34. Iglauer A, Reinhardt D, Schöter W, et al. Cryohemolysis test as a diagnostic tool for hereditary spherocytosis. Ann Hematol 1999;78:555–557.
35. Delaunay J. The molecular basis of hereditary red cell membrane disorders. Blood Rev 2007;21:1–20.
36. Walker RH, Jung HH, Dobson-Stone C, et al. Neurologic phenotypes associated with acanthocytosis. Neurology 2007;68:92–98.
37. Ramos MC, Schafernak KT, Peterson LC. Hereditary pyropoikilocytosis: a rare but potentially severe form of congenital hemolytic anemia. J Pediatr Hematol Oncol 2007;29:128–129.
38. Bisharat N, Omari H, Lavi I, et al. Risk of infection and death among post-splenectomy patients. J Infect 2001;43:182–186.

4

Hemolytic Anemia:
Thalassemias and Sickle Cell Disorders

Matthew M. Hsieh, John F. Tisdale, and Griffin P. Rodgers

Normal hemoglobin within red blood cells is composed of two α and two β chains with α to β synthesis ratio of 1:1. Thalassemias are a group of *quantitative* disorders with insufficient production of α or β chains, leading to an imbalanced accumulation of β or α chains, respectively. In contrast, hemoglobinopathies (or abnormal hemoglobin structural variants) are a separate group of *qualitative* disorders, with abnormal β or α chains in normal quantity, of which sickle cell disease (SCD) is best recognized. While these two disorders share features of variable degree of hemolytic anemia and transfusion-related complications, they differ in their pathophysiology, clinical manifestations, and management (Table 4.1).

The hemoglobinopathies and thalassemias are commonly encountered in areas where malaria is endemic, presumably because abnormal genes offer protection against malaria. However, there are observations that the malaria theory does not explain well. One is that thalassemia exists where there is little or no malaria, such as the Pacific; this may be explained in part by population migration and genetic drift. Another is why certain region contains only one type or pattern of hemoglobinopathy, such as hemoglobin (Hb) E in Southeast Asia, Hb C in West Africa, or only a few β-thalassemia mutations in a particular geographic location. Perhaps these regional differences are temporary, and over time, the different mutation patterns will be distributed globally.

PATHOPHYSIOLOGY

Thalassemias

Normally there arc four copies of α-globin gene, two copies on each chromatid of chromosome 16 (Table 4.2). α-Globin chains are essential in the synthesis of both fetal and adult hemoglobin. α-Thalassemia syndromes result from deletions of a large α-globin gene segment from unequal crossover or recombination, and less frequently from mutations. The deleted segments of DNA vary in size and can involve one ($-+$, or $\alpha+$) or both ($--$, or $\alpha 0$) alleles on the same chromatid. Deletion of one gene ($-+/++$) confers a silent carrier. Two-gene deletion ($--/++$ or $-+/-+$) is commonly referred as α-thalassemia minor or trait with microcytosis, hypochromia, but little or no anemia. Deletion of three genes ($--/-+$) leads to Hb H (β4), which is an unstable form of hemoglobin. Hb H disease is manifested by hypochromia, moderately severe hemolytic anemia, and splenomegaly. Absence of all four genes leads to hydrops fetalis with Hb Bart's (γ4). Hb Bart's transports O_2 poorly, causes profound tissue hypoxia, leads to heart and liver failure, and is almost always incompatible with life (Fig. 4.1).

Both α-globin gene deletion haplotypes, ($-+$) and ($--$), occur equally in Southeast Asians, whereas the ($--$) haplotype is much less common in Mediterraneans and rare in Africans. Hence all the α-thalassemic syndromes are seen in Southeast Asians, but hydrop fetalis is uncommon to rare in Mediterraneans and Africans. In addition to α-globin gene deletions, there are α-globin structural variants that may occur alone or in combination with α-gene deletions and lead to further reduction of α-globin synthesis. The best characterized α-globin variant is Hb Constant Spring.

TABLE 4.1. *General Features of Thalassemia and Sickle Cell Disease*

	α-Thalassemia	β-Thalassemia	Sickle Cell Disease
Geographic	Equatorial Africa; Mediterranean, Middle East; Arab peninsula; Caribbean; India; southeast Asia; South China		Africa; some Mediterranean, Middle Eastern countries; parts of India
Pathophysiology	Quantitative Hb defect: Gene deletion(s) leading to reduced α-chain production and hemolytic anemia	Quantitative Hb defect: Mutations leading to reduced β-chain production and hemolytic anemia	Qualitative Hb defect: Hb S polymerization leading to vaso-occlusion and hemolytic anemia
Therapy	Simple transfusions Iron chelation	Simple transfusions Iron chelation Hydroxyurea in selected individuals Transplantation	Simple and exchange transfusions Analgesia Hydroxyurea Transplantation

Hb, hemoglobin.

Similar to α-thalassemia, β-thalassemia syndromes also arise from genetic alterations that significantly reduce β-globin chain production. In contrast to the α-globin genes, there are only two β-globin genes, one on each chromatid of chromosome 11. While there are almost 200 mutations described, only about 20 mutations account for the majority of β-thalassemic individuals. Mutations are grouped by regional ethnic locations: Mediterranean basin, Southeast Asia, Africa, and Asian India. All disease-causing mutations alter β-globin gene mRNA transcription, processing, or translation. Some mutations decrease β-globin production by as little as 10% and some by as much as 90%. Homo- or heterozygosity of mildly or severely affected alleles explains the wide range of clinical syndromes. Patients with one abnormal and one normal β allele have β-thalassemia minor or trait: the synthesis of β chain is reduced by about one half. Although normal hemoglobin A (α2β2) is mildly decreased, there is no accumulation of excess α-chains. There is hypochromia and microcytosis but no clinically significant anemia, hemolysis, or ineffective erythropoiesis. The phenotype of two severe β-chain alleles is referred as β-thalassemia major or Cooley's anemia: β-chain synthesis and Hb A is virtually absent with α-chains in great excess and consequently severe hemolytic anemia.

TABLE 4.2. *Normal and Variant Hemoglobin*

Name	Designation	Molecular Structure	Proportion in
Adult hemoglobin	A	α2 β2	Adults: 97% Newborns: 20%–25%
Adult hemoglobin	A$_2$	α2 δ2	Adults: 2.5% Newborns: 0.5%
Fetal hemoglobin	F	α2 γ2	Adults: <1% Newborns: 75%–80%
	Hb H	β4	Adults: 0% Newborns: 15%–25% in Hb H disease
	Hb Barts	γ4	Adults: 0% Newborns: 15%–25% in Hb H disease, 100% in hydrop fetalis

Hb, hemoglobin.

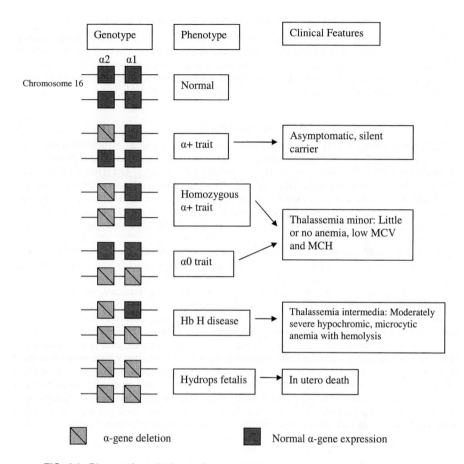

FIG. 4.1. Diagram for α-thalassemia gene deletion and corresponding phenotypes.

While the thalassemic syndromes are highly variable, severity is directly related to the imbalance of α to β chain ratio. Higher α to β chain ratio, 2–3:1, correlates with more severe β-thalassemia. In the severe thalassemic phenotype, excess unpaired α or β chains precipitate in erythrocyte precursors, resulting in their early death and ineffective erythropoiesis. Excess unpaired α or β chains also damage the red cell membrane and denature intracellular hemoglobin, promoting splenic sequestration and hemolysis and eventual splenomegaly and anemia. Chronic hemolytic anemia and tissue hypoxia stimulate bone marrow expansion and produce skeletal and metabolic derangements: bony deformities, fractures, extramedullary hematopoiesis, and increased gastrointestinal iron absorption. In addition, red cell membrane damage, activation of platelets and endothelium, and abnormal levels of coagulation inhibitors (antithrombin III, protein C and S) all contribute to increased risk of thromboembolism.

In β-thalassemia, the compensatory increase in Hb A_2 and F is inadequate to offset the α to β chain imbalance. Any genetic conditions that reduce α-chain excess (co-inheritance of α-thalassemia or increase in δ- or γ-chain production) or preserve some β-chain synthesis (a mild or silent β-thalassemic allele) ameliorate the severity of β-thalassemia. Thalassemia intermedia refers to patients with a lesser degree of hemolytic anemia, usually secondary to compound heterozygosity of two mild β-thalassemia alleles, δ- and β-thalassemia, or Hb E and β-thalassemia; β-thalassemia with hereditary persistence of fetal hemoglobin (HPFH); or co-existence of α- and β-thalassemia.

Hemoglobinopathies: Hemoglobin Structural Variants

Hemoglobin variants of α or β chains, or the hemoglobinopathies, are caused by point mutations (most common), frameshift mutations, chain elongations, or chain fusions. The nomenclature of hemoglobinopathies employs alphabetic letters (S, C, or E) and sometimes with locations of first discovery (O^{Arab} or D ^{Punjab}) or name of the index case (Lepore or Constant Spring), then followed by the chain, location, and amino acid substitution in that hemoglobin chain ($\beta6^{Glu \rightarrow Val}$).

Hemoglobin S

Sickle hemoglobin (Hb S) is the best characterized and the most important hemoglobinopathy. SCD is an inherited disorder in which normal glutamic acid is substituted by valine in the sixth codon of β-globin chain ($\beta6^{Glu \rightarrow Val}$), which favors bonding of hemoglobin molecules. As a result, Hb S is less soluble when deoxygenated (in the normal oxygenation-deoxygenation cycle), precipitates and polymerizes quickly in red cells, and causes a morphologic change to a crescent shape. These rigid sickle cells lead to hemolytic anemia and vaso-occlusion, which together cause all complications of SCD.

The life span of sickle cells is about 10 to 20 days, compared with 120 days for normal red cells. In the absence of clinically significant pain episodes, there is a chronic hemolytic anemia with mean hemoglobin of 6–8 g/dL, despite compensatory reticulocytosis of greater than 5% or 150 k/uL. Most sickle erythrocytes are removed in the spleen; some are destroyed intravascularly by mechanical forces or oxidative stress. Hemolysis has been implicated to activate inflammatory mediators, such as tumor necrosis factor-alpha (TNF-α), interleukin-2 (IL-2), thrombin, and platelet-activating factor (1). Leukocytosis is often associated with more frequent pain crises, stroke, and a shorter life expectancy in patients with homozygous sickle disease (Hb SS). Free hemoglobin, released by hemolysis, can consume nitric oxide and participate in endothelial dysfunction to promote vasoconstriction.

Vaso-occlusion begins with accumulation of sickle erythrocytes and can occur in any vascular bed. Bone marrow and spleen are particularly susceptible because of their slow venous blood flow and a high cell turnover rate. Pain crises in the long bones are the most common manifestation of SCD and repetitive vaso-occlusive episodes (VOE) eventually lead to marrow and splenic infarction. Although normal lung reoxygenates and potentially reverses polymerizations sickle erythrocytes, hypoxia or infection damages lung parenchyma, activates pulmonary endothelium, and promotes adherence of sickle erythrocytes. This process of vaso-occlusion in small and large pulmonary vessels can result in acute chest syndrome.

Other Hemoglobinopathies (E, C, Lepore, D, O^{Arab}, Constant Spring)

Hb E is a common hemoglobin variant, present in about 15% to 30% of the individuals in southern China and Southeast Asia. Hb E results from replacement of the normal glutamic acid to lysine in the twenty-sixth amino acid of the β-chain ($\beta26^{Glu \rightarrow Lys}$) and leads to only 50% of mRNAs being spliced normally. Individuals with heterozygous and homozygous Hb E have mild anemia, hypochromia, and microcytosis. When Hb E is combined with β-thalassemia, the clinical features resemble those of β-thalassemia intermedia.

Hb C results from substitution of the normal glutamic acid to lysine in the sixth amino acid of β-chain. Hb C is found mostly in individuals of African descent and is the second most common hemoglobinopathy in the United States and third most common worldwide. Carriers of Hb C are asymptomatic. Homozygous individuals (Hb CC) exhibit mild hemolytic anemia but are largely asymptomatic. Hb C combined with β-thalassemia produces mild to moderate hemolytic anemia with some features of β-thalassemia major. Compound heterozygosity with Hb C and S (Hb SC) leads to milder anemia with fewer leg ulcers, pain crises, and osteonecrosis than with homozygous SCD (Hb SS); there is also a slightly lower risk of infection from encapsulated organisms. Retinal proliferative disease and splenomegaly, however, manifest earlier and more frequently in Hb SC disease.

Hb Lepore is a fused globin chain consisting of N-terminal half of δ-chain and C-terminal half of β-chain and is produced at low levels (2.5%) compared with normal β-chains. Although typically seen in Greeks or Italians, this variant can occur in a many ethnic groups of northern European descent. Hb Lepore can occur alone or in combination with other β-thalassemic mutations, leading to symptoms similar to β-thalassemia. Hb D (same as Hb Los Angeles or Hb Punjab), another β-chain variant, is seen in Asian Indian population. When combined with β-thalassemia or SCD, the anemia is mild. Hb O^{Arab}, a rare β-chain variant when combined with SCD (Hb SO^{Arab}), behaves similarly to full sickle cell disease.

Hb Constant Spring, present in 5% to 10% of Southeast Asians, is caused by a point mutation in the stop codon of α-chain mRNA, leading to an elongated α-chain ($α^{CS}$). Because synthesis of $α^{CS}$ is reduced (only about 1% is made), Hb Constant Spring behaves like an α-chain deletion. When $α^{CS}$ is combined with a *cis* α-thalassemic defect, it resembles Hb H disease ($--/α^{CS} α$). Fortunately, $α^{CS}$ is typically coupled with a normal α-chain gene ($α^{CS} α$) on the same allele, and hydrop fetalis has not been observed.

DIAGNOSIS AND SCREENING

The diagnosis of SCD and thalassemias is now accomplished by neonatal or prenatal testing (2,3). The goal of postnatal testing is to identify α- or β-thalassemia carriers, Hb S, C, E, and other clinically important hemoglobinopathies. The process typically begins with a complete blood count (CBC). When red indices are suggestive (Table 4.3), peripheral blood smear and high performance liquid chromatography (HPLC) provide a provisional diagnosis (Fig. 4.2). HPLC has largely replaced traditional electrophoresis because it reliably quantitates the fraction of hemoglobin A_2, F, and S. Hemoglobinopathies are confirmed by isoelectric focusing or gel electrophoresis under alkaline (separates Hb S from Hb D/G) or acidic (separates Hb C, E, and O^{Arab}) conditions. Specific thalassemia mutations require polymerase chain reaction (PCR)-based DNA testing. Blood count indices vary widely and may deviate from typical values if there is concurrent iron deficiency or compound heterozygosity of other hemoglobinopathies. Any transfusion would also alter the hematologic parameters commonly found in each syndrome.

TABLE 4.3. *Hematologic Characteristics of Sickle Cell Disease and Thalassemias*

Normal	Total RBC: normal
	MCV >78 fl (or cubic microliter) or MCH >27 pg
	Hb A* >95%, F <1%, A_2 <3%
α- or β-thalassemia minor (trait)	MCV <78 fl or MCH < 25 pg, elevated total RBC
	Hb A,* F 1%–7%,† A_2 >3.5%‡
α-thalassemia major	MCV <70 fl or MCH < 25 pg, elevated total RBC
(Hb H disease)	Hb A,* F 1%–7%,† A_2 normal, Hb H 0.8%–40%
	Severe microcytosis, anisocytosis, hypochromia, and Hb H on peripheral smear
β-thalassemia major	MCV <70 fl or MCH <25 pg, elevated total RBC
	Hb A,* Hb F 1%–7%,† Hb A_2 >3.5%‡
	Severe microcytosis, anisocytosis, hypochromia on peripheral smear
Sickle cell trait	Hb A* near 50%, Hb S ≤40%
Sickle cell disease	Hb SS*: Hb S >70%, A_2 <4%, and variable % of Hb F; sickle cells in peripheral smear
	Hb SC: Hb S and C each 30%–40%; less sickle cells but more target cells and spherocytes in peripheral smear
Hb S/β+ thalassemia	Variable % of Hb A*, Hb S typically >50%
Hb S/β0 thalassemia	Hb S* typically >50%, <10% Hb A, A_2 >4%

*Screening hemoglobin electrophoresis or HPLC pattern.
† Hb F may be higher in individuals with concurrent δβ-thalassemia or hereditary persistence of fetal hemoglobin (HPFH).
‡Hb A_2 may be less than 3.5% in individuals with concurrent iron deficiency, some α-thalassemia, δβ-thalassemia, or certain β-chain mutations.
Hb, hemoglobin; MCH, mean corpuscular hemoglobin; MCV, mean corpuscular volume; RBC, red blood cell;

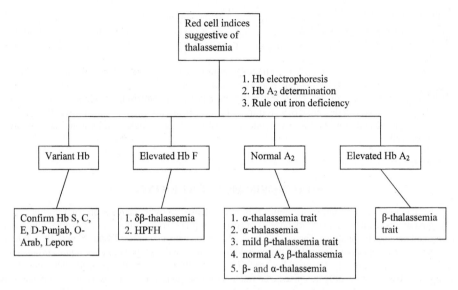

FIG. 4.2. Diagnostic schema for thalassemias.

α-Thalassemia Trait and Disease

Trans α-chain defect $(-+/-+)$ is more common in the Asian-Indian subcontinent, Africa, and Afro-Caribbean regions, and less likely to produce clinically severe thalassemic phenotypes (Hb H or hydrop fetalis). *Cis* α-chain defect $(--/++)$, in contrast, can be seen in individuals from China, Southeast Asia, Greece, Turkey, or Cyprus. Screening for the *cis* defect in at risk individuals is appropriate because the α-thalassemic phenotype may be moderate to severe. α-Thalassemia trait can been suspected with elevated total red blood cell number, normal or borderline Hb A_2, mean corpuscular volume (MCV) less than 78 micron, and mean corpuscular hemoglobin (MCH) less than 25 pg. The peripheral blood smear in Hb H disease can be stained with cresol blue to show Hb H precipitates in erythrocytes and reticulocytes.

β-Thalassemia Trait and Major

β-Thalassemia trait can be present in individuals of any ethnic group of northern European descent. Trait can be suspected from an elevated total red blood cell number, MCV less than 78 fl, MCH less than 27 pg, and normal or slightly low hemoglobin. On HPLC, there is a characteristic elution pattern of variably elevated Hb F (higher in the Mediterranean variant and lower in the African variant), normal Hb A, and greater than 3.5% Hb A_2. However, Hb A_2 may be normal (less than 3%) in individuals with concurrent iron deficiency or α-thalassemia; compound heterozygous δ- and β-thalassemia, or those with certain β-chain mutations. With β-thalassemia major, the MCV is usually less than 70 fl, MCH less than 25 pg, variably low hemoglobin (5–9 g/dL), and no Hb A on HPLC.

Sickle Cell Trait and Disease

Sickle cell trait or disease can be diagnosed by the combination CBC, HPLC, and the sickle solubility test. Sickle cell trait has near normal red cell indices; hemoglobin may be slightly low to normal, and the MCH and red cell distribution width (RDW) may be slightly elevated. Hb S will comprise 35% to 40% on HPLC. Conversely, in SCD, hemoglobin will range from 6 to 8 g/dL, and sickle erythrocytes will be seen on peripheral blood smear. Hb S will comprise >60% (typically 70% to 80%) of total hemoglobin with slightly elevated Hb A_2 on HPLC (because of co-elution of Hb S with Hb A_2).

Trait or SCD is then confirmed by sickle solubility test and acidic or alkaline gel electrophoresis to screen for other concurrent hemoglobinopathies, such as Hb D or G. Sickle SC disease is easily distinguished by HPLC. Additionally, the peripheral smear in Hb SC disease shows fewer sickle cells, more spherocytes and target cells, and an uneven distribution of hemoglobin among red blood cells.

CLINICAL SYNDROMES AND TREATMENT OF SICKLE CELL DISEASE

Vaso-Occlusive Episodes (Pain Crises)

Vaso-occlusive episode (VOE) is the most frequent clinical manifestation of SCD (4) and can occur spontaneously or precipitated by infection, stress, or dehydration. Frequent assessment and modification of therapy, involvement of a pain management service, and other consultations are important to address the complex etiology of pain in SCD. Evaluation begins by obtaining a full history of current and prior VOEs. Physical examination and vital signs identify any signs or symptoms related to a pain episode. Acute pain can affect multiple sites: bones, joints, the cardiopulmonary system, central nervous system (CNS), or abdominal visceral organs. Chronic pain is typically confined to leg ulcers and the skeletal system.

Mild acute pain can often be managed in the outpatient setting with a combination of nonsteroidal anti-inflammatory drugs (NSAIDs), acetaminophen, and/or an oral opioid. Moderate to severe acute pain typically requires intervention in a day-hospital or emergency department, which begins with rapid assessment of the pain; hydration using 5% dextrose in half normal saline (D5 ½ NS) and 20 mEq KCl, not exceeding 1 ½ times maintenance; and an opioid analgesic (typically morphine, hydromorphone, or fentanyl). The choice, dose, and frequency of medication depend on the patient's outpatient drug regimen and prior responses. Severe pain is managed by bolus and continuous infusion of an opioid analgesic, often with patient-controlled delivery (PCA) pumps. In those with poor intravenous access, subcutaneous injection is an acceptable short-term alternative; however, intramuscular injection should be avoided because the absorption varies. Parenteral meperidine should not be used as first-line treatment because the metabolite, normeperidine, has a long half life and increases the risk of mood disturbances and seizures. Opioid agonists are metabolized by the liver and excreted variably by the kidney, and dose reduction may be necessary in those with hepatic impairment. Meperidine and morphine have active metabolites and should be used with great caution in patients with renal impairment and avoided in patients with renal failure. Common side effects of all opioids—nausea, vomiting, pruritus, constipation, and respiratory depression—should be monitored and treated accordingly.

Nonopioid analgesics such as acetaminophen and NSAIDs have a ceiling effect and are often used with an oral opioid agonist. The total acetaminophen dose should not exceed 6 g daily in adults with normal hepatic function. Gastrointestinal, renal, and hematologic toxicities should be monitored. Benzodiazepines, antidepressants, anti-emetics, and opioid agonist-antagonists, such as pentazocine, nalbuphine, and butorphaol, are useful adjuncts to opioid agonists and potentiate their analgesic effects. Gabapentin can be used for neuropathic pain.

In a recent review of chronic opioid therapy (5), failure to achieve desired analgesia may result from (i) opioid tolerance, where the number of opioid receptors is reduced; (ii) opioid-induced hypersensitivity, where an individual experiences increased tenderness from known noxious stimuli; or (iii) worsening pain from progressive tissue damage. Prolonged, high-dose opioid therapy is associated with testosterone deficiency and suppression of immunity. Opioid dose escalation every 6 to 8 weeks or opioid rotation with a period of opioid abstinence may improve desired analgesia and minimize adverse effects in long-term analgesic therapy (Table 4.4).

Blood transfusions are not routinely administered during VOEs. Transfusions are important for concurrent complications, such as acute chest syndrome, stroke, or other organ ischemia and damage.

Infections

Because of functional asplenia, patients with SCD are at an increased risk of infection with encapsulated organisms: *Streptococcus pneumoniae*, *Hemophilus influenza,* and *Neisseria meningitides*. Several changes in patient management have reduced mortality rates. Neonatal diagnosis enables

TABLE 4.4. *Comparative Profiles of Common Opioid Agonists for Acute Pain*

	Equivalent Analgesic Dosing	Site of Metabolism and Excretion*	Dose Adjustment in Hepatic Impairment	Dose Adjustment in Renal Impairment
Fentanyl	IV or transdermal: 25 μg every hr	Liver: inactive metabolites Kidney: 75% of metabolites	No	GFR 10–50 mL/min: 75% of normal dosing GFR <10 mL/min: 50% of normal dosing
Hydromorphone	Every 3–4 hrs IV: 1.5–2 mg PO: 6–7.5 mg IV: PO ratio 1:5	Liver: inactive metabolites Kidney: little excretion	Consider	Consider
Meperidine	Every 3–4 hrs IV: 100 mg PO: 250 mg IV: PO ratio 1:3	Liver: several active metabolites Kidney: >70% excretion	Yes	Use of meperidine with renal impairment should be avoided
Morphine	Every 3–4 hrs IV: 10 mg PO: 30 mg IV: PO ratio 1:3	Liver: active and inactive metabolites Kidney: >90% excretion	Yes	Use of morphine in renal impairment should use caution GFR 10–50 mL/min: 75% normal dosing GFR <10 mL/min: avoid morphine or 50% of normal dosing with caution
Oxycodone	Every 4 hrs IV: not available PO: 20–30 mg	Liver: active metabolites Kidney: variable excretion of metabolites	Yes, start ⅓ to ½ of normal dose	GFR 10–50 mL/min: 33% to 50% of normal dosing GFR <10 mL/min: 33% of normal dosing

*Opioid agonists are typically metabolized in the liver into active or inactive products and are variably excreted by the kidneys.
IV, intravenous; GFR, glomerulai filtration rate; PO, per oral.

penicillin prophylaxis and family education. In a placebo-controlled clinical trial (6), prophylactic penicillin prevented 84% of life-threatening infections caused by *S. pneumoniae.* Penicillin may be discontinued in those older than 5 years of age who have been vaccinated against *S. pneumoniae*, because there was no statistically significant benefit compared with placebo. Patients allergic to penicillin can receive erythromycin. Additionally, fever should be evaluated and managed promptly as a potential sepsis event and empiric antibiotics administered while awaiting blood or urine culture and chest radiograph results. Finally, pneumococcal vaccination should begin in children and be renewed periodically. Influenza vaccinations should also be given yearly (Table 4.5).

Human parvovirus B19 is commonly spread among school-age children. B19 infects erythroid progenitors and causes transient red cell aplasia. While there is a wide range of clinical severity, influenza-like symptoms, fever, pain, and splenic sequestration can accompany an acute infection. Laboratory testing may reveal acute anemia, reticulocytopenia, and IgM antibody to parvovirus. Milder forms of SCD (e.g., Hb SC or Hb S/β+ thalassemia, hydroxyurea treatment, or chronic transfusions) do not protect individuals with SCD from developing severe complications related to B19 (7). Parvovirus infection is also known as fifth disease, but in patients suffering transient aplastic crisis, the characteristic facial rash is absent. B19 can cross the placenta and cause hydrop fetalis and stillbirths; thus, pregnant staff should be strictly isolated.

TABLE 4.5. *Suggested Antibiotic Prophylaxis and Vaccination Schedule for Sickle Cell Patients*

2 Months to 2 Years of Age	2 to 3 Years of Age	3 to 5 Years of Age	Older than 5 Years of Age	Adults
Penicillin VK 125 mg BID or erythromycin 10 mg/kg BID		Penicillin 250 mg BID or erythromycin	May discontinue antibiotic if vaccinated against *S. pneumoniae*	
Prenar (7 valent) 2–4 doses every 2 months	Pneumovax (23 valent) one dose Yearly influenza vaccination	Yearly influenza vaccination	Yearly influenza vaccination	Repeat pneumovax every 5 years Yearly influenza vaccination

BID, twice a day.

CENTRAL NERVOUS SYSTEM AND EYE DISEASE

Central Nervous System (Stroke)

Stroke is a major complication more frequently observed in Hb SS than Hb SC (8,9). Children tend to have thrombotic strokes, and adults hemorrhagic strokes. Because the incidence of stroke is 11% up to 20 years of age, children with Hb SS should be screened with transcranial Doppler (TCD) every 6 to 12 months from age 2 to18 years. For primary stroke prevention, the Stroke Prevention (STOP) trial showed that children (ages 2 to 16 years old) who had a TCD velocity greater than 200 cm/sec in the internal carotid or middle cerebral artery had improvement in the TCD velocity and a much lower incidence of brain infarction when managed on long-term transfusions to maintain Hb S less than 30% compared with supportive care (penicillin prophylaxis, vaccinations, folate supplementation, treatment of acute crises, and transfusions as needed) (8). A follow-up study to the original STOP trial showed that when long-term transfusions were discontinued, TCD velocity quickly returned to abnormal, and a few children developed acute strokes (10). Individuals 18 years and older tend to have lower transcranial velocities; thus, TCD may not be a good screening tool.

Children with suspected stroke or TIAs are evaluated promptly, and hydration, therapy for hypoxia or hyperthermia, and blood pressure stabilization should follow immediately. Tissue plasminogen activator (t-PA) has not been extensively used in children and therefore is not routinely recommended. The use of antiplatelet agents, aspirin, or clopidogrel, is uncertain but may be appropriate in selected circumstances. If a thrombotic stroke is present, exchange transfusions are initiated to reduce the Hb S level to less than 30%. If a hemorrhagic stroke is present, the source and the extent of bleeding are identified and the treatments are individualized; exchange transfusions may be indicated to reduce the Hb S level to less than 30%. If imaging studies do not identify any abnormality, the next steps may involve observation, simple transfusions, and/or participation in clinical trials.

As the recurrence rate for thrombotic strokes is high, long-term transfusion therapy to maintain Hb S less than 30% until 16 to 18 years of age should be planned. Long-term transfusions can also be considered in hemorrhagic stroke or vasculopathy (aneurysm or arterial stenosis). There is an ongoing multicenter Stroke with Transfusion Changing to Hydroxyurea (SWiTCH) trial that compares long-term transfusions with iron chelation to hydroxyurea and phlebotomy therapy for secondary prevention of stroke. There is also another international Silent Infarct Transfusion (SIT) trial that will compare long-term transfusion with no transfusions in children who had silent infarct on brain magnetic resonance imaging (MRI) with normal TCD velocities. The results of these two trials will no doubt improve the care of children with strokes.

Adults with acute strokes or TIAs are managed similarly to children (4). If a thrombotic stroke is identified, t-PA, antiplatelet therapy, and/or exchange transfusions can be considered. If a hemorrhagic stroke is identified, treatment is based on the source and the extent of bleeding; exchange transfusion to reduce the Hb S level to less than 30% may be indicated. For long-term therapy or secondary prophylaxis, antiplatelet therapy may be continued, with or without chronic transfusions to maintain the Hb S level less than 30%. Warfarin or dipyridamole may add to or substitute antiplatelet therapy for patients with recurrent strokes.

There is currently no single best screening method to identify adults who are at high risk for stroke. MRI/magnetic resonance angiography (MRA) of brain can be considered in those who have general risk factors of thrombotic strokes (age, prior transient ischemic attacks, and systemic hypertension) or risk factors specific to SCD (prior history of acute chest syndromes, dactylitis, severe anemia, and leukocytosis).

EYE DISEASE

Neovascularization results from repetitive vaso-occlusive episodes within the eye and leads to visual impairment. These proliferative changes are often asymptomatic early in the disease process; clinically detectable retinal changes are typically discovered between 15 to 30 years of age. Patients with Hb SC and sickle-thalassemia are disproportionately more prone to develop clinically significant ophthalmologic problems. Annual eye examinations starting in adolescence, carefully evaluating visual acuity, papillary reactivity, and anterior and posterior structures are important. In stage I eye disease, there is peripheral arteriolar occlusion; in stages II and III, vascular remodeling and neovascularization; in stage IV, vitreous hemorrhage; and in stage V, retinal detachment. These can be managed by observation, laser phototherapy, or surgical correction.

In patients with SCD or sickle cell trait, direct eye trauma that causes bleeding into anterior chamber requires urgent evaluation. Sickle erythrocytes can occlude the trabecular channels, increase intraocular pressure, and cause acute glaucoma.

CARDIOVASCULAR MANIFESTATIONS

Individuals with SCD have lower blood pressures compared with individuals with other types of chronic anemia. Renal sodium wasting is postulated as one possible cause, although other mechanisms may be present. Blood pressures in SCD correlate with age, hemoglobin, and body-mass index. When systolic or diastolic blood pressures approach those of age-, sex-, and race-matched normal individuals, the risk of stroke and mortality increases.

There are other cardiac manifestations in SCD. Systolic flow murmurs are frequent and related to the degree of anemia. On echocardiograms, pericardial effusions are found in approximately 10% of all studies; cardiac output, cardiac chamber size, and myocardial wall thickness are increased to improve the stroke volume without increasing the heart rate. With long-term and consistent increases in cardiac output, the ability to perform physical work is reduced by half in adults and by one third in children. Given the larger heart chamber sizes, congestive heart failure is uncommon. For individuals receiving chronic transfusion therapy, there may be additional cardiac damage from iron overload, leading to more severe dilated cardiomyopathy and heart failure.

Myocardial infarction because of large vessel occlusion (in the left anterior descending, circumflex, or right coronary artery) is rare, but cardiac damage from small vessel diseases may occur. Sudden death because of unexplained arrhythmia or autonomic dysfunction also has been described in adults with SCD.

PULMONARY COMPLICATIONS

Acute Complications

Acute chest syndrome (ACS) is typically defined by temperature higher than 38.5°C, cough, a new pulmonary infiltrate on chest radiograph or rales on auscultation (often in multiple lobes), chest pain, and other respiratory symptoms (11). Children tend to have more respiratory symptoms (wheezing, cough, and fever), while adults manifest symptoms of musculoskeletal pain and dyspnea and have a more severe course. Risk factors for ACS are Hb SS, low Hb F, high baseline hemoglobin (11 g/dL or greater), high white blood cell count (greater than 15 k/uL), and prior episodes of ACS. ACS is a frequent cause of death in both children and adults with SCD, the second most common cause of hospitalization, and the most frequent complication following surgery and anesthesia. Complications from ACS include CNS injury (anoxia, infarct, or hemorrhage), seizure, and respiratory failure. Frequent ACS episodes are associated with shortened survival.

While the cause of ACS is often unknown (less than half of events had an identifiable cause), it can be triggered by pneumonia, pulmonary infarction from vaso-occlusion within pulmonary vasculature, fat embolism from bone marrow infarction, or pulmonary thromboembolism. Microbiologic culture of sputum may reveal a variety of atypical organism (chlamydia or mycoplasma), viruses (respiratory syncytial virus), and bacteria (*S. aureus, S. pneumoniae,* or *H. influenza*); up to 30% of microbiologic cultures are negative (12).

Evaluation of ACS includes vital signs, pulse oximetry or arterial blood gas, microbiologic culture of sputum and blood, nasopharyngeal swab for viral culture, chest radiograph, and complete blood count, liver and renal function tests. Bronchoscopy may be indicated when patients do not respond to initial therapy.

Treatment for ACS includes oxygen, broad spectrum intravenous antibiotics (including coverage for atypical organisms), simple and/or exchange transfusions as needed to improve oxygen saturation, bronchodilators (as airway hyperreactivity often accompanies ACS), and analgesia for pain. All these efforts are aimed at reducing the percentage of sickle erythrocytes and minimizing sickle polymerization. Nitric oxide or acute pulmonary vasodilators are used for chronic pulmonary hypertension and may be beneficial in ACS (13). After an episode of ACS is successfully managed, strategies to prevent future episodes may include vaccinations (especially against *S. pneumoniae*), hydroxyurea, transfusions, or bone marrow transplantation.

Systemic fat embolism syndrome is a rare acute complication of SCD. Embolization occurs when there is a large bone marrow infarction and necrosis, and necrotic fat and marrow are released into systemic circulation and lodge in the pulmonary vasculature. Fat embolization can precipitate or develop concurrently with ACS. Multiorgan failure may result. Risk factors for developing systemic fat embolism syndrome are Hb SC genotype, pregnancy, and prior corticosteroid treatment.

Chronic Complications

Screening cohorts of children and adults with echocardiograms has estimated pulmonary hypertension to be about 20% to 30% (14). While the exact cause is unknown, one or more of the following may contribute to its pathogenesis: sickle cell-related vasculopathy, pulmonary damage from recurrent ACS, high blood flow from anemia, and chronic hemolysis. Clinically, pulmonary hypertension can manifest as dyspnea, clubbing, loud second heart sound (P_2), an enlarged right side of the heart on chest radiograph, and 95% or less oxygen saturation on room air at rest. Pulmonary hypertension can be documented on echocardiogram by a tricuspid regurgitation jet velocity (TRV) of greater than 2.5 m/sec or mean pulmonary arterial pressure (MPAP) of greater than 25 mmHg.

There is currently no single preferred treatment for patients with pulmonary hypertension. Simple transfusion to maintain hemoglobin at approximately 9 g/dL can reduce pulmonary pressure in some, but the possible development of red cell antibodies limits the applicability of this approach. Hydroxyurea reduces the frequency and severity of vaso-occlusive crises and ACS but may only delay the onset of pulmonary hypertension. Calcium channel blockers, sildenafil, anticoagulation with warfarin (target INR 2–3), prostacyclin, endothelin antagonist, and nitric oxide are adjunctive agents to consider; continuous or nocturnal oxygen can be considered for hypoxemic patients.

GALL BLADDER, HEPATIC, AND SPLENIC MANIFESTATIONS

Sickle cell disease can affect the hepatobiliary and splenic systems in multiple ways (Table 4.6). Hyperbilirubinemia (typically less than 4 mg/dL of unconjugated bilirubin) from chronic hemolysis is common. Other factors that increase total bilirubin level include cholesterol intake, presence of Gilbert's syndrome, and cephalosporin antibiotic use. Biliary sludge and cholethiasis can occur as

THERAPY

Transfusions

Transfusions are an important therapy for SCD (Table 4.7) and are commonly used acutely but also chronically for primary or secondary prevention of a specific complication (20–23). Transfusions can be separated into simple episodic, simple chronic, or exchange. It is important to notify blood bank of the type (simple or exchange), indication, and duration (episodic or chronic) of therapy. A detailed transfusion history should be maintained that includes the total number of prior red cells units, presence of any red cell antibodies, percent Hb S, and the hemoglobin or hematocrit.

Red cell antigen difference between patients with sickle cell and blood donors (mostly Caucasians) is the major reason for the high rate of alloimmunization. Alloimmunization can be minimized by typing for other Rh (D, E/e, and C/c) and Kell (K) antigens in addition to the usual ABO typing. When a patient has a prior transfusion history, other minor antigens (Kidd, S, and Duffy) should also be typed. Prestorage leukocyte depletion is now commonly used in blood banks. Other potential complications include the usual transfusion reactions that can occur in patients without SCD: volume overload, acute

TABLE 4.7. *Indications for Transfusions in Sickle Cell Disease*

Indications for *Simple Episodic* Transfusions	Consider In
1. Acute chest syndrome (mild to moderate) 2. Severe anemia (hgb <5 g/dL) or a decrease of >20% from baseline 3. Preoperatively for major surgery with general anesthesia (target hgb 9–10 g/dL and Hb S ≤60%) (20) 4. Symptomatic patients with heart failure, dyspnea, hypotension, or other organ failure 5. Infection-related anemia (parvovirus B19) or hemolysis-related anemia (concomitant G-6-PD deficiency) 6. Hepatic sequestration 7. Splenic sequestration (more in children, drop in Hb by 2 g/dL, acute splenomegaly, with thrombocytopenia)	1. Prolonged priapism 2. Nonhealing leg ulcers
Indications for *Simple Chronic* Transfusions	**Consider In**
1. Primary or secondary stroke prevention (8) 2. Complicated pregnancy (by progressive anemia, preeclampsia, increased pain episodes, prior pregnancy loss, multiple gestations)—starting at 20 weeks (21)	1. In children following acute chest syndrome (22) 2. Pulmonary hypertension, moderate or severe 3. Silent, hemorrhagic, or vasculopathic stroke 4. Chronic heart failure 5. Splenic sequestration in children; transfuse until 5–6 years of age 6. Chronic debilitating pain 7. Renal failure related anemia 8. Recurrent priapism
Indications for *Exchange* Transfusions	
1. Acute chest syndrome (moderate or severe) 2. Stroke (thrombotic, consider in hemorrhagic) 3. One or multiple organ failure 4. Hb SC patients with any of following: —Preoperatively for major surgery requiring general anesthesia (23) —Hepatic sequestration	

hemolytic reactions, transfusion transmitted infections (hepatitis B/C, human immunodeficiency virus [HIV], West Nile virus, Creutzfeldt-Jacob disease), and iron overload.

Fetal Hemoglobin Induction

The beneficial effect of fetal hemoglobin was first recognized from the observations that neonates with Hb SS do not develop SCD-related symptoms in the first 6 months, and patients with co-inheritance of SCD and hereditary persistence of fetal hemoglobin (HPFH), such as in Saudi Arabia and India, have milder symptoms. In vitro, Hb F inhibits Hb S polymerization. Currently hydroxyurea is the only Food and Drug Administration (FDA) approved drug for Hb F induction. Hydroxyurea is a cell cycle (S-phase)-specific agent that blocks the conversion of ribonucleotides to deoxyribonucleotides. Its primary clinical impact is Hb F induction, but other benefits may include reduced leukocyte and platelet counts, less hemolysis, decrease in bone marrow cellularity, and generation of nitric oxide.

The MSH study was a randomized placebo-controlled clinical trial that confirmed the beneficial effects and the safety of hydroxyurea. The 150 hydroxyurea-treated patients had fewer pain episodes and ACS, required less transfusions, and experienced minimal toxicity (19,24). Since the MSH, hydroxyurea has been used widely. Approximately 70% of patients with SCD are likely hydroxyurea-responsive: steady state Hb F should increase twofold from baseline or approximately 10% to 15%, and total hemoglobin should increase by 1 to 2 g/dL (Table 4.8). Whether hydroxyurea will prevent or reverse end organ damage is unknown.

Hydroxyurea can be started at 10 to 15 mg/kg daily and adjusted by 5 mg/kg per day increment every 6 to 8 weeks, to a maximum of approximately 25 mg/kg daily. Compromised hepatic or renal function may require lower dosing. Within a week of therapy, Hb F-containing reticulocytes will rise; at the end of 2 to 3 weeks, Hb F-containing red cells will increase. Other hematologic effects include increase in MCV and decrease in leukocytes (especially neutrophils), platelets, and reticulocytes. Two to 3 months are usually required before the effects on Hb F and blood counts are stabilized; a trial of 6 to 12 months is adequate to assess clinical benefit. Hydroxyurea in several cohorts of children has appeared safe (25), and adverse effects on growth and development have not been reported; the long-term effects of hydroxyurea in children, however, still remain largely unknown.

While there are other inducers of fetal hemoglobin available in research studies—5-azacytadine, decitabine, and butyrates—their nonoral formulation, unknown long-term effects of DNA methylation (5-azacytadine and decitabine), nonsustained increases in Hb F (arginine butyrates), and inconvenience (phenylbutyrates) make them less attractive (26).

TABLE 4.8. *Use of Hydroxyurea*

Indications	• Adults, adolescent, or children • Hb SS or Hb S/β^0 thalassemia with frequent pain, history of ACS, severe vaso-occlusive events, severe anemia
Dosing	• Start with 10–15 mg/kg per day • Adjust by 5 mg/kg per day increment every 6–8 weeks; maximum of 25–35 mg/kg per day • Duration: 6–12 months trial
Monitoring	• Initially: CBC every 2 weeks, chemistry every 2–4 weeks, Hb F every 6–8 weeks • At stable dose of hydroxyurea, CBC and chemistry every 4–8 weeks, Hb F every 8–12 weeks • Keep ANC >2000/μL, reticulocytes >100K/μL, and platelet >100k/μL • If marrow toxicity occurs, stop for 2 weeks and start at a lower dose when blood counts recover
Treatment Endpoint	• Less pain • Increased Hb F to 10%–20% or 2–2.5-fold increase from baseline • Increased hemoglobin if severely anemic • Improved well being, weight gain
Cautions	• Dose reduction in hepatic or renal insufficiency • Contraception for men and women

ACS, acute chest syndrome; ANC, absolute neutrophil count; CBC, complete blood count; Hb, hemoglobin.

Other Drugs

Agents that modify the pathophysiology of SCD are based on their ability to reduce Hb S polymerization in vitro. These include Hb S modifiers (urea, organic compounds), inhibitors of Gardos channel (clotrimazole, ICA 17403), chloride and cation channel blocker (dipyridamole, magnesium pidolate, NS-3623), and anti-adherence agents (Poloxamer 188, pentoxifylline). Many of these drugs are in preclinical testing; some are used in therapeutic trials. Erythropoietin, at doses two to five times those used in renal failure, in combination with hydroxyurea, can increase total hemoglobin.

SPECIAL TOPICS

Contraception and Pregnancy

Hydroxyurea is a teratogen in animal models. There is little published data on the effect of hydroxyurea on the developing fetus; therefore, both male and female patients with SCD should use contraception and discontinue the drug if pregnancy is planned. There are reports of normal neonates delivered from women receiving hydroxyurea therapy throughout pregnancy, but outcomes of any unplanned pregnancy should be discussed. Hydroxyurea is also secreted into breast milk, and breast feeding should be avoided.

Hydroxyurea is also an oral chemotherapeutic drug; thus, it is not surprising that there is a perceived risk of developing malignancy. While there are case reports of patients with SCD who have developed leukemia while receiving hydroxyurea, whether this rate is above that expected in the population is not known. No definitive risk increase has been directly attributed to hydroxyurea for individuals with myeloproliferative diseases or cyanotic heart disease.

Pregnant women with SCD are at an increased risk of preeclampsia, sickle pain crises, acute anemia or hemolysis, and postpartum infections (endometritis or pyelonephritis) (27,28). Miscarriage rate is at least 6%. Maternal mortality rate is low, and the overall outcome of the pregnancies is favorable; more than 90% of infants have Apgar scores of 7 or greater. At least 20% of infants will be small for gestation age (less than tenth percentile), and at least 25% would be born prematurely (average at 34 to 37 weeks). Women with Hb SS tend to have more frequent or severe complications than women with Hb SC. Transfusions are usually reserved for pregnancies complicated by progressive anemia, increased pain episodes, preeclampsia, prior pregnancy loss, or multiple gestations; prophylactic transfusions are generally discouraged.

Anesthesia and Surgery

Surgery and general anesthesia have higher morbidity and mortality in SCD compared with the general population. The risk is higher in those with Hb SS or Hb S/β^0 thalassemia than those with Hb SC or Hb S/β^+ thalassemia (20). Complications may be more frequent in those receiving regional anesthesia. ACS and postoperative infection are the most common, followed by pain crisis and stroke (Table 4.9).

TABLE 4.9. *Perioperative Considerations for Sickle Cell Patients*

Preoperative
1. Simple transfusions to achieve hemoglobin of 10 g/dL in Hb SS and Hb S/β^0 thalassemia. Individuals with Hb SC may require exchange transfusion, especially prior to abdominal surgery.
2. Bloodtyping for additional antigens, such as C, E, Kell, Kidd (Jk), S, and Duffy (Fy), to minimize alloimmunization
3. Hydration.

Postoperative
1. Hydration, oxygen, and monitoring respiration and peripheral perfusion.
2. Monitoring for acute chest syndrome, infection, pain crisis, or stroke.

Hb, hemoglobin.

SICKLE CELL TRAIT

Approximately 8% of African Americans have sickle cell trait (SCT). Under physiologic conditions, vaso-occlusion does not occur. Carriers have normal life expectancy, and many participate successfully in competitive sports or rigorous military training. There are exercise-related mortality reported in these individuals, which can be minimized by avoiding heat stress, dehydration, and sleep deprivation and with gradual heat acclimation and exercise endurance.

Compared with the general population, persons with SCT have normal risk of developing heart disease, stroke, leg ulcers, or arthritis. They are not more likely to develop complications from anesthetic agents. However, SCT is associated with increased risk for traumatic eye injury, hyposthenuria, hematuria, and splenic infarction. If traumatic eye injury occurs with hemorrhage into anterior chamber, erythrocytes may clog the trabecular outflow channels, increase intraocular pressure, and lead to acute glaucoma, requiring urgent evaluation and treatment. Changes in urinary frequency, pattern, and color should be closely evaluated. There have been reports of increased splenic infarction in SCT associated with hypoxemia; this risk appears to be small. Pregnant women with SCT are at an increased risk for urinary tract infections, preeclampsia, and postpartum endometritis; their infants also tend to be smaller.

CLINICAL SYNDROMES AND TREATMENT OF THALASSEMIAS

Anemia, Transfusions, and Splenomegaly

α-Thalassemia (mainly Hb H phenotype) and β-thalassemia are clinically characterized by chronic hemolytic anemia, hepatosplenomegaly, skeletal deformities, leg ulcers, gallstones, and folate deficiency. There are also two rare forms of α-thalassemia with mental retardation and developmental abnormalities, ATR 16 and ATR X syndromes. Transfusions and iron chelation are the mainstay of therapy and have improved the quality of life and extended life expectancy in thalassemia individuals. After the diagnosis in infancy or childhood, the decision to start transfusion depends on the degree of impact anemia has on the child: fatigue, reduced growth velocity, skeletal dysmorphism, poor weight gain, or organomegaly. Once started, the target hemoglobin of 10 g/dL is reasonable, although others have used a higher target. Transfusions are maintained every 2 to 4 weeks and are continued through adulthood. Improvements in the clinical signs and symptoms can be seen in adequately transfused individuals. Red cell alloimmunization can be minimized as in SCD by typing for major and minor blood group antigens (ABO, Rh, Kell, Kidd, and Duffy) and prestorage leukocyte depletion.

Splenomegaly can be seen in those with inadequate transfusions or red cell alloimmunization and is associated with worsening anemia, leukopenia, and thrombocytopenia. Hemoglobin will typically drop about 1.5 g/dL per week in nonsplenectomized individuals; in hypersplenism, this rate of decline will be higher, and eventually there will be an inadequate rise in posttransfusion hemoglobin. Splenectomy will improve these hematologic parameters and transfusion effectiveness but should be performed after vaccination for encapsulated organisms (*S. pneumoniae*, *H. influenza*, and *N. meningitidis*) and in children older than 5 years of age. Postsplenectomized transfusions should produce a 1 g/dL per week decrease in hemoglobin. Penicillin prophylaxis is appropriate. Postsplenectomy thrombocytosis can be variable but generally does not require antiplatelet therapy.

Iron Overload and Chelation

Early diagnosis and chronic transfusions have shifted the major complications of thalassemia from those secondary to the hemolytic anemia to the sequalae of iron overload. Excess iron from cumulative transfusions overwhelms the transferrin system and accumulates in the heart, liver, and various endocrine organs. The most serious result is heart failure and sudden unpredictable ventricular arrhythmia, which account for the majority of deaths in individuals with thalassemia. Nonuniform deposition of iron in the cardiac myocytes leads to the loss of normal cardiac architecture and fibrosis, resulting in the dilated cardiomyopathy and life-threatening arrhythmia. Excess iron also accumulates in the liver, producing hepatic inflammation, dysfunction, and fibrosis. While computed tomographic or MRI imaging, superconducting susceptometry (SQUID), and serum ferritin are helpful in estimating the amount of iron in liver, biopsy remains the standard. Furthermore, iron overload also affects various endocrine organs and can cause reduced growth velocity in children: hypothyroidism; hypogonadisim with pubertal delay or arrest; hypoparathyroidism leading to hypocalcemia and osteoporosis, and diabetes. All are managed in collaboration with endocrinologists.

The toxic effects of excess iron can be minimized by iron chelation. Desferrioxamine (deferoxamine or Desferal [Novartis Pharmaceuticals Corporation, East Hanover, NJ]) and desferasirox (Exjade [Novartis]) are FDA approved in the United States for this purpose. Desferal can be administered as early as 2½ years of age at 20 to 60 mg/kg (or 1.5 to 4 g per adolescent or adult) per day, delivered by subcutaneous or intravenous injection over 8 to 12 or 24 hours (29,30), and typically for at least 5 days a week. There is also evidence that twice a day subcutaneous bolus injection may also be efficacious (31). Side effects of Desferal are infrequent; they include impaired vision or hearing, motor-sensory neuropathy, changes in renal or pulmonary function, joint pain, metaphyseal dysplasia, or growth retardation. The other chelator, desferasirox (Exjade, Novartis), is administered orally at 10 to 20 mg/kg per day. Side effects include abdominal pain, diarrhea, rash, arthralgia, and mild increases in liver enzymes and serum creatinine. Oral deferiprone was used in clinical trials and appeared promising, but the enthusiasm of investigators has diminished because of common side effects of gastrointestinal discomfort, joint pain, and agranulocytosis, and controversy regarding effectiveness in iron removal and the possibility of hepatic fibrosis (32).

Fetal Hemoglobin Induction

The major endpoint for Hb F induction in thalassemia is an increase in total hemoglobin. Unfortunately, hydroxyurea has not been able to achieve this goal in most patients with thalassemic major receiving chronic transfusions, possibly because of a loss of Hb F response with transfusion or to certain mutations that are resistant to Hb F induction. Hydroxyurea, however, has had some effect in Hb Lepore/β-thalassemia, Hb E/β-thalassemia, and β-thalassemia intermedia (33). Erythropoietin also can be used with hydroxyurea, but the response is variable. Other inducers of Hb F, such as butyrates, have increased Hb F but not total hemoglobin.

THERAPY WITH CURATIVE INTENT

Hematopoietic Stem Cell Transplantation

Myeloablative hematopoietic stem cell transplantation (HSCT) is currently the only cure for SCD and thalassemia (34). The lack of available HLA-matched sibling donors and transplant-related complications has limited its wide applicability. For SCD, HSCT is generally reserved for patients less than 17 years of age, nonresponsive to hydroxyurea, who have had prior SCD-related organ damage (stroke, ACS, frequent pain crises, and multiple sites of osteonecrosis). For thalassemia, HSCT is also generally reserved for those less than 17 years of age with signs of liver dysfunction from iron damage (Pesaro class II and III). There are encouraging animal and clinical data that suggest reduced-intensity (nonmyeloablative) transplantations can achieve mixed donor and host hematopoiesis and ameliorate disease complications. If confirmed, this approach may be a reasonable alternative for older individuals who otherwise meet criteria for a standard myeloablative HSCT. Related umbilical cord blood transplantation is also an alternative.

Gene Therapy

Autologous transplantation following the insertion of a normal or therapeutic globin gene into hematopoietic stem cells is a rational approach to SCD and thalassemia (35). While problems in attaining reliable expression of globin constructs in erythroid progeny of hematopoietic stem cells proved seemingly insurmountable for a number of years, significant advances have been made toward this goal using lentiviral vector based on HIV. Therapeutic correction of murine models of both β-thalassemia and SCD has been achieved using this approach. These advances are coupled with progress in the ability to achieve moderate levels of engraftment of genetically modified cells in the nonhuman primate autologous transplant model. These preclinical studies should allow better assessment of the recently documented risk of insertional mutagenesis as well as optimization of gene transfer techniques to increase the likelihood of ultimate clinical success while minimizing risks (36). Summaries for SCD and thalassemias are provided in Tables 4.10 and 4.11.

TABLE 4.10. *Clinical Features of Two Common Severe β-Globin Disorders*

Sickle Cell Disease and Thalassemia Syndromes

Common features related to pathophysiology:
1. Hemolytic anemia (variable degree)
2. Gallstones
3. Leg ulcers (less common in thalassemia)
4. Pulmonary hypertension (less common in thalassemia)

Common features related to chronic transfusion (more common in thalassemia):
1. Red cell alloimmunization
2. Infections (HIV, hepatitis, WNV, CJD)
3. Iron overload
   - Dilated cardiomyopathy and arrhythmia
   - Endocrinopathy (hypothyroidism, hypogonadism, diabetes, osteoporosis)
   - Liver dysfunction and cirrhosis

SCD-Specific Manifestations	Thalassemia-Specific Manifestations
1. Vaso-occlusive pain	1. Splenomegaly
2. Stroke, retinal diseases	2. Thromboembolism
3. Acute chest syndrome	3. Infections: Yersinia sp
4. Avascular necrosis (osteonecrosis), fat embolism, osteomyelitis	
5. Splenic sequestration and eventual infarct in Hb SS or Hb S/β^0 thalassemia; splenomegaly in Hb SC	
6. Priapism	
7. Hyposthenuria; renal damage by glomerular or tubular damage or papillary necrosis in some individuals	
8. Infections: Parvovirus B19, salmonella sp, *S. pneumoniae, H. influenza*	
9. Hepatic sequestration or crisis	

CJD, Creutzfeldt-Jakob disease; Hb, hemoglobin; HIV, human immunodeficiency virus; WNV, West Nile virus.

TABLE 4.11. *Suggested Health Maintenance Schedule*

	Routine Health Maintenance	Supplement	Blood tests	Special Studies
Sickle Cell Disease				
Age 0–2 yr	Penicillin prophylaxis; Prevnar (7 valent), routine vaccinations	Folate, multi-vitamin, iron if appropriate	CBC every 3–6 months	
Age 2–18 yr	Penicillin prophylaxis until age 5; Pneumovax (23 valent), routine vaccinations, influenza vaccination yearly; Eye exam yearly	Folate; iron if appropriate	CBC every 6 months, renal and hepatic function and iron studies yearly	TCD and O_2 saturation every 6–12 months

(continued)

TABLE 4.11. *Suggested Health Maintenance Schedule (continued)*

	Routine Health Maintenance	Supplement	Blood tests	Special Studies
Age >18 yr	Pneumovax, influenza vaccination yearly; hepatitis A and B vaccination; Eye exam yearly	Folate; iron if appropriate	CBC, Hb F (if on hydroxyurea) every 3–6 months; UA for proteinuria, B$_{12}$, renal and hepatic function every 6 months	RUQ ultrasound every 1–2 yrs for biliary sludge; Echo and PFTs yearly
Thalassemia				
Age 0–2 yr	Routine vaccinations; Possible iron chelation; Growth velocity curve	Folate, multi-vitamin	CBC every 3–6 months	
Age 2–18 yr	Routine vaccinations; vaccinations for possible splenectomy in those >5 yr; Possible iron chelation; Growth velocity curve	Folate, multi-vitamin	CBC, hepatic, renal functions, iron studies every 3–6 months	Evaluate for iron overload; endocrine consultation every 6–12 months; Echo yearly
Age >18 yr	Vaccinations for possible splenectomy	Folate, multi-vitamin	CBC, hepatic, renal functions, iron studies every 6 months.	Evaluate for iron overload; endocrine consultation yearly; Echo yearly

CBC, complete blood count; PFTs, pulmonary function tests; RUQ, right upper quadrant;
SC heterozygous hemoglobin S and C; TCD, transcranial Doppler.

REFERENCES

1. Steinberg MH, Rodgers GP. Pathophysiology of sickle cell disease: role of cellular and genetic modifiers. Semin Hematol 2001;38:299–306.
2. Cao A, Galanello R, Rosatelli MC. Prenatal diagnosis and screening of the haemoglobinopathies. Baillieres Clin Haematol 1998;11:215–238.
3. The laboratory diagnosis of haemoglobinopathies. Br J Haematol 1998;101:783–792.
4. National Institutes of Health: National Heart, Lung, and Blood Institute. The Management of Sickle Cell Disease, 4th Ed. NIH Pub. 02-2117. Bethesda, MD: National Institutes of Health;2002.
5. Ballantyne JC, Mao J. Opioid therapy for chronic pain. N Engl J Med 2003;349:1943–1953.
6. Gaston MH, Verter JI, Woods G, et al. Prophylaxis with oral penicillin in children with sickle cell anemia. A randomized trial. N Engl J Med 1986;314:1593–1599.
7. Smith-Whitley K, Zhao H, Hodinka RL, et al. Epidemiology of human parvovirus B19 in children with sickle cell disease. Blood 2004;103:422–427.
8. Adams RJ, McKie VC, Hsu L, et al. Prevention of a first stroke by transfusions in children with sickle cell anemia and abnormal results on transcranial Doppler ultrasonography. N Engl J Med 1998;339:5–11.
9. Ohene-Frempong K, Weiner SJ, Sleeper LA, et al. Cerebrovascular accidents in sickle cell disease: rates and risk factors. Blood 1998;91:288–294.
10. Adams RJ, Brambilla D. Discontinuing prophylactic transfusions used to prevent stroke in sickle cell disease. N Engl J Med 2005;353:2769–2778.
11. Platt OS. The acute chest syndrome of sickle cell disease. N Engl J Med 2000;342:1904–1907.

12. Vichinsky EP, Neumayr LD, Earles AN, et al. Causes and outcomes of the acute chest syndrome in sickle cell disease. N Engl J Med 2000;342:1855–1865.
13. Gladwin MT, Schechter AN. Nitric oxide therapy in sickle cell disease. Semin Hematol 2001;38:333–342.
14. Gladwin MT, Sachdev V, Jison ML, et al. Pulmonary hypertension as a risk factor for death in patients with sickle cell disease. N Engl J Med 2004;350:886–895.
15. Mantadakis E, Ewalt DH, Cavender JD, et al. Outpatient penile aspiration and epinephrine irrigation for young patients with sickle cell anemia and prolonged priapism. Blood 2000;95:78–82.
16. Styles LA, Vichinsky EP. Core decompression in avascular necrosis of the hip in sickle-cell disease. Am J Hematol 1996;52:103–107.
17. Koshy M, Entsuah R, Koranda A, et al. Leg ulcers in patients with sickle cell disease. *Blood* 1989;74:1403–1408.
18. Eckman JR. Leg ulcers in sickle cell disease. Hematol Oncol Clin North Am 1996;10:1333–1344.
19. Charache S, Terrin ML, Moore RD, et al. Effect of hydroxyurea on the frequency of painful crises in sickle cell anemia. N Engl J Med 1995;332:1317–1322.
20. Vichinsky EP, Haberkern CM, Neumayr L, et al. A comparison of conservative and aggressive transfusion regimens in the perioperative management of sickle cell disease. The Preoperative Transfusion in Sickle Cell Disease Study Group. N Engl J Med 1995;333:206–213.
21. Koshy M, Burd L, Wallace D, et al. Prophylactic red-cell transfusions in pregnant patients with sickle cell disease. A randomized cooperative study. N Engl J Med 1988;319:1447–1452.
22. Miller ST, Wright E, Abboud M, et al. Impact of chronic transfusion on incidence of pain and acute chest syndrome during the Stroke Prevention Trial (STOP) in sickle-cell anemia. J Pediatr 2001;139:785–789.
23. Neumayr L, Koshy M, Haberkern C, et al. Surgery in patients with hemoglobin SC disease. Preoperative Transfusion in Sickle Cell Disease Study Group. Am J Hematol 1998;57:101–108.
24. Steinberg MH, Barton F, Castro O, et al. Effect of hydroxyurea on mortality and morbidity in adult sickle cell anemia: risks and benefits up to 9 years of treatment. JAMA 2003;289:1645–1651.
25. Wang WC, Helms RW, Lynn HS, et al. Effect of hydroxyurea on growth in children with sickle cell anemia: results of the HUG-KIDS Study. *J Pediatr* 2002;140:225–229.
26. Bank A. Regulation of human fetal hemoglobin: new players, new complexities. *Blood* 2006;107:435–443.
27. Smith JA, Espeland M, Bellevue R, et al. Pregnancy in sickle cell disease: experience of the Cooperative Study of sickle cell disease. Obstet Gynecol 1996;87:199–204.
28. Sun PM, Wilburn W, Raynor BD, et al. Sickle cell disease in pregnancy: twenty years of experience at Grady Memorial Hospital, Atlanta, Georgia. Am J Obstet Gynecol 2001;184:1127–1130.
29. Giardina PJ, Grady RW. Chelation therapy in beta-thalassemia: an optimistic update. *Semin Hematol* 2001;38:360–366.
30. Davis BA, Porter JB. Long-term outcome of continuous 24-hour deferoxamine infusion via indwelling intravenous catheters in high-risk beta-thalassemia. Blood 2000;95:1229–1236.
31. Franchini M, Gandini G, de Gironcoli M, et al. Safety and efficacy of subcutaneous bolus injection of deferoxamine in adult patients with iron overload. Blood 2000;95:2776–2779.
32. Olivieri NF, Brittenham GM, McLaren CE, et al. Long-term safety and effectiveness of iron-chelation therapy with deferiprone for thalassemia major. N Engl J Med 1998;339:417–423.
33. Atweh GF, Loukopoulos D. Pharmacological induction of fetal hemoglobin in sickle cell disease and beta-thalassemia. Semin Hematol 2001;38:367–373.
34. Sullivan KM, Parkman R, Walters MC. Bone marrow transplantation for nonmalignant disease. Hematology Am Soc Hematol Educ Program 2000:319–338.
35. Sadelain M, Boulad F, Galanello R, et al. Therapeutic options for patients with severe beta-thalassemia: the need for globin gene therapy. Hum Gene Ther 2007;18:1–9.
36. Bank A, Dorazio R, Leboulch P. A phase I/II clinical trial of beta-globin gene therapy for beta-thalassemia. Ann N Y Acad Sci 2005;1054:308–316.

5

Porphyrias

Peiman Hematti

The porphyrias are a diverse group of uncommon metabolic disorders caused by inherited deficiencies of the enzymes involved in the heme biosynthetic pathway. Mutations of the genes of all of these hemasynthetic enzymes have been identified. An exception is porphyria cutanea tarda, in which the enzyme deficiency in most cases is acquired. In all these ecogenic disorders, it is the interaction of genetic, physiologic, and environmental factors that cause disease in affected individuals. Each defective enzyme results in a characteristic clinical phenotype of porphyria, although disease mechanisms are not fully understood. Any patient with a long history of undiagnosed abdominal pain and/or atypical neuropsychiatric symptoms should have porphyria in their differential diagnosis (1).

EPIDEMIOLOGY

Porphyria cutanea tarda is the most prevalent of porphyrias, both genetic and acquired combined, but acute intermittent porphyria is the most common of genetic porphyrias. Acute intermittent porphyria has an estimated incidence of 5 in 100,000 in the United States and northern European countries. Approximately 90% of patients with this inherited enzyme deficiency remain symptom free throughout their life. In contrast, only rare cases of d-aminolevulinic acid dehydratase deficiency (ALAD) have been thus far reported (2,3).

PATHOPHYSIOLOGY

Heme is a complex of an iron atom and protoporphyrin IX. Heme is produced in a multistep biosynthetic pathway that functions mostly in the erythroid bone marrow and hepatocytes. Approximately 85% of the heme produced in the body is synthesized in erythroid cells to provide for hemoglobin formation; most of the remainder is produced in the liver to provide heme for cytochrome P-450 and other enzymes. Eight enzymes are involved in this tightly regulated pathway that sequentially converts glycine and succinyl CoA into heme (Fig. 5.1). Sequences of the genes for all these enzymes and their molecular defects have been well characterized (4).

Mutations of the first enzyme, δ-aminolevulinic acid (ALA) synthase, results in X-linked sideroblastic anemia. Mutations of the other seven enzymes result in porphyria because of overproduction of metabolic precursors and intermediates and/or their accumulation in tissues. All of these intermediate products are potentially toxic, and their overproduction causes the neurovisceral and/or photocutaneous symptoms characteristic of porphyria syndromes.

Despite the characterization of these disorders at the molecular level, the exact pathophysiologic mechanisms responsible for the specific organ manifestations are not fully understood.

Porphyrias are heterogeneous at the molecular level with numerous mutations found for each gene. There is a significant interaction between specific inherited genetic defects and acquired or environmental factors that result in a spectrum of clinical manifestations in affected patients. Patients with gene mutations for the acute hepatic forms of porphyrias may remain asymptomatic unless they are exposed to certain medications (Table 5.1) or hormones or are stressed by starvation, infection,

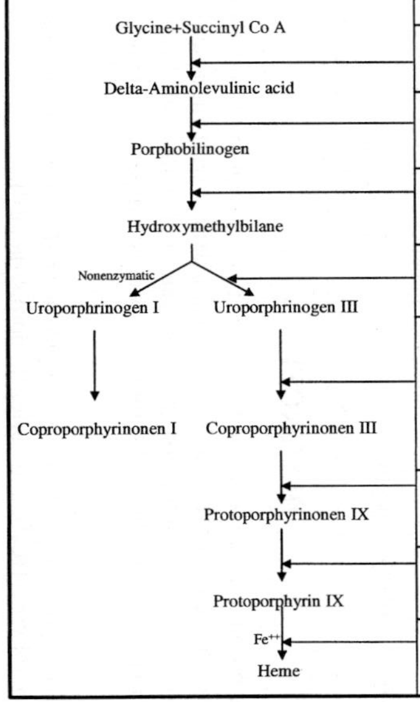

Enzyme Deficiency	Disease	Inheritance	Symptomatology	Hematological symptoms	Accumulated products
ALA synthase (ALAS)	Sideroblastic anemia (XLSA)	X-linked sideroblastic anemia	Hypochromic anemia	Hypochromic anemia	Ring Sideroblasts
ALA dehydratase (ALAD)	δ-Aminolevulinic acid dehydratase-deficient porphyria (ADP)	Autosomal recessive	Neurovisceral	None	Urinary ALA & coproporphyrin; RBC Zn protoporphyrin
Porphobilinogen Deaminase (PBGD)	Acute intermittent porphyria (AIP)	Autosomal dominant	Neurovisceral	None	Urinary ALA & PBG
Uroporphyrinogen III cosynthase (UCoS)	Congenital Erythropoietic porphyria (CEP)	Autosomal recessive	Photocutaneous	Hemolytic anemia, Splenomegaly	Urinary and RBC Uroporphyrin I and, Copprporphyrin I
Uroporphyrinogen Decarboxylase (UROD)	Porphyria cutanea tarda (PCT)	Acquired (type I) Autosomal dominant (type II & III)	Photocutaneous	None	Urinary uroporphyrin & 7-carboxylic porphyrin; Fecal isocoproporphyrin
	Hepatoerythropoietic porphyria (HEP)	Autosomal recessive	Photocutaneous	Hemolytic anemia, Splenomegaly	Urinary uroporphyrin; Fecal isocopropoprhyrin, RBC Zn protoporphyrin
Coproporphyrinogen oxidase (CPO)	Hereditary coproporphyria (HCP)	Autosomal recessive	Neurovisceral & Photocutaneous	None	Urinary ALA & PBG; Fecal coproporphyrin
Protoporphyrinogen oxidase (PPO)	Variegate porphyria (VP)	Autosomal dominant	Neurovisceral & Photocutaneous	None	Urinary ALA &PBG; Urinary & fecal coproporphyrin
Ferrochelatase (FeC)	Erythropoietic protoporphyria (EPP)	Autosomal dominant	Photocutaneous	Anemia	RBC protoporphyrin; Fecal protoporphyrin

Glycine+Succinyl Co A → Delta-Aminolevulinic acid → Porphobilinogen → Hydroxymethylbilane → Uroporphyrinogen I / Uroporphyrinogen III (Nonenzymatic) → Coproporphyrinogen I / Coproporphyrinogen III → Protoporphyrinogen IX → Protoporphyrin IX → (Fe^{2+}) Heme

FIG. 5.1. Classification of porphyrias based on their corresponding enzymatic deficiencies, their mode of inheritance, and their major symptoms. Deficiency of the first enzyme in the heme biosynthetic pathway does not cause a porphyria but X-linked sideroblastic anemia. Modified from Sassa S, Shibahara S. Disorders of heme production and Catabolism. In: Handin RI, Lux SE, Stossel TP, eds. Blood: Principles and Practice of Hematology, 2nd Ed. Philadelphia: Lippincott Williams & Wilkins; 2003, with permission.

TABLE 5.1. *Drugs Considered Unsafe or Safe in the Acute Porphyrias*

Unsafe Drugs	Safe Drugs
Alcohol	Acetaminophen
Barbiturates	Allopurinol
Calcium channel blockers	Aspirin
Carbamazepine	Atropine
Danazol	Cimetidine
Diclofenac	Corticosteroids
Erythromycin	Coumadin
Metoclopramide	Gabapentin
Isoniazid	Gentamycin
Phenytoin	Insulin
Progesterone	Narcotic analgesics
Rifampin	Peniciliin and derivatives
Sulfonamide antibiotics	Phenothiazines
Valproic Acid	Propanalol

This list is not comprehensive and does not reflect all information and opinions. Please refer to available texts and Web sites for a more extensive list of drugs and their updated status for use in porphyrias.

surgery, or other intercurrent disorders. Under these environmental circumstances, affected patients develop characteristic neurologic disturbances.

Photocutaneous hypersensitivity and resultant skin damage occurs after exposure to ultraviolet light. When porphyrins absorb light of this wavelength, they produce free radicals that can induce oxidant tissue damage. Consequently, avoidance of precipitating factors is key in the therapy of porphyrias.

CLASSIFICATION AND CLINICAL MANIFESTATIONS

For clinical purposes, porphyrias can be classified into hepatic and erythropoietic types depending on the major tissue site of production and accumulation of the heme precursors. The major manifestations of the hepatic porphyrias are neurovisceral symptoms, including abdominal pain, neurologic symptoms, and psychiatric disorders, whereas the erythropoietic porphyrias usually present primarily with cutaneous photosensitivity and hemolytic anemia. Porphyrias can be also classified as acute porphyrias presenting with life-threatening neurovisceral manifestations and nonacute porphyrias characterized by photosensitivity syndromes, but there can be some overlap in clinical manifestations. Because the porphyrias are well characterized at the molecular genetic level, they should be specifically classified by their unique enzyme deficiencies (4).

DIAGNOSIS

Many symptoms of the porphyrias are nonspecific, and diagnosis requires a high index of suspicion. However, although the porphyrias are often suspected in a patient with vague and unexplained complaints, actual diagnosis is rare. A useful first step is to determine which one of the three major manifestations of the porphyrias—neurovisceral symptoms, photosensitivity, or hemolytic anemia—is present.

- δ-Aminolevulinic Acid Dehydratase Deficiency Porphyria (ADP), acute intermittent porphyria (AIP), hereditary coproporphyria (HCP), and variegate porphyria (VP).
- Photosensitivity is present in congenital erythropoietic porphyria (CEP), porphyria cutanea tarda (PCT), hepatoerythropoietic porphyria (HEP), HCP, VP, and erythropoietic protoporphyria (EPP).
- Neurovisceral symptoms and photosensitivity are present in HCP and VP.
- Hemolytic anemia is present in CEP, HEP, and EPP.

Laboratory testing is then required to confirm or exclude the various types of porphyrias. The diagnosis is made initially by detection of the metabolite(s) produced and/or excreted in excess in red cells, plasma, urine, and/or feces. Porphyrin precursors in urine and total porphyrins in plasma are the initial diagnostic tests for acute and cutaneous porphyrias, respectively. Today the diagnosis of many of porphyrias can be confirmed by measuring the enzymatic activity in the appropriate tissue directly or by specific molecular genetic testing (4).

SPECIFIC TYPES OF PORPHYRIAS

δ-Aminolevulinic Acid Dehydratase Deficiency Porphyria

ADP is an autosomal recessive porphyria caused by markedly deficient activity of ALA dehydratase, the second enzyme in the heme biosynthetic pathway. The diagnosis has been unequivocally confirmed only in a few cases. Clinical manifestations are primarily neurovisceral, and their treatment and prevention are the same as for other acute porphyrias. Lead poisoning should be excluded, because it also diminishes activity of ALA dehydratase, may present as a clinical phenocopy, and is far more common.

Acute Intermittent Porphyria

AIP is inherited as autosomal dominant condition resulting from a partial deficiency of porphobilinogen deaminase (PBGD) activity, the third enzyme of the pathway. Approximately 90% of heterozygotes remain biochemically normal and clinically asymptomatic throughout life. Clinical expression of the disease is usually the result of exposure to factors such as endogenous and exogenous corticosteroid hormones, a low-calorie diet, certain drugs (barbiturates and sulfonamide antibiotics are most commonly implicated), alcohol ingestion, and stresses such as intercurrent illnesses, infection, and surgery. Symptoms usually develop after puberty and are more frequent in women. The pathophysiologic hallmark of the disease is neurologic dysfunction affecting peripheral, autonomic, and/or central nervous systems occurring as intermittent acute attacks. The most common symptom is acute abdominal pain (in 90% of cases), which may be generalized or localized, but tenderness, fever, and leukocytosis are absent because the symptoms are neurologic in origin from the visceral autonomic nervous system involvement. Gastrointestinal manifestations also include abdominal distention, nausea, vomiting, diarrhea, or constipation. Peripheral sensory or motor neuropathy is another common feature of AIP. Psychiatric symptoms including hysteria, anxiety, apathy, depression, phobia, psychosis, agitation, disorientation, hallucinations, and schizophrenic-type behaviors can be the only manifestations of the disease. Acute attacks may be accompanied by seizures, either a manifestation of the porphyria itself or caused by hyponatremia. Hyponatremia commonly occurs during attacks as a consequence of inappropriate secretion of antidiuretic hormone. Sympathetic hyperactivity results in tachycardia (in 80% of cases), hypertension, tremors, and sweating. Because of the nonspecific nature of symptoms and signs, use of highly sensitive and specific laboratory tests is essential to the diagnosis.

During acute attacks, symptomatic treatment may include narcotic analgesics, phenothiazines, low-dose benzodiazepines, and propranolol for hypertension and tachycardia. Although intravenous glucose (at least 300 g per day) can be effective in acute attacks of porphyria, intravenous heme is now considered the treatment of choice to reduce excretion of porphyria. Infusion of heme should be initiated as soon as possible after onset of an attack, but the rate of recovery depends on the degree of neuronal damage and may take days to months. Any intercurrent infection or disease should also be treated immediately. Identification and avoidance of precipitating factors is also essential for prevention. Cyclical attacks in some women associated with fluctuations in estrogen and progestins can be prevented with a long-acting gonadotropin-releasing hormone analogue (5).

Congenital Erythropoietic Porphyria

CEP, an autosomal-recessive disorder also known as Gunther's disease, is caused by deficient activity of uroporphyrinogen III cosynthase (the fourth enzyme of the pathway) and is associated with hemolytic anemia and cutaneous lesions. Severe cutaneous photosensitivity usually begins in early infancy as blistering of sun-exposed areas of the skin. Recurrent vesicles, bullae, and secondary infection can lead to cutaneous scarring and deformities. Porphyrin deposition may also occur in bones, leading to brownish discoloration of teeth. Protecting skin from sunlight is essential.

Mild to severe hemolytic anemia and secondary splenomegaly are features of CEP, and anemia can be severe. Transfusion is effective but results in iron overload if chronic. Splenectomy may reduce hemolysis and decrease the transfusion requirement. In transfusion-dependent children, allogeneic stem cell transplantation can be considered.

Porphyria Cutanea Tarda

Porphyria cutanea tarda, the most common of the porphyrias, is caused by acquired or inherited deficiency of uroporphyrinogen decarboxylase (the fifth enzyme of the pathway). The disease occurs worldwide, but its exact incidence is not known. The disease can be *sporadic* (noninherited or type I, most common) or *familial* (types II and III), although these subtypes are not distinguishable clinically. The frequency of disease varies in relation to risk factors such as alcohol use, smoking, hepatitis C, and human immunodeficiency virus (HIV) infection. The hallmark of PCT is cutaneous photosensitivity presenting as chronic blistering lesions on sun-exposed areas of skin without neurologic manifestations. Chronic changes including cutaneous thickening, scarring, and calcification can mimic systemic sclerosis. Also common are facial hypertrichosis and hyperpigmentation. PCT is almost always associated with abnormalities in liver function tests, and the risk of developing hepatocellular carcinoma is significantly increased in this disease (6).

Alcohol ingestion, estrogens, iron supplements and, if possible, any drugs that may exacerbate the disease and sun exposure should be avoided. A complete response can usually be achieved by repeated phlebotomy to reduce hepatic iron and is still considered standard treatment. Low-dose chloroquine or hydroxychloroquine is also effective, especially when phlebotomy is contraindicated. In contrast, similar skin lesions in VP, HCP, CEP, and HEP are unresponsive to these therapeutic interventions.

Hepatoerythropoietic Porphyria

This rare form of porphyria has been recently described. HEP is clinically indistinguishable from CEP and is caused by homozygous defect of the same enzyme involved in porphyria cutanea tarda. Patients usually present after birth with dark urine in the diapers followed by severe photosensitivity with blistering skin lesions and scleroderma-like scarring. Hemolytic anemia is often present with splenomegaly. The avoidance of sunlight is essential.

Hereditary Coproporphyria

HCP is an autosomal-dominant porphyria resulting from deficiency of coproporphyrinogen oxidase (the sixth enzyme of the pathway). The neurovisceral symptoms and other manifestations as well as the precipitating factors are virtually identical to those of AIP, but photosensitivity similar to PCT may also occur in one third of the patients. Avoidance of precipitating factors as in AIP is important. Neurologic symptoms are treated as in AIP, but in contrast to PCT, phlebotomy or chloroquine is not effective for cutaneous lesions.

Variegate Porphyria

This hepatic porphyria, the result of a mutation of the protoporphyria oxidase gene (the seventh enzyme in the pathway), is transmitted as an autosomal-dominant disorder and is particularly common in South African whites (prevalence of 3 in 1000) because of a genetic founder effect from a couple who emigrated from Holland to South Africa in late 1600s. The disease was termed variegate because it can present with either neurovisceral symptoms, cutaneous photosensitivity, or both. Neurovisceral symptoms are very similar to those of AIP and are provoked by the same precipitates. Acute attacks are treated with glucose and heme infusion as in AIP. Occurrence of skin manifestations is usually separate from the neurovisceral symptoms, and avoiding sun exposure is the only effective preventative measure for cutaneous photosensitivity.

Erythropoietic Protoporphyria

EPP, also known as protoporphyria, results from deficiency of ferrochelatase activity, the last enzyme in the heme biosynthetic pathway. EPP is the most common erythropoietic porphyria and third most common porphyria in general. Skin photosensitivity beginning in childhood is typical of the disease, but the skin lesions are different from other porphyrias. Erythema, burning, and itching accompanied by swelling can develop within minutes of sun exposure, but sparse vesicles and bullae are seen in only a minority of the cases. Chronic skin changes may occur, but severe scarring is rare. Treatment involves avoidance of sun exposure and the use of topical sun screens. Oral β-carotene (120 to 180 mg per day) can be effective in many patients with EPP, in contrast to those with photosensitivity from other forms of porphyria. The mechanism of action of β-carotene is not clear but is attributed to its antioxidant effect. In some patients, accumulation of protoporphyrin causes chronic liver disease that can progress to hepatic failure and death. Neurovisceral symptoms are seen only in patients with severe hepatic complications. Protoporphyrin-rich gallstones may occur. Mild anemia is sometimes seen in patients with EPP, but hemolysis is either infrequent or very mild. Splenectomy may be helpful when the disease is accompanied by hemolysis and significant splenomegaly. Caloric restriction, drugs, and exogenous sex hormones should be avoided. Intravenous heme therapy is sometimes beneficial. Liver transplantation has been performed, but the protoporphyrin-induced damage can recur in the donor liver (7).

REFERENCES

1. Anderson KE, Bloomer JR, Bonkovsky HL, et al. Recommendations for the diagnosis and treatment of the acute porphyrias. Ann Intern Med 2005;142:439–450.
2. Foran SE, Abel G. Guide to porphyrias. A historical and clinical perspective. Am J Clin Pathol 2003;119(Suppl):86–93.
3. Kauppinen R. Porphyrias. Lancet 2005;365:241–252.
4. Sassa S. Modern diagnosis and management of the porphyrias. B J Haematol 2006;135:281–292.
5. Dombeck TA, Satonik RC. The porphyrias. Emerg Med Clin N Am 2005;23:885–899.
6. Poblete-Gutierrez P, Wiederholt T, Merk HF, et al. The porphyrias: clinical presentation, diagnosis, and treatment. Eur J Dermatol 2006;16:230–240.
7. Sassa S. Hematologic aspects of the porphyrias. Int J Hematol 2000;71:1–17.

6

Bone Marrow Failure Syndromes: Acquired and Constitutional Aplastic Anemia, Paroxysmal Nocturnal Hemoglobinuria, Pure Red Blood Cell Aplasia, and Agranulocytosis

Neal S. Young, Phillip Scheinberg, and Johnson M. Liu

The bone marrow failure syndromes are characterized by inadequate blood cell production leading to low red blood cell, white blood cell, and/or platelet counts in the peripheral blood. Marrow failure can be acquired or constitutional and may affect all three blood cell lines, resulting in pancytopenia. In most, the bone marrow shows a simple deficiency of the related precursor cells, but marrow failure can also occur with relatively cellular marrows, presumably because of ineffective hematopoiesis, and be associated with cytogenetic abnormalities (see Chapter 7) or a genetically altered cell, as in paroxysmal nocturnal hemoglobinuria (PNH), discussed in this chapter because of its intimate relationship to aplastic anemia (AA) (1). Even the paradigmatic syndrome of AA clinically and pathophysiologically shows overlap with related diseases (Fig. 6.1A).

ACQUIRED APLASTIC ANEMIA

Acquired AA is characterized by pancytopenia with a hypocellular, often "empty" bone marrow.

AA is uncommon in the West; its incidence in Europe is about two new cases per million. However, the disease is two- to threefold more frequent in East Asia and probably elsewhere in the developing world. In most series, most patients are young, the majority presenting between 15 and 25 years of age. Historically, chemicals (benzene) and drugs (chloramphenicol) were implicated as causative but without satisfactory mechanisms of pathogenesis. The most important current associations are with nonsteroidal anti-inflammatory drugs, antithyroid drugs, penicillamine, allopurinol, and gold (Table 6.1) (2). Nonetheless, most AA is idiopathic or without a presumed environmental factor in an individual patient.

Etiology and Pathophysiology

Hematopoiesis is severely reduced in all AA, as observed in bone marrow specimens, CD34 cell counts, magnetic resonance imaging, or in functional studies of progenitors. Clinical and laboratory studies suggest that most acquired AA is secondary to *immunologically* mediated destruction of hematopoietic cells by cytotoxic lymphocytes and their cytokine products, especially interferon-γ and tumor necrosis factor-α. Marrow failure rarely can follow infectious mononucleosis (Epstein-Barr virus [EBV] infection) and is a component of the stereotypical post-hepatitis

AA syndrome, which is unassociated with any known hepatitis virus. EBV and the putative agent of seronegative hepatitis behave as triggers for immune system activity. In contrast, parvovirus B19 directly infects and kills erythroid progenitor cells and causes pure red cell aplasia but not AA. Direct killing of marrow cells by cytotoxic agents occurs following cancer chemotherapy, producing transient marrow aplasia, but is probably unusual as a mechanism of idiosyncratic drug-associated AA.

Clinical Features

Anemia leads to fatigue, weakness, lassitude, headaches, and in older patients dyspnea and chest pain, and these symptoms are most commonly responsible for the clinical presentation.

Thrombocytopenia produces mainly mucosal bleeding; petechiae of the skin and mucous membranes, epistaxis, and gum bleeding are frequent and early complaints. Bleeding is not brisk from low platelets unless in the presence of accompanying physical lesions, as in gastritis and fungal infection of the lungs. The most feared complication of thrombocytopenia is intracranial hemorrhage.

Infection can occur at presentation in the setting of neutropenia. Dark urine suggests PNH. Occasionally moderate cytopenias are identified serendipitously by routine blood work or at preoperative evaluation. Constitutional symptoms (malaise, anorexia and weight loss) should be absent.

Physical findings range from a well-appearing patient with minimal findings to an acutely ill patient with signs of systemic toxicity. Cachexia, lymphadenopathy, and splenomegaly are not seen and suggest an alternative diagnosis.

Anemia is reflected in pallor of the skin mucous membranes and nail beds. Constitutional AA is suggested by areas of hyper- or hypopigmentation of the skin, abnormal hands and thumbs, short stature (Fanconi anemia), nail dystrophy, and oral leukoplakia (dyskeratosis congenita).

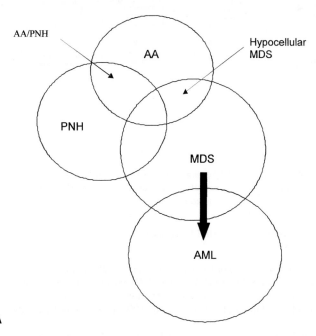

FIG. 6.1. (A) Venn diagram of the relationship among bone marrow failure syndromes. *(continued)*

A

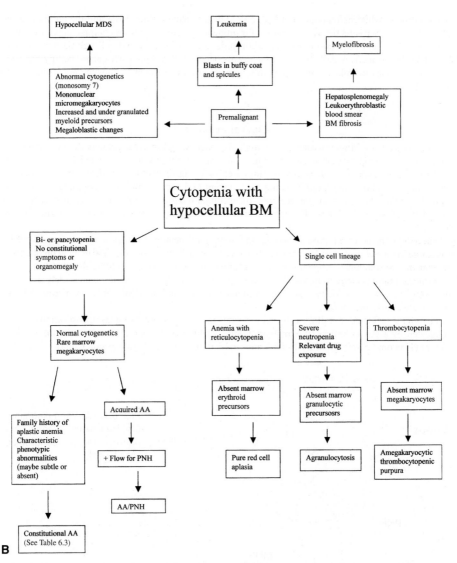

FIG. 6.1. *(continued)* **(B)** Differential diagnosis of cytopenias. AA, aplastic anemia; AML, acute myelogenous leukemia; BM, bone marrow; DKC, dyskeratosis congenita; MDS, myelodysplasia; PNH, paroxysmal nocturnal hemoglobinuria; SDS, Shwachman-Diamond syndrome.

Diagnosis and Differential Diagnosis

At diagnosis:

- Marked pancytopenia or reduction in two of three or less commonly one of three cell lines.
- Peripheral blood smear shows reduced platelets, neutrophils, and red cells (with normal morphology).
- Microspherocytes and giant platelets suggestive of peripheral destruction are not present.
- Bone marrow markedly hypocellular on biopsy (1-cm core); residual lymphocytes, plasma cells, mast cells on aspirate smear can be seen.
- Overall marrow biopsy cellularity is low (<30%, excluding lymphocytes), but there may be pockets of cellularity, so-called hot-spots.

TABLE 6.1. *Drugs Associated with Aplastic Anemia in the International Aplastic Anemia and Agranulocytosis Study*

Drug	
Nonsteroidal analgesics	Cardiovascular Drugs
Butazones	Furosemide
Indomethacin	Psychotropic drugs
Piroxicam	Phenothiazines
Diclofenac	Corticosteroids
Antibiotics	Penicillamine
Sulfonamides*	Allopurinol
Antithyroid drugs	Gold

*Other than trimethoprim-sulfonamide combination.

- Myeloblasts and megakaryocytes are almost always absent.
- Marrow cytogenetics should be normal.

In secondary marrow failure, the degree of pancytopenia is usually moderate, and the underlying illness is usually obvious from history and physical examination (e.g., stigmata of alcohol liver disease, presence of other autoimmune disease or infection). However, pancytopenia has many causes, of which AA is not the most common (Table 6.2).

TABLE 6.2. *Differential Diagnosis of Pancytopenia*

Pancytopenia with Hypocellular Bone Marrow
    Acquired aplastic anemia
    Inherited aplastic anemia
    Some myelodysplastic syndromes
    Rare aleukemic leukemia
    Some acute lymphoblastic leukemia
    Some lymphomas of the bone marrow

Pancytopenia with Cellular Bone Marrow
Primary Bone Marrow Diseases
    Myelodysplastic syndromes
    Paroxysmal nocturnal hemoglobinuria
    Myelofibrosis
    Hairy cell leukemia
    Some aleukemic leukemia
    Myelophthisis
    Bone marrow lymphoma
Secondary to Systemic Diseases
    Systemic lupus erythematosus, Sjögren's syndrome
    Hypersplenism
    Vitamin B12, folate deficiency (familial defect)
    Overwhelming infection
    Alcoholism
    Brucellosis
    Ehrlichiosis
    Sarcoidosis
    Tuberculosis and atypical mycobacteria

Hypocellular Bone Marrow with or without Cytopenia
    Q fever
    Legionnaire's disease
    Toxoplasmosis
    Mycobacteria
    Tuberculosis
    Anorexia nervosa, starvation
    Hypothyroidism

TABLE 6.3. *Diseases Easily Confused with Aplastic Anemia*

Disease	Distinguishing Characteristics	Diagnostic Test
Constitutional*		
Fanconi Anemia	Younger patients; family history and physical anomalies (short stature, café au lait spots, anomalies of the upper limb or thumb)	**Chromosome analysis of stressed blood lymphocyte cultures**
Dyskeratosis Congenita	Younger patients; family history and physical anomalies (nail changes, leukoplakia)	**Short telomeres mutations in TERC, TERT, DKC1**
Acquired		
Myelodysplasia	Older patients, insidious onset, marrow usually normo- or hypercellular	**Marrow morphology Marrow cytogenetics**
Aleukemic leukemia	Very young or very old patients	**Blasts in buffy coat and spicules**
PNH	Hemolysis (high LDH, low haptoglobin, hemoglobinuria), venous thrombosis	**Deficient GPI-anchored proteins on flow cytometry**
Myelofibrosis	Hepatosplenomegaly Leukoerythroblastic blood smear	**Fibrosis on marrow biopsy**
Large granular lymphocytosis	**Older age, insidious, neutropenia**	**Large granular lymphocytes in peripheral smear Flow cytometry T-cell receptor rearrangement**

*Phenotypic abnormalities may be subtle or absent.
LDH, lactate dehydrogenase; GPI, glycosylphosphatidylinositol; PNH, paroxysmal nocturnal hemoglobinuria.

Most important is to distinguish among primary marrow diseases (Table 6.3, Fig. 6.1B).

With constitutional AA presenting in adults, a family history is highly suggestive. Patients under 40 years of age (or older if the history or examination are suggestive) should be tested for Fanconi anemia. Although phenotypic abnormalities have been classically described in both Fanconi anemia and dyskeratosis congenita, patients with adult onset constitutional AA may have subtle signs on routine physical examination or no characteristic findings at all (3).

Myelodysplasia (MDS) is hypocellular in about 20% of cases. Dysplastic changes in AA when present are mild and limited to erythrocytes. In MDS, megaloblastic changes are more extreme; megakaryocytes are preserved and can be aberrantly small and mononuclear, and myeloid precursors may be increased and often poorly granulated. Chromosomal analysis of bone marrow cells is almost always normal in AA, while MDS is often associated with cytogenetic abnormalities. Nonetheless, the distinction may be so difficult that some patients are best labeled AA/MDS.

Small PNH expanded clones are common—as many as 50% of cases at presentation—in the setting of marrow failure now that flow cytometry has replaced the Ham test. Growth of clone size over time may lead to clinical hemolysis. Thrombosis is rare.

Acute lymphocytic leukemia in children and acute myelogenous leukemia in the elderly can occasionally present with pancytopenia and marrow hypocellularity.

Myelofibrosis has a characteristic leukoerythroblastic blood picture, marrow is dry tap (rather than watery, as in AA), and hepatosplenomegaly is common.

Large granular lymphocytosis is characterized by prolonged periods of neutropenia, less frequently anemia or thrombocytopenia, and increased numbers of large granular lymphocytes in the peripheral blood. Marrow is usually cellular; diagnosis rests on flow cytometry or molecular evidence of rearrangement of the T-cell receptor.

Severe AA is defined by two of the following three peripheral blood count criteria:

- absolute neutrophil count <500 /uL
- platelet count <20,000 /uL
- reticulocyte count (automated) <60,000 /uL

Definitive Treatments

Definitive therapy of AA consists of allogeneic hematopoietic stem cell transplantation (HSCT) or immunosuppression; both have dramatically changed the natural course of this illness, with 5-year survival of 75% in patients undergoing either treatment (4). Support with growth factors alone or in combination with transfusion are used but are of uncertain long-term benefit and unlikely to change the natural history of the disease. The main distinctions between immunosuppression and HSCT are shown in Table 6.4.

HSCT cures AA. Most transplants are performed using a histocompatible sibling donor, and most recipients are young. Overall long-term survival is about 70% (5). HSCT is almost always preferred in children to about age 20 who have an appropriate donor. With current cyclophosphamide-based conditioning, major toxicities are related to graft-versus-host disease (GVHD) and infection (not always easily separable). GVHD risk increases with recipient age. The source of donor cells may be important: in one recent retrospective study, granulocyte colony-stimulating factor (G-CSF)-mobilized stem cells produced a higher rate of chronic GVHD and mortality in younger patients than did bone marrow cells (6). Modest numbers of erythrocyte and platelet transfusions do not appear to increase the risk of graft rejection, especially with leukocyte-depleted products (7).

Seventy percent of patients will lack a suitable matched sibling donor. Transplantation from matched unrelated donors (MUD) is now more feasible with the development of large donor registries and an effective network. Overall results are about half as good as with human leukocyte antigen (HLA)-matched family members but likely to improve with modifications of conditioning regimens and high-resolution molecular typing for donor selection (8,9); in some small studies, outcomes with alternative donor approximate that of standard transplant outcomes (10,11). Donor searches should be initiated early for younger patients who might be eligible later for a MUD. For unclear reasons, umbilical cord blood transplantation has been associated with poor results in marrow failure states. In current practice, unrelated transplant is offered for children who have failed a single course of immunosuppression and to adults who are refractory to multiple courses of antithymocyte globulin (ATG) and alternative therapies such as androgens.

Immunosuppression using regimens combining ATG and cyclosporine is standard therapy. About two thirds of patients improve to transfusion independence, and overall survival rates at 5 years are comparable with HSCT. Immunosuppression is almost always preferred in older patients, especially if the neutrophil count is not severely decreased. One frequently used protocol for horse ATG is 40 mg/kg/d

TABLE 6.4. *Bone Marrow Transplantation Versus Immunosuppression*

	HSCT	Immunosuppression
Applicability	HLA-matched sibling	All
Cost	High	Moderate
Age limits	Best in children Adults <40	All ages
Outcome	65%–90% long-term survival	70% hematologic response
Short-term toxicity	10%–30% die of GVHD, infection, pneumonitis, veno-occlusive hepatic disease, or graft failure	Rare anaphylaxis
Long-term effects	Hematologic cure; modest increase in risk of solid tumors	Incomplete cure with possibility of development of PNH, MDS, AML

AML, acute myeloid leukemia; HLA, human leukocyte antigen; GVHD, graft-versus-host disease; MDS, myelodysplastic syndrome; PNH, paroxysmal nocturnal hemoglobinuria.

for 4 days. Rabbit ATG is administered at 3.5 mg/kg/d for 5 days (there is no evidence that one preparation is superior to the other). Corticosteroids, such as methylprednisolone at 1 mg/kg, are usually administered during the first 2 weeks to ameliorate serum sickness. In patients who are refractory to initial horse ATG, hematologic recovery can be achieved with a second course of ATG (12); in our institutional experience, about 30% of patients who are treated showed a hematologic response (13).

Major toxicities of ATG include immediate allergic reaction, serum sickness, and transient blood count depression. Anaphylaxis is rare but has been fatal and may be predictable by skin testing. Treatment of ATG allergy is mainly symptomatic: intravenous hydration, antihistamines (for urticaria) and meperidine (for rigors), and increased doses of corticosteroids (for symptomatic serum sickness). Cyclosporine is begun at 10 mg/kg in adults and 15/mg/kg in children, with dose adjustment to maintain blood levels about 200 ng/ml. We administer cyclosporine for 6 months following ATG. Renal and liver function monitoring is required to avoid nephrotoxicity; hypertension, gingival hypertrophy, and tremulousness are common side effects.

Prognosis is strongly correlated to hematologic response at 3 months, especially the robustness of blood count recovery (14). Even after hematologic response to ATG, blood counts may fall, especially on withdrawal of cyclosporine. Reinstitution of cyclosporine usually suffices, but retreatment with ATG may be necessary, and relapse is sometimes irreversible and fatal. Evolution to a clonal hematologic disease occurs in about 15% of patients over the decade after initial therapy and manifests as dysplastic bone marrow or cytogenetic abnormalities, especially monosomy 7 and trisomy 8.

Other therapies that are occasionally successful include growth factor combinations (erythropoietin and G-CSF); androgens; high-dose cyclophosphamide (controversial because of prolonged neutropenia it induces) (15). Our approach to treatment is shown in Figure 6.2.

PAROXYSMAL NOCTURNAL HEMOGLOBINURIA

Paroxysmal nocturnal hemoglobinuria (PNH) is a rare clonal disease of the bone marrow, which can produce a clinical triad of (i) hemolysis, (ii) venous thrombosis, and (iii) aplastic anemia (16).

Etiology and Pathophysiology

A somatic *mutation* in a gene called *PIG-A* occurs in a hematopoietic stem cell. This leads to deficient *synthesis* of a glycolipid moiety called the *glycosylphosphoinositol anchor (GPI)*. There is lack of cell surface presentation of a large family of *GPI-linked proteins*. The absence of one of these proteins, *CD59*, on the cell surface of erythrocytes leads to their susceptibility to complement and to intravascular hemolysis. PIG-A mutant cells are probably present in normal adult marrow, but clonal expansion of these cells is unusual, except in AA (about 40%–50% of cases) and in MDS (about 20%), where they may range in size from small to large. Which GPI-anchored proteins are important in permitting clonal expansion in AA and MDS and in the thrombotic proclivity is unknown.

Clinical Features

Clinical features include:

- *Intravascular hemolysis,* classically as periodic bouts of dark urine in the morning but also as continuous red cell destruction and without evident hemoglobinuria.
- *Venous thrombosis in unusual sites*, especially hepatic, mesenteric, portal, and intracranial veins.
- *Marrow failure*, frank AA or poor marrow function despite a relatively cellular histology.

Diagnosis

PNH should be considered in the setting of a suggestive history, hemoglobinuria, and elevated LDH. There may be accompanying iron deficiency and neutropenia/thrombocytopenia.

PNH patients can present with abdominal pain because of Budd-Chiari syndrome or symptoms of stroke. PNH clonal expansion should be sought in patients of AA and MDS.

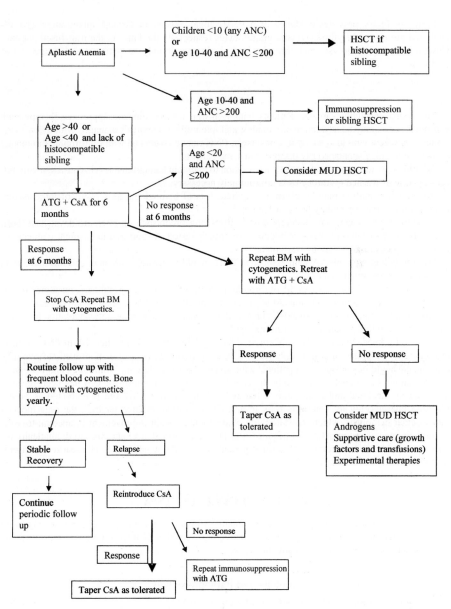

FIG. 6.2. Treatment of severe aplastic anemia. ANC, absolute neutrophil count; ATG, anti-thymocyte globulin; BM, bone marrow; CsA, cyclosporine A; HSCT, hematopoietic stem cell transplantation; MUD, matched unrelated donor.

Flow cytometry provides evidence of a PNH clonal expansion through quantitation of GPI-anchored proteins on erythrocytes and granulocytes (especially the latter in the transfused patient). However, severe hemolysis and thrombosis typically occur only in patients with large clones (>50%).

Treatment

The course is highly variable. Patients with AA who receive immunosuppressive therapy with expanded clones may be asymptomatic; modest and intermittent hemolysis managed with transfusions alone is consistent with long survival. Conversely, PNH can be associated with catastrophic thrombotic events. Clones may spontaneously disappear in some patients.

Additional treatment methods include transfusion to maintain hemoglobin levels consistent with full activity. Use of washed erythrocytes is not routinely necessary.

Iron supplementation may be given as required; loss of hemoglobin as a result of intravascular destruction prevents secondary hemochromatosis.

Corticosteroids, usually in moderate doses (30–50 mg prednisone on alternate days) have been frequently used to control hemolysis but never rigorously tested. A short trial in a patient with continuous red cell destruction may be warranted.

Marrow failure as frank AA with associated PNH should be treated with stem cell transplantation or immunosuppression (see above).

Most patients in Western series die of thrombotic complications, and thromboses, once they occur, may be refractory to anticoagulation. At least one uncontrolled trial has suggested that coumadin prophylaxis is effective, but the relative risk of hemorrhage secondary to chronic anticoagulation for years, even decades, in this population remains unclear (17).

Stem cell transplantation is the only curative therapy but may carry a higher risk in PNH because of comorbid conditions; nonmyeloablative conditioning regimens may offer improved survival (7). Transplant should be considered in patients with severe marrow failure or thrombotic complications.

Eculizumab (a monoclonal antibody directed to the active component of C5) has been recently approved by the Food and Drug Administration for patients with PNH and is marketed as Soliris (Alexion Pharmaceuticals, Cheshire, CT). In a large prospective multicenter trial, the drug blocked intravascular hemolysis, which translated to a clinically significant improvement in anemia, transfusion requirements, and in quality of life measures (18). Eculizumab also appeared to dramatically reduce the risk of clinical thromboembolism in patients with PNH, which is the major cause of morbidity and mortality in this disease (19).

PURE RED CELL APLASIA

Pure red cell aplasia (PRCA) is defined as anemia with absent reticulocytes and marrow erythroid precursor cells (20). This rare aregenerative anemia has a number of interesting clinical associations and is also usually responsive to treatment.

Etiology and Pathophysiology

Constitutional PRCA is Diamond-Blackfan anemia (DBA).

Acquired PRCA often behaves as an immunologically mediated disease. Clinical associations include thymoma (probably <10% of PRCA cases), collagen-vascular syndromes, myasthenia gravis, chronic lymphocytic leukemia, and large granular lymphocytic leukemia. PRCA may also be seen in MDS, especially with 5q- syndrome.

Parvovirus B19 infection is often asymptomatic but may cause erythema infectiosum (fifth disease) in children and transient aplastic crisis in patients with underlying hemolysis. Virus infection is ordinarily terminated by production of neutralizing antibodies. Persistence of parvovirus results from failure to mount a neutralizing antibody response, leading to chronic erythroid precursor destruction and anemia. Persistence of parvovirus B19 can occur in an immunodeficient host: in congenital immunodeficiencies

(Nezelof's syndrome), iatrogenic (immunosuppressive drugs and cytotoxic chemotherapy), and human immunodeficiency virus infection-induced immunodeficiency.

Clinical Features and Diagnosis

Reticulocytes are severely depressed; erythroid precursor cells are usually absent, but a few normoblasts may be present in the marrow. Giant pronormoblasts signal parvovirus, and uninuclear micromegakaryocytes indicate 5q- syndrome. Other blood counts are normal, as are cytogenetics (except for PRCA associated with MDS). Thymoma should be excluded by computed tomography scan.

Parvovirus B19 antibodies are usually absent, or only IgM may be observed; virus can be detected in the blood by DNA hybridization.

Treatment

For DBA, corticosteroids are standard. Patients may be dependent on exquisitely low doses, and relapse may not always be responsive to reinstitution of treatment. Despite transfusions and adequate iron chelation, patients may develop fatal late complications, including neutropenia and pulmonary hypertension.

For acquired PRCA, corticosteroids in moderate doses are usually first therapy, followed by either other immunosuppressives such as cyclosporine, ATG, and more recently (in a few case reports) monoclonal antibodies to CD20 (rituximab), or cytotoxic drugs such as moderate doses of azathioprine or cyclosphosphamide, administered orally. Anti-interleukin-2 receptor (daclizumab) has been shown to be safe and effective in a case series of 15 patients, in which hematologic response was observed in six (21).

Thymomas should be excised because they are locally invasive; surgery does not necessarily resolve the anemia.

Persistent parvovirus B19 infection responds to intravenous immunoglobulins at 0.4 g/kg daily for 5 to 10 days. Patients with large viral loads, especially in the acquired immunodeficiency syndrome, may relapse and require periodic retreatment.

AGRANULOCYTOSIS

Severe neutropenia with either complete or partial absence of myeloid precursor cells is agranulocytosis.

Etiology and Pathophysiology

Most agranulocytosis is drug-associated (Table 6.5). Idiopathic pure white cell aplasia (without exposure to a suspicious drug) is exceedingly rare (and like PRCA may also be associated with thymoma) (22,23).

Mechanisms of drug destruction of granulocyte precursors include direct effects (as with thorazine) and immune (antibody)-mediated (as with dipyrone) (Table 6.6).

Diagnosis and Treatment

The patient is usually older with a history of clear exposure to an incriminated agent, usually with introduction of the drug in the preceding 6 months. Absent neutrophils on smear should lead to a confirmatory bone marrow examination.

The classic presentation is fever and sore throat. Recovery occurs spontaneously but over a highly variable time period, from a few days to several weeks. G-CSF or granulocyte monocyte colony stimulating factor (GM-CSF) is almost always administered without clear evidence of efficacy. Fever and signs of infection require prompt administration of broad spectrum antibiotics by a parenteral route. Mortality remains substantial (about 10%) because of the combination of patient age, comorbid conditions, and lethal sepsis.

TABLE 6.5. *Drugs Associated with Agranulocytosis*

Heavy Metals	Antibiotics
Gold	Sulfa antibiotics
Arsenic compounds	Pyrimethamine
Analgesics	Penicillins
Aminopyrine, dipyrone	Cephalosporins
Butazones	Macrolides
Indomethacin	Vancomycin
Ibuprofen	Clindamycin
Acetaminophen	Aminoglycosides
Para-aminosalicylic acid	Antituberculosis agents
Sulindac	Levamisole
Antipsychotics, sedatives,	Antimalarials
antidepressants	Mebendazole
Phenothiazines	Antifungals
Trycyclics	Fluconazole
Chlorodiazepoxide	Antiviral
Barbiturates	Zidovudine
Serotonin reuptake inhibitors	Antihistamines
Anticonvulsants	Cimetidine
Phenytoin	Ranitidine
Ethosuximide	Chlorpheniramine
Carbamazepine	Miscellaneous
Antithyroid drugs	Isotretinoin
Propylthiouracil	Omeprazole
Methimazole	Colchicine
Cardiovascular drugs	Allopurinol
Procainamide	Aminoglutethimide
Captopril	Metoclopramide
Nifedipine	Ticlopidine
Quinidine	Tamoxifen
Propranolol	Penicillamine
Methyldopa	Insecticides
Propafenone	Hair dye
Aprindine	Chinese herbal medicines
Sulfa drugs	
Thiazide diuretics like	
spironolactone and	
acetazolamide	
Oral hypoglycemics	
Sulfasalazine	
Dapsone	
Sulfa antibiotics	

TABLE 6.6. *Immune Versus Toxic Agranulocytosis*

	Immunologic	Toxic
Paradigm drug	Aminopyrine	Phenothiazine
Time to onset	Days to weeks	Weeks to months
Clinical	Acute, often explosive symptoms	Often asymptomatic or insidious onset
Rechallenge	Prompt recurrence with small test dose	Latent period, high dose required
Laboratory	Leucoagglutinins	Evidence of direct or metabolite mediated toxicity to cells

CONSTITUTIONAL BONE MARROW FAILURE SYNDROMES

Marrow Failure Affects All Three Lineages (Erythrocytes, Granulocytes, Platelets)

Among the constitutional disorders that present with aplastic anemia, it is important to consider Fanconi anemia (FA) and dyskeratosis congenita (DC). Genes mutated in FA and in DC have been identified and are important in "housekeeping functions" in the cell; they have a key role in genomic stability and the maintenance of telomeres, respectively. An algorithm for laboratory testing to exclude FA and DC is presented below (Fig. 6.3).

FANCONI ANEMIA

FA is the most common of the constitutional syndromes, and inheritance may be autosomal recessive or x-linked. It is seen in all races and diagnosed on the basis of positive chromosome breakage test (see below).

Mutations can be seen in any of 13 genes: *FANCA, FANCB, FANCC, FANCD1/BRCA2, FANCD2, FANCE, FANCF, FANCG, FANCI, FANCJ/BACH1/BRIP1, FANCL, FANCM, FANCN/PALB2*.

Chief criteria are pancytopenia, hyperpigmentation, malformation of the skeleton, small stature, and hypogonadism. Malformations of the eye, ear, genitourinary and gastrointestinal tracts, cardiopulmonary and central nervous systems can occur.

FA is notoriously heterogeneous in the degree and number of clinical manifestations, and patients presenting solely with either congenital malformations or hematologic abnormalities may either be misdiagnosed or go unrecognized entirely.

Clinical Features

The diagnosis is suggested when a child presents with hyper- or hypopigmented skin lesions; short stature (poor growth); anomalies of the upper limb or thumb; male hypogonadism; microcephaly; characteristic facial features, including a broadened nasal base, epicanthal folds, and micrognathia; and structural renal abnormalities. When this constellation of physical anomalies is accompanied by bone marrow failure (which may often trigger initial medical evaluation), confirmation of the diagnosis can be made by standard diepoxybutane (DEB) or mitomycin C (MMC) chromosome breakage analysis (see below). The mean age at diagnosis is usually 8 or 9 years.

Diagnostic Tests

Diagnosis is made with a chromosome breakage test with DEB or MMC. Based solely on definition by the DEB test, nearly 40% of patients may be free of major physical anomalies. These patients with normal-appearing FA may go unrecognized unless there is a high index of suspicion for familial disease.

Another challenge is the diagnosis of FA in older patients. Although the mean age of diagnosis is in the first decade of life, FA has been described recently in a 56-year-old woman.

Hematologic Presentations and Cancer Predisposition

The symptoms and signs of FA typically relate to the hematologic presentation of cytopenias from marrow failure. Often, thrombocytopenia or leukopenia is noted before full pancytopenia; furthermore, the pancytopenia typically worsens with time. Almost all patients with FA will develop hematologic abnormalities in their lifetime. Erythropoiesis is usually macrocytic.

Classically, the bone marrow is hypocellular and fatty, indistinguishable from that seen in acquired aplastic anemia. Microscopic examination of the marrow may show dyserythropoiesis and dysplasia. Some patients may develop or even present with a morphologically defined MDS or frank acute myeloid leukemia (AML).

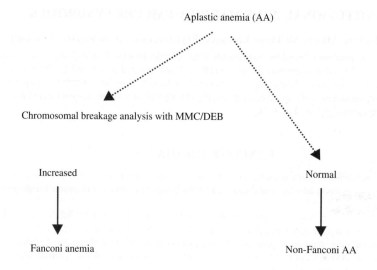

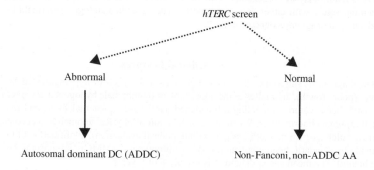

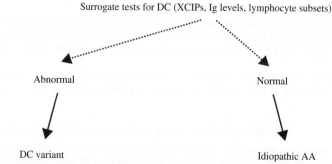

FIG. 6.3. Constitutional marrow failure. Figure courtesy of I. Dokal.

The crude risk of leukemia (exclusive of MDS) is ~5% to 10%, while the cumulative incidence of leukemia is about 10% by age 25. Less commonly recognized is the probability of developing MDS, approximately 5%, which appears also to correlate with a poor prognosis for patients with FA. Clonal karyotypic abnormalities, identical to those seen in non-FA MDS and secondary AML, are frequently found in patients with FA, whether or not they meet marrow morphologic criteria for a defined MDS. The prognostic significance of these clonal chromosomal abnormalities in patients with FA is not entirely clear, however, because cytogenetic abnormalities can fluctuate over time. Certain clonal abnormalities may be associated with poor prognosis, such as gains of chromosome 3q.

Solid organ malignancies have been noted, with a crude risk of 5% to 10% of patients overall (the risk increases with age, because those patients who have survived into adulthood develop solid tumors). Particularly common are vulvar, esophageal, and head and neck cancers. In addition to these (presumed) de novo tumors, a subset of long-term survivors of stem cell transplantation will develop secondary malignancies, typically head and neck.

For *FANCD1/BRCA2* and *FANCN/PALB2*, as has been demonstrated thus far, affected family members with monoallelic mutations are predisposed to breast cancer, whereas those with biallelic mutations present with an FA phenotype associated with childhood cancers and leukemia.

Stem Cell Transplantation and Supportive Care

Allogeneic stem cell transplantation (SCT) from an HLA-matched sibling donor is the only curative therapy for the hematologic manifestations of FA (aplasia or myelodysplasia). Typically, decreased doses of cyclophosphamide and irradiation must be used in order to avoid severe toxicity because of increased chemo- and radiosensitivity of patients with FA. Transplantation centers, which generally adopted this modified conditioning regimen with or without thoracoabdominal irradiation (TAI), have reported good results for patients with FA who did not present with leukemia or preleukemic transformation.

Umbilical cord blood transplantation from related donors has also been successfully applied to a small number of patients with FA. A few patients with FA have also undergone successful stem cell transplantation with cord blood from unrelated donors.

Clearly, young patients with an HLA-compatible sibling should be treated by SCT at the earliest stages of marrow failure in preference to other therapies. However, most patients do not have an HLA-identical donor and are dependent on the identification of a suitably matched nonsibling relative or unrelated donor. A smaller number of patients with FA have undergone BMT from such alternative sources (matched unrelated and haploidentical family donors) to treat either aplasia or myelodysplasia, with or without clonal chromosomal abnormalities. The results from these alternative donor transplants have generally been inferior to those from matched sibling donor transplants but are improving.

Patients lacking a suitable HLA-compatible donor (either sibling or matched unrelated) may benefit from chronic administration of androgens or hematopoietic growth factors (HGFs), which may serve as temporizing measures.

Androgens

Androgens have been shown to induce hematologic responses in approximately 50% of patients with FA, although their effectiveness in raising blood counts may be neither durable nor complete in all lineages. Typically, androgen therapy is initiated when the platelet count is consistently below 30,000/μl and/or the hemoglobin less than 7 gm/dl. Orally administered oxymetholone, at a dose of 2 to 5 mg/kg/day, is usually combined with prednisone, 5 to 10 mg every other day, to counterbalance the anabolic properties of oxymetholone with catabolic actions of corticosteroids.

Androgen therapy is associated with liver toxicities including transaminase enzyme elevation, cholestasis, peliosis hepatitis, and hepatic tumors. Injectable androgens are associated with a decreased risk of hepatotoxicity, but pediatricians have sometimes objected to their use over concerns of pain and local bleeding. One standard formulation is nandrolone decanoate, administered by intramuscular injection at a dose of 1–2 mg/kg/week.

Hematopoietic Growth Factors

Levels of most growth factors are markedly increased in FA as they are in acquired aplastic anemia, likely as a compensatory physiologic response. One worrisome aspect of chronic growth factor administration is the theoretical risk of stimulating a leukemic clone, particularly in patients prone to developing MDS or AML, or speeding the process of stem cell exhaustion. However, chronic administration of G-CSF may have transient beneficial effects on multiple hematopoietic lineages in some patients.

DYSKERATOSIS CONGENITA

Classical DC is an inherited bone marrow (BM) failure syndrome characterized by the mucocutaneous triad of abnormal skin pigmentation, nail dystrophy, and mucosal leukoplakia. It has been observed in many races, and estimated prevalence of DC is approximately 1 per million persons.

X-linked recessive (mutations in *DKC1*), autosomal dominant (some cases due to heterozygous mutations in the RNA component of telomerase, *hTERC*), and autosomal recessive (some cases due to *NOP10* gene mutations) forms of the disease are recognized. Heterozygous mutations in the reverse transcriptase component of telomerase (*TERT*) can lead to variable phenotypes. A variety of other (dental, gastrointestinal, genitourinary, hair greying/loss, immunologic, neurologic, ophthalmic, pulmonary, and skeletal) abnormalities have also been reported.

Bone marrow failure is the principal cause of early mortality with an additional predisposition to malignancy and fatal pulmonary complications.

Clinical manifestations in DC often appear during childhood, although there is a wide age range. The skin pigmentation and nail changes typically appear first, usually by the age of 10 years. BM failure usually develops before the age of 20 years; 80% to 90% of patients will have developed BM abnormalities by the age of 30 years. In some patients, the BM abnormalities may appear before the mucocutaneous manifestations and can lead to an initial diagnosis of "idiopathic aplastic anemia." The clinical features of these disorders are very heterogeneous, and this makes diagnosis based on clinical criteria alone difficult and unreliable.

Oxymetholone can produce durable hematologic responses in more than 50% of patients with DC and FA, but patients have to be monitored carefully for side effects. The current definitive treatment is allogeneic SCT. In patients with DC and FA, low-intensity transplant protocols are producing prompt engraftment, reduced toxicity, and have the potential to reduce the risk of secondary malignancies.

DIAGNOSTIC TESTING ALGORITHM FOR APLASTIC ANEMIA DUE TO *FANCONI ANEMIA* AND *DYSKERATOSIS CONGENITA*

Because the genes mutated in the X-linked recessive (*DKC1*) and autosomal-dominant (*hTERC*) DC subtypes are now known, it is possible to substantiate the diagnosis in a significant proportion of patients with DC. However, as these tests are complicated, it is necessary to be selective in screening. We suggest it is appropriate to screen for the *DKC1* gene if patients are male and have two out the following: abnormal skin pigmentation, nail dystrophy, leukoplakia, BM failure. The situation regarding the *hTERC* screen is different for two reasons. First, we already know that a subgroup of patients with AA have mutations in *hTERC*. Second, the screen for *hTERC* is relatively easy to perform. Therefore, it is reasonable to undertake analysis of the *hTERC* gene in all patients presenting with aplastic anemia. There is as of yet no easy universal functional test for DC. In patients presenting with AA, it is also important to undertake chromosomal breakage analysis for FA.

DIAMOND-BLACKFAN ANEMIA

DBA is most likely the second most common constitutional marrow failure syndrome after FA Most patients present with anemia in the neonatal period or in infancy. Approximately 30% of affected children present with a variety of associated physical anomalies. Thumb and upper limb malformations and craniofacial abnormalities are common. Other defects include atrial or ventricular septal defects, urogenital anomalies, and prenatal or postnatal growth retardation. There is a moderately increased risk of developing hematologic and solid organ malignancies. Most cases are sporadic, with an equal sex ratio, but 10% to 25% of patients have a positive family history for the disorder. Heterozygous mutations in the ribosomal protein genes *RPS19, RPS24,* and *RPS17* account for some cases.

Hematological Findings

Minimal diagnostic criteria for DBA include normochromic anemia in infancy (<2 years), low reticulocyte counts, absent or decreased bone marrow red cell precursors (<5% of nucleated cells), and a normal chromosome breakage test (to rule out FA). Additional features include the presence of malformations, macrocytosis, elevated fetal hemoglobin, and elevated erythrocyte adenosine deaminase (eADA) level. Some patients are identified after the age of 2 years after a more severely affected family member is first diagnosed.

Anemia is usually severe at the time of diagnosis (usually macrocytic). The bone marrow aspirate is usually normocellular, but erythroblasts are markedly decreased or absent. The other cell lines are normal, but mild to moderate neutropenia, thrombocytopenia, or both may occur later in the course. Progression of the single-lineage erythroid deficiency of DBA into pancytopenia and aplastic anemia is rare but may occur.

Differential diagnosis includes transient erythroblastopenia of childhood (TEC). Both TEC and DBA show similar marrow morphology, but TEC is self-limited, with a recovery within 5 to 10 weeks.

Treatment Modalities

Initial treatment in DBA is transfusions, but long-term administration of red cells may cause secondary hemochromatosis. Corticosteroids are the mainstay of treatment, and at least 50% of patients respond. There is no known predictor of steroid responsiveness, and later relapses occur. During treatment, some patients may recover sensitivity to corticosteroids or even proceed to a spontaneous remission.

Allogeneic BMT is a treatment option for DBA in steroid-resistant patients. Likewise, HGF therapy with interleukin-3 (IL-3) or EPO has been attempted for DBA. Only IL-3 has shown some effect in a subgroup of patients, and it has been suggested that IL-3 may play a role early in treatment.

SHWACHMAN-DIAMOND SYNDROME

SDS is presumably the third most common constitutional marrow failure syndrome after FA. This autosomal-recessive disorder usually manifests in infancy and is characterized by exocrine pancreatic insufficiency, short stature, and bone marrow dysfunction. Mutations in *SBDS* gene account for most cases. Additional clinical features include metaphyseal dysostosis, epiphyseal dysplasia, immune dysfunction, liver disease, growth failure, renal tubular defects, insulin-dependent diabetes mellitus, and psychomotor retardation.

Hematologic manifestations include neutropenia, raised fetal hemoglobin (HbF) levels, anemia, thrombocytopenia, and impaired neutrophil chemotaxis. There is a predilection for malignant myeloid transformation and MDS.

Clinical Diagnostic Criteria

Exocrine pancreatic dysfunction is defined by at least one of the following:

1. Serum cationic trypsinogen or amylase below normal range
2. Abnormal 72-hour fecal fat analysis plus evidence of pancreatic lipomatosis by ultrasonogram or CT scan
3. Abnormal quantitative pancreatic stimulation test

Hematologic abnormalities include at least one of the following:

1. Chronic (on two occasions at least 6 weeks apart) single lineage or multilineage cytopenia with bone marrow findings consistent with a defect in production
   a. Neutrophil counts $<1.5 \times 10^9/l$
   b. Hemoglobin concentration <2 standard deviations below mean, adjusted for age
   c. Thrombocytopenia $<150 \times 10^9/l$
2. Myelodysplastic syndrome

Supportive data include short stature, skeletal abnormalities, and liver dysfunction. Cystic fibrosis, Pearson syndrome, cartilage hair hypoplasia, and celiac disease need to be excluded.

Treatment Modalities

Treatment of hematologic manifestations (neutropenia, bone marrow failure) may involve HGF therapy with G-CSF. For neutropenia unresponsive to G-CSF, SAA, MDS, or leukemia, hematopoietic SCT may be considered.

KOSTMANN SYNDROME OR SEVERE CONGENITAL NEUTROPENIA

KS is now considered a subgroup of SCN with autosomal recessive inheritance that is associated with HAX-1 gene mutations. The majority of SCN cases have autosomal dominant or sporadic inheritance patterns with mutations in the neutrophil elastase (ELA2) gene or in the protooncogene GFI1, which targets and represses ELA2. SCN is characterized by severe neutropenia and an early-stage maturation arrest of myelopoiesis, leading to bacterial infections from early infancy

More than 90% of these patients respond to G-CSF (filgrastim, lenograstim) with absolute neutrophil count (ANC) that can be maintained around $1.0 \times 10^9/L$. Adverse events include mild splenomegaly, moderate thrombocytopenia, osteoporosis, and malignant transformation into myelodysplastic syndrome/leukemia. Development of additional genetic aberrations (G-CSF-receptor or *RAS* gene mutations, monosomy 7) during the course of the disease indicates an underlying genetic instability. Hematopoietic SCT is still the only available treatment for patients refractory to G-CSF.

CONGENITAL AMEGAKARYOCYTIC THROMBOCYTOPENIA

CAMT is characterized by severe thrombocytopenia because of a lack of megakaryocytes in the bone marrow from birth. The diagnosis is based mainly on the exclusion of other forms of congenital thrombocytopenia with ineffective megakaryopoiesis such as FA. The molecular basis for this autosomal recessive disorder may be homozygous or compound heterozygous mutations in the *c-mpl* gene coding for the thrombopoietin receptor. At time of diagnosis, the bone marrow of patients with CAMT is generally normocellular with a normal representation of all hematopoietic lines except for megakaryocytes. During the course of CAMT, the disease usually evolves into aplastic anemia. SCT has been shown to be the only curative therapy.

REFERENCES

1. Young NS, Calado RT, Scheinberg P. Current concepts in the pathophysiology and treatment of aplastic anemia. Blood 2006;108:2511–2521.
2. Kaufman DW, Kelly JP, Levy M, et al. The Drug Etiology of Agranulocytosis and Aplastic Anemia. New York: Oxford; 1991.
3. Fogarty PF, Yamaguchi H, Wiestner A, et al. Late presentation of dyskeratosis congenita as apparently acquired aplastic anaemia due to mutations in telomerase RNA. Lancet 2003;362: 1628–1630.

4. Bacigalupo A, Brand R, Oneto R, et al. Treatment of acquired severe aplastic anemia: bone marrow transplantation compared with immunosuppressive therapy—The European Group for Blood and Marrow Transplantation experience. Semin Hematol 2000;37:69–80.
5. Deeg HJ, Leisenring W, Storb R, et al. Long-term outcome after marrow transplantation for severe aplastic anemia. Blood 1998;91:3637–3645.
6. Schrezenmeier H, Passweg JR, Marsh JCW, et al. Worse outcome and more chronic GVHD with peripheral blood progenitor cells than bone marrow in HLA-matched sibling donor transplants for young patients with severe acquired aplastic anemia. Blood 2007;110:1397–1400.
7. Srinivasan R, Takahashi Y, McCoy JP, et al. Overcoming graft rejection in heavily transfused and allo-immunised patients with bone marrow failure syndromes using fludarabine-based haematopoietic cell transplantation. Br J Haematol 2006;133:305–314.
8. Margolis DA, Casper JT. Alternative-donor hematopoietic stem-cell transplantation for severe aplastic anemia. Semin Hematol 2000;37:43–55.
9. Passweg JR, Perez WS, Eapen M, et al. Bone marrow transplants from mismatched, related, and unrelated donors for severe aplastic anemia. Bone Marrow Transplant 2006;37:641–649.
10. Kennedy-Nasser AA, Leung KS, Mahajan A, et al. Comparable outcomes of matched-related and alternative donor stem cell transplantation for pediatric severe aplastic anemia. Biol Blood Marrow Transplant 2006;12:1277–1284.
11. Maury S, Balere-Appert ML, Chir Z, et al. Unrelated stem cell transplantation for severe acquired aplastic anemia: improved outcome in the era of high-resolution HLA matching between donor and recipient. Haematologica 2007;92:589–596.
12. Di Bona E, Rodeghiero F, Bruno B, et al. Rabbit antithymocytic globulin (r-ATG) plus cyclosporin and granulocyte colony stimulating factor is an effective treatment for aplastic anemia patients unresponsive to a first course of intensive immunosuppressive therapy. Gruppo Italiano Trapianto di Midollo Osseo (GITMO). Br J Haem 1999;107:330–334.
13. Scheinberg P, Nunez O, Young NS. Retreatment with rabbit antithymocyte globulin and cyclosporine for patients with relapsed or refractory severe aplastic anemia. Brit J Haem 2006;133:622–627.
14. Rosenfeld S, Follman D, Nunez, O, et al. Antithymocyte globulin and cyclosporine for severe aplastic anemia. Association between hematologic response and long-term outcome. JAMA 2003;289:1130–1135.
15. Tisdale JF, Dunn DE, Geller NL, et al. High-dose cyclophosphamide in severe aplastic anemia: a randomized trial. Lancet 2000;356:1554–1559.
16. Rosse WF, Nishimura J. Clinical manifestations of parosxysmal nocturnal hemoglobinuria: present state and future problems. Int J Hematol 2003;77:113–120.
17. Hall C, Richards S, Hillmen P. Primary prophylaxis with warfarin prevents thrombosis in paroxysmal nocturnal hemoglobinuria (PNH). Blood 2003;102:3587–3591.
18. Hillmen P, Hall C, Marsh JC, et al. Effect of eculizumab on hemolysis and transfusion requirements in patients with paroxysmal nocturnal hemoglobinuria. N Eng J Med 2004;350:552–559.
19. Hillmen P, Muus P, Duhrsen U, et al. Effect of the complement inhibitor eculizumab on thromboembolism in patients with paroxysmal nocturnal hemoglobinuria. Blood 2007;110:4123–4128.
20. Kang EM, Tisdale J. Pure red cell aplasia. In: NS Young, ed. Bone Marrow Failure Syndromes. Philadelphia: W.B. Saunders; 2000:135–155.
21. Sloand EM, Scheinberg P, Maciejewski JP, et al. Brief communication: successful treatment of pure red-cell aplasia with an anti-interleukin-2 receptor antibody (Daclizumab). Ann Intern Med 2006;144:181–185.
22. Andersohn F, Konzen C, Garbe E. Systematic review: agranulocytosis induced by nonchemotherapy drugs. Ann Intern Med 2007;146:657–665.
23. Young NS, Young NS. Agranulocytosis. In: NS Young, ed. Bone Marrow Failure Syndromes. Philadelphia: W.B. Saunders; 2000:156–182.

7

Myelodysplastic Syndromes

Aarthi Shenoy, Minoo Battiwalla, and Neal S. Young

The myelodysplastic syndromes (MDS) are a heterogeneous group of clonal stem cell disorders characterized by ineffective hematopoiesis and a variable tendency to progress to acute myelogenous leukemia (AML). Increasingly, MDS is diagnosed incidentally when modestly abnormal blood counts trigger a bone marrow examination.

MDS is a disease of older adults; the median age is in the mid-60s. Estimates of its incidence range from 10 to 100 per million people, and in the elderly the rate may be 2- to 8-fold higher, making MDS a relatively common hematologic disease. Death because of MDS occurs from the complications of cytopenias and/or progression to AML, but many patients will succumb first to comorbidities of the elderly.

Myelodysplasia of the marrow can be seen in aplastic anemia, especially as a late event after immunosuppressive treatment; in the course of Fanconi anemia; with paroxysmal nocturnal hemoglobinuria (PNH) and T-large granular lymphocyte lymphoproliferative states (T-LGL) disorders; and preceding AML (Fig. 7.1).

ETIOLOGY AND PATHOGENESIS

MDS is related to the accumulation of somatic mutations in a hematopoietic stem cell. In secondary MDS, prior chemotherapy (alkylating agents and toposisomerase inhibitors) and ionizing radiation are clearly etiologic; the latency period between exposure and the development of secondary MDS is typically 2 to 10 years. Radiation has been implicated in the marrow failure syndromes historically reported in occupationally and accidentally exposed individuals and in atomic bomb victims; solvents and smoking are also associated. For most MDS, age is the dominant risk factor. Indeed, childhood MDS is exceedingly rare (incidence rate = 0.01/100,000); it can be seen de novo or in patients with a history of acquired or constitutional aplastic anemia, especially Fanconi anemia.

The bone marrow is typically hypercellular, implying that ineffective hematopoiesis rather than absence of stem cells results in the cytopenias. In general, early MDS (refractory anemia) is characterized by an increased susceptibility to apoptosis, while late MDS (in transition to leukemia) is associated with reduced apoptosis. Although the principal defect is in the hematopoietic stem cells, immunological factors and the bone marrow microenvironment contribute to the bone marrow failure (Fig. 7.2). There are significant abnormalities in apoptosis, cytokine profiles, angiogenesis, and the T-cell repertoire. Specific mutations, in particular, abnormalities in chromosomes 7 and a complex karyotype, predispose to leukemic transformation. In contrast, 5q-, del (20q), and -Y are recurrent chromosomal abnormalities not associated with a high risk of transformation. Ras mutations and platelet-derived growth factor-β receptor translocations are more common in CMMoL.

In recent years, great advances have been made in the understanding of the molecular mechanisms underlying specific MDS subtypes. These include the identification of haploinsufficiency of the RPS14 gene for the phenotype of del(5q) MDS, the recognition of aberrant signaling through the G-CSF receptor in monosomy 7, the importance of cyclin D1 in trisomy 8 and the high frequency of uniparental disomy by array single nucleotide polymorphism (SNP) analysis in patients with normal metaphase cytogenetics (1–4).

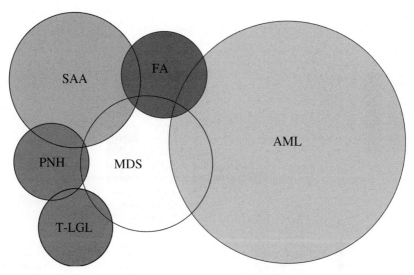

FIG. 7.1. AML, acute myelogenous leukemia; FA, Fanconi anemia; MDS, myelodys-plastic syndrome; SAA, severe aplastic anemia; T-LGL, T-cell large granular lympho-cytic leukemia.

CLINICAL FEATURES

Patients present with symptoms due to cytopenias, usually anemia. "Anemia of the elderly" may be unrecognized MDS. Lymphadenopathy and splenomegaly are absent. The clinical course is variable: patients may be asymptomatic or have mild anemia progressing to transfusion-dependence over many years, while others have an aggressive course with multilineage involvement and rapid evolution to acute leukemia.

DIAGNOSTIC STUDIES

Minimum diagnostic criteria for MDS require unexplained persistent cytopenia(s), and either evidence of clonality (such as with a cytogenetic abnormality) or unambiguous dysplastic marrow morphology (such as excess blasts or dysplasia in the megakaryocytic lineage) (5).

- Peripheral blood smear typically shows macrocytosis; hypogranular neutrophils; sometimes with Pelger-Huet nuclei and other abnormal nuclear patterns; and circulating micromegakyarocytes. Significant numbers of large granular lymphocytes should raise suspicion of a T-LGL/MDS overlap syndrome.
- Bone marrow biopsy is frequently hypercellular but is frankly hypocellular in about 20% of MDS. Abnormal localization of immature precursors (ALIPs) near bony trabeculae is characteristic. Increase in myeloblasts and dysplastic morphology in the white cell and/or the megakaryocytic lineages can be seen on the aspirate smear. Mononuclear, small, or dysplastic megakarytocytes are evidence of MDS. Erythroid dysplasia alone is less specific, but large numbers of ringed sideroblasts identify a specific MDS subtype.
- Chromosome analysis of marrow cells is critical; abnormal cytogenetics strongly suggest MDS and influence prognosis. Karyotyping should be repeated because chromosome patterns can evolve. Fluorescent in situ hybridization (FISH), while not now routine, may provide more subtle information than karyotyping alone. A stress test for Fanconi anemia is recommended for younger patients even if physical examination is normal.

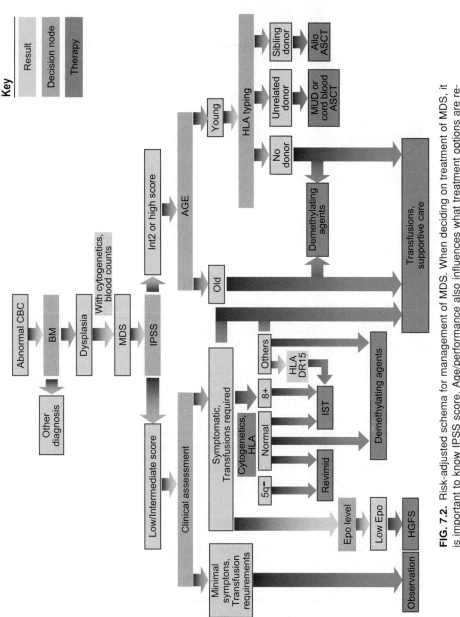

FIG. 7.2. Risk-adjusted schema for management of MDS. When deciding on treatment of MDS, it is important to know IPSS score. Age/performance also influences what treatment options are realistic. Note that azacytidine is approved for use in patients with all FAB types and IPSS scores. Decitabine is approved for patients with IPSS scores that are intermediate-1 or higher.

TABLE 7.1. *French-American-British Subtypes*

Type		BM blast (%)	Frequency (%)	Median Survival
Refractory anemia	RA	<5	30–40	35 mo.
Refractory anemia with ring sideroblasts	RARS	<5	15–25	35 mo.
Chronic myelomonocytic leukemia	CMMoL	<20	15	12 mo.
Refractory anemia with excess blasts	RAEB	5–20	15–25	18 mo.
Refractory anemia with excess blasts in transformation	RAEB-t	20–30	5–15	6 mo.

- Flow cytometry has limited utility; blast enumeration, critical to prognosis, can be assessed by routine morphology. Nevertheless, expert flow cytometry can be highly specific in diagnosing MDS, and, in the future, may offer useful phenotypic information
- HLA typing is needed to evaluate younger patients for allotransplantation and may provide predictive information for responsiveness to immunosuppression.
- Array-based genomic studies, currently investigational, may help in assessing clonality in patients with a normal metaphase cytogenetics.

CLASSIFICATIONS

- Accurate classification and prognosis for this highly heterogeneous disorder is necessary to individualize therapy.
- The first validated classification, the French-American-British (FAB; expanded in 1982) was based on morphology (Table 7.1). This scheme, in use for the past 20 years, recognized that the risk of leukemic progression was proportional to the blast count in the marrow.
- The International Prognostic Scoring System (IPSS; Table 7.2), derived from analyses of outcomes in large series of patients, combined information from cytogenetics, cytopenias, and blast count to generate a prognostic score (6). These values separate out median survivals for patients with low risk (5.7 years), intermediate-1 (3.5 years), intermediate-2 (1.2 years), and high-risk (0.4 years) MDS.
- The World Health Organization (WHO) classification (Table 7.3) attempts to better define risk and separate individual syndromes (7). Some of the deficiencies of the FAB are addressed by including the prognostic relevance of cytopenias and karyotypic information in addition to blast counts (Table 7.3). RAEB-t is discarded, and the threshold for defining AML is lowered to 20%. Multilineage dysplasia is recognized to produce worse outcomes than single lineage dysplasia. Proliferative CMMoL is now appropriately classified as a myeloproliferative disorder.
- 5q- syndrome is one of several specific MDS syndromes. Deletion of 5q, between bands q31 and q33, is separate in the WHO classification. 5q- usually manifests as anemia, with or without mild neutropenia and platelet counts either preserved or elevated. The prognosis is relatively good. Several cytokines, growth factors, and their receptors are found at the 5q locus, but their pathophysiologic importance is unknown. Lenalidomide (Celegene Corporation, Summit, NJ), a thalidomide analog, is especially efficacious in 5q- syndrome.

TABLE 7.2. *International Prognostic Scoring System*

	0	0.5	1.0	1.5
Blasts %	<5	5–10		11–20
Karyotype*	Good	Intermediate	Poor	
Cytopenias	0 or 1	2 or 3		

*Good, normal, -Y, del(5q), del(20q); Poor, complex (>3 abnormalities) or chromosome 7 anomalies; Intermediate, other abnormalities.
Scores: Low, 0; INT-1, 0.5–1.0; INT-2, 1.5–2.0; and High, ≥2.5.
Patients with 21% to 30% blasts may be considered as MDS or AML.
AML, acute myelogenous leukemia; MDS, myelodysplastic syndrome.

TABLE 7.3. *World Health Organization Classification*

Category	MDS Cases %	Peripheral Blood	Bone Marrow	Rate of AML Progression %
RA	5–10	Anemia <1% blasts $<1 \times 10\,e^9$ per liter monocytes	Erythroid dysplasia *only* <5% blasts <15% ringed sideroblasts	6
RARS	10–15	Anemia <1% blasts $<1 \times 10\,e^9$ per liter monocytes	Erythroid dysplasia *only* <15% ringed sideroblasts <5% blasts	1–2
RCMD	24	Bicytopenia or Pancytopenia <1% blasts No Auer rods $<1 \times 10\,e^9$ per liter monocytes	Dysplasia in >10% of cells in = 2 cell lines <5% blasts in marrow No Auer rods <15% ringed sideroblasts	11
RCMD – RS	15	Bicytopenia or pancytopenia No or rare blasts No Auer rods $<1 \times 10\,e^9$ per liter monocytes	Dysplasia in >10% of cells in $\geq$ 2 cell lines >15% ringed sideroblasts <5% blasts No Auer rods	11
RAEB –1&2	40	Cytopenias $<1 \times 10\,e^9$ per liter Monocytes	Unilineage or multilineage dysplasia	
		RAEB–1: <5% blasts, no Auer rods	5%–9% blasts, no Auer rods	25
		RAEB–2: 5%–19% blasts, Auer rods $\pm$	10%–19% blasts, Auer rods $\pm$	33
MDS – U		Cytopenias No or rare blasts No Auer rods	Unilineage dysplasia in granulocytes or megakaryocytes <5% blasts No Auer rods	Unknown
5q-syndrome		Anemia <5% blasts Platelets normal or increased	Normal to increased megakaryocytes <5% blasts No Auer rods Isolated del(5q)	Uncommon

AML, acute myelogenous leukemia; BM, bone marrow; MDS, myelodysplastic syndrome; MDS-U, unclassified; RA, refractory anemia; RAEB, refractory anemia with excess blasts; RARS, refractory anemia with ringed sideroblasts; RCMD, refractory cyteopenia with multileage dysplasia.
From Komkroji R, Bennet JM. The myelodysplastic syndromes: classification and prognosis. Curr Hemotol Rep 2003;2:179–185, with permission.

- Hypocellular MDS, while not categorized in any schema, may be easily confused with aplastic anemia, and patients may respond more favorably to immunosuppression with ATG.
- Chronic myelomonocytic leukemia (CMML) is biologically distinct, now classified as a myeloproliferative disease by the WHO although often associated with a dysplastic marrow. Angiogenesis, autocrine vascular endothelial growth factor stimulation, tyrosine kinase overactivity, and ras mutations appear to figure in the pathogenesis of the proliferation. Standard therapy of CMML is hydroxyurea and transfusions; patients with the PDGF-β receptor-associated mutations benefit from imatinib and demethylating agents have potential activity.

- Therapy-related (or secondary) MDS is an important subtype, constituting about 15% of cases in most series. This subtype has the highest rate of progression (75%) to acute leukemia, is difficult to treat, and is rapidly fatal. Almost all patients have recurrent chromosomal abnormalities: deletions in chromosomes 5 and/or 7 occur at a mean interval of 4 to 5 years after exposure to alkylating agents, and 11q23 abnormalities follow in a shorter time period after topoisomerase II inhibitors. A very high frequency of therapy-related MDS is seen in patients who have undergone high-dose chemotherapy (up to 19% at 10 years), more likely because of the cumulative prior therapy, especially alkylating agents, rather than the autotransplant. Overall, median survival is only 9 months.
- MDS can be associated with large granular lymphocytosis (LGL). Significant numbers of circulating T-LGLs should prompt suspicion of this overlap syndrome; the diagnosis is confirmed by a clonal pattern of T-cell receptor gene rearrangement. Cases of T-LGL/MDS may have hematological responses to therapy directed against the T-LGL component, such as cyclosporine or monoclonal antibody to CD52 (Campath); HLA-DR4 is a strong predictor of responsiveness.
- Pediatric MDS is unusual and should lead to evaluation for genetic syndromes, such as Fanconi anemia, Bloom syndrome, neurofibromatosis type 1, Schwachman syndrome, Pearson disease, Kostmann syndrome, familial monosomy 7, and constitutional chromosomal abnormalities.

THERAPY

Therapeutic strategies combine supportive care, suppression of the MDS clone and its leukemic progeny, efforts to improve bone marrow function, and curative attempts with allogeneic stem cell transplantation. Optimum management often requires the application of some or all of these approaches, preferably in the context of a research protocol (Table 7.4). Evidence-based decisions may be constrained by the clinical heterogeneity of MDS and the paucity of adequate data from clinical trials.

Supportive Care

Cytopenias are the single most important contributor to mortality.

Supportive care to maintain adequate peripheral counts and to prevent or treat infections is critical to the patient with MDS. Even moderate degrees of anemia may not be well tolerated by the elderly,

TABLE 7.4. *Therapeutic Strategies for Myelodysplastic Syndrome*

Therapeutic Strategies for Myelodysplastic Syndrome
Supportive Care
Transfusion
Antimicrobials
Iron Chelation
Treatments aimed at improving bone marrow function
Growth factors (erythropoietin, G-CSF, GM-CSF)
Immunosuppression (ATG, cyclosporine)
Anticytokine approaches (thalidomide and analogs)
Antiapoptosis
Treatments directed at the abnormal clone
Low-intensity chemotherapy (hydroxyurea, melphalan, low-dose ara-C, VP-16)
Induction regimens (anthracycline/ara-C combinations, FLAG, ADE)
DNA methyltransferase inhibitors (5-azacytidine, decitabine)
Farnesyl transferase inhibitors
Remission induction/autologous stem cell transplant
Antiangiogenesis (arsenic trioxide, anti-VEGF, RTK-Is, thalidomide)
Curative attempts (Stem cell transplantation)
Myeloablative transplantation
Reduced intensity conditioning

ADE, daunorubicin, cytarabine, etoposide; ATG, antithymocyte globulin; FLAG, fludarabine, cytarabine and granulocyte colony-stimulating factor; RTK-Is, receptor tyrosine kinase inhibitors; VEGF, vascular endothelial growth factor.

especially in the presence of cardiopulmonary disease, and maintenance of higher hemoglobin levels (>9 g/dL) can improve the quality of life without altering transfusion frequency. Iron chelation should be instituted in patients who are younger, without serious comorbidities, and who are in favorable diagnostic categories.

- Leukodepletion of blood products and single-donor platelet transfusions reduce the risk of eventual alloimmunization to platelets. If a prophylactic regimen is adopted, 10,000/uL is usually an adequate platelet transfusion threshold. Aminocaproic acid is a useful adjunct in patients who are refractory to platelet transfusions.
- Neutrophils may be dysfunctional in MDS. Infections in the setting of neutropenia must be treated promptly and aggressively.
- Growth factors are frequently used in MDS and are used at the lowest doses that maintain a response (8). Combinations of erythropoietin and G-CSF are synergistic, with hematological improvements in 40% of low-grade MDS patients (9). Growth factor combinations can be effective even when individual factors have failed to improve blood counts. Patients with low erythropoietin serum levels and more modest degrees of anemia appear to be most responsive. Growth factor therapy does not appear to hasten leukemic progression, but there is also little evidence for a positive impact on survival.

Stem Cell Transplant

Allotransplant is the only curative therapy. Favorable transplant outcomes are more likely in younger patients, those with a short interval between diagnosis and transplant, and patients with HLA identical siblings (10). Generally, patients with IPSS risk of Int-2 or High would benefit from allogeneic transplant as soon as a donor is identified whereas those with IPSS risk of Low or Int-1 would benefit from waiting till progression (11). In recent reports, survival outcomes after transplant from HLA-matched unrelated donors have been similar to conventional allotransplant from matched siblings; the improvement is in part attributed to use of high resolution HLA typing to screen for HLA disparity at the allele level (10). Data from the Center for International Blood and Marrow Transplant Research (CIBMTR) document that survival rates decrease precipitously in advanced stage MDS; survival is approximately 30% for both HLA-matched related and unrelated transplants, which is comparable or slightly worse than transplant outcomes for a similar age group with acute myelogenous leukemia. The IPSS score also predicts relapse and survival; patients with low-risk disease (low risk/Int-1 by IPSS) have significantly lower relapse rates (13% vs. 43%) and better disease-free survival (55% vs. 28%) than do patients with high-risk MDS (12). Therefore, the decision for transplantation requires balancing the probability of disease progression and complications against the morbidity and mortality incurred with transplant (highest in the first year following the procedure). While allotransplant remains the treatment of choice in younger patients, until recently transplant was not feasible for older adults because of higher treatment-related mortality with advanced age; as most patients with MDS are diagnosed in their 60s, the age limit eliminated the only curative option. With the advent of reduced intensity conditioning regimens (RIC) that use less myelosuppression with more intense immunosuppression, older patients with MDS are now being transplanted. RIC regimens offer less treatment-related mortality but at the expense of more disease relapse. The disease-free survival of younger high-risk patients undergoing myeloablative transplant is similar to that of older patients transplanted with an RIC regimen.

Specific Therapies: DNA Methyltransferase Inhibitors

The DNA methyltransferases function to hypermethylate the CpG promoter regions of many tumor suppressor genes and to decrease their gene expression. Hypermethylation is one of many epigenetic modifications that can influence gene expression. In malignancy (such as in MDS), acquired hypermethylation of tumor suppressor genes downregulates expression, increasing the potential for dysplastic growth. Two agents that inhibit hypermethylation are 5-azacytidine (Vidaza, Celgene Corporation, Summit, NJ) and its active metabolite 5-aza-2'-deoxyazacytidine (Decitabine or Dacogen, Eisai Inc. Woodcliff Lake, NJ). At low doses they induce cellular differentiation by inhibiting DNA methyltransferase, while at higher doses these analogs of cytidine can be incorporated into DNA (decitabine) or both RNA and DNA (azacytidine) to exert a direct cytostatic effect.

Azacytidine is currently approved for use in patients with all FAB subtypes. The landmark trial that demonstrated efficacy of azacytidine, CALGB 9221, was a randomized trial of 5-azacitidine versus best supportive care. The data from this trial were recently re-analyzed using the WHO classification for MDS and the International Working Group response criteria (13). Overall response rate was 47% (14). Although the complete remission and partial remission rates were low (10% and 1%, respectively), there was a significant improvement in overall survival, time to leukemia progression, and quality of life (15,16). In responders, median time to first response was 3 cycles, and 90% responded by the sixth cycle. While worsening cytopenias were seen in many patients, there was no increase in infection or bleeding. A definitive phase III trial (Aza-001) compared Azacytidine (75 mg/m^2/d × 7 days q4 weeks) versus a choice of three conventional care regimens (best supportive care, low dose Ara-C or Ara-C + Daunorubicin) for Int-2 to High IPSS risk patients (17). Patients were treated until disease progression. A significant survival benefit for azacytidine treatment was seen over conventional care regimens (24.5 months vs. 15 months median overall survival).

Decitabine is FDA approved for the treatment of IPSS scored intermediate-1 or higher risk patients. At the FDA-approved dose of 15 mg/m^2 given intravenously inpatient every 8 hours for 3 days every 6 weeks, a phase III randomized trial demonstrated a statistically significant overall response rate (17% vs. 0%) and improvement in quality of life compared to supportive care alone but only a nonstatistically significant trend towards overall survival or time to leukemogenesis (18). Among responders the median time to first response was 3.3 months or after two cycles of therapy. Unfortunately 48% of patients enrolled on this intent to treat analysis received suboptimal therapy, less than or equal to two cycles of therapy. A subsequent EORTC trial using the FDA-approved dosing schedule without maintenance also failed to demonstrate a survival benefit (19). Alternative outpatient dosing schedules for decitabine have demonstrated hematological response rates similar to azacytidine but have not been studied for their impact on survival (20).

Dose and schedule optimization of the demethylating agents are ongoing. Maintenance therapy is important and hematological responses are not a precondition for a survival benefit. Demethylating agents should now be considered a standard of care in Int-2 and high IPSS risk patients who are not transplant candidates or as a bridge to allogeneic BMT (21).

Specific Therapies: Immunomodulatory Agents (Thalidomide, Lenalidomide)

Thalidomide inhibits angiogenesis, interferes with cellular adhesion, alters inflammatory cytokine profiles, and is capable of producing hematological responses in about 20% of transfusion dependent patients. However, cumulative toxicities limit its use. Lenalidomide is an oral analog of thalidomide with far greater potency, superior safety, and established efficacy in MDS. Currently, lenalidomide is approved for use in patients with transfusion-dependent anemia and low or intermediate-1 risk MDS with deletion 5q with or without other cytogenetic abnormalities. One hundred and forty-eight patients with refractory anemia associated with deletion 5q were treated with 10mg of lenalidomide daily or for 21 days every 28 days (22). Rapid responses were noted (median time to response was 4.6 weeks), and complete transfusion independence was achieved in 67% of patients. Favorable results were obtained in patients with isolated deletion 5q as well as further complex karyotypes. Seventy-three percent achieved a cytogenetic response, including 45% complete cytogenetic response. Patients who lack deletion 5q demonstrated a 26% transfusion-independence response rate (23).

Immunosuppression

Horse antithymocyte globulin (hATG) at 40mg/kg/d × 4 days produces hematological responses in about one-third of patients with low-risk MDS (24). Subjects who are less than 50 years of age, with a shorter duration of red cell transfusion dependence and who are HLA-DR15+ are most likely to respond to immunosuppression (25). In a retrospective analysis of 129 MDS patients treated with antithymocyte globulin (ATG) and/or cyclosporine (CsA), younger age was the most significant factor favoring response to therapy (26). Other favorable factors affecting response were HLA-DR15 positivity and combination ATG plus CsA treatment. Cyclosporine (5 mg/kg/d for 3 months, tapered to a low maintenance dose thereafter) may be effective especially in T-LGL/MDS patients who are HLA-DR4 positive.

Specific Therapies: Histone Deacetylase (HDAC) Inhibitors

HDAC inhibitors inhibit deacetylation of histone lysine tails, resulting in relaxation of chromatin and decreased transcription of the involved DNA. The compounds have activity in AML and MDS. HDAC inhibitors currently under investigation include valproic acid, suberoylanilide hydroxamic acid (vorinostat), depsipeptide, phenylbutyrate, MGCD0103, MS-275, and LBH589. HDAC inhibitors as single agent therapy do not have a strong favorable impact on disease, but early results from phase I/II trials suggest a synergistic response with the combination of DNA methyltransferase inhibitors and HDAC inhibitors. Dosing regimens, toxicity, and impact on disease are under ongoing investigation (27).

Chemotherapy

Many guidelines have suggested a role for standard chemotherapy to eliminate the neoplastic clone, and popular agents are cytosine arabinoside and topotecan. However, no prospective studies show long-term survival benefit. Unlike de novo AML, advanced MDS often demonstrates high response rates to induction chemotherapy, only to be followed by the virtual certainty of relapse (up to 90%). Likely futile efforts to eradicate an MDS clone have to be balanced against the risk of further reduction of the marrow reserve. Some chemotherapy (hydroxyurea or etoposide) may be useful for leukemia reduction with a palliative goal once MDS transforms, especially in the aged patient.

SUMMARY

The past decade has seen a significant growth in treatment options for MDS. When evaluating a patient, many factors need to be considered in the decision to treat, including age, comorbidities, karyotype, HLA status, IPSS, and availability of sibling and unrelated donor matches (Fig. 7.2). Targeted therapies have not yet made a clear long-term impact on survival. Clinical and laboratory research in MDS is robust and may continue to yield therapeutic advances.

REFERENCES

1. Ebert BL, Pretz J, Bosco J, et al. Identification of RPS14 as a 5q- syndrome gene by RNA interference screen. Nature 2008;451(7176):335–339.
2. Maciejewski JP, Mufti GJ. Whole genome scanning as a cytogenetic tool in hematologic malignancies. Blood 2008;112(4):965–974.
3. Sloand EM, Pfannes L, Chen G, et al. CD34 cells from patients with trisomy 8 myelodysplastic syndrome (MDS) express early apoptotic markers but avoid programmed cell death by up-regulation of antiapoptotic proteins. Blood 2007;109(6):2399–2405.
4. Sloand EM, Yong AS, Ramkissoon S, et al. Granulocyte colony-stimulating factor preferentially stimulates proliferation of monosomy 7 cells bearing the isoform IV receptor. Proc Natl Acad Sci U S A 2006;103(39):14483–14488.
5. Valent P, Horny HP, Bennett JM, et al. Definitions and standards in the diagnosis and treatment of the myelodysplastic syndromes: Consensus statements and report from a working conference. Leuk Res 2007;31(6):727–736.
6. Greenberg P, Cox C, LeBeau MM, et al. International scoring system for evaluating prognosis in myelodysplastic syndromes. Blood 1997;89:2079–2088.
7. Harris NL, Jaffe ES, Diebold J, et al. The World Health Organization classification of neoplasms of the hematopoietic and lymphoid tissues: report of the Clinical Advisory Committee meeting—Airlie House, Virginia, November, 1997. Hematol J 2000;1:53 T-LGL/MDS 66.
8. Rizzo JD, Somerfield MR, Hagerty KL, et al. Use of epoetin and darbepoetin in patients with cancer: 2007 American Society of Clinical Oncology/American Society of Hematology clinical practice guideline update. J Clin Oncol 2008;26:132–149.
9. Hellstrom-Lindberg E, Ahlgren T, Beguin Y, et al. Treatment of anemia in myelodysplastic syndromes with granulocyte colony-stimulating factor plus erythropoietin: results from a randomized phase II study and long-term follow-up of 71 patients. Blood 1998;92:68–75.

10. Runde V, de Witte T, Arnold R, et al. Bone marrow transplantation from HLA-identical siblings as first-line treatment in patients with myelodysplastic syndromes: early transplantation is associated with improved outcome. Chronic Leukemia Working Party of the European Group for Blood and Marrow Transplantation. Bone Marrow Transplant 1998;21:255–261.

11. Cutler CS, Lee SJ, Greenberg P, et al. A decision analysis of allogeneic bone marrow transplantation for the myelodysplastic syndromes: delayed transplantation for low-risk myelodysplasia is associated with improved outcome. Blood 2004;104(2):579–585.

12. de Witte T, Hermans J, Vossen J, et al. Haematopoietic stem cell transplantation for patients with myelodysplastic syndromes and secondary acute myeloid leukaemias: a report on behalf of the Chronic Leukaemia Working Party of the European Group for Blood and Marrow Transplantation (EBMT). Br J Haematol 2000;110:620–630.

13. Cheson BD, Greenberg PL, Bennett JM, et al. Clinical application and proposal for modification of the International Working Group (IWG) response criteria in myelodysplasia. Blood 2006;108(2):419–425.

14. Silverman LR, McKenzie DR, Peterson BL, et al. Further analysis of trials with azacitidine in patients with myelodysplastic syndrome: studies 8421, 8921, and 9221 by the Cancer and Leukemia Group. B J Clin Oncol 2006;24:3895–3903.

15. Kornblith AB, Herndon JE, Silverman LR, et al. Impact of azacytidine on the quality of life of patients with myelodysplastic syndrome treated in a randomized phase III trial: a Cancer and Leukemia Group B study. J Clin Oncol 2002;20:2441–2452.

16. Silverman LR, Demakos EP, Peterson BL, et al. Randomized controlled trial of azacitidine in patients with the myelodysplastic syndrome: a study of the cancer and leukemia group. B J Clin Oncol 2002;20:2429–2440.

17. Fenaux P, Mufti GJ, Santini V, et al. Azacitidine (AZA) Treatment Prolongs Overall Survival (OS) in Higher-Risk MDS Patients Compared with Conventional Care Regimens (CCR): Results of the AZA-001 Phase III Study. ASH Annual Meeting Abstracts. Blood 2007;110(11):817.

18. Kantarjian H, Issa JP, Rosenfeld CS, et al. Decitabine improves patient outcomes in myelodysplastic syndromes: results of a phase III randomized study. Cancer 2006;106:1794–1803.

19. WijerMans P, Suciu S, Baila L, et al. Low dose decitabine versus bests care in elderly patients with intermediate or high risk MDS not eligible for intensive chemotherapy: final results of the randomized phase III study (06011) of the EORTC Leukemia and German MDS Study Groups. ASH Annual Meeting Abstracts. Blood 2008;112(11):226.

20. Kantarjian H, Oki Y, Garcia-Manero G, et al. Results of a randomized study of 3 schedules of low-dose decitabine in higher-risk myelodysplastic syndrome and chronic myelomonocytic leukemia. Blood 2007;109(1): 52–57.

21. Greenberg PL, Battiwalla M, Bennett JM, et al. Myelodysplastic syndromes. J Nat Compr Cancer Network 2008;6(9):902–926.

22. List A, Dewald G, Bennett J, et al. Lenalidomide in the myelodysplastic syndrome with chromosome 5q deletion. N Engl J Med 2006;355(14):1456–1465.

23. Raza A, Reeves JA, Feldman EJ, et al. Phase 2 study of lenalidomide in transfusion-dependent, low-risk, and intermediate-1 risk myelodysplastic syndromes with karyotypes other than deletion 5q. Blood 2008;111:86–93.

24. Molldrem JJ, Leifer E, Bahceci E, et al. Antithymocyte globulin for treatment of the bone marrow failure associated with myelodysplastic syndromes. Ann Intern Med 2002;137:156–163.

25. Saunthararajah Y, Nakamura R, Nam JM, et al. HLA-DR15 (DR2) is overrepresented in myelodysplastic syndrome and aplastic anemia and predicts a response to immunosuppression in myelodysplastic syndrome. Blood 2002;100(5):1570–1574.

26. Sloand EM, Wu CO, Greenberg P, et al. Factors affecting response and survival in patients with myelodysplasia treated with immunosuppressive therapy. J Clin Oncol 2008;26(15):2505–2511.

27. Griffiths EA, Gore SD. DNA methyltransferase and histone deacetylase inhibitors in the treatment of myelodysplastic syndromes. Semin Hematol 2008;45(1):23–30.

pathogenesis of PV. Splicing defects in the EPO receptor RNA in some patients with PV are of unclear significance (7).

At diagnosis, 10% to 20% of patients with PV have abnormal cytogenetics including trisomy 8, trisomy 9, and deletion 20q. Loss of heterozygosity at chromosome 9p, undetectable on routine cytogenetics, is found in 33% of patients. The frequency of chromosomal abnormalities increases with disease progression (5).

Clinical Features

The elevated red cell mass in PV may result in a myriad of clinical signs and symptoms including:

- Hypertension
- Thrombosis, venous or arterial
- Pruritus
- Erythromelalgia
- Ulceration of fingers and toes
- Joint pain
- Epigastric pain
- Weight loss
- Headache
- Weakness
- Paraesthesias
- Visual disturbances
- Vertigo
- Tinnitus
- Ruddy cyanosis
- Conjunctival plethora

Pruritus aggravated by bathing is a distinctive feature of PV and is present in almost 50% of patients. PV is the most common cause of erythromelalgia and often responds to aspirin therapy. Increased cellular turnover in PV may result in gout or kidney stones. Palpable splenomegaly is found in 70% of patients.

Both bleeding and thrombosis can occur in PV. Less than 10% of patients experience major bleeding episodes, and hemorrhage is the cause of death in only 2% to 10% of PV. A variety of platelet defects are detectable and acquired von Willebrand disease exists in 33% of patients.

Thrombotic events (coronary events, cerebral vascular accidents, deep venous thrombosis [DVT], pulmonary embolism [PE], mesenteric thrombosis, and many others) are a major complication of PV. Multiple series have documented the incidence of major thrombosis to be 34% to 39% at diagnosis. Sixty-six percent of these are arterial events and one third are venous (8–11). Increased risk of thrombosis is associated with age >65, a Hct >45% (12), and a leukocytosis of $\geq 15 \times 10^9$/L (13). Patients at high risk of thrombosis and thrombocytosis (i.e., older individuals, patients with a history of thrombosis or atherosclerotic disease), should be treated with hydroxyurea to ensure platelet counts of less than 600,000 cells/uL (14).

While erythrocytosis distinguishes PV from the other MPN, only 20% of patients with PV present with erythrocytosis alone, while 40% have trilineage hyperplasia at the onset of disease. PV can also present with isolated leukocytosis or thrombocytosis. Typical bone marrow findings in PV include hypercellularity, atypical megakaryocyte hyperplasia and clustering, and decreased stainable iron. Laboratory abnormalities include elevated leukocyte alkaline phosphatase, lactate dehydrogenase (LDH), uric acid, and elevated serum B12 (40% of patients).

The risk of transformation to acute leukemia is 1.5% in patients treated with phlebotomy alone. Patients with PV have a 10% to 25% risk of transforming into the spent phase (postpolycythemic myeloid metaplasia) at 10 and 25 years of follow-up, respectively. The spent phase is characterized by normalization of the red cell mass associated with cytopenias, increasing splenomegaly because of extramedullary hematopoiesis, and collagen fibrosis of the bone marrow.

Diagnostic Criteria

The WHO criteria for the diagnosis of PV are shown in Table 8.2 (15). In the new 2008 WHO guidelines, an elevated red cell mass is not an absolute requirement for diagnosis. Additionally, JAK2V617F or a similar mutation can be used to diagnose PV. While erythrocytosis distinguishes PV from the other myeloproliferative neoplasms, not all patients with PV have elevated hematocrits and not all patients with elevated hematocrits have PV. Although dehydration can cause spurious elevation of the hematocrit, resulting in apparent erythrocytosis, a hematocrit greater than 60% in men or 55% in women is usually caused by an elevated red cell mass. Direct determination of blood volume and red cell mass is usually required. On the other hand, erythrocytosis may be masked by expanded plasma volume secondary to splenomegaly or by occult blood loss. Iron deficiency can also cause a decrease in the hematocrit in patients with PV. Secondary erythrocytosis caused by elevation of serum EPO must also be excluded.

Conditions associated with physiologically appropriate production of EPO caused by hypoxemia as well as diseases associated with inappropriate EPO production that result in erythrocytosis are listed below:

EPO overproduction secondary to hypoxia
Lung disease
High altitude
Smoking (carboxyhemoglobin)
Cyanotic heart disease
Methemoglobinemia
High oxygen affinity hemoglobin
Cobalt

EPO overproduction
Tumors—renal, brain, hepatoma, uterine fibroids, pheochromocytoma
Renal artery stenosis
Neonatal
Inappropriate EPO secretion
Bartter's syndrome
Renal cysts, hydronephrosis

Other causes
EPO receptor hypersensitivity
Congenital erythrocytosis
Androgen therapy
Adrenal tumors
Autotransfusion (blood doping), self injection of EPO
Polycythemia vera
Note that EPO levels in PV may be either low or normal; high EPO levels are not consistent with PV.

Laboratory studies that may be useful in evaluation of erythrocytosis are:
• Arterial blood gas measurement
• Iron studies
• Serum EPO level
• Liver and kidney function studies
• Abdominal ultrasound or computed tomography (CT) scan
• Bone marrow aspirate and biopsy
• Red cell mass

Table 8.3 shows clinical findings and assay results other than JAK2 mutational status that can be useful for distinguishing secondary polycythemia from PV. Specialized studies may be required in equivocal cases. For example, a recently described polymerase chain reaction (PCR)-based assay for overexpression of PRV1 (CD177) mRNA in peripheral granulocytes is positive in most patients with PV but not in secondary erythrocytosis (16). Large prospective trials are in progress to assess the role

TABLE 8.2. *World Health Organization Criteria for Diagnosis of Polycythemia Vera*

	2008 WHO Diagnostic Criteria		
	Polycythemia Vera[a]	Essential Thrombocythemia[a]	Primary Myelofibrosis[a]
Major criteria	1. Hgb >18.5 g dl^{-1} (men) >16.5 g dl^{-1} (women) or Hgb or Hct >99th percentile of reference range for age, sex, or altitude of residence or Hgb >17 g dl^{-1} (men), or >15 g dl^{-1} (women) if associated with a sustained increase of ≥2 g dl^{-1} from baseline that cannot be attributed to correction of iron deficiency or Elevated red cell mass >25% above mean normal predicted value	1. Platelet count ≥450 × 10^{9}l^{-1}	1. Megakaryocyte proliferation and atypia[b] accompanied by either reticulin and/or collagen fibrosis, or In the absence of reticulin fibrosis, the megakaryocyte changes must be accompanied by increased marrow cellularity, granulocytic proliferation, and often decreased erythropoiesis (i.e., prefibrotic PMF).
	2. Presence of *JAK*2V617F or similar mutation	2. Megakaryocyte proliferation with large and mature morphology. No or little granulocyte or erythroid proliferation.	2. Not meeting WHO criteria for CML, PV, MDS, or other myeloid neoplasm
		3. Not meeting WHO criteria for CML, PV, PMF, MDS, or other myeloid neoplasm	3. Demonstration of *JAK*2V617F or other clonal marker or no evidence of reactive marrow fibrosis
		4. Demonstration of *JAK*2V617F or other clonal marker or no evidence of reactive thrombocytosis	
Minor criteria	1. BM trilineage myeloproliferation 2. Subnormal serum Epo level 3. EEC growth		1. Leukoerythroblastosis 2. Increased serum LDH 3. Anemia 4. Palpable splenomegaly

CML, chronic myelogenous leukemia; EEC, endogenous erythroid colony; Epo, erythropoietin; Hct, hematocrit; Hgb, hemoglobin; LDH, lactatedehydrogenase; MDS, myelodysplastic syndrome; WHO, World Health Organization.
[a]Diagnosis of polycythemia vera (PV) requires meeting either both major criteria and one minor criterion or the first major criterion and 2 minor criteria. Diagnosis of essential thrombocythemia requires meeting all four major criteria. Diagnosis of primary myelofibrosis (PMF) requires meeting all three major criteria and two minor criteria.
[b]Small to large megakaryocytes with an aberrant nuclear/cytoplasmic ratio and hyperchromatic and irregularly folded nuclei and dense clustering.

TABLE 8.3. *Features Distinguishing Polycythemia Vera from Secondary Polycythemia and Apparent Polycythemia**

Findings	Polycythemia Vera	Secondary Polycythemia	Apparent Polycythemia
Splenomegaly	+	−	−
Leukocytosis	+	−	−
Thrombocytosis	+	−	−
Red blood cell volume	↑	↑	Normal
Arterial oxygen saturation	Normal	↓	Normal
Serum vitamin B12 level	↑	Normal	Normal
Leukocyte alkaline phosphatase	↑	Normal	Normal
Marrow	Panhyperplasia	Erythroid hyperplasia	Normal
EPO level	↓	↑	Normal
Endogenous CFU-E growth	+	−	−

*The differences listed are not present in all patients. CFU-E, colony forming units-erthryocytes. (From Ernest Beutler, et al. Williams Hematology. New York: McGraw Hill, 2001, with permission).

of PRV1 in clinical diagnosis. Reduced thrombopoietin (TPO) receptor (c-mpl) levels have been described in PV megakaryocytes and platelets and in some patients with ET and MMM. Production of endogenous erythroid colonies in vitro is seen in PV but not in secondary erythrocytosis (17). When it is impossible to make a definitive diagnosis, laboratory evaluation should be repeated in 3 months.

Staging and Prognostic Features

In untreated PV, median survival is only 6 to 18 months; death most frequently results from thrombosis (9). Age greater than 65 and a previous history of thrombosis are the major risk factors for thrombosis (18). Other causes of mortality include transformation to acute leukemia or to the spent phase.

Treatment

Treatment goals are to (i) relieve the clinical symptoms that result from an elevated red cell mass, (ii) decrease thrombotic risk, and (iii) slow or prevent leukemic transformation. The efficacy of therapies must be balanced against their toxicities.

The international Polycythemia Vera Study Group (PSVG) began to organize a series of large randomized trials in 1967. Four hundred and 31 patients were randomly assigned to phlebotomy, chlorambucil, or P32. The thrombosis rate for patients treated with phlebotomy alone was 37.3%, significantly higher than for those treated with chlorambucil or P32. However, there were an excess number of deaths secondary to leukemia in the chlorambucil and P32 arms of the study. The PSVG08 study showed that hydroxyurea significantly lowered the risk of thrombosis compared with phlebotomy alone, but patients who received hydroxyurea exhibited a trend toward increase in the risk of leukemic transformation. The ECLAP trial followed a cohort of 518 patients with PV without a contraindication to aspirin therapy who received low-dose aspirin and were undergoing phlebotomy; major thrombosis was decreased by 60% in this cohort compared with controls without a significant increase in bleeding (13).

Therapy in PV is based on risk of thrombohemorrhagic complication. Risk stratification is outlined below:

Low risk
Age, less than 60 years, and
No history of thrombosis, and
Platelet count less than 1.5 million/ul, and
No cardiovascular risk factors (smoking, obesity)

High risk
Age older than 60 years, or
Previous history of thrombosis, or
Cardiovascular risk factors (smoking, atherosclerosis, hyperlipidemia)
Intermediate risk
Neither high risk nor low risk

Phlebotomy is the treatment of choice for most patients. The hematocrit should be maintained at less than 45% in men, 42% in women, and less than 37% in late pregnancy. Additionally, for patients aged 60 years or older, myelosuppression is recommended to decrease the thrombotic risk. Paradoxically, the initiation of phlebotomy is transiently associated with an increase in thrombotic risk and is greatest in the elderly. Interferon-α has also been used for cytoreduction in younger patients. Busulfan or P32 may be used in the elderly who may be unable to tolerate hydroxyurea. A suggested treatment algorithm is seen in Figure 8.2.

Additional therapies may be required for other complications related to PV. Low-dose aspirin appears effective for alleviation of microvascular sequelae including headache, vertigo, visual disturbances, distal paraesthesias, and erythromelalgia. The safety and benefits of low-dose aspirin in PV have been investigated in a multicenter project (ECLAP) (7,19): aspirin lowered the risk of cardiovascular death, nonfatal myocardial infarction, nonfatal stroke, and total mortality; treatment nonsignificantly increased

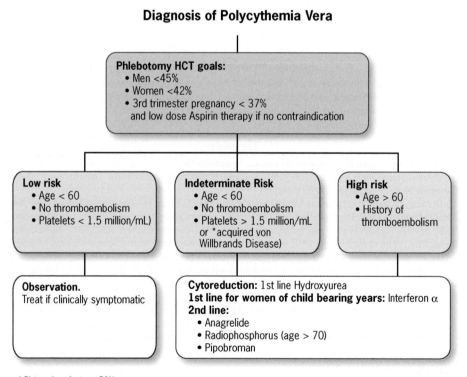

FIG. 8.2. Treatment algorithm for polycythemia vera.

major bleeding. Aspirin should not be used if there is a history of hemorrhage or with extreme thrombocytosis (more than 1 million/ul).

Pruritus is a problem in 40% to 50% of patients with PV. Variably effective measures include reduction of water temperature and use of antihistamines. Other agents of uncertain efficacy for these symptoms include cholestyramine, PUVA, and interferon-α. The selective serotonin reuptake inhibitors paroxetine (20 mg every day) or fluoxetine (10 mg every day) provide some relief in many patients experiencing pruritis (20).

Patients with PV undergoing surgery are at high risk of postoperative complications. Elective procedures should be postponed until the hematocrit has normalized for more than 2 months.

Transformation to a spent phase occurs on average 10 years after the initial diagnosis and is heralded by the development of cytopenias and splenomegaly. Hydroxyurea and interferon-α may alleviate cytopenias because of splenomegaly. Although splenectomy may provide some relief from these symptoms, hepatomegaly secondary to extramedullary hematopoiesis may be a consequence. Low-dose splenic irradiation usually provides only short-term relief.

Stem cell transplantation remains an option for advanced PV and can be curative. Outcomes are more favorable in those transplanted in spent phase than in after evolution to acute leukemia (21).

ESSENTIAL THROMBOCYTOSIS

Essential thrombocytosis was first described by Epstein and Goedel in 1934 and was called hemorrhagic thrombocythemia. Dameshek classified it as one of the MPN in 1951 (4).

Epidemiology

The annual incidence of ET is estimated at 1 to 2.5 per 100,000. Most patients are between age 50 and 60 at presentation, and there is no gender predilection. A second peak occurs around age 30 when women are more often affected. Prevalence is higher in women than men 1.5–2:1. The median survival of ET is more than 10 years (5). The etiology of the disease is unknown.

Pathophysiology

Although ET has been traditionally described as a clonal disorder, X-chromosome inactivation studies suggest polyclonal hematopoiesis in some patients (22). JAK2V617F is found in 30% to 50% of patients with ET; the mutation is associated with elevated hemoglobin and neutrophil counts, lower erythropoietin levels, more venous thromboses, and increased progression to polycythemia (23). Familial cases associated with molecular abnormalities of the thrombopoietin gene have been reported. One percent of patients with ET have a mutation in the gene encoding for the thrombopoietin receptor (MPL 515), and in many cases this is found with the JAK2 mutation. Patients with ET tend to have normal to high thrombopoietin levels and many have low thrombopoietin receptor (c-MPL) levels (24). The rate of clonal cytogenetic abnormalities in ET is approximately 5%.

Clinical Features

As many as half of patients are asymptomatic at presentation. Vasomotor symptoms occur in approximately 40% of patients and include visual disturbances, lightheadedness, headaches, palpitations, atypical chest pain, erythromelalgia, livedo reticularis, and acral paraesthesias. Thrombosis occurs in 15% of cases at presentation and in 10% to 20% during the course of the disease. Associated thrombotic events include DVT and PE, digital ischemia, portal vein thrombosis, and cerebrovascular and coronary ischemia. Major hemorrhage occurs in 5% to 10% of patients during the disease course. Other disease associations include recurrent first trimester abortions and palpable splenomegaly, which is present in less than 50% of patients. The risk of leukemic transformation is low in the first decade after diagnosis but increases with each subsequent decade, but overall, is less than for other MPNs.

with anagrelide and interferon-α used as the second line. Intermediate-risk patients are generally not given cytoreductive therapy unless they develop extreme thrombocytosis associated with bleeding or vasomotor symptoms unresponsive to aspirin.

As in PV, low-dose aspirin is safe in and may even lower thrombotic complications in patients who do not have a significant bleeding risk (27,28). Aspirin is efficacious for treating vasomotor symptoms. Aspirin is contraindicated in patients who have experienced bleeding episodes or if the platelet count exceeds 1.5 million.

Alkylating agents are generally avoided because of the risk of leukemia but are useful in the very elderly whose comorbidities make them intolerant to other therapies.

Hydroxyurea decreases thrombotic complications in patients with ET (14) but can cause bone marrow suppression. Questions remain as to its leukemogenic potential in the absence of controlled randomized clinical trials. Hydroxyurea is contraindicated in women of childbearing age.

Anagrelide interferes with platelet maturation but is associated with toxicities including fluid retention, headache, and palpitations and is extremely expensive compared to hydrea. Most abate within 2 to 4 weeks after initiation of therapy, so it is prudent to slowly titrate the dose. Anagrelide should be avoided in patients with cardiovascular comorbidities because of its side effect profile. In a trial where randomized patients received aspirin plus hydroxyurea or anagrelide, there were lower rates of venous thromboembolism in the anagrelide arm, but arterial thrombosis, hemorrhage, and marrow fibrosis were increased (29).

Interferon-α is effective in reducing platelet count but is associated with significant side effects including flulike symptoms and depression.

Plateletpheresis is used in emergent thrombosis where abrupt decrease in platelet count is mandated.

All patients with ET should be instructed to avoid smoking and to avoid nonsteroidal anti-inflammatory drugs.

MYELOFIBROSIS WITH MYELOID METAPLASIA

Myelofibrosis was first described in 1879 by Hueck and was first included as one of the MPN in 1951 (4).

Epidemiology

The annual incidence of MMM is 0.5 to 1.5 per 100,000. The median age at presentation is 65 years. The male to female ratio is 1:1. Median survival is only 3 to 5 years, so MMM has the worst outcome of all the MPNs. The etiology of the disease is unknown, but a familial occurrence has been reported in rare kindreds (5). A high incidence of MMM was observed in individuals exposed to radiation at Hiroshima.

MMM that develops in late stage PV or ET is referred to as postpolycythemic metaplasia (PPMM) or postthrombocythemic myeloid metaplasia (PTMM), respectively. De novo MMM is often referred to as agnogenic myeloid metaplasia (AMM) or idiopathic myelofibrosis.

Pathophysiology

MMM is characterized by marrow fibrosis and extramedullary hematopoiesis. The marrow fibroblasts in MMM are not derived from the abnormal clone. Increased levels of PDGF, transforming growth factor (TGF)β, and other cytokines produced by megakaryoctyes may be responsible for the marrow fibrosis. Cytogenetic abnormalities are present in approximately 50% of patients and include 13q, 20q, 12p, trisomy 8, and trisomy 9. High levels of CD34$^+$ cells may be present in the circulation of patients with MMM and appear to correlate with the extent of myeloproliferation (30).

The JAK2V617F mutation is found in approximately 50% of patients with MMM and is associated with poorer overall survival (31). The MPL 515 mutation, also identified in ET, is present in approximately 5% of these patients.

Clinical Features

Approximately one third of patients are asymptomatic at diagnosis. Presenting complaints include profound fatigue, symptoms of anemia, abdominal discomfort, early satiety, or diarrhea caused by splenomegaly, bleeding, weight loss, and peripheral edema. The constitutional symptoms of fever and night sweats occur in most patients during the course of the disease. Splenomegaly is common in MMM and may be marked. Episodic left upper quadrant pain may occur secondary to splenic infarction. Palpable hepatomegaly is found in the majority of cases. Extramedullary hematopoiesis may occur in almost any organ.

Laboratory abnormalities in patients with MMM may include leukocytosis or leukopenia and thrombocytosis or thrombocytopenia. The classic blood smear shows leukoerythroblastosis but bone marrow morphologic findings vary from mild to marked fibrosis (32). Osteosclerosis and periostitis can cause severe bone pain. Elevations of LDH, serum B12, and alkaline phosphatase are commonly seen. Transformation to acute leukemia occurs in approximately 20% of patients during the first decade after diagnosis.

Diagnostic Testing

There is no standard for the diagnosis of MMM. The bone marrow is often inaspirable, leading to a "dry tap." The classic peripheral smear shows teardrop-shaped red cells, nucleated red cells and granulocyte precursors (leukoerythroblastosis). However, other marrow infiltrative processes can cause a similar picture and must be excluded (Table 8.5). Absence of splenomegaly makes a diagnosis of MMM suspect. Many benign and malignant conditions may mimic MMM, including metastatic cancer, granulomatous disease, connective tissue disease, lymphoma, systemic mast cell disease, hypereosinophilic syndrome, and other myeloid disorders. Both ET and PV can transform to MMM. Cytogenetics and FISH or PCR for BCR/ABL should be performed to exclude fibrotic CML.

Staging and Prognostic Features

MMM often progresses to marrow failure. Features associated with decreased survival include the following:

- Advanced age
- Hypercatabolic symptoms*

TABLE 8.5. *Causes of Marrow Fibrosis*

Nonhematologic	Hematologic
Infections	Myeloproliferative disorders
TB	ET, PV, MMM
Leishmaniasis	Hypereosinophilic syndrome
Histoplasmosis	Systemic mastocytosis
HIV	CML
Connective tissue disease	AML-M7
Renal osteodystrophy	MDS
Metastatic cancer	Multiple myeloma
Vitamin D deficiency	Hairy cell leukemia
Hypothyroidism	Lymphoma
Hyperthyroidism	ALL
Paget disease	Grey platelet syndrome
Gaucher's disease	

ALL, acute lymphocytic leukemia; AML-M7, acute megakaryoblastic leukemia; CML, chronic myelomonocytic anemia; ET, essential thrombocytosis; HIV, human immunodeficiency virus; MDS, myelodyplastic syndrome; MMM, myelofibrosis with myeloid metaplasia; PV, polycythemia vera; TB, tuberculosis.

- Anemia (hemoglobin less than 10 g/dL)**
- Leukopenia (white cell count less than 4,000/mm^2)**
- Leukocytosis (white cell count higher than 30,000/mm^2)
- Abnormal cytogenetics or the presence of circulating granulocyte precursors or blasts*

(*May be an indication for splenectomy or **transplantation.)

Splenic irradiation may provide short-term improvement in patients with symptoms referable to organomegaly who are not surgical candidates.

Median survival in high-risk patients is less than 2 years, while patients with low risk features have median survivals of over 10 years. Up to 30% of patients may progress to AML, and this is thought to be more common after splenectomy.

Treatment

Treatment in MMM is largely palliative. Approximately 30% of patients with anemia will show improvement with a combination of androgen (oxymethalone 50 mg four times per day or fluoxymesterone 10 mg three times per day) and prednisone (30 mg/day) therapy. Responses are usually brief in duration. EPO is most often ineffective. In patients with a more favorable prognosis who require transfusions for symptomatic anemia, timely initiation of chelation therapy is warranted.

Hydroxyurea, busulfan, interferon, or melphalan may be used to control thrombocytosis, leukocytosis, or organomegaly. Lower doses of hydroxyurea are used in MMM than in ET or PV (start at 20 to 30 mg/kg two or three times per week). None of these agents is effective in preventing disease progression or improving survival. Anagrelide and imatinib are not effective, and ongoing studies are assessing the efficacy of thalidomide in MMM.

Allogeneic stem cell transplantation for patients with poor prognosis remains the only treatment with curative potential (33). Debate continues as to the value of splenectomy prior to transplantation. Concerns about graft failure because of marrow fibrosis have proven unwarranted and, in fact, successful transplantation is associated with resolution of marrow fibrosis. In both the European multicenter cooperative studies and Seattle single institution trials, overall survival after myeloablative transplantation was 60% (34,35). Reduced intensity conditioning is under exploration for older patients and for those who are not candidates for myeloablative protocols (21).

CHRONIC MYELOMONOCYTIC LEUKEMIA

Epidemiology

The annual incidence of CMML is estimated at 4 cases per 100,000. There is a male predominance of 1.5–3:1. The median age at presentation is 70 years. Median survival is estimated at 12 to 18 months. The etiology of the disease is unknown.

Pathophysiology

The WHO classification places CMML in the category labeled myelodysplastic/myeloproliferative, which is appropriate because the marrow cells in this disease show dysplastic features, and there are many characteristics of myeloproliferation as well. The spleen, liver, and lymph nodes are the most common sites of extramedullary involvement. Clonal cytogenetic abnormalities are present in 20% to 40% of CMML and include trisomy 8, deletion 7q, and translocations involving 5q31–35; the latter activate the PDGFRβ and are associated with eosinophilia (5,36,37).

Clinical Features

CMML frequently presents with fatigue, fever, weight loss, or night sweats. There is risk of infection because of neutropenia and of bleeding secondary to thrombocytopenia. In approximately 50% of patients, the white count at presentation may be normal or decreased, while in the remainder it is elevated.

In all cases there is persistent peripheral blood monocytosis, the defining feature of the disease. Progression to acute leukemia occurs in 15% to 30% of cases (38).

Diagnostic Testing

WHO diagnostic criteria include the following:

- Persistent peripheral blood monocytosis (greater than 1×10^9 per liter for more than 3 months).
- Absence of the Philadelphia chromosome or BCR/ABL fusion gene.
- Less than 20% blasts in the blood or bone marrow.
- Dysplasia of one or more myeloid lineages.
- Clonal cytogenetic abnormality.

If dysplasia is absent, the diagnosis can be made if there is a clonal abnormality and no other causes of monocytosis.

Staging and Prognostic Features

Based on peripheral blood leukocyte counts, the FAB group proposed dividing CMML into a dysplastic and a proliferative form with a white count over $13,000/mm^2$. Attempts to evaluate the prognostic value of these distinctions have yielded disparate results. Recent analysis of patients with CMML diagnosed based on FAB classification identified the following factors as independently associated with shorter survival: hemoglobin less than 12 g/dL; lymphocyte count greater than $2500/mm^2$; medullary blast count 10% or more, and presence of circulating immature myeloid cells. Median survival was 12 months (39).

Treatment

Treatment approaches are all experimental, and none has proven effective in modifying the natural course of the disease. Evaluation of treatment responses of patients with CMML specifically is difficult, because they have historically been grouped under the myelodysplastic syndromes. Growth factors have been used to attempt to treat cytopenias and low-dose chemotherapy during the preleukemic phase of the disease. Hydroxyurea is effective in controlling cell counts in the proliferative phase. Although many patients respond initially to chemotherapy, complete responses are rare and remissions generally short lived (40). A variety of low-dose chemotherapeutic agents including cytarabine, topotecan, fludarabine, oral idarubicin, and oral etoposide have shown little success in altering long-term survival rates. Imatinib mesylate is effective in the rare patients with CMML who have PDGFRβ translocations (41,42). Stem cell transplantation has proved successful in a small number of cases.

REFERENCES

1. Parganas E, Wang D, Stravopodis D, et al. Jak2 is essential for signaling through a variety of cytokine receptors. Cell 1998;93:385–395.
2. Levine RL, Pardanani A, Tefferi A, et al. Role of JAK2 in the pathogenesis and therapy of myeloproliferative disorders. Nat Rev Cancer 2007;7:673–683.
3. Baxter EJ, Scott LM, Campbell PJ, et al. Acquired mutation of the tyrosine kinase JAK2 in human myeloproliferative disorders. Lancet 2005;365:1054–1061.
4. Tefferi A. The history of myeloproliferative disorders: before and after Dameshek. Leukemia 2007;22:3–13.
5. Jaffe E, Harris LH, Stein H. Tumors of Hematopoietic and Lymphoid Tissues. Lyon, France: IARC Press; 2001.
6. Scott LM, Tong W, Levine RL, et al. JAK2 exon 12 mutations in polycythemia vera and idiopathic erythrocytosis. N Engl J Med 2007;356:459–468.
7. Spivak JL, Barosi G, Tognoni G, et al. Chronic myeloproliferative disorders. Hematology Am Soc Hematol Educ Program 2003;200–224.

8. Tefferi A, Elliot M. Thrombosis in myeloproliferative disorders: prevalence, prognostic factors, and the role of leukocytes and JAK2V617F. Semin Hematol 2007;33:313–320.

9. Gruppo Italiano Studio Policitemia. Polycythemia vera: the natural history of 1213 patients followed for 20 years. Ann Int Med 1995;123:514–515.

10. Marchioli R, Finazzi G, Landolfi R, et al. Vascular and neoplastic risk in a large cohort of patients with polycythemia vera. J Clin Oncol 2005;23:2224–2232.

11. Passamonti F, Brusamolino E, Lazzarino M, et al. Efficacy of pipobroman in the treatment of polycythemia vera: long-term results in 163 patients. Haematologica 2000;85:1011–1018.

12. McMullin MF, Bareford D, Campbell P, et al. Guidelines for the diagnosis, investigation, and management of polycythaemia/erythrocytosis. Br J Haematol 2005;130:174–195.

13. Landolfi R, Di GL, Barbui T, et al. Leukocytosis as a major thrombotic risk factor in patients with polycythemia vera. Blood 2007;109:2446–2452.

14. Cortelazzo S, Finazzi G, Ruggeri M, et al. Hydroxyurea for patients with essential thrombocythemia and a high risk of thrombosis. N Engl J Med 1995;332:1132–1136.

15. Tefferi A, Varian JW. Classification and diagnosis of myeloproliferative neoplasms: the 2008 World Health Organization criteria and point-of-care diagnostic algorithms. Leukemia 2008;22:14–22.

16. Klippel S, Strunck E, Temerinac S, et al. Quantification of PRV-1 mRNA distinguishes polycythemia vera from secondary erythrocytosis. Blood 2003;102:3569–3574.

17. Streiff MB, Smith B, Spivak JL. The diagnosis and management of polycythemia vera in the era since the Polycythemia Vera Study Group: a survey of American Society of Hematology members' practice patterns. Blood 2002;99:1144–1149.

18. Di NM, Barbui T, Di GL, et al. The haematocrit and platelet target in polycythemia vera. Br J Haematol 2007;136:249–259.

19. Landolfi R, Marchioli R, Kutti J, et al. Efficacy and safety of low-dose aspirin in polycythemia vera. N Engl J Med 2004;350:114–124.

20. Diehn F, Tefferi A. Pruritus in polycythaemia vera: prevalence, laboratory correlates, and management. Br J Haematol 2001;115:619–621.

21. Fruchtman SM. Transplant decision-making strategies in the myeloproliferative disorders. Semin Hematol 2003;40:30–33.

22. Harrison CN, Gale RE, Machin SJ, et al. A large proportion of patients with a diagnosis of essential thrombocythemia do not have a clonal disorder and may be at lower risk of thrombotic complications. Blood 1999;93:417–424.

23. Campbell PJ, Scott LM, Buck G, et al. Definition of subtypes of essential thrombocythaemia and relation to polycythaemia vera based on JAK2 V617F mutation status: a prospective study. Lancet 2005;366:1945–1953.

24. Cerutti A, Custodi P, Duranti M, et al. Thrombopoietin levels in patients with primary and reactive thrombocytosis. Br J Haematol 1997;99:281–284.

25. Kralovics R, Buser AS, Teo SS, et al. Comparison of molecular markers in a cohort of patients with chronic myeloproliferative disorders. Blood 2003;102:1869–1871.

26. Tefferi A. Recent progress in the pathogenesis and management of essential thrombocythemia. Leuk Res 2001;25:369–377.

27. Landolfi R, Marchioli R. European Collaboration on Low-dose Aspirin in Polycythemia Vera (ECLAP): a randomized trial. Semin Thromb Hemos 1997; 23:473–478.

28. van Genderen PJ, Mulder PG, Waleboer M, et al. Prevention and treatment of thrombotic complications in essential thrombocythaemia: efficacy and safety of aspirin. Br J Haematol 1997;97:179–184.

29. Harrison CN. Essential thrombocythaemia: challenges and evidence-based management. Br J Haematol 2005;130:153–165.

30. Barosi G. Myelofibrosis with myeloid metaplasia. Hematol Oncol Clin North Am 2003;17:1211–1226.

31. Campbell PJ, Griesshammer M, Dohner K, et al. V617F mutation in JAK2 is associated with poorer survival in idiopathic myelofibrosis. Blood 2006;107:2098–2100.

32. Tefferi A. Myelofibrosis with myeloid metaplasia. N Engl J Med 2000;342:1255–1265.
33. Guardiola P, Anderson JE, Bandini G, et al. Allogeneic stem cell transplantation for agnogenic myeloid metaplasia: a European Group for Blood and Marrow Transplantation, Societe Francaise de Greffe de Moelle, Gruppo Italiano per il Trapianto del Midollo Osseo, and Fred Hutchinson Cancer Research Center Collaborative Study. Blood 1999;93:2831–2838.
34. Deeg HJ, Gooley TA, Flowers MED, et al. Allogeneic hematopoietic stem cell transplantation for myelofibrosis. Blood 2003;102:3912–3918.
35. Guardiola P, Anderson JE, Bandini G et al. Allogeneic Stem Cell Transplantation for Agnogenic Myeloid Metaplasia: A European Group for Blood and Marrow Transplantation, Societe Francaise de Greffe de Moelle, Gruppo Italiano per il Trapianto del Midollo Osseo, and Fred Hutchinson Cancer Research Center Collaborative Study. Blood 1999;93:2831–2838.
36. Gunby RH, Cazzaniga G, Tassi E, et al. Sensitivity to imatinib but low frequency of the TEL/PDGFRbeta fusion protein in chronic myelomonocytic leukemia. Haematologica 2003; 88:408–415.
37. Magnusson MK, Meade KE, Brown KE, et al. Rabaptin-5 is a novel fusion partner to platelet-derived growth factor beta receptor in chronic myelomonocytic leukemia. Blood 2001;98: 2518–2525.
38. Cortes J. CMML: a biologically distinct myeloproliferative disease. Curr Hematol Rep 2003;2: 202–208.
39. Onida F, Kantarjian HM, Smith TL, et al. Prognostic factors and scoring systems in chronic myelomonocytic leukemia: a retrospective analysis of 213 patients. Blood 2002;99:840–849.
40. Bennett J. Chronic myelomonocytic leukemia. Curr Treat Options Oncol 2002;3:221–223.
41. Apperley JF, Gardembas M, Melo JV, et al. Response to imatinib mesylate in patients with chronic myeloproliferative diseases with rearrangements of the platelet-derived growth factor receptor beta. N Engl J Med 2002;347:481–487.
42. Magnusson MK, Meade KE, Nakamura R, et al. Activity of STI571 in chronic myelomonocytic leukemia with a platelet-derived growth factor beta receptor fusion oncogene. Blood 2002;100:1088–1091.

9

Neutrophil Disorders and Neutropenias

Matthew M. Hsieh and Harry L. Malech

Neutrophil or polymorphonuclear cells (PMN) are 5 μm in diameter with a distinctive multilobed nucleus and many small granules. Neutrophil maturation begins with myeloblasts in the bone marrow. These differentiate into promyelocytes characterized by the appearance of primary (azurophil) granules containing myeloperoxidase, followed by myelocytes characterized by the formation of secondary granules containing lactoferrin and gelatinase, and progress through metamyelocytes, band form, and finally mature neutrophils. This process is typically 10 to 14 days but may be accelerated in the setting of infection, in some cases leading to forms retaining excessive numbers of large azurophil granules (toxic granulation). Once mature neutrophils exit bone marrow, they remain in circulation for about 6 to 12 hours. At sites of infection or inflammation, neutrophils adhere to and migrate between postvenule endothelial cells to exit blood vessels into the tissues where they last about 1 to 3 days. In the absence of overt infection, most neutrophils in the circulation progress to apoptosis and are taken up by macrophages in the spleen. Even without infection there is a baseline rate of neutrophil migration into the mouth and gastrointestinal tract where, together with the barrier function of the mucosa, they prevent entry of bacteria into tissues at those sites. This is why in the setting of severe neutropenia, the gastrointestinal tract is often the first site of invasive bacterial infection.

Neutrophils circulate in a metabolically quiescent state. When stimulated by inflammation or infection-related cytokines or chemotactic factors, they exit the circulation by adherence to endothelial cells and migrate to sites of inflammation. Neutrophils are one of the first cells to migrate to sites of inflammation and thus represent the first line of defense against microbes. They internalize microbial particles by phagocytosis via Fc receptors and complement C_3, and granule contents and reactive oxidants are released into phagosomes to kill microbes. Increased numbers of life-threatening bacterial infections occur in association with inherited or acquired disorders characterized by abnormal granule formation, poor neutrophil adherence, failure to produce microbicidal oxidants, or where there is very low production or increased destruction of neutrophils (1) (Table 9.1). The summary of neutrophil disorders and neutropenia is provided in Table 9.2.

NEUTROPHIL DISORDERS

Leukocyte Adhesion Deficiency

The β_2 integrins in neutrophils are particularly important for normal neutrophil egress from blood postcapillary venules, for migration through tissues, and for complement mediated phagocytosis. There are three leukocyte β_2 integrins adhesion molecules that share the CD18 protein antigen as a common subunit: CD11a/CD18 (lymphocyte function associated antigen-1), CD11b/CD18 (macrophage 1 antigen), and CD11c/CD18 (also known as p150/95). Mutations in the gene encoding CD18 are responsible for a disease known as leukocyte adhesion deficiency 1 (LAD-1). LAD-2 and -3 have been described in a handful of individuals and relate to an abnormality of fucose glycosylation (ligand required for selectin binding) and G-protein coupled receptor mediated integrin activation, respectively (2,3). In general, "LAD" used without the numerical identification refers to LAD-1, because this is the defect responsible for the great majority of cases. LAD has an autosomal recessive inheritance pattern and affects only a few individuals per million. LAD is associated with recurrent life-threatening infections and other

TABLE 9.1. Definition of Severity of Neutropenia

Disease	Molecular or Genetic Defect	Pathogenic Organisms and Sites Affected	Clinical Presentation
LAD	CD18	Gram-negative enteric bacteria, S. aureus, candida species, aspergillus species	Leukocytosis; recurrent infections of skin, soft tissue, respiratory, and GI tract; periodontal disease; delayed separation of umbilical cord
MPO deficiency	Reduced MPO from multiple defects	Candida species in those with diabetes	Typically with no or mild clinical disease
CGD	Defective NADPH oxidases	Catalse-positive organisms: S. aureus, B. cepacia, aspergillus species, nocardia species, S. marcescens	Cellulitis, lymphadenitis, pneumonia; abscess formation in lungs, liver, brain, and bone; granuloma in gastrointestinal or genitourinary tract
CHS	LYST mutation → giant granules	S. aureus, oropharyngeal organisms	Albinism, peripheral neuropathy, recurrent bacterial infections, peridontitis, easy bruising
SGD	C/EBPε	S. aureus, S. epidermidis, enteric bacteria	Recurrent skin and lung infections
Drug-induced neutropenia	Peripheral clearance or marrow suppression	Not applicable	Infection severity dependent on degree of neutropenia
Infection-related neutropenia	Immune clearance or marrow suppression	Nonspecific	Nonspecific; anemia and thrombocytopenia may also occur
Severe congenital neutropenia	Unknown, some with ELA2 or HAX1 mutation	S. aureus, P. aeruginosa, cellulitis, stomatitis, meningitis, perirectal abscess	Recurrent infections starting at 3–6 mo of age; responsive to G-CSF injections; increased risk of MDS/AML
Cyclic neutropenia	Unknown, some with ELA2 19p13.3 mutation	Aphthous ulcers, gingivitis, stomatitis, cellulitis	21-day pattern of neutropenia; some may require G-CSF; no risk of MDS/AML
Autoimmune neutropenia	Antineutrophil antibodies	Nonspecific	Co-existing autoimmune disorders
Idiopathic neutropenia	Unknown	Skin and oropharynx	Usually mild infections; rare severe infections; negative antineutrophil antibodies
Benign ethnic neutropenia	Unknown	Asymptomatic	Seen mostly in those of African descent, neutrophil count may range from 1000–1500/uL

Adapted from Lekstrom-Himes JA, Gallin JI. Immunodeficiency diseases caused by defects in phagocytes. N Engl J Med 2000;343:1704 and Klempner MS, Malech HL. Phagocytes: normal and abnormal neutrophil host defenses. In Infectious Diseases. 3rd Ed. Gorbach SL, Bartlett JG, Blacklow NR, eds. Philadelphia: Lippincott, Williams & Wilkins; 2004:24, with permission.
AML, acute myelogenous leukemia; CGD, chronic granulomatous disease; CHS, Chediak-Higashi syndrome; G-CSF, granulocyte-colony stimulating factor; LAD, leukocyte adhesion deficiency; MDS, myelodysplastic syndrome; MPO, myeloperoxidase; SGD, specific granule deficiency.

TABLE 9.2. *Summary of Neutrophil Disorder and Neutropenia*

Degree of Neutropenia and ANC	Neutrophil Reserve	Duration of Neutropenia
Normal: >1500 /mm³ Mild: 1000–1500 /mm³ Moderate: 500–1000 /mm³. Some increased risk for infections Severe: <500 /mm3. Significant risk for infections	Normal if: –no prior cytotoxic therapy –appropriate ANC increases in response to infection or stress –normal bone marrow biopsy	Periodic or episodic (e.g., following chemotherapy) Chronic

ANC, absolute neutrophil count.

characteristic clinical manifestations. Diagnosis is usually made by flow cytometry measurement of the amount of CD11b or CD18 on the surface of neutrophils using specific antibodies. The severity of disease manifestations, including risk of early death from infection, appears to be correlated with the amount of β_2 integrins present. Moderate phenotype has 1% to 10% of normal levels of β_2 integrins, while the severe phenotype is associated with presence of less than 1% detectable β_2 integrins. On the cellular level, there is poor neutrophil adhesion to endothelial and other immune cells, and neutrophils do not egress from vasculature and migrate to sites of inflammation. Baseline peripheral neutrophil count even in the absence of infection is characteristically about 2 to 3 times normal, and when infections are present, neutrophil counts can exceed 60 k/uL. Sometimes this is mistaken for a leukemic condition. Despite the very high circulating levels of neutrophils, there may be only mild erythema or pain at sites of infection and the patients fail to form pus, a condition that has been called "tissue neutropenia." One of the hallmarks of severe LAD is delayed separation of umbilical cord indicating a role for neutrophils in providing the proteases and hyaluronidases required for that event. A prominent manifestation of severe LAD is recurrent infections with large nonhealing ulcers of the skin, particularly on the lower abdomen, perineum, and legs. Patients also have recurrent infections of the oral cavity (gingivitis and peridontitis with early loss of primary and secondary teeth), respiratory tract (sinusitis, otitis media, and pneumonia), gastrointestinal tract, and genital mucosa. Infection of the wall of the small bowel or colon complicated by perforation is a particular risk that often leads to a fatal outcome. Infections are commonly caused by *Staphylococcus aureus,* enteric organisms, candida, and aspergillus species. In patients with milder forms of LAD who are not transplanted and survive past the first decade, the chronic large nonhealing ulcers of the lower extremities and groin become a particularly characteristic chronic problem and are very difficult to control or treat. Treatments include bacterial prophylaxis with trimethoprim/sulfamethoxazole (TMP/SMX), supportive antibiotics during acute infections, and surgical débridement of skin when necessary, and skin grafting. There is a high mortality rate (~75%) of severe LAD in the first year of life. Successful bone marrow transplant is curative and should be considered for all patients with severe LAD.

Myeloperoxidase Deficiency

Myeloperoxidase (MPO) is the most abundant protein in neutrophil granules. It resides in the primary (azurophilic) granules and has antimicrobial functions (catalyzes the production of hypochlorous acid from chloride and the hydrogen peroxide product of the phagocyte NADPH oxidase). MPO deficiency is the most common neutrophil abnormality, at an incidence of about one per 2000 for partial deficiency and one per 4000 for complete deficiency (4). Most individuals with MPO deficiency do not manifest any clinical problems, although ex vivo assays of bacterial and fungal killing demonstrate a defect associated with MPO deficiency. MPO deficiency is inherited through an autosomal recessive pattern, although it can also be manifested as an acquired abnormality associated with leukemia or myelodysplasia. Specific mutations in the MPO gene have been identified that may affect transcription, translation, and/or insertion of the heme group. Neutrophils with MPO deficiency mature, migrate, and phagocytose normally, but as noted there are defects in microbial killing. Some individuals do appear to have mildly increased frequency in bacterial infections, and in the setting of cofactors like diabetes may have particular difficulty in clearance of infection by candida species (*albicans, tropicalis, stelatoidea,* and *krusei*). Diagnosis of MPO deficiency may be made by measuring peroxidase activity using flow cytometry or by using certain types of automated blood count devices that use peroxidase activity to perform differential counts of blood leukocytes. Because most of these patients have clinically mild disease, antimicrobial and supportive therapy is sufficient. Prophylactic antibiotics should be limited to those with recurrent infections or with another disorder predisposing to infections, such as diabetes.

Chronic Granulomatous Disease

Chronic granulomatous diseases (CGD) are a group of closely related inherited disorders characterized by defective phagocyte NADPH oxidase manifested by a failure of stimulated neutrophils, monocytes, eosinophils, and macrophages to produce superoxide and hydrogen peroxide (3). CGD affects approximately 5 individuals per million appearing to equally affect all nationalities and ethnic groups. CGDs are caused by mutations in any of four subunit components of the phagocyte NADPH oxidase. The clinically most severe is the X-linked, gp91phox subunit deficient form of CGD usually associated with total absence of any oxidant production and affecting almost 70% of patients with CGD. The other three types of CGD are inherited in an autosomal-recessive pattern and consist mostly of p47phox deficient CGD patients (25% of CGD patients) with the remainder comprising the much less common p67phox or p22phox deficient forms of CGD. Clinical manifestations of CGDs involve both recurrent infections and formation of inflammatory granulomas where the severity and individual manifestations can vary widely. The average age of diagnosis of X-linked CGD is 3 years of age, but the average age of diagnosis of females with the p47phox form of CGD is 9 years of age. Thus, some patients with no family history may reach young adulthood before the disease is recognized. Unlike patients with severe neutropenia or LAD who get infected primarily with commensal organisms (such as enteric bacterial normally found in the gastrointestinal tract), CGD patients are generally not susceptible to commensal organisms such as *E. coli*, for example. They are particularly susceptible to a defined group of environmental organisms that generally have the characteristic of being catalase positive. The usual bacterial pathogens are *Staphylococcus aureus*, nocardia, *Burkholderia cepacia* (and other Burkholderia species), and *Serratia marcescens*. Fungal pneumonia and other fungal infections are primarily aspergillus species, with *Aspergillus nidulans* being a problem particular to CGD patients. However, infections with paecilomyces and other fungi including dematiaceous molds are an increasing problem and must be considered because they may be resistant to voriconazole but sensitive to posaconazole. Interestingly, CGD patients do not seem to be particularly susceptible to *Candida albicans* infections, although other candida species such as glabrata are a problem. While infections are usually recurrent and prolonged, the infections are episodic, meaning that CGD patients who are on appropriate effective prophylaxis may go many months or even years between severe infection. In infancy, *Serratia marcescens* osteomyelitis or soft-tissue infection is a very common first-presenting infection leading to diagnosis. In older children and adults with CGD, the most common life-threatening infections are bacterial or fungal pneumonias, although local soft-tissue infections and lymph node infections are more common. All other tissues can be infected including sites as diverse as osteomyelitis or brain abscess. After pneumonia, the most common severe infections are liver abscesses. It is noteworthy that in CGD patients taking trimethoprim-sulfamethoxazole daily prophylaxis, severe staphylococcal deep tissue infections are relatively uncommon, yet almost 90% of liver abscesses appear to be caused by *S. aureus*. Methicillin-resistant *S. aureus* liver abscess is an increasing problem. Also of note is that liver abscess is generally not an easily drained pustular lesion but most often consists of a solid granulomatous mass with micro-abscesses that requires surgical extirpation together with prolonged antibiotic therapy for most effective cure. In some individuals with CGD, granuloma formation may be the predominant problem rather than the infection, and in some cases the granulomatous inflammation can cause gastroesophageal junction or gastric outlet obstruction, bladder outlet obstruction, or chronic abdominal pain with diarrhea. In some cases the gastrointestinal granulomatous process may be indistinguishable from Crohn's disease and appears to respond to similar treatments as those used for Crohn's disease. CGD granulomas are distinguished from granulomas of autoimmune diseases in that the CGD granulomas in some cases are

ANC less than 0.1 per liter or 100/uL) but usually requires only that the sensitizing drug be discontinued. Neutrophil counts usually begin to recover within 5 to 10 days after the offending drug is stopped. Re-administration of the sensitizing drug may decrease neutrophil counts abruptly. It is important to note that while some drugs (see an abbreviated list in the box below) have more often been cited as a cause of drug-related neutropenia, severe immune-mediated, drug-induced neutropenia can be associated with any drug including such unlikely agents as aspirin or acetaminophen.

Infection-Related Neutropenia

Neutropenia following infections is common and can result from one or more of the following: destruction, margination, sequestration, or marrow suppression. Neutropenia from viral infections can be seen as early as a few days and can persist for the duration of viremia. The degree and duration of viral-induced neutropenia is usually mild and short, but neutropenia from Epstein-Barr virus, hepatitis, and human immunodeficiency virus (HIV) can be severe and protracted. Gram-negative bacterial infections can cause neutropenia in those with impaired marrow neutrophil reserve, such as neonates, the elderly, and the chronically immunosuppressed. Protozoal (Leishmania) and rickettsial (RMSF and Ehrlichia) infections can also cause neutropenia, often with accompanying anemia and/or thrombocytopenia.

Immune-Related Neutropenia

This form of neutropenia is typically associated with specific antibodies directed to neutrophil antigens (these are not to be confused with antinuclear antibodies). These antibodies may occur with or without autoimmune disorders. Many syndromes appear clinically similar and will be briefly discussed below.

In *alloimmune (or isoimmune) neonatal neutropenia* (9), maternal IgG antibodies are directed toward paternal antigens on fetal neutrophils causing moderate neutropenia that is self-limiting, lasting only a few weeks to a few months. These neonates have increased risk of infections and can develop pulmonary, skin, or urinary tract infections from gram-positive or -negative organisms. The treatment is supportive with antibiotics, intravenous immunoglobulin (IVIg), and sometimes granulocyte-colony stimulating factor (G-CSF).

Autoimmune neutropenia of infancy/childhood (9) is typically seen in those less than 2 years of age. The degree of neutropenia is variable, and infections in the oropharynx, ear, sinus, and upper respiratory tract can occur. The neutropenia may resolve spontaneously over many months or years and typically does not require treatment. Antibiotics and G-CSF are given during acute infections, and TMP/SMX is often given for prophylaxis.

Autoimmune neutropenia (9) in adults is best described in those with systemic lupus erythematosus, rheumatoid arthritis, or collagen vascular disease. Felty syndrome is manifested by the triad of neutropenia, rheumatoid arthritis, and splenomegaly. The degree of these neutropenias is variable, and the treatment of the underlying autoimmune disorder will generally improve neutropenia. While autoimmune neutropenia can occur *without* concurrent autoimmune disorders, the clinical syndromes are less well described.

Large granular lymphocytosis (10) is caused by abnormally expanded T or NK cells infiltrating the bone marrow, spleen, and liver, resulting in variable degree of pancytopenia and splenomegaly. This may be an oligoclonal or monoclonal disease and in its more aggressive form is considered a form of leukemia. It is typically described in individuals older than 55 years. Laboratory evaluation will reveal multiple abnormalities: 60% of affected individuals will have lymphocytosis $>5 \times 10^9/\text{mm}^3$, 80% with ANC $<1.5 \times 10^9/\text{mm}^3$, 50% with hemoglobin <11 g/dL, 20% with platelet $<150/\text{mm}^3$; 40% will have LGL count of $1-4 \times 10^9/\text{mm}^3$, and 40% with LGL count of $4-10 \times 10^9/\text{mm}^3$. LGL can also occur with other autoimmune disorders, myeloid and B-cell malignancies, or solid tumors. Bone marrow examinations are also variable, but the majority will have hypercellular marrow. No treatment is necessary until there are recurrent infections or symptomatic anemia. Corticosteroids and cyclosporine have been used with generally good response rates. However, aggressive monoclonal LGL disease should be considered a form of leukemia requiring specific chemotherapies appropriate to control the disease.

Congenital Neutropenias

Severe Congenital Neutropenia (Kostmann Syndrome and Autosomal Dominant Forms)

Dr. Kostmann in 1956 described severe neutropenia associated with recurrent bacterial infections in several families in northern Sweden (11). This syndrome was later observed in other geographic locations. Kostmann syndrome is an autosomal recessive form of severe congenital neutropenia that is a rare clinical entity with an incidence rate of about 1 to 2 per million (12). Very recent studies have shown that Kostmann syndrome is caused by mutations in the HAX1 gene (13). Neutrophil elastase (ELA 2) mutations appear to be responsible for almost half of the individuals with the autosomal dominant or sporadic forms of severe congenital neutropenia. Mutations in ELA 2 have been hypothesized to cause defective signal transduction and cause programmed cell death (apoptosis) at the myelocyte level (14). These effects may be a result of cellular mechanisms that detect protein misfolding. There are additional abnormalities that can be acquired that may lead to myelodysplasia and/or acute myeloid leukemia: G-CSF receptor mutation, RAS oncogene mutation, or chromosome 7 monosomy. An autosomal-dominant form of neutropenia has been reported to result from heterozygous mutations in the GFI1 gene that may affect ELA 2 (15).

Clinically, these individuals are infected at as early as 2 to 3 months of age by gram-positive or -negative bacteria in one or more of the following sites: skin, ears, oral, or gastrointestinal mucosa, upper or lower respiratory tract, urinary tract, or blood. Blood counts usually reveal neutrophil count less than 500 per uL ($<0.5 \times 10^9$ per liter) with compensatory monocytosis and eosinophilia. Bone marrow biopsies show maturation arrest at the promyelocyte-myelocyte level and absent band forms or mature neutrophils. Treatment includes supportive therapy and antibiotics for acute infections. G-CSF between 3 and 10 μg/kg has been used successfully to increase neutrophil count and reduce the frequency of infections. A minority of individuals will require an excess of 30 μg/kg/day. G-CSF is not currently thought to be associated with acquisition of G-CSF mutations and is not itself thought to be a cause of the leukemia associated with this disorder. However, individuals requiring longer duration or high cumulative doses of G-CSF may have a more severe form of the disorder and therefore are at higher risk of malignant transformation to leukemia. Side effects of chronic G-CSF administration include bone pain from marrow expansion, osteopenia or osteoporosis, and splenomegaly. Bone marrow transplant is a curative option for those with HLA-matched sibling donors.

Cyclic Neutropenia

The incidence of inherited cyclic neutropenia is not known (14,16). Its cause is also not completely understood, although neutrophil elastase 19p13.3 mutations are associated with this disorder and have been hypothesized to cause neutrophil apoptosis and thus to initiate the cycling. Clinically neutrophil count oscillates predictably between very low or agranulocytic to low normal range; the average cycle length is 21 days with neutropenic duration of 3 to 6 days. The nadir neutrophil count can go to zero or can be as low as 200/uL (0.2×10^9 per liter). Platelet, reticulocytes, lymphocyte, and monocytes counts may also "counter-cycle" between normal to high range, coinciding or not with the neutrophil cycles. Serial bone marrow examinations will appear normal with normal neutrophil count and will show decreased myeloid precursors in neutropenic phase. Individuals with cyclic neutropenia may be asymptomatic during periods of normal neutrophil count and may have fever, lymphadenopathy, mild skin infections, and/or oral mucosal ulcers during periods of neutropenia. Mild skin infections and/or mouth ulcers are treated symptomatically. G-CSF, at 2 to 3 ug/kg per one or two days, appears to improve the neutrophil nadir, shorten the cycles, and thus reduce infections. GM-CSF does not effectively treat inherited cyclic neutropenia.

Other Inherited Disorders Associated with Clinically Significant Neutropenia

There are a number of inherited disorders where clinically significant neutropenia is observed but where neutropenia is not considered the most prominent feature of the inherited syndrome. Three examples are provided. There is a specific mutation responsible for Wiskott-Aldrich syndrome that can be associated with neutropenia (17). Patients with Wart, Hypogammaglobulinemia, Infection, and Myelokathexis (WHIM) syndrome, which is caused by inherited C-terminal truncations in CXCR4, suffer from clinically significant neutropenia that is responsive to treatment with G-CSF (18). A third example is that a subset of patients with CD40 ligand deficiency (X-linked Hyper-IgM syndrome) has clinically significant neutropenia (19).

Other Neutropenias

Idiopathic Neutropenia

Idiopathic neutropenia, or chronic idiopathic neutropenia, affects about two to four individuals per million and can be seen in both children and adults (20). Clinically, it behaves very similar to autoimmune neutropenia, except antineutrophil antibodies were not detected and other studies are nondiagnostic. A majority of these individuals have moderate neutropenia with mild symptoms. There is a small subset of individuals that have severe neutropenia, recurrent fevers, oropharyngeal infections (mucosal ulcers, gingivitis), or severe systemic infections. Treatments are largely tailored for symptomatic relief and antibiotics dictated by sites of infection. G-CSF, 1 to 3 μg/kg per dose weekly or on alternate day, is used in those with severe clinical syndromes. Development of myelodysplastic syndrome or leukemias has not been observed. Generally patients who increase their neutrophil count with infection or other stress setting have a benign clinical course.

Benign Ethnic Neutropenia

Benign ethnic neutropenia (BEN) is a condition seen mostly in individuals of African descent, including African Americans, Yemenite Jews, and certain populations in the Caribbean and Middle East. Prior studies showed that up to 25% of non-U.S. individuals of African descent and about 4% of African Americans have neutrophil counts less than 1.5×10^9 per liter (21). The cause for this observation is unknown, but several investigators earlier have excluded stem cell disorder, excessive margination, and differentiation defect, suggesting that this may be a normal population-based variant. The physiologic mechanisms controlling the normal set point for circulating levels of neutrophils is unknown, but there is some suggestion that the CXCR4 chemokine receptor for the SDF-1 chemokine may play a role in egress of neutrophils from the marrow, and at least theoretically differences in expression or function of this cytokine/cytokine receptor could affect this set point. Perhaps normal variants in this or other receptors may be responsible for these population differences observed in average circulating neutrophil counts. Clinically, individuals with this ethnically based neutropenia variant are asymptomatic, without recurrent oral, skin, or systemic infections. When these individuals acquire typical viral or bacterial infections, these infections are not more severe and do not need longer period of treatment. Laboratory evaluations will show many blood counts that are abnormal over many years, and the bone marrow examinations will be normal. Other than usual symptomatic treatment and antibiotics as needed (as for a normal healthy adult), no additional treatment is required, but it is important to note this variation to avoid unnecessary medical evaluation.

REFERENCES

1. Lekstrom-Himes JA, Gallin JI. Immunodeficiency diseases caused by defects in phagocytes. N Engl J Med 2000;343:1703–1714.
2. Bunting M, Harris ES, McIntyre TM, et al. Leukocyte adhesion deficiency syndromes: adhesion and tethering defects involving beta 2 integrins and selectin ligands. Curr Opin Hematol 2002; 9:30–35.
3. Malech HL, Hickstein DD. Genetics, biology, and clinical management of myeloid cell primary immune deficiencies: chronic granulomatous disease and leukocyte adhesion deficiency. Curr Opin Hematol 2007;14:29–36.
4. Lanza F. Clinical manifestation of myeloperoxidase deficiency. J Mol Med 1998;76:676–681.
5. Ott MG, Schmidt M, Schwarzwaelder K, et al. Correction of X-linked chronic granulomatous disease by gene therapy, augmented by insertional activation of MDS1-EVI1, PRDM16, or SETBP1. Nat Med 2006;12:401–409.

6. Ward DM, Shiflett SL, Kaplan J. Chediak-Higashi syndrome: a clinical and molecular view of a rare lysosomal storage disorder. Curr Mol Med 2002;2:469–477.

7. Gombart AF, Koeffler HP. Neutrophil specific granule deficiency and mutations in the gene encoding transcription factor C/EBP(epsilon). Curr Opin Hematol 2002;9:36–42.

8. Andersohn F, Konzen C, Garbe E. Systematic review: agranulocytosis induced by nonchemotherapy drugs. Ann Intern Med 2007;146:657–665.

9. Palmblad JE, von dem Borne AE. Idiopathic, immune, infectious, and idiosyncratic neutropenias. Semin Hematol 2002;39:113–120.

10. Lamy T, Loughran TP Jr. Clinical features of large granular lymphocyte leukemia. Semin Hematol 2003;40:185–195.

11. Kostmann R. Infantile genetic agranulocytosis. Acta Paediatrica Scandinavia 1956;45:1–78.

12. Welte K, Zeidler C, Dale DC. Severe congenital neutropenia. Semin Hematol 2006;43:189–195.

13. Klein C, Grudzien M, Appaswamy G, et al. HAX1 deficiency causes autosomal recessive severe congenital neutropenia (Kostmann disease). Nat Genet 2007;39:86–92.

14. Horwitz MS, Duan Z, Korkmaz B, et al. Neutrophil elastase in cyclic and severe congenital neutropenia. Blood 2007;109:1817–1824.

15. Person RE, Li FQ, Duan Z, et al. Mutations in proto-oncogene GFI1 cause human neutropenia and target ELA2. Nat Genet 2003;34:308–312.

16. Dale DC, Bolyard AA, Aprikyan A. Cyclic neutropenia. Semin Hematol 2002;39:89–94.

17. Devriendt K, Kim AS, Mathijs G, et al. Constitutively activating mutation in WASP causes X-linked severe congenital neutropenia. Nat Genet 2001;27:313–317.

18. Hernandez PA, Gorlin RJ, Lukens JN, et al. Mutations in the chemokine receptor gene CXCR4 are associated with WHIM syndrome, a combined immunodeficiency disease. Nat Genet 2003;34:70–74.

19. Winkelstein JA, Marino MC, Ochs H, et al. The X-linked hyper-IgM syndrome: clinical and immunologic features of 79 patients. Medicine (Baltimore) 2003;82:373–384.

20. Dale DC, Cottle TE, Fier CJ, et al. Severe chronic neutropenia: treatment and follow-up of patients in the Severe Chronic Neutropenia International Registry. Am J Hematol 2003;72:82–93.

21. Hsieh MM, Everhart JE, Byrd-Holt DD, et al. Prevalence of neutropenia in the U.S. population: age, sex, smoking status, and ethnic differences. Ann Intern Med 2007;146:486–492.

10

Childhood Hematologic Diseases

Kristin Baird and Alan S. Wayne

Despite some overlap with disorders encountered in adults, many congenital and acquired hematologic diseases manifest primarily during childhood. In addition, pediatric hematology is distinguished by developmental differences in normal physiology and blood parameters (1). The purpose of this chapter is to highlight unique features in the evaluation, diagnosis, and treatment of common pediatric hematologic conditions. The reader is referred to other chapters in this edition for additional details of the management of specific disorders.

ANEMIA

Normal red blood cell (RBC) values vary with age and are affected by such factors as race, sex, and altitude (Table 10.1). The RBC count is highest at birth and continues to decrease gradually to a physiologic nadir at 2 to 4 months (earlier for premature infants), at which point erythropoiesis is stimulated. Anemia is defined as an overall reduction in red cell mass or hemoglobin (Hb) concentration, usually set at two standard deviations below the mean normal value for the specific population.

Pediatric anemia is commonly classified according to RBC size (Table 10.2). Microcytic anemias account for the majority of cases of anemia in early childhood (Table 10.3). Current recommendations include screening for anemia between the ages of 9 to 12 months with additional screening between the ages of 1 and 5 years for patients at risk (Table 10.4) (2–4).

The initial diagnostic evaluation of a child with anemia should consist of a detailed history and physical examination and the following minimal laboratory testing: complete blood count (CBC), reticulocyte count, and examination of the peripheral smear (3). Consideration of the physiologic basis for anemia can be helpful in guiding further investigation (Table 10.5).

Microcytic Anemias

Iron deficiency is the most common cause of anemia during childhood and may result from a combination of low stores at birth, high requirements because of growth and blood volume expansion, inadequate nutrition, and poor bioavailability of dietary iron. Iron deficiency because of blood loss is most commonly a result of gastrointestinal tract irritation and occult hemorrhage associated with introduction of cow's milk before the first year of life or menstruation during adolescence. On history, additional risk factors for iron deficiency may include prematurity, limited or prolonged breastfeeding, non-iron–fortified formula, or excessive intake of whole milk (generally more than 1 quart per day). Early iron deficiency may result only in a low ferritin. This is followed by a decrease in serum iron and transferrin saturation and an increase in total iron-binding capacity (TIBC) and free erythrocyte protoporphyrin (FEP). With frank deficiency, there is hypochromia, microcytosis, and anisocytosis on the blood smear. The platelet count also may be increased. A response to a trial of elemental iron (3 mg/kg per day) is often helpful in differentiating iron deficiency from thalassemia trait: an Hb increase of more than 1 g/dL at 1 month and reticulocyte peak at 10 to 14 days is diagnostic. Iron supplementation (3 mg/kg per day for mild anemia, 6 mg/kg per day for moderate to severe anemia) should be provided for 3 to 6 months (3–6). The most common cause for lack of response to oral iron therapy is lack of compliance.

Lead toxicity (7) often coexists with iron deficiency in at-risk populations and may further inhibit gastrointestinal absorption of iron. Lead poisoning should be suspected if there is a history of pica or

TABLE 10.1. *Normal Hematologic Parameters in Children*

Age	Hemoglobin (g/dL) Mean	-2 SD	Hematocrit (%) Mean	-2 SD	MCV (fL) Mean	-2 SD	Neutrophils ($10^3/\mu L$) Mean	Range
Birth	16.5	13.5	51	42	108	98	11	6–26
1 mo	14	10	43	31	104	85	3.8	1–9
3–6 mo	11.5	9.5	35	29	91	74	3.8	1–8.5
0.5–2 yr	12	10.5	36	33	78	70	3.5	1.5–8.5
2–6 yr	12.5	11.5	37	34	81	75	4.3	1.5–8
6–12 yr	13.5	11.5	40	35	86	77	4.4	1.8–8
12–18 yr								
Female	14	12	41	36	90	78	4.4	1.8–8
Male	14.5	13	43	37	88	78	4.4	1.8–8

Modified from Dallman PR Normal hematologic values children. In: Rudolph A, ed. Pediatrics, 16th ed. New York: Appleton-Century-Crofts; 1977:1111, 1178.
MCV, mean cell volume; mo, month; SD, standard deviation; yr, year.

TABLE 10.2. *Classification of Childhood Anemia*

Microcytic	Normocytic	Macrocytic
Iron deficiency	Acute chronic inflammation, infection	Reticulocytosis
Lead poisoning	Bone marrow suppression or infiltration	Vitamin B12, folate deficiency
Thalassemia syndromes	Congenital hemolytic anemias	Congenital pure red cell aplasia
Sideroblastic anemias	Acquired hemolytic anemia (auto or alloimmune, microangiopathic)	(Diamond-Blackfan)
Chronic inflammation	Acute or subacute blood loss	Bone marrow failure (aplastic anemia, Fanconi)
Hypoproteinemia	Splenic sequestration/ hypersplenism	Liver disease
	Transient erythroblastopenia of childhood (TEC)	Hypothyroidism
		Drug-related
		Normal newborn

TABLE 10.3. *Evaluation of Microcytic Anemia*

	Iron Deficiency	Thalassemia Trait	Thalassemia Major	Lead Toxicity	Chronic Disease
RDW	↑	NL	↑↑	NL	NL
MCV	↓	↓	↓	↓	↓
RBC #	↓	NL	↓	↓	↓
FEP	↑	NL	NL	↑↑	↑
Iron	↓	NL	↑	NL	↓
TIBC	NL ↑	NL	NL ↑	NL	NL ↓
% Sat	↓	NL	↑	NL	↓
Ferritin	↓	NL	↑	NL	NL ↑
Hgb A₂	↓	β > 3.5%	β > 3.5%	NL	NL

FEP, free erythrocyte protoporphyrin; MCV, mean cell volume; RBC, red blood cells; RDW, red cell distribution width; TIBC, total iron binding capacity.

TABLE 10.4. *Recommendations for Anemia Screening*

American Academy of Pediatrics (AAP) recommendations*:
Option 1: Universal screening (communities with high-risk populations)
9–12 months, 15–18, months, yearly until 5 if risk factors
Adolescents: Males at peak growth, females at routine exams
Option 2: Selective screening (communities with low-risk populations)
Screen high-risk patients at 9–12 months, 15–18 months, yearly until 5
Adolescents: Males at peak growth, females at routine exams
Center for Disease Control (CDC)[†]:
High-risk populations: 9–12 months, 15–18 months, yearly until 5
Adolescent females every 5–10 years, yearly if risk factors
Adolescent males at peak growth

*American Academy of Pediatrics Committee on Nutrition. Iron deficiency. In: Kleinman RE, ed. Pediatric Nutrition Handbook, 4th Ed. Elk Grove Village, IL: American Academy of Pediatrics; 1998.
†Centers for Disease Control and Prevention. Recommendations to prevent and control iron deficiency in the United States. MMWR 1998;47:1–29.

exposure to lead-based paint, particularly in children with developmental delay or autism because these are common comorbid conditions (8). An elevated FEP and basophilic stippling on peripheral smear may be seen. Therapy should include oral treatment with succimer or, in severe cases, parenteral treatment with dimercaprol (BAL) or calcium-sodium ethylenediaminetetraacetic acid (EDTA). Center for Disease Control (CDC) recommendations for management of children with elevated lead levels can be found in Table 10.6.

Thalassemia syndromes are common causes of microcytic anemia in childhood. The α-thalassemias present in utero or at birth, whereas β-thalassemias are not evident until 6 months of age, when β-globin synthesis becomes predominant. Thalassemia trait is often mistaken for iron deficiency (9). In contrast to iron deficiency, β-thalassemia trait is associated with a normal red cell distribution width (RDW), basophilic stippling and targeting on the blood smear, and an elevated Hb A2 on electrophoresis. α-Thalassemia trait is associated with a normal Hb electrophoresis outside of the newborn period, although Hb Bart's (γ_4) is present on newborn screening samples. In the evaluation of thalassemias, ethnic heritage is often suggestive, and microcytosis should be seen in at least one parent. Thalassemia trait (heterozygous β- and 1 and 2 gene deletion α-thalassemias) requires no therapy. In contrast, in thalassemia major, aggressive packed RBC transfusion should be initiated early in life to eliminate the increased erythropoietic drive and to allow normal linear growth and bone development. In utero transfusion has been used to prevent hydrops fetalis in 4-gene–deletion α-thalassemia (Hb Bart's disease), which is otherwise fatal. Care should be given to address iron overload and chelation therapy in transfusion-dependent children to prevent end organ damage later in life. As an alternative to lifelong transfusion and chelation therapy, allogeneic hematopoietic stem cell transplantation (SCT) is a curative approach for children with thalassemia major who have human leukocyte antigen (HLA)-matched sibling donors.

TABLE 10.5. *Characteristics of Anemia Based on Pathophysiology*

Decreased Production	Increased Destruction	Blood Loss	Mixed Pathophysiology
↓ Reticulocytes +/– ↓ WBC, platelets Erythroid Bone marrow hypoplasia	↑ Reticulocytes ↑ Indirect bilirubin, LDH ↓ Haptoglobin Hemoglobinuria Abnormal morphology on smear May have splenomegaly	Acute or subacute blood loss (may be occult) ↑ Reticulocytes Evolving iron deficiency	↓ Reticulocytes in setting of increased destruction (as in parvovirus B19 associated aplastic crisis in sickle cell disease or other congenital hemolytic anemia)

LDH, lactate dehydrogenase; WBC, white blood cells.

TABLE 10.6. *Summary of Recommendations for Children with Confirmed Elevated Venous Blood Lead Levels*

Blood Lead Level (μg/dL)				
10–14	15–19	20–44	45–69	>70
Lead education –Dietary –Environmental	Lead education –Dietary –Environmental	Lead education –Dietary –Environmental	Lead education –Dietary –Environmental	Hospitalize and commence chelation therapy
Follow-up blood lead monitoring (3 months)	Follow-up blood lead monitoring (1–3 months) Proceed according to actions for 20–44 μg/dL if: –follow-up blood level is in this range at least 3 months after initial venous test or –blood level increases	Follow-up blood lead monitoring (1–3 months if level 20–24; 2–4 weeks if level 25–44) Complete history and physical exam Lab work: –Hemoglobin or hematocrit –Iron status Environmental investigation Lead hazard reduction Neurodevelopmental monitoring Abdominal x-ray (if particulate lead ingestion is suspected) with bowel decontamination if indicated	Follow-up blood lead monitoring (as soon as possible) Complete history and physical exam Lab work: –Hemoglobin or hematocrit –Iron status –Free Erythrocyte Porphyrin or Zinc Proto-orphyrin Environmental investigation Lead hazard reduction Neurodevelopmental monitoring Abdominal x-ray with bowel decontamination (if indicated) Chelation therapy	Proceed according to actions for 45–69 μg/dL

*Modified from the National Center for Environmental Health, Centers for Disease Control and Prevention. Managing elevated blood lead levels among young children: recommendations from the Advisory Committee on Childhood Lead Poisoning Prevention. Atlanta (GA): 2002. Available at: http://www.cdc.gov/nceh/lead/CaseManagement/caseManage_chap3.htm, accessed December 7, 2008.

Normocytic Anemias

Anemia is a common manifestation of numerous systemic conditions in pediatrics. The anemia of acute inflammation and chronic disease is frequently mild and usually normocytic, although the mean corpuscular volume (MCV) is occasionally low. Transferrin is frequently diminished (Table 10.3). Treatment is aimed at the primary condition. Viral infection is the most common cause of transient bone marrow suppression in children and may result in both anemia and leukopenia. The hallmark of viral suppression is failure of the reticulocyte count to increase in the face of anemia. Usually, only close observation is required because the bone marrow suppression is self-limited.

Transient erythroblastopenia of childhood (TEC) is an acquired pure red cell aplasia that can also follow viral illness in previously healthy children (10). The median age for presentation is 2 years, in contrast to congenital pure red cell aplasia, which commonly presents in infancy. Reticulocytopenia and, occasionally, leukopenia and thrombocytopenia are seen. Most children with TEC recover in 1 to 2 months. Observation alone is usually sufficient, although short-term transfusion therapy may be required for cardiovascular compromise associated with severe anemia.

Hemolysis usually results in normocytic anemia. There are a large number of congenital and acquired hemolytic conditions of childhood including membrane disorders, hemoglobinopathies, metabolic defects, enzymopathies, and immune-mediated hemolysis. Immune-mediated hemolysis, either isoimmune or alloimmune, may present in neonates; autoimmune hemolytic anemia is seen in older children. Hemoglobinopathies such as sickle cell disease, enzyme deficiencies such as glucose-6-phosphate dehydrogenase deficiency, and membrane disorders such as hereditary spherocytosis (HS) should be considered in the differential diagnosis of hemolysis. Microangiopathic hemolysis may be seen in hemolytic uremic syndrome (HUS) and disseminated intravascular coagulation (DIC). Laboratory features consistent with hemolysis include reticulocytosis, elevated lactate dehydrogenase (LDH), indirect hyperbilirubinemia, decreased serum haptoglobin, and, in severe cases, hemoglobinuria. A direct Coomb's test indicates immune-mediated hemolysis. Examination of the peripheral smear may reveal characteristic red cell morphology. Thrombocytopenia and renal impairment are additional features of HUS. Treatment of hemolysis should be directed toward the underlying cause, with transfusions reserved for severe anemia and cardiovascular compromise. Immune hemolysis often requires corticosteroids and/or other immunosuppressive medications.

The diagnosis of sickle cell disease is usually made on the newborn screen by hemoglobin electrophoresis. Children diagnosed with sickle cell disease should be cared for by practitioners with specific expertise in the management and prevention of complications of sickle cell disease. Consultation with a pediatric hematologist is strongly recommended if possible. Early presentation of sickle cell crisis seen in pediatric patients includes dactylitis (vasoocclusive crisis of the hands and feet). Children should receive influenza vaccine annually starting at six months of age. Penicillin prophylaxis should begin at diagnosis and continue until age 5 years and completion of pneumococcal vaccination series. Importantly, the risk of pneumococcal sepsis is lifelong, and children require immediate medical attention for fever or signs of infection. Children should also undergo annual transcranial Doppler ultrasound between the ages of 2 and 16 years (11).

Macrocytic Anemias

Vitamin B12 deficiency is associated with megaloblastic changes in the bone marrow (12). In infants, vitamin B12 deficiency may be the result of maternal depletion and decreased stores at birth. In older children and adolescents, causes include pernicious anemia, malabsorption, dietary deficiency, and inborn errors of metabolism. Unrecognized, severe deficiency early in life may cause failure to thrive and even permanent neurologic damage. Symptoms in older children may include anorexia, weight loss, diarrhea, constipation, weakness, glossitis, peripheral neuropathy, ataxia, and dementia. Anemia is commonly accompanied by neutropenia, hypersegmented neutrophils, and thrombocytopenia. A low serum B12 level and a response to replacement therapy are confirmatory.

Folate deficiency is also associated with a megaloblastic bone marrow (12). The newborn infant has increased demands for folate. Risk factors for early deficiency include prematurity, low levels in maternal breast milk, and a predominance of goat's milk intake. In older children, folate deficiency is usually the result of malnutrition, although it may also be caused by certain medications, chronic hemolysis, malabsorption, and inborn errors of metabolism. Serum and erythrocyte folate levels will be low, and the anemia should respond to small replacement doses of folic acid.

Diamond-Blackfan anemia (DBA) or congenital pure red cell aplasia is usually noted soon after birth or during the first year of life. The main other entity in the differential diagnosis is TEC, which more commonly presents after the first year of life. Twenty-five percent of patients with DBA have associated anomalies, such as short stature and/or abnormalities of the head, face, and upper limbs. Laboratory features include reticulocytopenia, high MCV (often only mildly elevated), increased Hb F, normal or decreased white blood cell (WBC) count, and normal or increased platelet count. The bone marrow shows erythroid hypoplasia. In considering the differential diagnosis, a normal CBC in the past supports TEC, and an abnormal chromosomal breakage study confirms Fanconi anemia (FA).

The majority of children with DBA respond to corticosteroids. Prednisone is begun at a dosage of 2 mg/kg per day, with a response usually seen within 1 month. Once the Hb has reached a satisfactory level, steroids should be tapered to the lowest possible dose (ideally on an alternate day schedule). Although spontaneous remissions have occurred, corticosteroid dependence is the rule, and chronic transfusion and chelation therapy should be considered for those with associated toxicity. Allogeneic SCT may be curative (13).

Fanconi anemia can often be differentiated from acquired aplastic anemia by characteristics such as impaired growth and/or anomalies of the thumbs, radii, kidneys, head, eyes, ears, skin, and/or genitourinary system. Inheritance is autosomal recessive, and the family history may be positive for marrow failure and leukemia. There is a 10% to 35% risk of developing leukemia or myelodysplastic syndrome (14). Although the mean age of diagnosis is between 8 and 9 years, the first hematologic signs of FA may develop in infancy and often include macrocytosis, elevated Hb F, and/or mild cytopenia(s). Severe pancytopenia usually develops later in life. The differential includes other familial or acquired bone marrow failure syndromes. Abnormal chromosomal breakage analysis or FA genotyping confirms the diagnosis. Anemia is commonly androgen-responsive. Only SCT is curative for the hematologic manifestations of FA, but modified pretransplant conditioning is required to avoid severe toxicity caused by chemotherapy and radiation sensitivity.

BLEEDING

Many congenital and acquired disorders of hemostasis, including platelet abnormalities, present in infancy and childhood. Bleeding disorders that present in infancy may manifest as bleeding from the umbilicus, circumcision site, unusually large cephalohematomas, and the more serious but rare intracranial hemorrhages. Importantly, normal ranges for coagulation assays are age-dependent and differ greatly from the neonatal period to infancy and later childhood (Table 10.7). Most coagulation proteins increase in parallel with gestational age. Because physiologic levels of many clotting factors are low at birth, it is often difficult to diagnose disorders of hemostasis in newborns.

Acquired Factor Deficiencies

Hemorrhagic disease of the newborn (HDN) is a complication of physiologic low levels of vitamin K-dependent factors in the newborn (15). Classic HDN presents on days 2 to 7 of life in otherwise healthy, full-term infants and occurs in 1/10,000 live births without vitamin K prophylaxis. Risk factors include poor placental transfer of vitamin K, marginal levels in breast milk, inadequate milk intake, and the sterile newborn gut. Although rarely necessary, diagnosis can be confirmed by screening coagulation tests and vitamin K-dependent factor levels. Determination of decarboxylated forms of vitamin K-dependent factors induced by vitamin K antagonists may also be helpful. HDN should be prevented in all newborns by prophylactic administration of vitamin K at birth with a single dose of 0.5 to 1 mg intramuscularly (preferred route) or an oral dose of 2 to 4 mg, followed by continued supplementation in breast-fed infants.

Vitamin K deficiency can also be seen in children with liver disease, chronic antibiotic use, inadequate intake, or disorders that interfere with vitamin K absorption, such as chronic diarrhea, cystic fibrosis, or other fat malabsorption syndromes. Therapy should include vitamin K administration as well as disease-specific measures.

DIC can be differentiated from vitamin K deficiency and liver disease by assaying coagulation factor levels. DIC results in a decrease in all clotting factors because of consumption. In contrast, factor VIII, the only clotting protein not synthesized solely in the liver, is normal or elevated in liver disease. Therapy should be directed at the underlying cause, although supportive measures may include treatment with fresh-frozen plasma (FFP).

Inherited Factor Deficiencies

Hemophilia A and B often present in early childhood. Newborns with hemophilia can bleed with circumcision and rarely manifest intracranial hemorrhage after delivery. In the absence of a family

TABLE 10.7. *Normal Age-Specific Coagulation Values*

Coagulation Test	30–36 wk Gestation at Birth	Term Infant at Birth	1–5 Yr	6–10 Yr	11–16 Yr	Adult
PT (sec)	13 (10.6–16.2)	13 (10.14–15.9)	11 (10.6–11.4)	11.1 (10.1–12.1)	11.2 (10.2–12)	12 (11–14)
aPTT (sec)	53.6 (27.5–79.4)	42.9 (31.3–54.5)	30 (24–36)	31 (26–36)	32 (26–37)	33 (27–40)
Fibrinogen (g/L)	2.43 (1.5–3.73)	2.83 (1.67–3.99)	2.76 (1.7–4.05)	2.79 (1.57–4)	3 (1.54–4.48)	2.78 (1.56–4)
II (U/ml)	0.45 (0.2–0.77)	0.48 (0.26–0.7)	0.94 (0.71–1.16)	0.88 (0.67–1.07)	0.83 (0.61–1.04)	1.08 (0.7–1.46)
V (U/ml)	0.88 (0.41–1.44)	0.72 (0.36–1.08)	1.03 (0.79–1.27)	0.9 (0.63–1.16)	0.77 (0.55–0.99)	1.06 (0.62–1.5)
VII (U/ml)	0.67 (0.21–1.13)	0.66 (0.28–1.04)	0.82 (0.55–1.16)	0.85 (0.52–1.2)	0.83 (0.58–1.15)	1.05 (0.67–1.43)
VIII (U/ml)	1.11 (0.5–2.13)	1.0 (0.22–1.78)	0.9 (0.59–1.42)	0.95 (0.58–1.32)	0.92 (0.53–1.31)	0.99 (0.5–1.49)
IX (U/ml)	0.35 (0.19–0.65)	0.53 (0.15–0.91)	0.73 (0.47–1.04)	0.75 (0.63–0.89)	0.82 (0.59–1.22)	1.09 (0.55–1.63)
X (U/ml)	0.41 (0.11–0.71)	0.4 (0.12–0.68)	0.88 (0.58–1.16)	0.75 (0.55–1.01)	0.79 (0.5–1.17)	1.06 (0.7–1.52)
XI (U/ml)	0.3 (0.08–0.52)	0.38 (0.1–0.66)	0.97 (0.56–1.5)	0.86 (0.52–1.2)	0.74 (0.5–0.97)	0.97 (0.67–1.27)
XII (U/ml)	0.38 (0.1–0.66)	0.53 (0.13–0.93)	0.93 (0.64–1.29)	0.92 (0.6–1.4)	0.81 (0.34–1.37)	1.08 (0.52–1.64)
XIIIa (U/ml)	0.7 (0.32–1.08)	0.79 (0.27–1.31)	1.08 (0.72–1.43)	1.09 (0.65–1.51)	0.99 (0.57–1.4)	1.05 (0.55–1.55)
vWF (U/ml)	1.36 (0.78–2.1)	1.53 (019–2.87)	0.82 (0.6–1.2)	0.95 (0.44–1.44)	1 (0.46–1.53)	0.92 (0.5–1.58)
ATIII (U/ml)	0.38 (0.14–0.62)	0.63 (0.39–0.87)	1.11 (0.82–1.39)	1.11 (0.9–1.31)	1.05 (0.77–1.32)	1.0 (0.74–1.26)
Protein C (U/ml)	0.28 (0.12–0.44)	0.35 (0.17–0.53)	0.66 (0.4–0.92)	0.69 (0.45–0.93)	0.83 (0.55–1.11)	0.96 (0.64–1.28)
Protein S, Total (U/ml)	0.26 (0.14–0.38)	0.36 (0.12–0.6)	0.86 (0.54–1.18)	0.78 (0.41–1.14)	0.72 (0.52–0.92)	0.81 (0.6–1.13)
Protein S, Free (U/ml)	N/A	N/A	0.45 (0.21–0.69)	0.42 (0.22–0.62)	0.38 (0.26–0.55)	0.45 (0.27–0.61)

Values expressed in units per milliliter are compared with pooled plasma, which contains 1.0 U/ml. However, pooled plasma contains 0.4 U/ml of free protein S.

Modified from Andrew M, Vegh P, Johnston M, et al. Maturation of the hemostatic system in childhood. Blood 1992;80:1998–2005. Andrew M, Paes B, Milner R, et al. Development of the coagulation system in the healthy premature infant. Blood 1988;72:1651–1657. Andrew M, Paes B, Milner R, et al. The development of the human coagulation system in the fullterm infant. Blood 1987;70:165–170.

history, the diagnosis of hemophilia is most often made when a child with moderate to severe factor deficiency begins to crawl or walk. Common symptoms include easy bruising, hemarthrosis in weight-bearing joints, and deep intramuscular hemorrhage. Central nervous system (CNS) bleeding is the most common cause of early mortality. Laboratory evidence for hemophilia includes a prolonged partial thromboplastin time (PTT), which corrects on mixing studies. An abnormally low factor VIII or IX level confirms the diagnosis. Care should be taken to evaluate and treat hemarthroses aggressively in children to prevent later development of chronic arthropathy. The treatment of hemophilia in children is similar to that in adults and includes factor replacement dosed according to the site, type, and severity of hemorrhage. The availability of recombinant factor concentrates has increased the safety and feasibility of prophylaxis in children with frequent hemorrhagic episodes (16). In patients with mild hemophilia A, desmopressin is often effective for short-term management of mild bleeding. As in adults, routine screening for inhibitors should be used.

Von Willebrand disease (vWD) usually presents with less severe bleeding, primarily mucocutaneous, compared with hemophilia. Because recurrent bruising and epistaxis are common complaints in children, history should be directed toward the presence of prolonged, unusual, or severe bleeding. A careful family history may reveal similar symptoms in parents or siblings. The diagnosis is confirmed by abnormal assays for factor VIII, von Willebrand factor (vWF) antigen and activity, and multimer analysis. Factor VIII and vWF are acute phase reactants and, in children, falsely elevated levels caused by interval illnesses may obscure the diagnosis. Thus, repeat testing should be considered if the diagnosis of vWD is suspected. Therapy is as in adults.

Platelet Disorders

Neonatal alloimmune thrombocytopenia (NAIT) results from the placental transfer of maternal alloantibodies against paternally inherited antigens (most commonly HPA-1a) on fetal platelets. Newborns present with transient, isolated but severe thrombocytopenia that must be distinguished from other causes, including maternal immune thrombocytopenic purpura (ITP), severe infection, DIC, hypersplenism, and Kasabach-Merrit syndrome. Approximately 15% of affected neonates experience intracranial hemorrhage, either in utero or in the immediate postnatal period. Unlike Rh disease of the newborn, prior sensitization is not required, and thus NAIT may occur with the first pregnancy. A normal platelet count in the mother helps to differentiate NAIT from maternal ITP. Immunophenotyping of maternal and paternal platelets is useful to confirm the diagnosis. The treatment of choice in severe NAIT is transfusion of maternal platelets. When they are not readily available, platelets obtained from a known HPA-1a–negative donor or from random donors may be used for active bleeding. Intravenous immunoglobulin (IVIg) or corticosteroids may also be used as a temporary measure either in the antenatal or postnatal periods, with dosing as in ITP.

Immune thrombocytopenic purpura affects approximately 1 in 10,000 children annually in the United States (17). In contrast to adults, ITP in childhood is usually a self-limited, benign condition. Children typically present under the age of 10. Eighty percent have spontaneous resolution within 6 months. Infants and older children are more likely to have prolonged thrombocytopenia. The typical presentation in acute ITP is the abrupt onset of mucosal bleeding, petechiae, and bruising in healthy children, often preceded by a viral illness. Most children present with severe thrombocytopenia (platelet counts less than 20,000 per microliter) and an otherwise normal CBC. Large platelets are commonly seen on peripheral blood smear. Acute ITP is a diagnosis of exclusion, although otherwise healthy children with no other significant medical history or findings on physical examination rarely require extensive laboratory testing. Human immunodeficiency virus (HIV) assay should be considered. The diagnostic utility of bone marrow examination for a child with suspected ITP is low. Evaluation for chronic ITP should include bone marrow studies and testing for immunodeficiency and autoimmune disease. The need for treatment in acute ITP is often debated; current guidelines recommend therapy for significant bleeding or a platelet below 10,000 per microliter (18). Although the risk of intracranial hemorrhage is small, precautions should be taken to prevent head trauma, and helmets are recommended for toddlers just learning to walk. There are several standard first-line therapeutic options (Table 10.8).

Inherited platelet disorders may be qualitative or quantitative; they are a rare cause of thrombocytopenia in infancy and childhood. The variety of qualitative disorders includes Glanzmann thrombasthenia (GT), Bernard-Soulier syndrome (BSS), platelet-type pseudo-vWD, and platelet storage granule defects. Quantitative defects are seen in congenital amegakaryocytic thrombocytopenia, thrombocytopenia-absent radii (TAR), X-linked thrombocytopenia, Wiskott-Aldrich syndrome (WAS), and May-Hegglin anomaly. Children with these disorders commonly present with petechiae, easy bruising, or

TABLE 10.8. *Treatment Regimens for Childhood Immune Thrombocytopenic Purpura*

IVIg: 1 g/kg × 1 day or 2 g/kg over 2–5 days *OR*
Anti-D: 50–75 mcg/kg × 1 day (Rh positive patients only) *OR*
Prednisone 4–8 mg/kg/day × 7–21 days with taper *OR*
Methylprednisolone 30 mg/kg/day × 3 days

Anti-D, anti-Rh(D) immune globulin; IVIg, intravenous immunoglobulin.

TABLE 10.9. *Heparin Therapy in Children*

Age	Heparin Bolus (U/kg)	Heparin Infusion (U/kg/hr)*	Enoxaparin (treatment)†	Enoxaparin (prophylaxis)
Infants	75–100	28	*<2 mos* 1.5 mg/kg q12 h	*<2 mos* 0.75 mg/kg q12 h
Children	75–100	20	*≥ 2 mos* 1 mg/kg q12 h	*≥ 2 mos* 0.5 mg/kg q12 h
Adults	80	18	1 mg/kg q12 h	30 mg q12 h

Modified from Monagle P, Michelson AD, Bovill E, et al. Antithrombotic therapy in children. Chest 2001;119:344–370. *Goal is aPTT of 1.5–2.5× control (60–85 sec). †Goal is antifactor Xa level of 0.5–1.0 U/ml 2–6 hours after injection.

mucocutaneous bleeding. Rarely, gastrointestinal or intracranial bleeding may occur. Screening for qualitative disorders requires platelet aggregation and/or flow cytometric studies. Characteristic features of specific disorders should be sought (forearm deformities in TAR, immunodeficiency in WAS, macrothrombocytes in May-Hegglin anomaly). Treatment for bleeding is usually supportive. Platelet transfusions should be avoided if possible in patients with BSS and GT, because of the risk of developing alloantibodies to the missing platelet antigens GPIb-IX and αIIb-β3, respectively.

THROMBOSIS

As with coagulation factor levels, normal ranges for endogenous antithrombotic proteins are age- and gestation-dependent (Table 10.7). Notably, venous thromboembolic events (TEE) are less common in children compared with adults, with the exception of specific at-risk patient populations (19). Unless specific risk factors are identified, arterial thrombosis is extremely infrequent.

Anticoagulant and thrombolytic therapy should be dosed according to age and weight (Tables 10.9 and 10.10). The duration, monitoring, efficacy, and long-term effects of anticoagulation in the management of TEE in children require further study. The treatment of children with oral anticoagulants is complicated by an increased risk of bleeding complications. As in adults, caution is required when instituting warfarin therapy. To avoid paradoxical thrombosis, heparinization should be continued until the international normalized ratio (INR) is therapeutic.

Congenital Prothrombotic Disorders

Children who are homozygous or compound heterozygous for deficiencies of anticoagulant proteins usually present in the neonatal or early childhood period. In the absence of additional risk factors, how-

TABLE 10.10. *Warfarin Therapy in Children**

Day 1	Days 2–4		Maintenance	
	INR	*Action*	*INR*	*Action*
Load 0.2 mg/kg po if baseline INR 1.0–1.3	1.1–1.4	Repeat initial loading dose	1.1–1.4	Increase by 20% of dose
	1.5–1.9	50% of loading dose	1.5–1.9	Increase by 10% of dose
	2.0–3.0	50% of loading dose	2.0–3.0	No change
	3.0–4.0	25% of loading dose	3.1–4.0	Decrease by 10% of dose
	>4.5	Hold until INR <4.5, restart at 50% less than previous dose	4.1–4.5	Decrease by 20% of dose
			>4.5	Hold until INR <4.5, restart at 20% less than previous dose

*Do not initiate warfarin until therapeutic heparinization. Heparin should not be discontinued until INR is therapeutic.
Modified from Michelson AD, Bovill E, Andrew M. Antithrombotic therapy in children. *Chest* 1995;108:506–22. INR, international normalized ratio.

ever, individuals who are heterozygous for thrombophilic conditions infrequently experience their first TEE early in life. In general, evaluation for possible inherited deficiency is recommended for children with a family history of congenital thrombophilia, and if thromboses are unexplained, occur in unusual sites, are particularly severe, and/or are recurrent.

Protein C and S deficiency, in the homozygous state, classically presents as purpura fulminans within hours or days of birth. Purpura fulminans is more common with protein C deficiency and is characterized by acute DIC with rapidly progressive hemorrhagic necrosis of the skin and other thrombotic/hemorrhagic complications, including death. Homozygous infants usually have undetectable levels of protein C or S, and their parents have heterozygous deficiency. Both functional and immunologic assays for protein C and S should be utilized. Acquired causes of protein C and S deficiency, such as liver disease and sepsis, should be excluded. Purpura fulminans should be treated with FFP and, if available, purified protein C concentrate. Warfarin-induced skin necrosis has been described in children with heterozygous protein C and S deficiency, and extreme caution is required when converting such individuals from heparin to warfarin anticoagulation.

Other inherited thrombophilic states including antithrombin III deficiency, factor V Leiden, prothrombin G20210A mutations, and homocysteinemia have also been associated with recurrent thromboembolism in children and adolescents. The incidence of deep vein thrombosis related to those conditions is low, and the value of an extensive evaluation of the first TEE has been questioned.

Acquired Prothrombotic Disorders

As in adult patients, thromboembolism in children is usually secondary; central venous catheters are the most common cause. Neonates are at particularly high risk, and the use of umbilical lines may be associated with portal system thrombosis. Other risk factors include malignancy, surgery, trauma, pregnancy, congenital heart disease, Kawasaki disease, nephrotic syndrome, and systemic lupus erythematosus. Complete evaluation for possible underlying conditions should be undertaken. The laboratory examination should be guided by clinical findings and risk factors and in most cases should include lupus anticoagulant or antiphospholipid antibody assay.

NEUTROPENIA

Normal neutrophil counts vary with age and are affected by race and other factors (Table 10.1). For example, the lower limit of normal in African Americans may be 200 to 600 per microliter less than in Whites.

Neutropenia is commonly encountered in pediatrics, most often caused by viral suppression. Children, like adults, are at increased risk for life-threatening bacterial infection when the absolute neutrophil count (ANC) falls below 500 per microliter. Common pyogenic infections seen in association with neutropenia include cellulitis, superficial or deep abscesses, pneumonia, sepsis, and recurrent or chronic otitis media and sinusitis.

General management recommendations include aggressive monitoring for and treatment of infection, judicious use of antibiotics, rapid institution of empiric broad-spectrum parenteral antibiotics for fever, and maintenance of good skin and oral hygiene. Granulocyte colony stimulating factor (G-CSF, filgrastim) is often effective in increasing the rate of ANC recovery in certain disorders.

Viral infections are the most common cause of transient neutropenia in childhood. Neutropenia usually develops during the first 24 to 48 hours of illness and commonly lasts up to a week or longer. Neutropenia may also occur with serious bacterial infections, especially in neonates.

Autoimmune neutropenia of childhood is the most common cause of chronic neutropenia in pediatrics, primarily affecting children younger than 3 years of age. The ANC at presentation is usually below 250 per microliter. Associated monocytosis is common, and antineutrophil antibodies can be detected in most patients (20). Other causes of neutropenia should be excluded, such as immunodeficiency, drug-related, transient postinfectious, and congenital neutrophil disorders. Although the ANC is often extremely low or absent, most children experience only minor infections and thus, this condition is sometimes referred to as chronic benign neutropenia of childhood. Nonetheless, empiric, broad-spectrum parenteral antibiotics are recommended for the first few episodes of fever. If a child appears to have a benign course, subsequent febrile episodes might be managed more routinely unless there is documented infection or signs of sepsis. Daily trimethoprim/sulfamethoxasole may be useful in preventing recurrent minor bacterial infections. G-CSF is usually effective in low doses (1 to 2 μg/kg per day) and should be considered for children with recurrent, severe neutropenic complications. Spontaneous remission within the first few years of diagnosis is common, especially in young children.

Cyclic neutropenia is characterized by periodic oscillations in the ANC. Cycles commonly occur every 3 to 4 weeks, and the nadir is usually below 200 per microliter. Symptoms typically begin in the first year of life and commonly include recurrent fever, gingivitis, stomatitis with oral aphthous ulcers, and pharyngitis. Diagnosis is confirmed by monitoring serial CBCs twice per week for 6 to 8 weeks to establish the periodicity of the neutropenia, which may also be accompanied by oscillations in other blood counts. Cyclic neutropenia is often an autosomal-dominant condition, so parental history and/or CBCs may be helpful. Although cyclic neutropenia is a benign condition in most cases, serious infectious complications may occur. G-CSF in low doses (2 to 3 μg/kg per dose) daily or every other day should be titrated to raise neutrophil levels.

Severe congenital neutropenia (Kostmann disease) is an autosomal-recessive disorder associated with severe (usually less than 200 per microliter), chronic neutropenia from birth. Recurrent bacterial infections include those commonly seen in more benign neutropenic conditions, as well as life-threatening sepsis, meningitis, and gastrointestinal tract infection. Neonates commonly present with omphalitis. Bone marrow examination reveals neutrophil developmental arrest. Standard therapy consists of daily G-CSF, but high doses may be required, and patients undergoing long-term therapy are at high risk for myelodysplastic syndrome and acute myelogenous leukemia (21). SCT should be considered as a curative approach.

Shwachman-Diamond syndrome and Chédiak-Higashi syndrome are both autosomal-recessive disorders that are associated with neutropenia. Shwachman-Diamond is characterized by progressive marrow failure, pancreatic exocrine insufficiency, short stature, and skeletal deformities. Two thirds of patients have a moderate neutropenia that can be intermittent and responsive to G-CSF. Chédiak-Higashi is also a multiorgan disease that includes oculocutaneous albinism, recurrent bacterial infection, a mild bleeding disorder, and neurologic dysfunction. The accumulation of giant granules in neutrophils leads to premature destruction. Affected individuals commonly progress to an accelerated phase characterized by hemophagocytic lymphohistiocytosis, which is usually fatal. Therapy is supportive, and SCT is the only known cure for the hematologic manifestations.

Other causes of neutropenia include drug-induced, inborn errors of metabolism, nutritional deficiency, or bone marrow infiltration. Treatment should be directed at the underlying cause.

LEUKOCYTOSIS

Leukocytosis refers to an increase in total WBC count for age. Neutrophilia is an increase in the ANC above 7,500 per microliter, although the upper limit of normal may be higher in newborns and infants (Table 10.1). Neutrophilia may result from increased production, mobilization from the bone marrow, or peripheral demargination. In children, neutrophilia in the acute setting is most often related to bacterial or viral infection. Absolute lymphocytosis usually indicates an acute or chronic viral process. The evaluation of leukocytosis should include a detailed history and physical examination, looking closely for symptoms and signs of infection and for lymphadenopathy and hepatosplenomegaly. Examination of the peripheral blood smear is essential to distinguish normal from atypical and malignant white blood cells.

Leukocyte adhesion deficiency type I (LAD I) is a disorder of impaired phagocyte adhesion, chemotaxis, and ingestion caused by partial or total deficiency of CD18-related surface glycoproteins. The hallmark of this disorder is the occurrence of repeated, severe bacterial or fungal infections in the absence of pus accumulation despite persistent neutrophilia. Infants typically present in the newborn period with omphalitis or delayed umbilical cord separation. The diagnosis of LAD can be confirmed by flow cytometry. LAD type II, which is caused by defective fucose metabolism, produces a less severe phenotype. The treatment for both LAD I and II should be directed at the underlying infection. SCT may be curative.

Infectious mononucleosis (IM) is classically associated with atypical lymphocytosis and is caused by infection with Epstein-Barr virus (EBV) (22). In adolescents and young adults, a prodrome of fatigue and anorexia usually precedes development of fever, lymphadenopathy, exudative pharyngitis, and hepatosplenomegaly. Young children commonly present with a mild respiratory illness only. Rash can occur, especially after treatment with penicillin or ampicillin. Hematologic complications, including immune-mediated hemolytic anemia, thrombocytopenia, aplastic anemia, and hemophagocytosis can be seen, as can other rare complications such as CNS involvement, myocarditis, orchitis, and splenic rupture. Children with acquired or congenital immunodeficiency states can develop EBV-associated lymphoproliferative syndrome, which can evolve into non-Hodgkin's lymphoma. EBV in boys with Duncan syndrome (X-linked lymphoproliferative syndrome) results in fatal IM in the majority of cases.

Atypical lymphocytosis and early immunologic evidence of EBV infection, either by heterophil or EBV-specific antibody testing, are the most consistent laboratory findings. Nonspecific heterophil antibody tests are often negative in children younger than 4 years of age. Other infections, such as cytomegalovirus (CMV), pertussis, and cat-scratch disease should be excluded in the setting of EBV-negative IM. Therapy of IM is supportive. Rarely, short course corticosteroids are used to manage life-threatening manifestations, such as upper airway obstruction from tonsillar/adenoidal hypertrophy. To avoid splenic rupture, contact sports should be avoided until splenomegaly resolves.

HEMATOLOGIC MANIFESTATIONS OF SYSTEMIC CONDITIONS

Many systemic conditions can result in secondary hematologic abnormalities. Evaluation of the CBC and peripheral smear may also provide important clues during the evaluation of a diagnostic dilemma. A number of systemic disorders that have prominent hematologic findings and present predominantly in childhood are detailed below.

Lysosomal storage diseases are caused by a deficiency in specific enzymes of the lysosomal metabolic pathway and result in pathologic accumulation of normal substrate. Dramatic changes in the central nervous and hematologic systems as well as enlargement of organs that comprise the reticuloendothelial system, including liver and spleen, result. Vacuolated lymphocytes and hypergranulated neutrophils in the peripheral blood and lipid-laden macrophages ("foam" or "storage" cells) in the bone marrow are commonly observed. Other characteristic cell types include the sea-blue histiocyte in Niemann-Pick disease and the Gaucher cell. Although specific enzyme replacement therapy has proven successful for some of these disorders, therapy is only supportive for others (23). SCT has proven curative in a limited number of the storage conditions.

Autoimmune lymphoproliferative syndrome (ALPS) is a rare disorder of early childhood caused by defective lymphocyte apoptosis (24). Symptoms include lymphadenopathy, splenomegaly, autoimmunity, and risk of lymphoma. Autoimmune cytopenias are common. The presence of increased numbers of double negative (CD4-/CD8-) T-cells on flow cytometry supports the diagnosis, which can be confirmed by the demonstration of diminished lymphocyte apoptosis. A number of molecular defects have been identified, most commonly mutations in Fas (*TNFRSF6*, CD95). Therapy is mainly supportive, although immunosuppressive medications may be needed to manage complications of autoimmunity and lymphoproliferation, and SCT can be curative.

Collagen vascular diseases commonly have hematologic manifestations, most often anemia of chronic illness and/or autoimmune-mediated cytopenias. Aplastic anemia has been described in systemic lupus erythematosus (SLE). Patients with autoimmune disorders are at increased risk for developing antiphospholipid antibodies; although such lupus anticoagulants result in prolongation of prothrombin time (PT) and PTT, they predispose to thromboembolism rather than bleeding.

TRANSFUSION SUPPORT

The indications for transfusion in infants and children are similar to that in adults. Patient size, blood volume, and underlying condition mandate special precautions in regard to dosing and risks. In all cases, careful consideration should be given to the indication for, appropriate dose of, and potential

17. Kühne T, Imbach P, Bolton-Maggs PH, et al; Intercontinental Childhood ITP Study Group. Newly diagnosed idiopathic thrombocytopenic purpura in childhood: an observational study. Lancet 2001;358:2122–2125.

18. Medeiros M, Buchanan GR. Idiopathic thrombocytopenic purpura: beyond consensus. Curr Opin Pediatr 2000;12:4–9.

19. Monagle P, Adams M, Mahoney M, et al. Outcome of pediatric thromboembolic disease: a report from the Canadian Childhood Thrombophilia Registry. Pediatr Res 2000;47:763–766.

20. Kobayashi M, Nakamura K, Kawaguchi H, et al. Significance of the detection of antineutrophil antibodies in children with chronic neutropenia. Blood 2002;99:3468–3471.

21. Freedman MH, Bonilla MA, Fier C, et al. Myelodysplasia syndrome and acute myeloid leukemia in patients with congenital neutropenia receiving G-CSF therapy. Blood 2000;96:429–436.

22. Krabbe S, Hesse J, Uldall P. Primary Epstein-Barr virus infection in early childhood. Arch Dis Child 1981;56:49–52.

23. Schiffmann R, Brady RO. New prospects for the treatment of lysosomal storage diseases. Drugs 2002;62:733–742.

24. Carter LB, Procter JL, Dale JK, et al. Description of serologic features in autoimmune lymphoproliferative syndrome. Transfusion 2000;40:943–948.

11

Acute Myelogenous Leukemia

Vijay S. Suhag, Scott R. Solomon, and Vera Malkovska

Acute myelogenous leukemia (AML) is a heterogeneous group of diseases characterized by uncontrolled proliferation of myeloid progenitor cells that gradually replace normal hematopoiesis in the bone marrow. The genetic changes arising in the neoplastic clone lead to cascades of molecular events that cause abnormal proliferation, aberrant differentiation, and inhibition of normal hematopoiesis by the malignant cells.

Characterization of transforming genetic events is increasingly important in establishing diagnosis, defining prognosis, and planning therapy in AML. Aggressive chemotherapy with optimal supportive treatment has improved outcomes in younger patients with AML: most achieve a complete remission but many relapse, and their five-year survival remains below 50% in large studies (1). Patients over the age of 60 have a median survival of less than a year and long-term survival rates below 10%; both the unfavorable biology of AML and poor tolerance of chemotherapy in the elderly are to blame (2). The current challenge is to understand the molecular mechanisms of AML and design leukemia-specific treatments effective in chemotherapy-resistant disease and applicable to older patients.

EPIDEMIOLOGY

The age-adjusted incidence rate of AML in the United States is 3.4 per 100,000, leading to approximately 10,000 deaths per year. AML accounts for about 15% to 20% of acute leukemias in children and adolescents and 90% in adults. The incidence of AML increases with age, and most patients are over 60 years of age at presentation (Fig. 11.1) (3).

ETIOLOGY

The molecular origins of AML are unknown. The pathophysiologic mechanisms are multiple, act in concert, and are distinct in different types of AML. Inherited genetic predisposition and environmental mutagens such as radiation, drugs, and other toxins all play a role in the development of AML (3). Genetic causes are suggested by the increased incidence of AML in identical twins, as well as the association of AML with a variety of congenital disorders. AML arising from pre-existing hematologic disorders, most commonly the myelodysplastic syndromes, have inferior prognosis. Resistance to treatment and short survival are characteristic of AML following exposure to chemotherapy and radiation (3).

Known risks factors for AML include:

1. Environmental exposures
   - Benzene and its derivatives, ethylene oxides, and herbicides
   - Ionizing radiation
2. Genetic Disorders
   - Down syndrome
   - Bloom syndrome
   - Fanconi anemia
   - Aataxia telangiectasia
   - Li-Fraumeni syndrome
   - Kostmann syndrome
   - Klinefelter syndrome

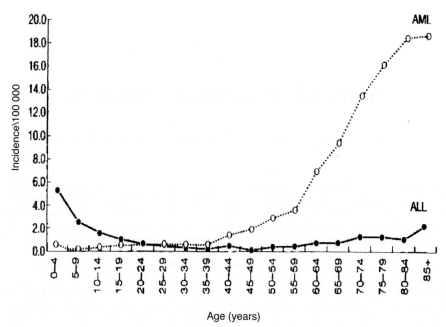

FIG. 11.1. The age-related incidence of acute myelogenous leukemia (AML) in the United States.

3. Pre-existing hematologic disorders
   - Myelodysplastic syndromes (MDS)
   - Myeloproliferative disorders
   - Paroxysmal nocturnal hemoglobinuria
4. Treatment-associated
   - Alkylating agents: AML usually arises from MDS, after a 3- to 10-year latency period and is associated with characteristic chromosomal abnormalities, mainly deletions involving chromosomes 5 or 7.
   - Topoisomerase II inhibitors: AML lacks preceding myelodysplasia, has a shorter latency, exhibits monocytic morphology, and is associated with characteristic cytogenetic changes involving the long arm of chromosome 11 (11q23).
   - Radiotherapy alone or in combination with chemotherapy.

PATHOGENESIS

At the molecular level, the pathogenesis of AML is a complex multistep process that results from the interaction of two different classes of mutations. The first class of mutations impairs cell differentiation resulting in clonal expansion of myeloid progenitors. The second class causes abnormal cell proliferation by constitutive activation of cellular proto-oncogenes, including FLT 3 tyrosine kinase, RAS, c-KIT, and others. The silencing of tumor suppressor genes also contributes to pathogenesis. Some molecular genetic alterations in AML are highlighted by distinct chromosomal changes, including translocations, inversions, and deletions, while others can be only identified by molecular analysis (Table 11.1). Common mutations found in AML that are thought to cooperate in the malignant transformation are shown in Table 11.1 (4). Analysis of cytogenetics and molecular

TABLE 11.1. *Common Cytogenetic Abnormalities and Mutations in Acute Myelogenous Leukemia*

Mutations That Impair Differentiation	Mutations That Promote Proliferation
Balanced translocations and inversions • t (8;21): AML-1 ETO • t (15;17): PML-RARA • Inv 16: CBFB-MYH 11 • 11q23: MLL PTD • Rare - t(6;11), t (9;11), t (6;9), inv 3	Proto-oncogene mutations • FLT 3 activating mutation • RAS mutations • c-KIT (CD 117) activating mutations • NPM 1 mutations • BAALC and ERG over expression
Point mutations in transcription factors • Core-binding factor mutations • CEBPA mutations • Wilms tumor (WT-1) mutation	Tumor suppressor gene mutations • P53, retinoblastoma

AML-1 ETO, acute myelogenous leukemia-eight twenty-one gene; BAALC, brain and acute leukemia, cytoplasmic; CBFB-MYH, core-binding factor gene–smooth muscle myosin heavy chain; CD, cluster designation; CEBPA, CCAAT/enhancer binding protein alpha; ERG, ETS-related gene; FLT 3, Fms-like tyrosine kinase 3; MLL-PTD, mixed lineage leukemia–partial tandem duplication; NPM, nucleophosmin; PML-RARA, promyelocytic leukemia–retinoic acid receptor; RAS, retinoic acid syndrome.

changes is used to predict clinical outcomes and formulating treatment paradigms in AML (Table 11.2). Studies are underway to understand the downstream molecular pathways triggered by these mutations that lead to the unrestricted growth of leukemic cells and suppression of normal hematopoiesis by the malignant clone.

CLINICAL FEATURES

Patients with AML usually present with bone marrow failure that causes symptoms of anemia, bleeding from thrombocytopenia, and neutropenic infections. Tissue infiltration with leukemic blasts involving gums, skin, meninges, and other organs is commonly associated with monocytic morphology. Striking bruising and life-threatening hemorrhage should raise suspicion of disseminated intravas-

TABLE 11.2. *Diagnostic Markers in Acute Myelogenous Leukemia*

FAB Class	Cytochemistry	Immunophenotype	Cytogenetics
MO Minimally differentiated	MPO <3%	CD34+, HLA DR+ CD33+/−, CD13+/−	11q13
M1 Without maturation	MPO <3%	CD34+, HLA DR+ CD33+, CD13+	−5, −7, −17 Del 3p, +21, +8
M2 With maturation	MPO >10%	CD34−, HLA DR + CD33+, CD13+	t (8;21), del3p or inv 3 −5, −7, +8, t (6;9)
M3 Promyelocytic	MPO + +	CD 34−, HLA DR-, CD 13+, CD 33+	t (15;17)
M4 Myelomonocytic	MPO +, Esterase +	CD 34−, HLA DR+, CD 13+, CD 33+ CD 11+, CD14+,	Inv 16, t(16;16) −5, −7, t(6;9)
M5 Monocytic	Esterase ++, PAS +	CD 34−, HLA DR+, CD 13+/−, CD 33+ CD11+, CD14+,	t (9;11) (p21;23), +8
M6 Erythroid	PAS ++ Esterase −	Glycophorin A +	−5q, −5, −7, −3. +8
M7 Megakaryocytic	PAS +/−	CD41+	+8, +21, inv or del 3p

CD, cluster designation; HLA-DR, human leukocyte antigens D-related; MPO, myeloperoxidase; PAS, periodic acid-Schiff. Myeloid Markers: CD 13, CD33; Monocytic Markers: CD 11, CD14

cular coagulation (DIC), which is frequent in acute promyelocytic leukemia, but DIC can occur in any type of AML. Leukostasis and hyperviscosity causing organ dysfunction usually occurs with blast cell counts over 100,000; manifested by confusion, visual impairment, and shortness of breath. Leukostasis can also lead to hemorrhage in the retina, brain, lungs, and other organs. Rare but striking manifestations of AML include the Sweet syndrome, a skin rash with neutrophilic infiltrates in the dermis, and chloromas, tumors of myeloid blasts. Extramedullary leukemia portends a worse prognosis.

Symptoms and signs on presentation include:

Marrow failure
- Fatigue
- Shortness of breath
- Fever
- Focal infections
- Petechiae
- Bruising
- Bleeding (if severe, suspect promyelocytic leukemia)

Tissue involvement
- Bone pain, tenderness
- Mild splenomegaly
- Gingival hyperplasia
- Central nervous system (CNS) and cranial nerve dysfunction
- Visual changes (retinal involvement, hemorrhage, papilledema)

Rare manifestations
- Sweet syndrome
- Chloromas

LABORATORY FINDINGS

Common laboratory findings in AML include anemia, thrombocytopenia, neutropenia, and myeloid blasts on the blood smear. The blasts have distinct immunophenotypes detected by flow cytometry. In aleukemic leukemia, blasts are seen only in the bone marrow. Coagulopathy resulting from DIC is frequent in promyelocytic leukemia. Hyperuricemia from high cell turnover is often seen on presentation and worsens during chemotherapy. Rapidly rising serum levels of uric acid, potassium, and phosphate with decreasing calcium herald a tumor lysis syndrome that can result in acute renal failure. Renal tubular dysfunction caused by muramidase released from leukemic blasts can add to the electrolyte abnormalities of AML. Lactic acidosis tends to occur with leukostasis, while high lactate dehydrogenase (LDH) is associated with CNS involvement. High numbers of leukemic blasts in blood samples can lead to spurious hypoglycemia, hypoxemia, hypokalemia, and other abnormalities resulting from cellular metabolic activity in vitro. Rapid processing of anticoagulated blood samples avoids this artifact.

In addition to routine chest radiographs, imaging studies including computerized tomography (CT) and magnetic resonance imaging (MRI) scans directed according to symptoms can reveal leukemic infiltrates, hemorrhage, or infection.

Laboratory findings in AML include:

Hematologic
- Increased white blood cell count with blasts in peripheral blood
- Anemia
- Granulocytopenia
- Thrombocytopenia
- DIC

Chemistry
- Hyperuricemia
- Elevated blood-urea nitrogen (BUN) and creatinine (urate nephropathy)

- High LDH
- Hypokalemia (tubular dysfunction)
- Lactic acidosis (leukostasis)
- Hypercalcemia, rarely hypocalcemia
- Spurious hypoxemia, hypoglycemia, hyperkalemia, or hypokalemia

Imaging studies
- Intracranial hemorrhage (often with hyperviscosity) (CT)
- Thickened nerve sheets (MRI)
- Lung infiltrates (CT)

CLASSIFICATION

There are two commonly used classifications of AML. The older French-American-British (FAB) classification based on morphology, cytochemical staining, and immunophenotype of the predominant cells divides AML into eight subtypes (M0–M7) (see below and Table 11.2):

M0   Minimally differentiated AML: negative peroxidase reaction, two or more myeloid markers by flow cytometry, frequently has complex cytogenetic abnormalities associated with poor prognosis.

M1   AML without maturation: less than 10% promyelocytes or more mature myeloid forms.

M2   AML with maturation: subset of patients have the t(8;21) translocation associated with favorable prognosis.

M3   Acute promyelocytic leukemia (APL): in most cases heavy granulation and bilobed nuclear contour; rarely microgranular variant with inconspicuous granules. Most cases have t(15;17) translocation and favorable prognosis.

M4   Acute myelomonocytic leukemia: monocytes and promonocytes in the marrow exceed 20%. M4Eo variant contains more than 5% abnormal eosinophils; associated with the inv(16) cytogenetic abnormality and favorable prognosis.

M5   Acute monocytic leukemia: 80% or more of nonerythroid cells are monoblasts, monocytes, or promonocytes. Nonspecific esterase stain is positive. Associated with extramedullary disease and abnormalities of the long arm of chromosome 11 (11q).

M6   Acute erythroleukemia: more than 50% nucleated marrow cells are erythroid, often severely dyserythropoietic. Erythroblasts are strongly periodic acid-Schiff (PAS)-positive and glycophorin A positive.

M7   Acute megakaryocytic leukemia: may have micromegakaryoblasts. Diagnosis is confirmed by immunophenotyping (CD41) or electron microscopy (platelet peroxidase).

The World Health Organization (WHO) classification takes into account molecular genetics, therapy-related leukemias, and biphenotypic leukemias:

AML with recurrent cytogenetic translocations
- AML with t(8;21)(q22;q22)
- AML with t(15;17)(q22;q11) + variants = APL (M3)
- AML with abnormal marrow eosinophils inv(16)(p13q22) or t(16;16)(p13;q11)
- AML with 11q23 (MLL) abnormalities

AML with multilineage dysplasia
- With prior myelodysplastic syndrome (MDS)
- Without prior MDS

AML and MDS: therapy-related
- Alkylating agent-related
- Epipodophyllotoxin-related
- Other

AML not otherwise categorized
- AML minimally differentiated
- AML with maturation
- AML without maturation
- Acute myelomonocytic leukemia
- Acute monocytic leukemia
- Acute erythroid leukemia
- Acute megakaryocytic leukemia
- Acute basophilic leukemia
- Acute panmyelosis with myelofibrosis

Acute biphenotypic leukemias

The classification of AML continues to evolve and incorporate newly detected molecular mutations with a defined impact on the biology of the different subtypes of the leukemia. Ultimately, better understanding of the signaling pathways in leukemogenesis will lead to a more sophisticated subclassification into disease entities, especially for sensitivity to different targeted therapies.

DIAGNOSTIC EVALUATION

Leukemic myeloblasts are usually seen on the blood smear and are always found in the bone marrow biopsy. According to the World Health Organization (WHO) consensus, the diagnosis of AML requires at least 20% myeloid blasts in the peripheral blood or bone marrow. The evaluation of a patient with AML at diagnosis includes blood count and inspection of blood smear, bone marrow aspirate and biopsy (morphology with Wright-Giemsa stain, immunophenotyping by flow cytometry, cytogenetics, and gene analysis [FLT3 internal tandem duplication; other mutations for clinical studies only]), and lumbar puncture (if there are CNS symptoms, monocytic morphology or high blast count [after blasts cleared from blood]).

The morphologic diagnosis of AML can be supported by the presence of Auer rods in the cytoplasm, positive cytochemistry with Sudan black, and staining for myeloperoxidase (MPO) and esterases (Table 11.2). Immunophenotyping with a panel of monoclonal antibodies is particularly useful for distinguishing AML from acute lymphoblastic leukemia (ALL) and for identification of the subtypes, including AML with minimal differentiation, erythroleukemia, and megakaryoblastic leukemia (Table 11.2). Cytogenetic abnormalities associated with the morphologic subtypes further support the diagnosis and help predict treatment outcomes (Table 11.2).

PROGNOSTIC FACTORS

The most powerful prognostic factors, established over decades of clinical study, include age, cytogenetics, prior MDS, and treatment-related AML; these factors have been recently supplemented by molecular genetic abnormalities (4,5). The independent prognostic variables associated with adverse treatment outcomes include clinical prognostic factors such as age, AML arising from pre-existing MDS, treatment-related AML, performance status, and comorbid conditions. Laboratory-based prognosis factors include white blood cell count >20,000/μl at presentation, cytogenetics, molecular genetic changes (e.g., FLT3 internal tandem duplication [ITD]), CD34 positive blasts, and multidrug resistance.

Cytogenetic findings at the time of diagnosis are, next to age, the most important independent prognostic indicators for response to treatment, risk of relapse, and overall survival. Cytogenetic analysis is used to stratify patients into three risk groups with different responses to therapy (Table 11.3) (4). For example, patients in the favorable group with core binding factor mutations are most likely to obtain a long remission after consolidation with high-dose cytosine arabinoside, while patients with unfavorable cytogenetics do not benefit from this treatment. Approximately 40% to 50% of all patients have a normal karyotype at the time of diagnosis and fall into the most heterogeneous intermediate risk category (Table 11.3). Molecular genetic changes in cytogenetically normal AML that correlate with prognosis have been used to subdivide this intermediate risk group and create more refined treatment

TABLE 11.3. *Prognostic Categories Based on Karyotype*

Risk Assessment	Karyotype	Incidence
Favorable Group	t (8;21) (q22;q22)	5%–10%
	t(15;17) (q22;q12–21)	5%–10%
	Inv (16)	5%–10%
Intermediate Group	Normal Karyotype	40%–50%
	−Y	
	Rare- Del 7q, 9q, 11q, 20q,	
	+8, +13, +21	
Unfavorable Group	Complex Karyotype	10%
	−5	7%
	−7	7%
	Inv 3	1%
	11q23, 20q-, t (6;9), t(6;11),	<1% each
	t(11;19)	

algorithms (Table 11.4) (5). The best studied mutations, the internal tandem duplications (ITD) of the FLT 3 gene that codes for a tyrosine kinase receptor, are found in approximately 20% of patients with AML; patients harboring such mutations respond poorly to treatment and have significantly shorter disease-free survival (DFS) and overall survival (OS) (6). In the absence of FLT 3 mutations, patients with nucleophosmin (NPM) 1 and CEBPA mutations have improved complete remission (CR) rates and OS (Table 11.4) (7,8). Several other genetic alterations, including MLL-PTD mutations, overexpression of BAALC and ERG genes, and mutations of p53, c-KIT, BCL2, and WT1, have prognostic significance. They also provide substantial insights into pathogenesis of AML and help identify molecular targets for treatment.

The outcome for younger patients with AML has markedly improved over the last three decades because of advances in both chemotherapy and supportive care. Approximately 40% of patients under the age of 60 can be cured with current treatments. Unfortunately, little progress has been made in the long-term survival of older adults with AML. Older patients have more unfavorable disease characteristics, a higher frequency of comorbid conditions, and poor tolerance of toxic therapy. Because the median age of AML patients is 65 to 70 years, novel treatment strategies are needed for the older majority (3).

TREATMENT

Because AML is strikingly heterogeneous, therapy must be individualized. Aside from age, the most important prognostic factors that impact treatment decisions are acquired genetic changes in

TABLE 11.4. *Genetic Mutations in Cytogenetically Normal Acute Myelogenous Leukemia Correlate with Prognosis*

Mutation	Incidence	Prognostic Effects
FLT 3 Internal Tandem Duplications (ITD) (6)	17%–25%	Presence significantly reduces CR rates, DFS, and OS; most important poor prognostic factor
NPM 1 mutations (7)	46%–62%	In absence of FLT 3 improves CR, DFS, and OS
CEBPA mutations (8)	15%–20%	Presence improves CR rates and OS
MLL–PTD (9)	5%–10%	Duration of CR shorter in presence of mutation
BAALC and ERG overexpression (4)		Shorter OS with overexpression

BAALC, brain and acute leukemia, cytoplasmic; CEBPA, CCAAT/enhancer binding protein alpha; CR, complete response; DFS, disease-free survival; ERG, ETS-related gene; FLT 3, Fms-like tyrosine kinase 3; MLL–PTD, mixed lineage leukemia–partial tandem duplication; NPM, nucleophosmin; OS, overall survival.

leukemia cells as detected by conventional cytogenetics and alternative techniques such as fluorescence in situ hybridization (FISH) and polymerase chain reaction (PCR) (4,5). Treatment plans in patients with AML depend on the prognostic categories based on cytogenetics (Table 11.2). Molecular analysis of genetic mutations is used to further subdivide these groups and direct new treatment approaches (Table 11.4). The first example of a targeted treatment directed against a specific mutation is the successful use of all-trans-retinoic acid (ATRA) for APL.

The treatment for AML is generally divided into two phases: remission induction and postremission therapy. The goal of the former is to achieve a CR defined by the following criteria: less than 5% blasts in a bone marrow that is 20% or more cellular, absent extramedullary leukemia, a neutrophil count greater than 1,000/uL, and a platelet count greater than 100,000/uL. Achievement of CR as defined by these simple criteria translates into improved survival. Disappearance of karyotypic or molecular abnormalities is not required by the definition of CR, and it is therefore not surprising that clinical trials confirm an almost 100% risk of relapse when patients receive only induction chemotherapy. Long-term survival requires postremission treatment. Intensive chemotherapy given after achievement of CR (similar to that given during induction) is termed consolidation therapy.

Initial Management

The initial management of patients with AML should be well organized and executed by an experienced team.

The initial evaluation should include:

- History and physical examination
- Complete blood count with differential
- Examination of the peripheral blood smear
- Coagulation studies: prothrombin time (PT), activated partial thromboplastin time (aPTT), fibrinogen, D-dimer
- Serum chemistries with uric acid, calcium, and phosphorus
- Evaluation of renal and liver function
- Hepatitis B and C, herpes simplex virus (HSV), cytomegalovirus (CMV), varicella, and human immunodeficiency virus (HIV) serologies
- Bone marrow aspirate for morphology, cytochemistry, cytogenetics, molecular genetic studies, and flow cytometry
- Bone marrow biopsy
- Human lymphocyte antigen (HLA) typing of patient and siblings if younger than 55 years
- Lumbar puncture delayed until blasts cleared from blood in patients at high risk for CNS involvement (CNS symptoms, elevated leukocyte count, extramedullary disease, and monocytic morphology-FAB M4 or M5)
- Chest radiograph and electrocardiogram
- Evaluation of cardiac function by echocardiogram or multigated acquisition scan (MUGA) in selected patients
- Central venous access catheter placement

The initial workup is typically followed by an unhurried discussion with the patient concerning diagnosis, prognosis, side effects of therapy, impact on lifestyle, and anticipated requirements for support by family and friends. In frail elderly patients, a decision to give only supportive treatment without chemotherapy may be reached jointly by the patient and the attending physician.

The final outcome depends not only on the choice of chemotherapy but also on close monitoring, prevention, and meticulous management of complications. Many events associated with AML therapy and their timing are predictable. For example, hyperleukocytosis, tumor lysis, and DIC tend to occur early while marrow aplasia with resulting complications can be expected from the second week of chemotherapy. Patients should be monitored for side effects such as cardiotoxicity because of anthracyclines or neurotoxicity from high doses of cytosine arabinoside. Infection prophylaxis includes meticulous care for indwelling central venous catheters and prevention of mucositis. Broad spectrum intravenous antibiotics should be administered immediately if the patient becomes febrile while neutropenic. A treatment algorithm for febrile neutropenia based on local microbial sensitivity should be implemented. Prompt treatment of oral and perianal herpetic ulcerations prevents discomfort and bacterial superinfection. Drug prophylaxis against herpes viruses can prevent these complications and decrease the severity of mucositis. Consideration should be also given to prophylactic antifungal therapy to decrease fungal infections. Transfusion support with irradiated and leukodepleted blood products should be provided to prevent symptoms of severe anemia and maintain the platelet count above 10,000 per microliter. Transfusions of blood products in AML are guided by the same principles as described for acute lymphoblastic leukemia (Chapter 12).

Induction Therapy

The most commonly used chemotherapy consists of a combination of conventional doses of cytarabine, 100 to 200 mg/m^2 given by continuous intravenous (IV) infusion over 7 days, and 3 days of an anthracycline, usually daunorubicin, at 45 to 60 mg/m^2/day given as IV bolus. This "3 + 7" regimen results in CR rates of approximately 60% to 80% in patients younger than 55 to 60 years (10). If leukemia persists in the bone marrow at day 14 to 21, a second identical or modified course of chemotherapy is usually given.

Several modifications of this standard induction regimen have not substantially changed the treatment outcomes (11). These included the addition of high-dose cytarabine (HIDAC), etoposide, or topotecan or the use of an alternative athracycline. Intensifying the induction regimen through the use of HDAC or the addition of etoposide does improve DFS but not OS in younger patients (10). The modest improvement probably does not outweigh the increased toxicity and myelosuppression that accompanies the intensified regimen, especially because similar intensification can be delivered during postremission therapy.

Three randomized trials suggest that idarubicin at 12 to 13 mg/m^2 is a superior anthracycline to daunorubicin at 45 to 60 mg/m^2, particularly in younger patients. The CR rates are higher, and fewer patients require two courses of induction to achieve CR (11). The event-free survival also appears longer in idarubicin-treated patients.

Postremission Treatment

Nearly all patients in CR after induction therapy have residual disease that, without further treatment, would lead to relapse. Multiple strategies have been explored to prevent relapse: low-dose maintenance chemotherapy, intensive consolidation chemotherapy, marrow ablative therapy with autologous stem cell rescue, and allogeneic stem cell transplantation (11). Low-dose maintenance therapy is generally not helpful and has shown minimal benefit only in patients who received suboptimal induction and consolidation.

Intensive consolidation treatment improves survival in younger patients with AML. A dose-dependent response to cytarabine has been shown in randomized controlled trials (Table 11.5) (12). Consolidation with HDAC-based therapy using daily doses of 1 to 6 g/m^2 (e.g., 2 to 3 g/m^2 twice daily on days 1, 3, and 5 or twice daily for 6 days) is now standard for patents younger than 60 years. The optimal number of courses of HDAC-based consolidation has not been determined, but the evidence suggests that two to four courses are reasonable. HDAC appears to be most beneficial to younger patients with favorable cytogenetics, especially those with core-binding factor mutations (t 8;21 and inv 16) (Table 11.5). Patients over age 60 years do not benefit from HDAC consolidation (Table 11.5).

Hematopoietic Stem Cell Transplantation

High doses of marrow ablative chemotherapy and total body radiation followed by autologous or allogeneic stem cell rescue have been widely used in AML (13–16). Autologous stem cell transplantation (auto-SCT) requires stem cell collection from a patient in CR. Allogeneic stem cells are usually obtained from HLA-matched siblings, unrelated donors, or less frequently cord blood. Allogeneic SCT (allo-SCT) confers an additional immune-mediated antileukemic activity, the so-called graft-versus-leukemia (GVL) effect. Multiple prospective randomized trials comparing standard consolidation

TABLE 11.5. *High-dose Cytarabine Consolidation in Different Prognostic Subgroups*

Prognostic Groups	Cytarabine Per Dose	DFS	OS
Age <60	100 mg/m^2	24%	35%
N = 496	400 mg/m^2	29%	40%
	3 gm/m^2	44%	52%
Age >60	100 mg/m^2	<16%	9%
N = 129	400 mg/m^2	<16%	9%
	3 gm/m^2	<16%	9%
Favorable	100 mg/m^2	16%	N/A
Cytogenetics	400 mg/m^2	57%	N/A
N = 57	3 gm/m^2	78%	N/A
Intermediate	100 mg/m^2	20%	N/A
Cytogenetics	400 mg/m^2	37%	N/A
N = 140	3 gm/m^2	40%	N/A
Unfavorable	100 mg/m^2	<21%	N/A
Cytogenetics	400 mg/m^2	<21%	N/A
N = 88	3 gm/m^2	<21%	N/A

Adapted from Mayer R, Davis R, Schiffer C, et al. Intensive postremission chemotherapy in adults with acute myeloid leukemia, Cancer and Leukemia Group B. N Engl J Med 1994;331:896–903.
DFS, disease-free survival at 4 year; N/A, not available; OS, overall survival.

chemotherapy with SCT have demonstrated that allo-SCT provides the best antileukemic therapy with the lowest risk of recurrence, followed by auto-SCT, which in turn is superior to conventional chemotherapy (Table 11.6) (13–16).

The excellent antileukemic activity of allo-SCT has not translated into better overall survival (OS) in several prospective randomized trials analyzed on an intention-to-treat basis (Table 11.7). The availability of a donor has been used as a surrogate for randomization in these protocols. In some studies, the lower relapse rate was offset by the higher treatment-related mortality (TRM) rate of allo-SCT (Table 11.7) (13–16,18,19). In the most recent trial, improvement in OS after allo-SCT was present in all AML patients except those with favorable cytogenetics, with benefit most pronounced in younger patients (16). Whether the negative prognostic effects of FLT3 ITD and other mutations can be overcome by allo-SCT is yet to be determined (17).

In patients who lack an available HLA-matched sibling donor, autologous SCT offers a theoretical benefit over conventional consolidation chemotherapy because of its associated lower relapse risk. Randomized studies do not support a clear benefit for autologous SCT because of high TRM (14% in the ECOG/SWOG study and 18% in the MRC AML 10 study) (14,15). The use of peripheral blood as the source of stem cells has decreased TRM to approximately 5%, raising questions about the relevance of earlier studies to current practice. As both transplantation technology and chemotherapy continue to improve, the best treatment approach remains uncertain. Moreover, because AML is a heterogenous malignancy, the most appropriate therapy will be ultimately determined by the cytogenetic and molecular characteristics of the disease.

TABLE 11.6. *Relapse Rates Following allo-SCT, auto-SCT, and Chemotherapy in Prospective Randomized Studies*

Study	Allo-SCT	Auto-SCT	Chemotherapy
GIMEMA 8 (13)	24	40	57
MRC 10 (14)	19	35	53
ECOG/SWOG (15)	29	48	61

SCT, stem cell transplant.

TABLE 11.7. *Trials of Allogeneic Stem Cell Transplant on an Intent-to-Treat Basis*

Trial	DFS (%)		OS (%)	
	Donor	No donor	Donor	No donor
GIMEMA 8	46	33	48	40
GOELAM	44	38	53	53
MRC AML 10	50	42	55	50
ECOG/ SWOG	43	35	46	52
GIMEMA 10	51	41	58	49
HOVON-SAKK	48	37	54	46

DFS, disease-free survival; OS, overall survival.
Donor, patient with human leukocyte antigen-matched donor; No Donor, patient without donor.

Risk-based Approach to Acute Myelogenous Leukemia Treatment in Younger Patients

Favorable-Risk Cytogenetics

Patients with a favorable karyotypes (core-binding factor AML with t[8;21] or inv[16]) do well with either multiple rounds of intensive consolidation chemotherapy or autologous SCT. Long-term DFS of 60% to 70% can be achieved with these approaches in younger patients. Allo-SCT, with its higher TRM, is generally not used in this subset of patients outside clinical studies (11).

Unfavorable-Risk Cytogenetics

If an HLA-matched donor is available, patients should be evaluated for SCT as soon as possible after diagnosis. Although the CR rate in this group of patients is approximately 50%, the long-term survival rate with chemotherapy or autologous SCT has been disappointingly low (18,19). Allo-SCT from unrelated donors matched by high-resolution HLA-typing has comparable outcomes to transplants from HLA-matched family donors (11). In younger, healthier patients without an HLA-matched donor, consideration should be given to allogeneic SCT from a haploidentical family member or from umbilical cord blood. Patients with significant comorbidity who achieve CR might undergo allo-SCT with reduced-intensity conditioning. New therapeutic agents given on clinical trials should be offered to the majority of patients without a donor.

Intermediate-Risk Cytogenetics

Treatment decisions are particularly complex in this largest and most heterogenous prognostic group of patients. Until outcome data are available for subgroups classified on the basis of molecular abnormalities such as FLT3, CEBPA, and NPM1, treatment decisions should be carefully individualized based on patient age, comorbidity, type of transplant donor, and risk of relapse. If an HLA-matched family donor is available, allo-SCT should be offered to patients less than 55 to 60 years of age who have a good performance status, given the superior antileukemic activity of this therapy. Auto-SCT, following intensive consolidation for in vivo purging, is another approach in patients without an HLA-matched donor. In general, the benefit of allo-SCT over auto-SCT or HDAC consolidation will be seen in subgroups of younger healthier patients, for whom the improvement in relapse risk outweighs the higher procedural mortality. A recent study suggests that patients with a risk of relapse greater than 35% benefit from allo-SCT (16). Meta-analysis of approximately 4000 patients showed a 12% OS survival benefit in patients undergoing allo-SCT (16). In the future, further risk stratification using newly defined molecular markers such as activating FLT3 mutations may help treatment decisions.

Treatment of Acute Promyelocytic Leukemia

Acute promyelocytic leukemia (APL) is the first example of leukemia in which therapy directed against the leukemogenic event (the t[15;17]) resulting in the PML-RARα fusion transcript) improved clinical outcome. With better management of the associated coagulopathy and the introduction of the differentiating agents ATRA and arsenic trioxide (ATO), APL now represents the most curable subtype of AML (11).

The current standard approach consists of a combination of ATRA and anthracycline-based chemotherapy for induction, followed by at least two courses of anthracycline-based chemotherapy and ATRA for consolidation, and maintenance therapy with intermittent ATRA alone (15 days every 3 months) or combined with 6-mercaptopurine and methotrexate. This regimen produced CR rates of over 80% and cure rates of over 70%. Recent data suggest that maintenance therapy may not be necessary after more intensive induction and consolidation (11). ATO has emerged as the most active drug in APL. ATO for induction and consolidation is currently explored in randomized trials. In a recent phase III randomized trial, arsenic trioxide used as first postremission therapy in addition to standard induction consolidation significantly prolonged DFS (81% vs. 66% at 3 years) and OS (86% vs. 79% at 3 years) (20). Early findings suggest that the combination of ATO and ATRA used as induction therapy can result in higher CR rates, lower relapse, and milder side effects than the same regimen used with chemotherapy. Thus, APL may become the first acute leukemia that can be successfully treated without chemotherapy.

The goal of induction and consolidation therapy should be PCR negativity for the PML-RARα rearrangement, because the persistence of such minimal residual disease predicts relapse. For patients with ATRA-resistant disease, ATO is the salvage therapy of choice. A U.S.-based multicenter study in 40 relapsed patients showed CR rates of 85%, molecular responses in 77%, and an OS of 66% (21). Consolidation strategies after ATO, such as combinations with chemotherapy, SCT, or gemtuzumab ozogamicin, are under investigation.

Despite the introduction of ATRA and improvement in the treatment of coagulopathy, bleeding remains an important early cause of death. For this reason, APL should be treated as a medical emergency. ATRA and aggressive supportive measures should be initiated as soon as the diagnosis is suspected, even before confirmatory genetic tests are available. The coagulopathy is treated with FFP, fibrinogen, and platelets with the goal to maintain fibrinogen level above 150 mg/dL and platelets well above 30×10^9/L until resolution of the coagulopathy (11). The APL differentiation syndrome emerged as a major toxicity associated with both ATRA and ATO, characterized by pleural and pericardial effusions, weight gain, edema, dyspnea, fever, episodic hypotension, and pulmonary infiltrates. The syndrome should be promptly treated with intravenous administration of dexamethasone at a dose of 10 mg twice a day. The incidence of this complication is reduced in patients receiving concomitant chemotherapy during induction. Patients receiving ATO should be also closely monitored for prolongation of QT interval, and their electrolytes should be maintained within normal range (11).

Treatment of Relapsed and Refractory Acute Myelogenous Leukemia

Unfortunately, AML relapses in the majority of patients. Moreover, approximately 25% of younger patients are refractory to standard induction chemotherapy. If a suitable HLA-matched donor is available, the first option should be allo-SCT (11). Patients transplanted at the time of relapse have similar outcomes to those treated in second CR. If a suitable donor is not available, management is guided by the duration of the first CR. For patients in CR more than 12 months, reinduction with HDAC-containing regimen can achieve a CR rate of 50% to 60% and a 5% to 10% long-term DFS. For patients with shorter CR durations, the priority should be treatment on a research protocol. Novel agents under investigation include clofarabine, farnesyltransferase inhibitors, and FLT3 inhibitors (Table 11.8). Clinical trials should be considered in all relapsed and refractory patients because response rates with current drugs remain dismal.

Hematopoietic Growth Factors

Colony-stimulating factors (CSFs) can shorten the duration of neutropenia during chemotherapy and can improve outcomes. Both granulocyte macrophage-colony stimulating factor (GM-CSF) and granulocyte-colony stimulating factor (G-CSF) accelerate neutrophil recovery after induction chemotherapy. G-CSF and GM-CSF have also been used to sensitize blasts to chemotherapy by recruiting cells into the cell cycle, but numerous clinical trials failed to show a reproducible survival benefit of such an approach. In general, CSFs administered during induction chemotherapy shorten the period of neutropenia by 2 to 7 days, reduce infections in some patients, but have no consistent beneficial effect on survival or CR rate (22).

TABLE 11.8. *Clinical Experience with Novel Agents in Acute Myelogenous Leukemia*

Drug Class and Examples	Clinical Outcomes
FLT 3 inhibitors: CEP 701, PKC 412, MLN 518	Trials of monotherapy produced very low CR rates (5%–10%) Combination with conventional chemotherapy shows early promising results, Phase III trials are in progress.
Farnesyl transferase inhibitors: Tipifarnib, Lonafarnib, BMS 214662, L 778	Phase II trial of Tipifarnib in older patients showed CR in 18% with OS of 5–6 months.
Hypomethylating agents: Azacytidine, Decitabine	Phase II trial of Azacytidine in 20 patients with AML showed RR 60%, CR 20%, and median OS of 15 months in responders. Phase II trial of Decitabine in high-risk MDS showed CR in 28% of patients. Combination with ATRA-CR 14%, median OS of 7.5 months.
Nucleoside analogue: Clofarabine	Combination with cytarabine for induction in 60 patients with age >50 yrs showed 52% CR, OS of 5.5 months.
Alkylating agent: Cloretazine	Elderly patients with AML had a CR rate of 49% with OS of 22% at 1 year.
Histone deacetylase inhibitors: Valproic acid	Phase I/II trial in combination with Decitabine in 10 patients showed 50% response rate, remission duration of 7 months, median OS of 15 months.
Proteosome inhibitor: Bortezomib	Small study of 12 patients with relapsed disease showed 33% CR.
Bcl-2 antisense: Oblimersen	Phase II study of 29 elderly patients showed 48% CR.
Toxin conjugated monoclonal antibody-: Gemtuzumab	Gemtuzumab with daunorubicin in 53 untreated patients less than 60 yrs of age produced CR of 83%.
m TOR inhibitors: Sirolimus	Showed modest activity as single agent, in trials with chemotherapy.
VEGF inhibitors: Bevacizumab	Phase II trial with chemotherapy showed 33% CR.
Vaccines: WT-1 and Proteinase 3	Phase I/II trials showed cytotoxic T-cell responses in the majority of patients that correlated with clinical responses, CRs were rare.
P glycoprotein inhibitor: Zosuquidar, PSC 833	Zosuquidar in combination with standard chemotherapy showed CR of 69% in 16 patients.

ATRA, all-trans-retinoic acid; Bcl, B-cell lymphoma; CR, complete remission; FLT 3, Fms-like tyrosine kinase 3; m TOR, mammalian target of Rapamycin; MDS, myelodysplastic syndrome; OS, overall survival; VEGF, vascular endothelial growth factor.

Acute Myelogenous Leukemia in Older Patients

Older adults have a dismal prognosis that has not changed significantly over the last three decades (1,2). Care of these patients is challenging because of the higher rates of unfavorable prognostic features including comorbidity, high-risk cytogenetics, and multidrug resistance of leukemic blasts (2). Patients over the age of 60 years who do not have significant comorbidities can receive standard "3 + 7" induction therapy. Their outcomes worsen with advancing age, because early death rate and treatment resistance increase. The group of patients who benefit most from standard chemotherapy can be reasonably selected by the following criteria: age 60 to 69 years, no secondary AML or pre-existing MDS, good performance status, no pretreatment infection, and normal bilirubin and creatinine (2). Results from MD Anderson Cancer Center in this small subgroup of patients show a 70% CR rate and a median survival of 14 months (2). Choice of postremission therapy for older patients remains problematic. In contrast to younger patients, no studies with HDAC-based therapy have demonstrated a survival advantage in patients over 60 years of age (12). As this population represents the majority of patients with AML, new strategies are needed to improve outcomes. For the majority of elderly patients, clinical trials with novel agents should be considered at the time of diagnosis because the poor results of conventional therapy (Table 11.8). Modestly successful options available outside the clinical trial setting include azacytidine, decitabine, and low-dose cytarabine. Azacytidine was used as outpatient therapy in a phase II trial of 20 patients with AML who were treated with 75 mg/m^2/day for 7 days every 4 weeks (23). Therapy was well tolerated (20% hospitalized during first cycle) with overall response rate of 60%, CR 20%, and median OS of 15 months in responders. Azacytidine has become a first-line option for patients who cannot tolerate intensive induction or for those who do not enter a research trial. Low-dose decitabine in patients with high-risk MDS and elderly patients with AML has produced CR rates of 14% to 28% and is better tolerated than standard induction (Table 11.8) (24). In the elderly unfit for more intensive treatment, low-dose cytarabine (20 mg subcutaneously twice daily for 10 days every 4 to 6 weeks) was superior to hydroxyurea or best supportive care (25). Choice among these regimens is based on individual preference, because any comparison of efficacy or toxicity is problematic across different studies. In some patients, especially those with poor performance status, abnormal organ function, or active infection, palliative care may be the best choice.

Acute Myelogenous Leukemia in Pregnancy

The management of pregnant patient with AML is daunting. Delaying chemotherapy until delivery may be detrimental to the mother, whereas chemotherapy, particularly in the first trimester, poses serious risk to the fetus. The results of one single institution study demonstrated an absence of congenital malformations in 17 live births after exposure to chemotherapy in the second and third trimester. CR rates were no different than that in nonpregnant patients. Furthermore, three of four mothers who delayed treatment until after delivery died shortly after the initiation of chemotherapy (26). Therefore, induction chemotherapy should be undertaken once the patient is beyond the first trimester.

Evaluation of Minimal Residual Disease

The detection of minimal residual disease (MRD) predicts outcome in some patients with AML. The quantitation of residual AML cells could allow individualization of therapy and thereby increase the likelihood of cure. The goal of MRD detection is to identify patients at higher risk for relapse and assign them to different therapeutic approaches. MRD assessment could also serve as a surrogate endpoint for evaluation of efficacy of new treatments. Both multiparametric flow cytometry and PCR have been used to monitor MRD in AML (27). Flow cytometry can detect one leukemic cell in up to 10^3 to 10^4 normal cells and is applicable to about 80% of patients with AML in whom malignant cells express a unique constellation of surface markers that is different from normal cells. PCR has greater sensitivity, detecting up to 1 in 10^6 cells, but because it depends on the presence of a known genetic marker, it is applicable to only about 40% of AML cases.

The significance of a positive MRD in AML varies depending on the type of leukemia, the therapy used, and the timing of detection. The levels of residual disease that have predictive value must always be determined in specific types of AML at defined time points during therapy. For example, the achievement of molecular remission in APL patients is critical to obtaining long-term DFS, whereas persistence of the PML-RARα rearrangement after consolidation predicts relapse. In contrast, a positive molecular result in patients with t(8;21) AML does not necessarily indicate impending relapse (27). Although very promising in APL, the clinical significance and utility of evaluating MRD in other subtypes of AML remains unproven. Caution should be taken in applying MRD detection techniques to clinical practice outside prospective clinical trials.

Novel Therapeutic Targets in Acute Myelogenous Leukemia

Standard treatment for AML is based on aggressive cytotoxic chemotherapy administered in repeated cycles to achieve disease eradication. However, only a minority of patients are cured by this approach. The success of ATRA and ASO in APL demonstrates that more selective and less toxic drugs can substantially increase cure rates of AML. The current challenge is to find new molecular targets that can be attacked by specific agents with favorable toxicity profiles (28). With improved understanding of the mechanisms underlying leukemogenesis, several novel classes of drugs have entered clinical trials (Table 11.8) (28). These include antibody-based therapies, FLT3 inhibitors and other tyrosine kinase inhibitors, farnesyltransferase inhibitors (FTIs), clofarabine, inhibitors of methylation, angiogenesis agents, and vaccines (Table 11.8) (28–31). Most appear to have limited activity as single agents, and their full potential may be only realized in combination therapies (28).

Gemtuzumab ozogamicin (Mylotarg, Wyeth, Madison, NJ) is a humanized anti-CD33 monoclonal antibody covalently linked to a semisynthetic derivative of the potent cytotoxic agent calicheamicin. Mylotarg has been approved by the Food and Drug Administration as a single agent for first-relapse AML in older patients in whom response rates approach 30% (32). Gemtuzumab ozogamicin used in combination with chemotherapy has been associated with high CR rates in phase II studies, and this promising approach is being tested in phase III trials (28). Although nonhematologic toxicities of gemtuzumab ozogamicin are mild, its association with hepatic veno-occlusive disease may limit its clinical applicability, especially in patients who are transplant candidates.

Farnesyltransferase Inhibitors (FTIs) represent a new class of small-molecule inhibitors that selectively inhibit farnesylation of a number of intracellular proteins such as Ras. The FTI tipifarnib is well tolerated and has activity as single agent in newly diagnosed and relapsed AML (30). Its efficacy in combination with chemotherapy is under investigation. FLT3 kinase inhibitors have generated interest because activating FLT3 mutations in AML confer poor prognosis. Similar to other targeted therapies, these agents appear to be well tolerated and are in trials in combination with chemotherapy (Table 11.8) (28,29). There is a plethora of new agents and drug combinations that need to be tested in AML. Patients with AML, including the elderly, should be encouraged to enroll in well-designed clinical trials.

SUMMARY

AML represents a genetically, morphologically, and clinically heterogeneous group of hematopoietic malignancies characterized by a rapid growth of myeloid blasts and suppression of normal hematopoiesis. The initiating genetic events and the pathways involved in the pathogenesis of AML are the subject of intense laboratory investigations. These events and pathways determine the type of AML, response to therapy, and, to some extent, the final outcome of the disease. The well-established prognostic factors including age and cytogenetic changes are being expanded by molecular characteristics. Mutation testing is now used to develop prognostic models and identify treatment targets. Unfortunately, less than half of younger patients and fewer than 10% of patients over 60 years are cured of AML by current therapies. In younger patients, the longest DFS can be achieved with repeated cycles of intensive chemotherapy containing anthracyclines and cytarabine. Postremission consolidation therapy is crucial, while maintenance is not necessary with the exception of APL. HDAC is the consolidation of choice for younger patients with favorable cytogenetics, while those with intermediate or unfavorable cytogenetics who have an HLA-matched donor may benefit from allo-SCT. Questions remain about the optimal drugs for induction and the length of consolidation, but it is unlikely that refining standard chemotherapy will result in dramatic improvement in survival. Aggressive chemotherapy is not suitable for older patients, who can derive modest benefit from hypomethylating agents or low-dose cytarabine. New targeted treatments including antibodies, tyrosine kinase inhibitors and other drugs targeting signal transduction, inhibitors of drug resistance, and vaccines have shown some activity and acceptable toxicity in clinical studies. Combinations of these agents based on studies of cell biology will hopefully lead to higher cure rates than the unselective cytotoxic therapy.

REFERENCES

1. Appelbaum FR, Gundacker H, Head DR, et al. Age and acute myeloid leukemia. Blood 2007;109:3481–3485.
2. Estey E. Acute myeloid leukemia and myelodysplastic syndromes in older patients. J Clin Oncol 2007;25:1908–1915.
3. Deschler B, Lubbert M. Acute myeloid leukemia: Epidemiology and etiology. Cancer 2006;107:2009–2107.

4. Frohling S, Scholl C, Gilliland DG. Genetics of myeloid malignancies—pathogenetic and clinical implications. J Clin Oncol 2005;23:6285–6295.

5. Bienz M, Ludwig M, Oppliger LE, et al. Risk assessment in patients with acute myeloid leukemia and a normal karyotype. Clin Cancer Res 2005;11:1416–1424.

6. Whitman SP, Archer KJ, Feng L, et al. Absence of the wild-type allele predicts poor prognosis in adult de novo acute myeloid leukemia with normal cytogenetics and the internal tandem duplication of FLT3: A Cancer and Leukemia Group B study. Cancer Res 2001;61:7233–7239.

7. Schnittger S, Schoch C, Kern W, et al. Nucleophosmin gene mutations are predictors of favorable prognosis in acute myelogenous leukemia with a normal karyotype. Blood 2005;106: 3733–3739.

8. Fröhling S, Schlenk RF, Stolze I, et al. CEBPA mutations in younger adults with acute myeloid leukemia and normal cytogenetics: prognostic relevance and analysis of cooperating mutations. J Clin Oncol 2004;22:624–633.

9. Schnittger S, Kinkelin U, Schoch C, et al. Screening for MLL tandem duplication in 387 unselected patients with AML identify a prognostically unfavorable subset of AML. Leukemia 2000;14:796–804.

10. Stone RM, O'Donnell MR and Sekeres MA. Acute myeloid Leukemia. Hematology Am Soc Hematol Educ Program 2004;98–117.

11. Tallman MS, Gilliland G, Rowe JM. Drug therapy for acute myeloid leukemia. Blood 2005; 106:1154–1163.

12. Mayer R, Davis R, Schiffer C, et al. Intensive postremission chemotherapy in adults with acute myeloid leukemia, Cancer and Leukemia Group B. N Engl J Med 1994;331:896–903.

13. Zittoun RA, Mandelli F, Willemze, et al. Autologous or allogeneic bone marrow transplantation compared to intensive chemotherapy for acute myeloid leukemia in first remission. EORTC and GIMEMA Leukemia Cooperative Groups. N Engl J Med 1995;332:217–223.

14. Burnett AK, Goldstone AH, Stevens RM, et al. Randomized comparison of addition of autologous bone-marrow transplantation to intensive chemotherapy for acute myeloid leukaemia in first remission: results of MRC AML 10 trial. Lancet 1998;351:700–708.

15. Cassileth PA, Harrington DP, Appelbaum FR, et al. Chemotherapy compared with autologous or allogeneic bone marrow transplantation in the management of acute myeloid leukemia in first remission. N Engl J Med 1998;339:1649–1656.

16. Cornelissen JJ, Van Putten WLJ, Verdonck LF, et al. Results of a HOVON/SAKK donor versus no-donor analysis of myeloablative HLA-identical sibling stem cell transplantation in first remission acute myeloid leukemia in young and middle-aged adults: benefits for whom? Blood 2007;109:3658–3666.

17. Gale R, Hills R, Kottaridis PD, et al. No evidence that FLT3 status should be considered as an indicator for transplantation in acute myeloid leukemia (AML): an analysis of 1135 patients excluding promyelocytic leukemia from the UK MRC AML10 and 12 trials. Blood 2005;106:3658–3665.

18. Harousseau JL, Cahn JY, Pignon B, et al. Comparison of autologous bone marrow transplantation and intensive chemotherapy as postremission therapy in adult acute myeloid leukemia. The Groupe Ouest Est Leucemies Aigues Myeloblastiques (GOELAM). Blood 1997;90:2978–2986.

19. Suciu S, Mandelli F, de Witte T, et al. EORTC and GIMEMA Leukemia Groups. Allogeneic compared with autologous stem cell transplantation in the treatment of patients younger than 46 years with acute myeloid leukemia (AML) in first complete remission (CR1): an intention-to-treat analysis of the EORTC/GIMEMA AML-10 trial. Blood 2003;102:1232–1240.

20. Powell BL, Moser B, Stock W. Effect of consolidation with arsenic trioxide (As_2O_3) on event-free survival (EFS) and overall survival (OS) among patients with newly diagnosed acute promyelocytic leukemia (APL): North American Intergroup Protocol C9710. J Clin Oncol 2007;25 18S 2007:2.

21. Soignet SL, Frankel SR, Douer D, et al. United States multicenter study of Arsenic Trioxide in Relapsed Acute Promyelocytic Leukemia. J Clin Oncol 2001;19:3852–3860.

22. Rowe JM, Andersen JW, Mazza JJ, et al. A randomized placebo-controlled Phase III trial of granulocyte macrophage colony-stimulating factor in adult patients with acute myelogenous leukemia: a study of the Eastern Cooperative Oncology Group (E1490). Blood 1995;86:457–462.

23. Sudan N, Rossetti JM, Shadduck RK, et al. Treatment of acute myelogenous leukemia with out-patient azacytidine. Cancer 2006;107:1839–1843.
24. Lubbert M, Ruter B, Schmid M, et al. Continued low-dose decitabine is an active first-line treatment of older AML patients: first results of a multicenter phase II study. Blood 2005;106:527.
25. Burnett AK, Milligan D, Prentice AG, et al. A comparison of low-dose cytarabine and hy-doxyurea with or without ATRA for acute myeloid leukemia and high-risk MDS in patients not considered fit for intensive treatment. Cancer 2007;109:1114–1124.
26. Greenlund LJ, Letendre L, Tefferi A. Acute Leukemia during pregnancy: a single institutional experience with 17 cases. Leuk Lymphoma 2001;41:571–577.
27. Yin JL, Grimwade D. Minimal residual disease evaluation in acute myeloid leukemia. Lancet 2002;360:160–162.
28. Aribi A, Ravandi F, Giles F. Novel agents in acute myeloid leukemia. Cancer J 2006;12:77–91.
29. Smith BD, Levis M, Beran M, et al. Single-agent CEP-701, a novel FLT3 inhibitor, shows bio-logic and clinical acitivity with relapsed or refractory acute myeloid leukemia. Blood 2004;103:3669–3676.
30. Harousseau JL, Lancet JE, Reiffers J, et al. A Phase 2 study of the oral farnesyltransferase inhibitor tipifarnib in patients with refractory or relapsed acute myeloid leukemia. Blood 2007;109:5151–5156.
31. Faderl S, Gandhi V, O'Brien S, et al. Results of a phase 1 to 2 study of clofarabine in combination with cytarabine (ara-C) in relapsed and refractory acute leukemias. Blood 2005;105: 940–947.
32. Giles F, Estey E, O'Brien S. Gemtuzumab ozogamicin in the treatment of acute myeloid leukemia. Cancer 2003;98:2095–2104.

12

Acute Lymphoblastic Leukemia

Alan S. Wayne

Approximately 5000 new cases of acute lymphoblastic leukemia (ALL) are diagnosed each year in the United States, more than half of these in children. ALL represents the most common pediatric malignancy, accounting for approximately 25% of childhood cancer. The peak prevalence of ALL is between the ages of 2 and 9 years. There is a slight male predominance, and Caucasians have a twofold increased risk compared with African Americans.

ETIOLOGY AND RISK FACTORS

There are a variety of conditions that predispose to ALL, most notably trisomy 21 (Down's syndrome) where the relative risk is increased 15-fold. Other predisposing conditions include immunodeficiency and chromosomal breakage syndromes, but most often no such underlying disorder is found. Epstein-Barr virus (EBV) infection is implicated in a minority of cases of mature B-cell ALL. Environmental exposure risks have been suggested, but few (radiation) have been shown to be causal. Acquired chromosomal abnormalities confined to the lymphoblasts are found in more than 90% of cases, including aneuploidy (most commonly hyperdiploidy) and/or translocations that in some cases have been shown to be prenatal in origin. The genes involved in leukemogenesis are frequently transcription factors expressed in hematopoietic tissues.

CLINICAL FEATURES

Presenting signs and symptoms are almost always caused by blast infiltration of the bone marrow with resultant blood count abnormalities (Table 12.1). Other organs may also be involved. T-cell ALL frequently presents with bulky adenopathy, mediastinal mass, pleural effusion, and/or hyperleukocytosis. Gastrointestinal presentation because of Peyer's patch involvement, usually ileocecal intussusception, is almost always confined to mature B-cell ALL. There are a number of life- or organ-threatening presentations that require emergent intervention (Table 12.2).

LABORATORY FEATURES

Diagnosis is readily confirmed by the demonstration of lymphoblasts in the blood and/or bone marrow. Blast morphology can be classified into three categories (L1, L2, L3) according to the French-American-British (FAB) system (Table 12.3). Only the latter is of clinical and prognostic significance, because L3 morphology is indicative of mature B-cell or Burkitt-type ALL. Routine hematopathologic staining, immunohistochemistry, flow cytometry, and cytogenetics are used to define the subtype and further identify prognostic factors. The majority of ALL is of precursor B-cell (pre-B) phenotype (CD10, CD19, CD22, HLA-DR, TDT+), 10% to 20% is T-cell (CD2, CD7+), and less than 5% is mature B-cell or Burkitt-type (CD20, surface-IgM κ or λ +). Certain cytogenetic abnormalities are not apparent on routine karyotyping and thus molecular testing may be required, most notably for t(12;21) in children (Table 12.4). Lumbar puncture is required to evaluate for the possibility of meningeal leukemia.

TABLE 12.1. *Presenting Features*

Common Presenting Signs and Symptoms	Sites of Involvement
70% Hepatosplenomegaly 60% Fever 50% Fatigue 50% Lymphadenopathy 40% Bleeding 40% Bone or joint pain 20% Anorexia 10% Abdominal pain	100% Bone marrow 10% Anterior mediastinal mass 5% Central nervous system (CNS) 2% Testicular <5% Other (e.g., eye, skin, pericardium, pleura, kidney, breast, ovary, priapism, intussusception)

TABLE 12.2. *Emergency Presentations*

Emergent Presentation	Intervention
Leukostasis	Oxygen, leukapheresis
Neutropenia with fever or infection	Broad spectrum IV antibiotics
Thrombocytopenia	Platelet transfusion
Disseminated intravascular coagulation	Fresh frozen plasma, cryoprecipitate
Tumor lysis syndrome	IV hydration, allopurinol or rasburicase, and supportive measures as clinically indicated (e.g., dialysis)
Airway obstruction	Oxygen, corticosteroids, and/or radiation
Superior vena cava syndrome	Corticosteroids and/or radiation
Pericardial tamponade	Pericardiocentesis, corticosteroids
Intussusception	Surgical decompression
CNS manifestations	Corticosteroids and/or radiation
Ocular involvement	Radiation
Spinal cord compression	Corticosteroids and/or radiation

CNS, central nervous system; IV, intravenous.

TABLE 12.3. *Classification*

FAB Morphology
L1: homogeneous blasts, minimal cytoplasm
L2: increased nuclear heterogeneity, prominent nucleoli
L3: basophilic cytoplasm with prominent vacuolization

Bone Marrow
M1: <5% blasts
M2: 5%–25% blasts
M3: >25% blasts

Cerebrospinal Fluid Cytology
CNS-1: no blasts
CNS-2: WBC <5/μL with blasts
CNS-3: WBC ≥5/μL with blasts
    or symptomatic CNS involvement (e.g., cranial nerve palsy)

CNS, central nervous system; FAB, French-American-British; WBC, white blood cell count.

TABLE 12.4. *Common Chromosomal Translocations*

t(12;21): *TEL/AML1* (25% childhood ALL)
t(1;19): *E2A/PBX1*
t(9;22): *BCR/ABL* p190 fusion (25% adult ALL)
11q23: *MLL*, multiple fusion partners (70% infant ALL)
14q11 or 7q35: *TCR*, T-cell phenotype
t(8;14), t(8;22), t(2;8): c-*myc/Ig*, mature B-cell (Burkitt) phenotype

ALL, acute lymphoblastic leukemia.

PROGNOSTIC FACTORS

Disease-free-survival (DFS) rates have improved steadily for children with ALL and currently approximately 80% will achieve cure. Results are inferior in infants and adolescents. In adults, cure rates decline with advancing age, with overall DFS rates of approximately 40%. T-cell and mature B-cell disease have historically faired poorer than pre-B phenotype; however, stratified treatment has minimized this difference. A number of clinical and biologic features are used to stratify risk-directed treatment for individuals with pre-B ALL (Table 12.5) (1). Recently, cDNA microarray gene expression analysis has been shown to allow further discrimination in regard to diagnostic subtype, risk classification, and treatment response prediction (2).

TREATMENT

Many chemotherapy regimens have been shown to be effective for children and adults with ALL. Therapy is stratified based on clinicopathologic features, and treatment should be directed by physicians familiar with subtype-specific regimens. The following core recommendations are based on results of large cooperative group clinical trials (3–11).

Therapy should be instituted as soon as possible after diagnosis. Treatment is stratified based on phenotype and prognostic factors and includes the following phases: induction, consolidation, central nervous system (CNS) sterilization, and maintenance for a total of 2 to 3 years (Table 12.6A). Initial induction therapy often consists of 3 to 5 drugs given as a 28-day cycle, although there are alternative approaches (12). There are a variety of consolidation and intensification regimens in common use, some of which are detailed below. Multiple consolidation/intensification blocks are often used for high-risk patients. A late reinduction phase, also known as delayed intensification, improves DFS for children who are slow early responders (SER) (Table 12.6B) (13). Randomized trials of various intensification blocks for adults have shown mixed results (14,15). Prolonged maintenance with total treatment duration of 24 to 36 months improves DFS for both adults and children.

TABLE 12.5. *Risk Group Assignment in B-Precursor Acute Lymphoblastic Leukemia*

	Standard Risk	High Risk	Very High Risk	Ultra High Risk
Age (years)	1–9	10–35	>35	< 1
WBC (/μL)	<50,000	≥50,000		
CNS	Negative	Positive		
Chromosomes	t(12;21), Double or Triple Trisomy 4/10/17	11q23, t(1;19)		t(9;22)
DNA Index	≥1.16, ≤1.60			<0.81
Treatment Response	RER		SER	Induction failure

CNS, central nervous system; RER, rapid early responder; SER, slow early responder; WBC, white blood cell count.

TABLE 12.6A. *Common Treatment Regimens for Pre-B-cell Acute Lymphoblastic Leukemia and T-cell Acute Lymphoblastic Leukemia**

A: Induction (weeks 1–4)

3-Drug (Standard Risk)
- Prednisone 40–60 mg/m^2/day *or* Dexamethasone 6 mg/m^2/day in divided doses PO × 21–28 days (Day 0–)
- Vincristine 1.5 mg/m^2/dose (maximum dose 2 mg) IV weekly × 4 doses (Days 0, 7, 14, 21)
- E. coli L-Asparaginase 6,000–10,000 IU/m^2/dose IM × 6–9 doses, QOD, 3 days per week × 2–3 weeks
- IT Methotrexate:
  - CNS-1: Every 2 weeks × 2 doses (Days 0, 14).
  - CNS-2 or CNS-3: Weekly × at least 4 doses and until 2 successive CNS-1 (Days 0, 7, 14, 21).

4-Drug (High Risk): Add the following to above
- Doxorubicin 25–30 mg/m^2/dose *or* Daunorubicin 25–45 mg/m^2/dose IV weekly × 4 doses (Days 0, 7, 14, 21) *or* IV daily × 2–3 doses (Days 0, 1, +/− 2)

5-Drug (Higher risk groups): Add the following to above
- Cyclophosphamide 800–1,200 mg/m^2/dose IV × 1 dose (Day 0)

Response Evaluation
Day 14 Bone Marrow
- M1: Rapid Early Responder
- M2 or M3: Slow Early Responder

Day 28 Bone Marrow
- M1: remission, continue as below
- M2 or M3: induction failure, salvage reinduction required

*A bcr/abl kinase inhibitor should be incorporated into the treatment regimen for individuals with Philadelphia chromosome-positive acute lymphoblastic leukemia. QOD, every other day.

Allogeneic Stem Cell Transplantation

Although relapse rates are lower after allogeneic tem cell transplantation (SCT) compared with chemotherapy, treatment-related mortality rates are higher after transplantation (16). Thus, SCT is rarely used for children in first remission (CR1). Given the relatively poor results of chemotherapy in older individuals, some groups recommend allogeneic SCT in CR1 for adults with human leukocyte antigen (HLA)-matched sibling donors.

Autologous Stem Cell Rescue

High-dose therapy followed by stem cell rescue can be used as consolidation therapy in ALL, but multiple randomized trials have shown no significant DFS advantage compared with chemotherapy. Because of the increased risks associated with autologous transplant, this approach is not frequently used.

Risk Group Assignment for B-Precursor ALL

Although there is some variability in the approach to risk-adapted therapy, the aforementioned designations are suggested based on published pediatric cooperative group data (Table 12.5). Age, white blood cell (WBC) count, central nervous system (CNS) involvement, DNA index, and phenotype are used for the initial risk group assignment (1). Subsequently, the risk group may be elevated based on cytogenetics and response to induction, the latter of which is defined by morphologic blast reduction (in peripheral blood on day 7 or bone marrow on day 7 or 14) and/or minimal residual disease determination (by flow cytometry or polymerase chain reaction amplification). Prognostic factors are similar in adults, although the strong adverse influence of older age has limited further refinements in treatment stratification. Patients with ultra-high-risk features require more intensive treatment, and allogeneic SCT in CR1 is commonly considered for those with HLA-matched siblings.

TABLE 12.6B. *Common Treatment Regimens for Pre-B-cell Acute Lymphoblastic Leukemia and T-cell Acute Lymphoblastic Leukemia**

B: Postinduction

Pretreatment criteria
- ANC $\geq$750/μL, platelets $\geq$75,000/μL
- ALT <20 times the upper limit of normal, direct bilirubin normal for age
- Serum creatinine normal for age
- No active infection or life-threatening organ dysfunction

Consolidation (Week 5)

Standard Berlin-Frankfurt-Munster Study Group (BFM)
- Cyclophosphamide 1,000 mg/m^2/dose IV $\times$ 2 doses (Days 0, 14)
- Mercaptopurine (6-MP) 60 mg/m^2/dose PO once daily (administer at bedtime on an empty stomach to improve absorption) $\times$ 28 days (Days 0–27)
- Vincristine 1.5 mg/m^2/dose (maximum dose 2 mg) IV $\times$ 4 doses (Days 14, 21, 42, 49)
- Cytarabine 75 mg/m^2/dose IV or SQ (Days 1–4, 8–11, 15–18, 22–25)
- IT Methotrexate weekly $\times$ 4 doses (Days 1, 8, 15, 22)

Augmented BFM
- Cyclophosphamide 1000 mg/m^2/dose IV $\times$ 2 doses (Days 0, 28)
- Mercaptopurine (6-MP) 60 mg/m^2/dose PO once daily (administer at bedtime on an empty stomach to improve absorption) $\times$ 28 days (Days 0–13, 28–41)
- Vincristine 1.5 mg/m^2/dose (maximum dose 2 mg) IV $\times$ 4 doses (Days 14, 21, 42, 49)
- Cytarabine 75 mg/m^2/dose IV or SQ (Days 1–4, 8–11, 29–32, 36–39)
- *E. coli* L-Asparaginase 6000 IU/ m^2/dose IM $\times$ 12 doses, every other day 3 doses per week (Days 14, 16, 18, 21, 23, 25, 42, 44, 46, 49, 51, 53)
- IT Methotrexate weekly $\times$ 4 doses (Days 1, 8, 15, 22)

High-Dose Methotrexate with Leucovorin Rescue
- Refer to protocol-specific dosing, administration, and leucovorin rescue guidelines

Capizzi
- Cytarabine (Ara-C) 3,000 mg/m^2/dose IV over 3 hours every 12 hours $\times$ 4 doses, weekly $\times$ 2 (Days 0, 1 and Days 7, 8)
- *E. coli* L-asparaginase 6,000 IU/m^2/dose IM at hour 42 following Ara-C (3 hours after the completion of the fourth Ara-C infusion on Days 1 and 8)

Ifosfamide/Etoposide
- Etoposide (VP-16): 100mg/m^2/dose IV $\times$ 5 doses (Days 1–5)
- Ifosfamide: 1.8 gm/m^2/dose IV $\times$ 5 doses (Days 1–5). Begin immediately upon completion of VP-16 infusion
- Mesna: 360 mg/m^2/dose IV prior to ifosfamide and every 3 hours $\times$ 8 doses/day (Days 1–5)

Interim Maintenance
- Commonly used between Consolidation and Delayed Intensification/Reinduction courses

Delayed Instensification/Reinduction
- Dexamethasone 10 mg/m^2/day in divided doses PO $\times$ 14–28 days (Day 0–)
- Vincristine 1.5 mg/m^2/dose (maximum dose 2 mg) IV weekly $\times$ 5 doses (Days 0, 14, 21, 42, 49)
- Doxorubicin 25–30 mg/m^2/dose IV weekly $\times$ 3 doses (Days 0, 7, 14)
- Cyclophosphamide 1,000 mg/m^2/dose IV (Day 28)
- 6-Thioguanine (6-TG) 60 mg/m^2/dose PO once daily $\times$ 14 days (Days 28–41)
- Cytarabine 75 mg/m^2/dose IV or SQ (Days 29–32, 36–39)
- IT Methotrexate $\times$ 2 doses (Days 29, 36)

With or Without:
- *E. coli* L-Asparaginase 6,000 IU/m^2/dose IM $\times$ 6–12 doses (Days 3, 5, 7, 10, 12, 14 +/− 42, 44, 46, 49, 51, 53)

ALT, alanine-aminotransferase; ANC, absolute neutrophil count; IM, intramuscular; IV, intravenous; PO, oral; SQ, subcutaneous.

Infant Acute Lymphoblastic Leukemia

Children younger than 1 year of age at diagnosis should be treated on age-specific protocols with certain agents dosed on a per-kilogram basis to decrease the risk of severe toxicity.

T-Cell Acute Lymphoblastic Leukemia

Patients with T-cell phenotype are treated similarly to higher risk group pre-B ALL. Improved outcome has been associated with the use of intensified therapy that commonly includes high-dose methotrexate and intensified L-asparaginase (17,18).

Mature B-Cell Acute Lymphoblastic Leukemia

Patients with mature B-cell phenotype ALL should be treated with Burkitt's lymphoma regimens. These are most commonly dose and sequence intensive, short course chemotherapy regimens that include hyperfractionated cyclophosphamide, high-dose methotrexate, and high-dose cytarabine (19,20).

Central Nervous System-Directed Therapy

All patients require CNS sterilization. Intensive intrathecal chemotherapy in combination with systemic agents that have good CNS penetration, most notably dexamethasone and high-dose methotrexate, are highly effective (Table 12.7). To minimize neurotoxicity, radiation is usually reserved for those with active meningeal leukemia or at high risk of CNS relapse (e.g., T-cell phenotype with hyperleukocytosis) (Table 12.8).

Testicular Leukemia

Males with testicular involvement should receive radiation to both testes (Table 12.8).

DOSE MODIFICATION

Improved outcome is associated with greater drug exposure; thus, attempts should be made to deliver protocol-specified doses unless toxicity prevents such. Importantly, 6-MP and methotrexate doses should be increased during maintenance to achieve a targeted degree of myelosuppression (Table 12.6C). In the event of significant chemotherapy-related toxicity, individual agents should be dose-reduced or discontinued as clinically indicated. Specific agents may require dose adjustment for renal or hepatic dysfunction. Patients with thiopurine S-methyltransferase deficiency (approximately 1:300 incidence) require significant dose reduction of 6-MP. Individuals with Down's syndrome tolerate methotrexate poorly.

TABLE 12.6C. *Common Treatment Regimens for Pre-B-cell Acute Lymphoblastic Leukemia and T-cell Acute Lymphoblastic Leukemia**

C: Maintenance/Continuation
Repeat cycles to complete 24–36 months of total treatment.
- Prednisone 40–60 mg/m^2/day *or* Dexamethasone 6 mg/m^2/day in divided doses PO × 5 days every 28 days
- Vincristine 1.5 mg/m2/day (maximum dose 2 mg) IV every 4 weeks
- Mercaptopurine (6-MP) 75 mg/m^2/dose* PO once daily (administer at bedtime on an empty stomach to improve absorption)
- Methotrexate 20 mg/m^2/dose* PO once weekly
- IT Methotrexate every 4–12 weeks for 1–2 years of treatment

*6-MP and methotrexate doses should be adjusted to maintain the ANC between 750–1500/μL and the platelet count >75,000/μL.
IM, intramuscular; IT, intrathecal; IV, intravenous; PO, oral; SQ, subcutaneous.

Transfusions

Blood transfusion should be used to prevent complications related to severe cytopenias. To decrease the risk of transfusion-associated complications, specialized products should be used.

To prevent bleeding, platelet counts should routinely be maintained above 10,000 per microliter. Higher levels are recommended for management of bleeding, prior to invasive procedures such as lumbar puncture, and to reduce the risk of leukostasis-induced CNS hemorrhage in the setting of hyperleukocytosis. Single donor platelets are recommended whenever possible to decrease donor exposure and the risk of HLA-alloimmunization (27).

Concomitant anemia partially offsets the hyperviscosity associated with severe hyperleukocytosis. Thus, RBC transfusion should be avoided if possible when the WBC is higher than 100,000 per microliter. If transfusion is necessary, the hemoglobin and hematocrit should be increased slowly using small aliquots of packed RBCs until the peripheral blast count is reduced.

To reduce the risk of transfusion associated graft-versus-host disease, all cellular blood products should be irradiated.

Platelets and red cells should be leukoreduced to decrease the risk of febrile reactions, HLA-alloimmunization with subsequent platelet-refractoriness, and transmission of cytomegalovirus (CMV) infection.

Infection Prophylaxis

Aggressive surveillance, prophylaxis, and treatment for bacterial, fungal, viral, and opportunistic infections are essential to prevent morbidity and mortality.

Pneumocystis Carinii *Pneumonia*

All patients should receive *Pneumocystis carinii* pneumonia (PCP) prophylaxis (e.g., trimethoprim/sulfamethoxazole) continuing until 6 months after chemotherapy is completed.

Management of Neutropenic Fever

Patients with an absolute neutrophil count (ANC) less than 500 per microliter and temperature of 38.3°C or higher should be evaluated for possible infection and treated empirically with parenterally administered broad-spectrum antibiotics. Antifungal therapy should be initiated for neutropenic fever that persists for 5 to 7 days. Antibiotics should be continued until the ANC rises to more than 500 per microliter, fever resolves, cultures are negative, and any suspected infection is fully treated.

Intravenous Immunoglobulin

Hypogammaglobulinemia is common during treatment for ALL. Immunoglobulin G (IgG) levels should be assayed for those with recurrent infections, and if low, intravenous immunoglobulin supplementation should be considered (approximately 500 mg/kg every 4 weeks as needed to maintain an IgG level of 500 mg/dL).

Myeloid Growth Factors

Granulocyte colony-stimulating factor (G-CSF) during induction has been shown to improve outcome for adults, although no benefit was demonstrated in a pediatric study. Myeloid growth factor support should be used during treatment of mature B-cell ALL (i.e., Burkitt's or L3) in both children and adults.

Chemotherapy Prophylaxis

Agent-specific prophylaxis should be utilized as clinically indicated. For example, gastritis prophylaxis is recommended during corticosteroid administration. To reduce the risk of conjunctivitis associated with high-dose Ara-C, corticosteroid ophthalmic solution should be administered during and for 24 to 48 hours after treatment. Mesna should be used in an attempt to prevent hemorrhagic cystitis associated with high-dose ifosfamide and cyclophosphamide.

Nutritional Support

Nutritional status should be monitored and supplementation provided as indicated. Routine folic acid use should be avoided with methotrexate administration because it may counteract the therapeutic efficacy of folate antagonism. (In contrast, leucovorin rescue is indicated to prevent severe toxicity after high-dose methotrexate.)

Psychosocial Support

Multidisciplinary support for the patient and family is an important part of successful treatment.

EVALUATIONS

Serial evaluations to monitor for response, relapse, complications, and therapy-associated toxicity should be conducted throughout all treatment phases.

Evaluations during Treatment

History, physical examination, and routine laboratory assessments including CBC and chemistry panel should be performed regularly throughout treatment. Bone marrow aspiration should be obtained at the following times:

- Induction day 7 or 14 to assess early response.
- Induction day 28 to assess remission status. If indeterminate, repeat weekly until recovery to confirm remission or induction failure.
- At the end of therapy.

Bone marrow should also be performed at suspicion of relapse.

Flow cytometry, cytogenetics, and/or molecular genetic studies can be used to monitor minimal residual disease, which is prognostic. CSF cell count and cytospin should be performed at the time of all intrathecal chemotherapy administrations. Lumbar puncture should also be performed for suspicion of CNS relapse.

Evaluations after Treatment

Follow-up evaluations to include history, physical examination, and routine laboratory studies (CBC, chemistry panel) should be conducted to monitor for toxicity and recurrent disease until at least 5 years posttreatment on the following schedule (or as clinically indicated):

- Every 1 to 2 months during the first year.
- Every 2 to 3 months during the second year.
- Every 3 to 4 months during the third year.
- Every 6 months during the fourth year.
- Yearly thereafter.

Late Effects

Lifelong follow-up to monitor for a variety of possible late complications of treatment is recommended (28,29). The following are among the most frequent late effects.

Cardiomyopathy

To decrease the risk of cardiotoxicity, cumulative anthracycline doses are usually limited to less than 400 mg/m^2. Echocardiograms for left ventricular function determination should be performed at baseline, at completion of treatment, every 1 to 2 years after treatment until serial studies remain normal, and as clinically indicated.

Neurologic Toxicity

Children are at especially high risk of neurotoxicity from chemotherapy and radiation. All patients should be monitored for neurologic toxicity including neurodevelopmental dysfunction.

Endocrinologic Dysfunction

Patients should be monitored for endocrinopathies including growth retardation and infertility.

Osteonecrosis

Corticosteroids, especially dexamethasone, are associated with a high incidence of osteonecrosis in survivors of ALL.

Secondary Malignancy

Patients should be monitored for secondary malignancies because these continue to develop even in the second decade after treatment (28,29).

REFERENCES

1. Smith M, Arthur D, Camitta B, et al. Uniform approach to risk classification and treatment assignment for children with acute lymphoblastic leukemia. J Clin Oncol 1996;14:18–24.
2. Holleman A, Cheok MH, den Boer ML, et al. Gene-expression patterns in drug-resistant acute lymphoblastic leukemia cells and response to treatment. N Engl J Med 2004;351:533–542.
3. Pui C-H, Crist WM. Acute lymphoblastic leukemia. In: Pui C-H, ed. Childhood Leukemias, 1st Ed. New York: Cambridge University Press; 1999:288–312.
4. Pui C-H, Rellins MV, Downing JR. Acute lymphoblastic leukemias. N Engl J Med 2004;350: 1535–1548.
5. Schrappe M, Reiter A, Ludwig W, et al. Improved outcome in childhood acute lymphoblastic leukemia despite reduced use of anthracyclines and cranial radiotherapy: results of trial ALL-BFM 90. Blood 2000;95:3310–3322.
6. Pui C-H, Boyett JM, Rivera GK, et al. Long-term results of Total Therapy studies 11, 12, and 13A for childhood acute lymphoblastic leukemia at St. Jude Children's Research Hospital. Leukemia 2000;14:2286–2294.
7. Silverman LB, Gelber RD, Dalton VK, et al. Improved outcome for children with acute lymphoblastic leukemia: results of Dana-Farber Consortium Protocol 91-01. Blood 2001;97: 1211–1218.
8. Faderl S, Jeha S, Kantarjian HM. The biology and therapy of adult acute lymphoblastic leukemia. Cancer 2003;98:1337–1354.
9. Gökbuget N, Hoelzer D. Recent approaches in acute lymphoblastic leukemia in adults. Rev Clin Exp Hematol 2002;6:114–141.
10. Larson RA, Dodge RK, Burns CP, et al. A five-drug induction regimen with intensive consolidation for adults with acute lymphoblastic leukemia: Cancer and Leukemia Group B Study 8811. Blood 1995;84:2025–2037.
11. Annino L, Vegna ML, Camera A, et al. Treatment of adults with acute lymphoblastic leukemia (ALL): long-term follow-up of the GIMEMA ALL 0288 randomized study. Blood 2002;99: 863–871.
12. Kantarjian HM, O'Brien S, Smith TL, et al. Results of treatment with hyper-CVAD, a dose-intensive regimen, in adult acute lymphocytic leukemia. J Clin Oncol 2000;18:547–561.
13. Nachman JB, Sather HN, Sensel MG, et al. Augmented post-induction therapy for children with high-risk acute lymphoblastic leukemia and a slow response to initial therapy. N Engl J Med 1998;338:1663–1671.

14. Richards S, Burrett J, Hann I, et al. Improved survival with early intensification: combined results from the Medical Research Council childhood ALL randomised trials, UKALL X, and UKALL XI. Leukemia 1998;12:1031–1036.

15. Durrant IJ, Prentice HG, Richards SM. Intensification of treatment for adults with acute lymphoblastic leukemia: results of U.K. Medical Research Council randomized trial UKALL XA. Br J Haematol 1997;99:84–92.

16. Barrett AJ, Horowitz MH, Pollock BH, et al. Bone marrow transplants from HLA-identical siblings as compared with chemotherapy for children with acute lymphoblastic leukemia in a second remission. N Engl J Med 1994;331:1253–1258.

17. Reiter A, Schrappe M, Ludwig WD, et al. Intensive ALL-type therapy without local radiotherapy provides a 90% event-free survival for children with T-cell lymphoblastic lymphoma: a BFM group report. Blood 2000;95:416–421.

18. Amylon MD, Shuster J, Pullen J, et al. Intensive high-dose asparaginase consolidation improves survival for pediatric patients with T-cell acute lymphoblastic leukemia and advanced stage lymphoblastic lymphoma: a Pediatric Oncology Group study. Leukemia 1999;13:335–342.

19. Thomas DA, Cortes J, O'Brien S, et al. Hyper-CVAD program in Burkitt's type adult acute lymphocytic leukemia. J Clin Oncol 1999;17:2461–2470.

20. Magrath I, Adde M, Shad A, et al. Adults and children with small non-cleaved-cell lymphoma have a similar excellent outcome when treated with the same chemotherapy regimen. J Clin Oncol 1996;14:925–934.

21. Wassmann B, Pfeifer H, Goekbuget N, et al. Alternating versus concurrent schedules of imatinib and chemotherapy as front-line therapy for Philadelphia-positive acute lymphoblastic leukemia (Ph+ALL). Blood 2006;108:1469–1477.

22. Wayne AS, Kreitman RJ, Pastan I. Monoclonal antibodies and immunotoxins as new therapeutic agents for childhood acute lymphoblastic leukemia. In: Govindan R, ed. American Society of Clinical Oncology 2007 Educational Book. Alexandria, VA: American Society of Clinical Oncology; 2007:596–601.

23. Buchanan GR, Boyett JM, Pollock BH, et al. Improved treatment results in boys with overt testicular relapse during or shortly after initial therapy for acute lymphoblastic leukemia. A Pediatric Oncology group study. Cancer 1991;68:48–55.

24. Ritchey AK, Pollock BH, Lauer SJ, et al. Improved survival of children with isolated CNS relapse of acute lymphoblastic leukemia: a pediatric oncology group study. J Clin Oncol 1999;17:3745–3752.

25. Hahn T, Wall D, Camitta B, et al. The role of cytotoxic therapy with hematopoietic stem cell transplantation in the therapy of acute lymphoblastic leukemia in children: an evidence-based review. Biol Blood Marrow Transplant 2005;11:823–861.

26. Coiffier B, Altman A, Pui CH, et al. Guidelines for the management of pediatric and adult tumor lysis syndrome: an evidence-based review. J Clin Oncol 2008,26(16):2767–2778.

27. Slichter SJ. Optimizing platelet transfusions in chronically thrombocytopenic patients. Semin Hematol 1998;35:269–278.

28. Pui C-H, Cheng C, Leung W, et al. Extended follow-up of long-term survivors of childhood acute lymphoblastic leukemia. N Engl J Med 2003;49:640–649.

29. Oeffinger KC, Mertens AC, Sklar CA, et al: Chronic health conditions in adult survivors of childhood cancer. New Engl J Med 2006;355:1572–1582.

13

Chronic Myelogenous Leukemia

John A. Barrett and Agnes S. M. Yong

Although chronic myelogenous leukemia (CML) is rare, it has achieved disproportionate prominence in the medical literature because its biologic basis has been elucidated in unprecedented detail. Furthermore, CML has become a model for developing effective molecularly targeted and immune-based treatments for leukemia. Nowell and Hungerford first reported the occurrence of a unique, unusually small G group chromosome in patients with CML and named it the Philadelphia (Ph) chromosome in 1960 (1)—the first association of a human malignant disease with a consistent chromosomal marker. In 1973, the Ph chromosome was identified as the truncated chromosome 22 consequent to a reciprocal translocation involving chromosome 9. It was not until the 1980s that the fusion partners of the translocation were identified as the c-*abl* oncogene on chromosome 9 and the breakpoint cluster region (BCR) on chromosome 22 (2–4). The BCR-ABL oncoprotein was found to have tyrosine kinase activity, and when the gene was inserted into mouse stem cells it induced leukemia in recipient animals (5). Until recently, allogeneic stem cell transplantation (SCT) was the preferred first-line treatment in eligible CML patients because the disease is highly susceptible to a graft-versus-leukemia effect from transplanted donor lymphocytes (6). The advent of imatinib mesylate (Gleevec, Novartis Pharmaceuticals Corporation, East Hanover, NJ), the first of a new class of small molecule drugs designed specifically to block the BCR-ABL tyrosine kinase, has supplanted SCT for many patients because these drugs seem to confer durable disease control, particularly in the earlier stages of CML (7,8). Despite progress in CML biology and treatment, fundamental questions about its origin remain unanswered. Evidence suggests that a predisposition to develop CML precedes the clonal expansion of BCR-ABL translocated stem cells (9), and the discovery of very low levels of BCR-ABL in the blood of individuals who do not develop CML raises the possibility that the BCR-ABL translocation is not alone sufficient to cause leukemia (10). The astounding success of imatinib has led to the development and availability of other drugs targeting tyrosine kinases (11). However, the emergence of drug resistance, only a proportion of which are attributable to mutations of the ABL kinase domain, is a serious clinical issue but also of great biologic interest. Unfortunately, advanced phases of CML still are largely refractory to available treatments.

EPIDEMIOLOGY

- Rare: incidence of 1 to 1.5 in 100,000.
- Represents 10% to 15% of all leukemias.
- Incidence increases with age (median age of diagnosis = 66); exceedingly rare in children.
- Male predominance (1.5:1).
- Worldwide distribution: no sociogeographic preponderance.
- Ionizing radiation is the only known causative factor; leukemia occurs usually within 6 to 8 years of exposure.
- No known genetic factors determine susceptibility to CML.

PATHOPHYSIOLOGY

Leukemic Hematopoiesis Originates in a Multipotent Stem Cell

BCR-ABL translocation is found in all cells of the myeloid lineage (erythroid and granulocyte precursors and megakaryocytes) as well as in B cells but not in T cells (12). There are two major hypotheses for this observation: first, the acquisition of BCR-ABL may occur in a multipotent stem cell with little or no T differentiation capacity; second, T cells bearing BCR-ABL may be systematically eliminated. Unregulated proliferation of BCR-ABL-positive stem cells is responsible for massive expansion, primarily in granulocyte production, that leads to leucocytosis.

Clonal Dominance

The BCR-ABL-positive clone outcompetes normal hematopoiesis. At diagnosis it is common to find a mixed population of Ph-positive and Ph-negative cells in the bone marrow. With time, normal stem cells are progressively replaced by CML stem cells. CML CD34+ progenitor cells require less hematopoietic growth factors than do normal progenitors for survival and proliferation, a characteristic that may be partially because of the presence of an autocrine production of hematopoietic growth factors by CML cells (13).

Molecular Basis of CML in the BCR-ABL Translocation

The BCR-ABL oncoprotein is a constitutively activated tyrosine kinase that phosphorylates intermediate molecules in several important pathways, affecting proliferation, maturation, resistance to apoptosis and cell adhesion, ultimately resulting in the typical leukemic phenotype (14).

Genomic Instability

CML is characterized by progression to refractory acute leukemia. CML usually starts as a relatively benign disorder that evolves to an accelerated phase (AP), when the leukemia is much more difficult to control and additional chromosomal abnormalities appear, followed by a progressive increase in blast cells in blood and marrow, termed the blastic phase (BP) or blast crisis, when the disease transforms to an acute myeloid or B lymphocytic leukemia. Clonal evolution, which is matched by increasing malignant behavior of the leukemia, has a variable pace but is inevitable.

PRESENTATION

Classic Presentation

Classic presentation includes insidious history of increasing fatigue, lassitude, weight loss, night sweats, massive splenomegaly, and gout. Some patients have leucocyte counts greater than 300,000/uL and experience symptoms of leucostasis with headache, focal neurologic deficits, and priapism.

Typical Presentation in the Developed World

Overt symptoms and signs are rarely encountered because the diagnosis is made earlier. Commonly, patients present with fatigue, with or without moderate weight loss, abdominal discomfort and early satiety from an enlarged spleen, or simply because the chance observation of an elevated leucocyte count. CML should be considered in the differential diagnosis of a patient at any age presenting with splenomegaly and with white blood cell count.

Rare Presentations

Rare presentations of CML include chloroma, petechiae, and bruising. These features suggest progression of CML to an accelerated or blastic phase.

Unlike other leukemias, CML seldom if ever presents with bacterial or fungal infection because neutrophil function is preserved.

DIAGNOSIS

While blood and bone marrow examinations share features with other myeloproliferative disorders, the typical presentation with high leucocyte count and a hypercellular marrow with basophilia is pathognomonic of CML. Chromosome and molecular analysis confirm the presence of a BCR-ABL translocation.

Blood Count

The leucocyte number varies between being slightly elevated to over 200,000 per cubic millimeter; counts as high as 700,000 per cubic millimeter are occasionally encountered. The platelet count is normal or elevated, and there is often a mild normochromic normocytic anemia.

Blood Film

Blood film is of great diagnostic value, because many of the typical features of CML are unique—a left shift with circulating myeloblasts, myelocytes, metamyelocytes, and band forms. The hallmark of CML is *basophilia*, with basophil counts often exceeding 1000 per cubic millimeter. Sustained basophilia is almost never encountered outside CML and some cases of mastocytosis. Eosinophilia and occasional nucleated red blood cells are also common findings. Platelet morphology is usually normal, but giant forms can be seen.

Bone Marrow

The bone marrow aspirate shows cellular spicules, and the biopsy is hypercellular with almost complete effacement of the fat spaces. There is granulocytic hyperplasia of the neutrophil, eosinophil, and basophil series. Megakaryocytes are normal or increased and may show reduced numbers of nuclei. Sea-blue histiocytes are commonly seen in CML marrows. Fibrosis of the marrow is a feature of accelerated phase CML, as is an increase in blasts over 15%. Blastic phase shows than 20% blasts.

Chromosome Analysis

The typical karyotype of CML shows the reciprocal translocation t(9;22)(q34;q11) (Fig. 13.1). Variants include three-way translocations between chromosomes 9, 22 and 11, or 19. An additional

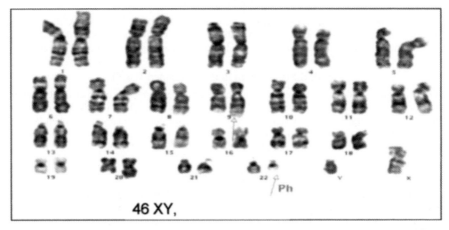

FIG. 13.1. The Philadelphia chromosome. G-banded metaphase preparation showing the diminutive Ph-positive chromosome and extra chromosomal material on the long arm of chromosome 9.

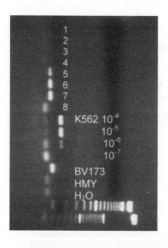

FIG. 13.2. Polymerase chain reaction for BCR-ABL. Patients 1, 2, 3, 4, and 8: negative for BCR-ABL at a sensitivity of less than 10^6 copies. Patients 5, 6, 7 BCR-ABL–positive (b2a2 translocation) *Positive control* K562 cell line (b3a2) and BV173 cell line (b2a2). *Negative control* HMY cell line and H_2O.

chromosome abnormality or Ph chromosome duplication indicates disease progression to accelerated or blastic phase. Fluorescence in situ hybridization (FISH) is a rapid and sensitive technique to detect the Ph chromosome directly in blood or marrow because it does not rely on dividing cells.

Molecular Diagnosis

More than 95% of patients presenting with the clinical and morphologic features of CML will have Ph chromosomes in the marrow. Of the 5% who are Ph-negative, half have a cryptic BCR-ABL transcript detected by Southern blot or by polymerase chain reaction (PCR) (Fig.13.2). The remaining patients are described as having atypical Ph-negative CML. A few such cases are morphologically indistinguishable from Ph-positive CML, but most have atypical features on careful examination and are considered to have a form of myelodysplastic syndrome or neutrophilic leukemia. Molecular analysis provides further information of the precise transcript. Depending on the BCR breakpoint, four common *BCR-ABL* transcript variants are possible: e13a2 and e14a2 [formerly b2a2 and b3a2], both encoding the 210 kD BCR-ABL oncoprotein (p210); e1a2, which is more common in Ph-positive acute lymphoblastic leukemia, encoding the 190 kD BCR-ABL oncoprotein (p190); and e19a2, which encodes the 230 kD BCR-ABL oncoprotein of chronic neutrophilic leukemia. No prognostic or diagnostic significance is attached to either the e13a2 or the e14a2 variant in CML. Rarely, unusual transcript variants, such as e1a3 or e6a2, have also been described (15).

Other Laboratory Features

Neutrophil alkaline phosphatase (NAP) stain is typically low or absent in CML, believed to be a consequence of low levels of G-CSF. Serum elastase levels, lactic dehydrogenase, and vitamin B_{12} are elevated.

DIFFERENTIAL DIAGNOSIS

The diagnosis of CML is made in three stages (Fig. 13.3):

- Persisting leucocytosis without any obvious infective cause suggests a myeloproliferative disease, prompting further examination of the blood and bone marrow.
- Morphology and blood count will show either typical features of CML (basophilia being especially significant) or suggest other myeloproliferative disorders (high platelet counts, essential thrombocythemia; high red cell count, polycythemia vera; teardrop red cells, myelofibrosis). Dysplasia suggests a hyperproliferative myelodysplastic syndrome.

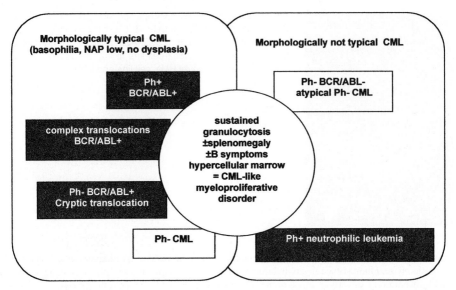

FIG. 13.3. Differential diagnosis of chronic myelogenous leukemia (CML) and related disorders.

- Definitive diagnosis requires chromosome analysis of the bone marrow. Cytogenetics will identify the Ph-positive chromosome and the BCR-ABL translocation in all but a small percentage of patients with a morphologic diagnosis of CML. Confirmation of the presence of *BCR-ABL* transcripts by PCR is advised because its aids in disease monitoring following treatment (16).

COURSE OF CHRONIC MYELOGENOUS LEUKEMIA

CML is a multistage disease that progresses from chronic phase (CP) to an accelerated phase (AP) and then to a blastic phase (BP) (Fig. 13.4).

Chronic Phase

Untreated patients in CP show a gradual rise in the leucocyte count with emergence of splenomegaly and ultimately the full picture of a myeloproliferative disorder with B symptoms, weight loss, and hyperleucocytosis.

The duration of CP is highly variable. Some patients progress within months of diagnosis directly to AP and BP, while others can remain for more than a decade in stable CP. Sometimes patients present in AP or BP without a clear preceding CP. In this circumstance, it is important to distinguish CML presenting as acute leukemia from de novo (Ph-negative) acute leukemia because the treatment approaches are distinct.

Median time to progression from CP to AP has been slowly increasing, in part because of better treatment (8) and in part because the diagnosis of CML tends to be made earlier.

Accelerated Phase

AP is characterized by one or more of the following (Table 13.1):

- Clonal evolution by a further mutation. Patients may acquire new chromosomal abnormalities such as a second Ph chromosome.
- Escape of the blood counts from treatment control.

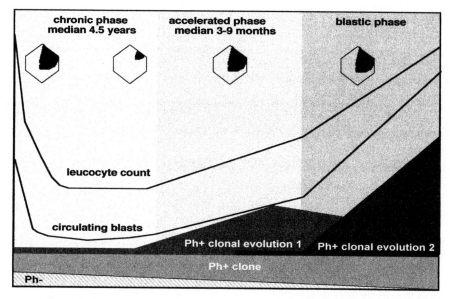

FIG. 13.4. Course and clonal evolution of chronic myelogenous leukemia (CML).

- Organomegaly.
- Leucocytosis, basophilia, thrombocytosis, or thrombocytopenia in a patient previously well controlled with therapy.
- Myelofibrosis with teardrop cells in the blood smear and increased marrow reticulin.
- Chloromas in external soft tissues, the retroperitoneal spaces, paraspinal areas (leading to nerve root compression), and in intramedullary spaces.

Blastic Phase

- Signs and symptoms of acute leukemia: bone pains, weight loss, and B symptoms, increasing numbers of blasts in the blood and marrow.
- Marrow failure: decreasing red cell count and platelets. (Neutrophil counts are better conserved.)
- Clonal evolution: further chromosomal abnormalities.

TABLE 13.1. *Characteristics Distinguishing Chronic Myelogenous Leukemia at Different Stages of Evolution*

	CP	AP	BP
Blasts in blood	<15%	>15%–30%	>30%
Blasts in marrow	<20%	>20%–50%	>50%
Basophils	<20%	>20%	
Karyotype	Ph+	Second Ph+	7q-, t(15;17), other
NAP score	Low	Low	Normal
Marrow fibrosis		+	+
Escape from control		+	+
Cytopenias			+

AP, acute phase; BP, blastic phase; CP, chronic phase; NAP, neutrophil alkaline phosphatase.

CHARACTERIZATION OF THE ACUTE LEUKEMIA IN BLASTIC PHASE

Approximately 60% of patients develop myeloid blastic phase resembling acute myeloid leukemia (AML); the remainder have lymphoid blastic phase reminiscent of acute lymphoblastic leukemia (ALL). In both phenotypes, blasts are poorly differentiated. Auer rods are not seen, and the lymphoid or myeloid origin of the leukemia is only reliably determined by cytochemical stains and surface phenotype, revealing either a pre-B ALL (PAS block-positive, TdT-positive, $CD10^+$, $CD19^+$, $CD33^\pm$, $CD34^\pm$) or an undifferentiated AML (peroxidase weak-positive, $CD33^+$, $CD34^+$, $CD13^\pm$). A peculiar feature of CML is the variability of its subsequent evolution. Patients achieving remission from AML can re-enter a chronic phase only to relapse again with ALL or vice versa.

PROGNOSTIC FACTORS

Poor prognosis (tendency to rapid progression to BP):

- High leucocyte counts ($>100,000$ per cubic millimeter)
- Massive splenomegaly and constitutional symptoms
- Patients of African origin
- High basophil counts

Of predictive scores using patient characteristics at diagnosis that were validated in the pre-imatinib era to determine outcome and survival (17,18), the Sokal score still appears to be prognostic in patients who are treated with imatinib (8,19,20).

TREATMENT OF CHRONIC MYELOGENOUS LEUKEMIA

Treatment of CML involves diverse, evolving approaches outlined in the algorithm in Figure 13.5 (16). The drugs commonly used to treat CML are detailed in Table 13.2.

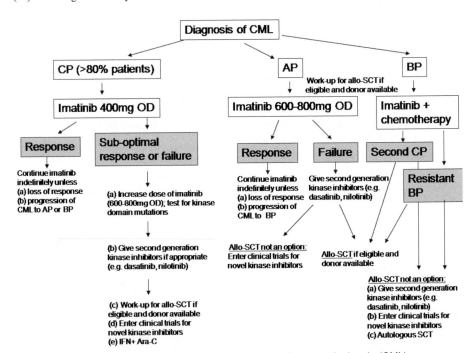

FIG. 13.5. Treatment algorithm for chronic myelogenous leukemia (CML).

TABLE 13.2. *Commonly Used Drugs to Treat CML*

Indication	Drug	Dose
Cytoreduction at presentation or for more advanced disease	Hydroxyurea	po 0.5–2.5 g daily
Standard treatment of CP	Imatinib	po 300–800 mg daily
Second line treatment CP/AP	Dasatinib	po 70 mg twice daily
	Nilotinib	po 400 mg twice daily
Remission induction BP (AML)	Daunorubicin	iv 45 mg/m^2 × 2–3 days
	Cytosine arabinoside	sc or iv 200 mg/m^2 12 hourly × 5–7 days
Remission induction BP (ALL)	Vincristine	iv 2 mg/m^2 weekly × 4
	Prednisone	60 mg/m^2 daily × 4 weeks
	+/− Daunorubicin	iv 45 mg/m^2 week 1

ALL, acute lymphoblastic leukemia; AML, acute myelogenous leukemia; AP, accelerated phase; BP, blastic phase; CP, chronic phase; iv, intravenous; po, oral; sc, subcutaneous.

CML treatment is guided by disease monitoring using regular blood counts and bone marrow examination to document hematologic changes, chromosome analysis of marrow or FISH analysis of blood or marrow to detect response or progression at the karyotypic level, and PCR for *BCR-ABL* mRNA transcripts in the blood to quantify response at the molecular level. The degree of disease bulk reduction determines the appropriate monitoring approach, and the degree of response is defined as hematologic response, cytogenetic response, and molecular response or molecular cure (16) (Fig. 13.6).

Treating Newly Diagnosed Chronic Myelogenous Leukemia in Chronic Phase

The large majority (>80%) of patients with CML are diagnosed in CP. Initial treatment is aimed at reducing disease bulk and obtaining hematologic remission (normalization of blood counts). Subsequent therapy is tailored towards achieving either a "cure" or "minimal residual disease" (MRD).

- Imatinib, 400 mg daily.
- Add hydroxyurea 1 to 2 g daily for patients with leucocyte counts over 100,000 per cubic millimeter or with massive splenomegaly.
- Allopurinol, 300 mg daily until blood counts normalize.

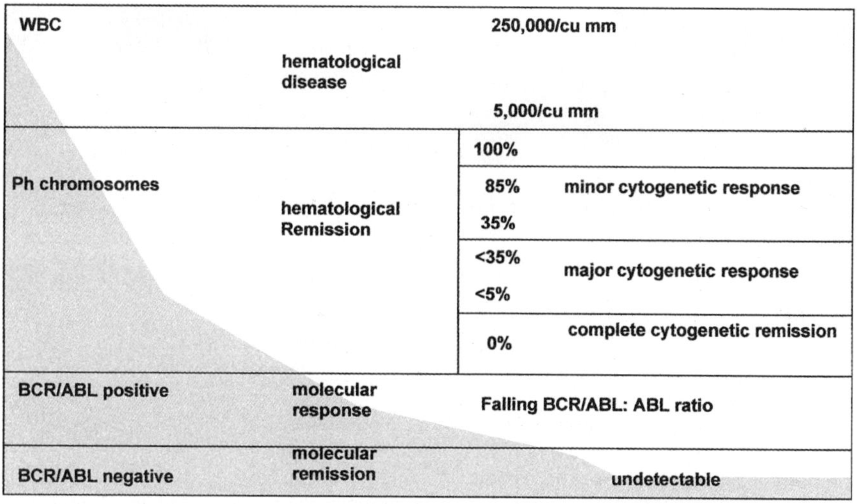

FIG. 13.6. Disease monitoring in chronic myelogenous leukemia (CML).

Monitoring Response to Imatinib

Full blood counts should be monitored every 2 weeks until complete hematologic response (HR), equivalent to normalization of blood counts, is achieved. Complete HR should be confirmed on two subsequent occasions (16).

Bone marrow aspiration should be performed every 6 months to assess cytogenetic response, analyzing at least 20 metaphases for the Ph chromosome. Patients who achieve complete cytogenetic response (0% Ph) have a prolonged period without disease progression (see definitions in Fig. 13.6). The cytogenetic response improves over time in responding patients, and once complete cytogenetic response is achieved and confirmed on 2 subsequent occasions, bone marrow examinations for cytogenetics can be performed every 12 months to detect possible onset of dysplasia or clonal changes in the Ph negative cells (21).

Quantitative PCR for *BCR-ABL* transcripts in the blood should be performed at least every 3 months. Serial *BCR-ABL* measurements are clinically useful to document if patients are responding to treatment with declining transcripts, have stable (plateau) levels of transcripts, or are losing their response as signaled by rising transcripts. Reduction of *BCR-ABL* transcripts by three or more logs below a standardized baseline value for untreated patients (major molecular response) is associated with particularly good outcome.

Achieving Minimal Residual Disease

Administer imatinib at the maximum tolerated dose (to 800 mg daily), and continue treatment indefinitely, unless loss of response occurs (see below).

Over 85% of patients with CML-CP treated with imatinib from diagnosis achieve a complete cytogenetic response (0% Ph), and of these, 80% have a 3 log reduction in *BCR-ABL* transcripts by 4 years follow-up (8). This MRD status is associated with longer survival. Upfront treatment with imatinib may reduce the number of leukemic progenitors at risk of clonal evolution and disease progression. Patients with CP-CML who are treated with imatinib from diagnosis and achieve complete cytogenetic response appear to have decreasing annual rates of disease progression to AP or BP with longer follow-up (8). Although the ultimate duration of imatinib treatment is still unclear, current recommendations are to continue treatment until relapse or progression of disease (16). A complete molecular remission (undetectable *BCR-ABL* transcripts in the blood by PCR) is achieved by less than 10% of patients in complete cytogenetic remission, and imatinib has been discontinued in a few such patients. But the majority of these patients have relapsed at variable intervals, suggesting that imatinib does not totally eradicate CML (22,23).

Suboptimal Response or Loss of Response to Imatinib Treatment

Failure to achieve a hematologic remission with a combination of imatinib and hydroxyurea is uncommon unless the disease has already progressed to AP.

Failure of imatinib treatment:

- No HR in 3 months
- No cytogenetic response (Ph >95%) in 6 months
- Less than partial cytogenetic response (Ph >35%) in 12 months
- No complete cytogenetic response (any Ph detected) in 18 months
- Loss of previously achieved responses—e.g., loss of complete HR, or complete cytogenetic response (16)

Suboptimal response to imatinib treatment:

- No complete HR in 3 months
- Less than partial cytogenetic response (Ph >35%) in 6 months
- No complete cytogenetic response (any Ph detected) in 12 months
- No major molecular response in 18 months
- Loss of previously achieved responses: loss of major molecular response; additional chromosomal abnormalities in Ph+ cells in serial bone marrow examinations (16)

Patients who lose an initial response to imatinib may have developed drug resistance because of point mutations of the *BCR-ABL* gene, which result in amino acid changes in the catalytic domain of the BCR-ABL protein ("kinase domain mutation"), resulting in impaired imatinib binding (11). Alternatively, CML may have progressed to AP or BP. A bone marrow aspirate is indicated to determine the status of the disease, and analysis for kinase domain mutations should be undertaken.

When stable MRD is not achieved or disease progression not responding to higher doses of imatinib is encountered, treatment with second-generation inhibitors of BCR-ABL tyrosine kinase such as dasatinib or nilotinib is indicated (11).

Patients who have not achieved a satisfactory cytogenetic response or who have progressed after an initial response to tyrosine kinase inhibitors should be offered an allogeneic SCT from a human leukocyte antigen (HLA)-identical sibling or a well-matched unrelated donor.

For patients unsuitable for SCT or without a matched donor, cytosine arabinoside (ARA-C) and interferon-α (IFN-α) improve the degree of response in a proportion of cases. Some patients may benefit from enrolling in clinical trials investigating the efficacy of combining tyrosine kinase inhibitors with ARA-C or IFN-α, or G-CSF. More experimental approaches with novel tyrosine kinase inhibitors, aurora kinase inhibitors, autologous SCT, and peptide vaccines are also being evaluated (11).

Allogeneic Stem Cell Transplation: Treatment with Curative Intent

SCT from an HLA-matched sibling in CP within a year of diagnosis achieve long-term disease control and survival of 70% (approximately 60% for patients with CP who undergo transplantation more than a year from diagnosis) (24). Age has a major impact on outcome, results being especially favorable for the minority pediatric CML population, while patients older than 40 years of age have lower disease-free survival. Disease stage is the other major variable affecting transplantation success. Both transplant-related mortality (TRM) and relapse are higher in transplants performed for AP and BP (Fig. 13.7); however, patients who achieve a second CP have a better chance of disease-free survival (DFS). Most reported results analyze survival in the first 5 years. Longer term follow-up indicates that late relapses and deaths from chronic graft-versus-host disease (GVHD) continue to cause late mortality many years after transplant. In evaluating outcome after transplant for CML, measuring DFS underestimates the final cure rate because donor lymphocyte infusions can cure relapsed disease. In summary, the long-term, allogeneic SCT from a matched sibling results in cure in approximately 65% of individuals in CML CP.

Unrelated Donor Transplants

There is now a large experience in transplants for CML using unrelated volunteer donors. Age, timing of transplant (early or late CP, more advanced disease), and degree of matching each strongly affects success of the transplant. For low-risk patients (defined as younger than 40 years, in first CP, less than 1 year from diagnosis and with an HLA-matched unrelated donor), DFS of approximately 60% can be achieved; poorer results can be anticipated from patients with less favorable presentations. However, reduced intensity transplants have improved the outlook for older patients. Thus, it is not inappropriate to offer lower intensity SCT to patients with CML up to the age of 70 who have no significant comorbidities.

Selecting Patients for Allogeneic Transplantation

Gratwohl et al. described a simple scoring system to predict the chance of a successful transplant outcome (Table 13.3) (25). SCT is no longer recommended as primary therapy for CP-CML for the majority of patients (16,26). However, because SCT has a definite curative potential with long-term survival documented over many decades, it is still appropriate to recommend it for young patients under the age of 30 who are expected to have a particularly low morbidity and mortality, and also in circumstances in which there is difficulty obtaining tyrosine kinase inhibitors because of economic reasons. For other patients, imatinib is the first-line treatment, followed by other tyrosine kinase inhibitors, and SCT is reserved for patients who fail to respond, progress, or present with CML beyond CP. Several studies have ascertained that prior therapy with imatinib does not jeopardize the results of SCT (16).

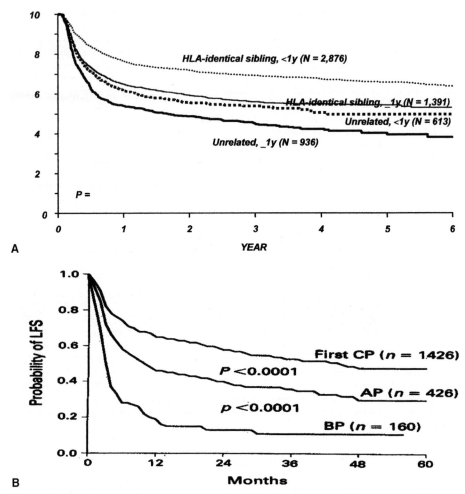

FIG. 13.7. (A) Probability of survival for CML in CP by donor type and time from diagnosis (International Blood and Marrow Transplant Registry data 1994–1999). **(B)** Probability of leukemia-free survival showing the impact of disease state on transplant outcome for 2012 patients with chronic myelogenous leukemia (CML) receiving human leukocyte antigen (HLA)-identical sibling transplants reported to the International Blood and Marrow Transplant Registry in the 1980s.

Treatment of Accelerated Phase

Allogeneic SCT is the most substantiated curative therapy for CML AP and should be offered to patients with a fully or partially-matched HLA-identical donor. However, up to 40% of patients with CML AP respond to imatinib 600 mg daily (16). Furthermore, second generation tyrosine kinase inhibitors are effective in imatinib-resistant disease (11). Alternatively, interferon in combination with cytosine arabinoside can achieve disease control. Experimental treatment approaches include SCT from a mismatched-related donor and high-dose chemotherapy or radiation followed by autologous SCT.

Treatment of Blastic Phase

The first step in managing CML BP is to determine whether the leukemia has developed into lymphoid or myeloid BP. The average survival upon progression to BP is between 6 and 10 months,

TABLE 13.3. *Gratwohl Score for Predicting Outcome
after Bone Marrow Transplantation*

Score	0	1	2	3	4	5	6
Survival at 5 years (%)	72	70	62	48	40	18	22
Transplant-related mortality (%)	20	23	31	46	51	71	73

Score	0	1	2
Donor type	HLA-id sibling	Matched unrelated	–
Disease stage	First CP	AP	BP, CP2+
Recipient age	<20 yr	20–40 yr	>40 yr
Donor/recipient gender	M/M, F/F, M/F	F/M	–
Diagnosis-to-transplantation	<12 months	12 months	–

AP, acute phase; BP, blastic phase; CP, chronic phase; F, female; HLA, human leukocyte antigen; M, male.

slightly longer for lymphoid BP (27). Patients who have not already developed resistance to imatinib should be treated immediately with 800 mg daily. Many patients treated de novo with imatinib will have a complete or at least a partial response. Imatinib-refractory patients may benefit from second generation BCR-ABL inhibitors such as dasatinib or nilotinib, but those with rapidly progressing leukemia require induction chemotherapy with standard regimens—ALL-like for lymphoid BP: daunorubicin 45 mg/m^2 day 1 and 2, vincristine 2 mg/m^2 weekly, prednisolone 60 mg/m^2 daily for 3 weeks, and AML-like for patients with myeloid BP: daunorubicin 50 mg/m^2 daily for 2 to 3 days with cytosine arabinoside 200 mg/m^2 daily for 5 to 7 days. Patients with lymphoid BP also require prophylactic central nervous system treatment to prevent meningeal leukemia. Up to 40% of patients achieve a second CP, but most relapse rapidly. Allogeneic SCT, although considered salvage therapy and associated with significant transplant-related mortality in patients who have progressed to BP, offers the only chance of cure and should be offered to eligible patients. A significant number of patients have prolonged cytopenia after successful eradication of blasts; for this reason moderate intensity remission induction chemotherapy is often used (such as "2 + 5" for myeloid BP and avoidance of high-dose cytosine arabinoside regimens such as hyper-CVAD [cyclophosphamide, vincristine doxorubicin, dexamethasone] for patients with lymphoid BP). Sometimes further remissions can be induced, especially when the relapse occurs in the alternate lineage. Patients who have few clinical options may benefit from entering clinical trials of several newer second-generation BCR-ABL tyrosine kinase inhibitors (11).

SPECIAL ISSUES IN CHRONIC MYELOGENOUS LEUKEMIA MANAGEMENT

Treatment of Relapse after Transplantation

Durable molecular remissions after donor lymphocyte infusion (DLI) are achieved between 3 and 12 months after DLI in as many as 80% of patients relapsing in CP and in more than 90% of molecular relapses. Predictably, the occurrence of GVHD results in a much higher probability of leukemic response, and the antileukemic effect of DLI is greatest in the absence of immunosuppression. While DLI is often effective, it may cause bone marrow failure and lethal GVHD. Bone marrow failure is a greater risk in patients with no detectable residual donor marrow cells at relapse. Marrow aplasia in these patients can be prevented or treated by infusing more donor stem cells. Despite concerns that DLI in the setting of unrelated donor transplants would result in excessive toxicity, response and durable remission rates are similar to those seen after matched sibling DLI. GVHD remains a hazard but does not appear to be more frequent or more severe than that encountered after matched-sibling DLI.

Other Issues

Leukostasis is an uncommon problem in CML and only occurs in a minority of patients with high leucocyte counts (over 300,000 per cubic millimeter). In patients with priapism or neurologic deficit, emergency leukapheresis can be effective but may require several large-volume apheresis sessions to lower the leucocyte count significantly. At presentation, such patients should receive high-dose hydroxyurea (up to 4 g daily) or cytosine arabinoside 1 g/m^2 daily for 2 to 3 days with allopurinol 300 mg daily, adequate hydration, and monitoring of blood chemistry. Imatinib may be started once control of the leucocyte count has been achieved.

Splenic infarcts usually occur when the disease is uncontrolled. Treatment is symptomatic, while attempts to lower the blood count are made. Splenectomy is not generally indicated.

Myelofibrosis causing significant cytopenias can be treated by splenectomy, but this maneuver is frequently followed by increasing symptomatic hepatomegaly. Myelofibrosis is not a contraindication for allogeneic SCT and diminishes after successful SCT.

Chloromas often respond poorly to chemotherapy and are best treated with local radiotherapy.

Psychological Responses of Patients with Chronic Myelogenous Leukemia to Their Disease

Patients presenting with CML are often asymptomatic and may have difficulty accepting that they have a potentially lethal disease. Perhaps for this motive some will explore alternative treatments and attempt psychosomatic techniques to control their leukemia. The complexity of disease evolution and the dilemmas of treatment in CML make it essential to educate patients about their leukemia to provide them with an informed basis for making treatment decisions.

REFERENCES

1. Nowell PC, Hungerford DA. A minute chromosome in human chronic granulocytic leukemia. Science 1960;132:1497.
2. Rowley JD. Letter: A new consistent chromosomal abnormality in chronic myelogenous leukaemia identified by quinacrine fluorescence and Giemsa staining. Nature 1973;243:290–293.
3. Groffen J, Stephenson JR, Heisterkamp N, et al. Philadelphia chromosomal breakpoints are clustered within a limited region, bcr, on chromosome 22. Cell 1984;36:93–99.
4. Heisterkamp N, Stephenson JR, Groffen J, et al. Localization of the c-abl oncogene adjacent to a translocation break point in chronic myelocytic leukaemia. Nature 1983;306:239–242.
5. Daley GQ, Van Etten RA, Baltimore D. Induction of chronic myelogenous leukemia in mice by the P210bcr/abl gene of the Philadelphia chromosome. Science 1990;247:824–830.
6. Kolb HJ, Schmid C, Barrett AJ, et al. Graft-versus-leukemia reactions in allogeneic chimeras. Blood 2004;103:767–776.
7. Druker BJ, Talpaz M, Resta DJ, et al. Efficacy and safety of a specific inhibitor of the BCR-ABL tyrosine kinase in chronic myeloid leukemia. N Eng. J Med 2001;344:1031–1037.
8. Druker BJ, Guilhot F, O'Brien SG, et al. Five-year follow-up of patients receiving imatinib for chronic myeloid leukemia. N Eng. J Med 2006;355:2408–2417.
9. Raskind WH, Ferraris AM, Najfeld V, et al. Further evidence for the existence of a clonal Ph-negative stage in some cases of Ph-positive chronic myelocytic leukemia. Leukemia 1993;7:1163–1167.
10. Biernaux C, Loos M, Sels A, et al. Detection of major bcr-abl gene expression at a very low level in blood cells of some healthy individuals. Blood 1995;86:3118–3122.
11. Weisberg E, Manley PW, Cowan-Jacob SW, et al. Second-generation inhibitors of BCR-ABL for the treatment of imatinib-resistant chronic myeloid leukaemia. Nat Rev Cancer 2007;7:345–356.
12. Takahashi N, Miura I, Saitoh K, et al. Lineage involvement of stem cells bearing the philadelphia chromosome in chronic myeloid leukemia in the chronic phase as shown by a combination of fluorescence-activated cell sorting and fluorescence in situ hybridization. Blood 1998;92:4758–4763.
13. Jiang X, Lopez A, Holyoake T, et al. Autocrine production and action of IL-3 and granulocyte colony-stimulating factor in chronic myeloid leukemia. Proc Natl Acad Sci U S A 1999;96:12804–12809.
14. Goldman JM, Melo JV. Chronic myeloid leukemia—advances in biology and new approaches to treatment. N Engl J Med 2003;349:1451–1464.

15. Melo JV. The diversity of BCR-ABL fusion proteins and their relationship to leukemia phenotype. Blood 1996;88:2375–2384.

16. Baccarani M, Saglio G, Goldman J, et al. Evolving concepts in the management of chronic myeloid leukemia: recommendations from an expert panel on behalf of the European LeukemiaNet. Blood 2006;108:1809–1820.

17. Sokal JE, Cox EB, Baccarani M, et al. Prognostic discrimination in "good-risk" chronic granulocytic leukemia. Blood 1984;63:789–799.

18. Hasford J, Pfirrmann M, Hehlmann R, et al. A new prognostic score for survival of patients with chronic myeloid leukemia treated with interferon alfa. Writing Committee for the Collaborative CML Prognostic Factors Project Group. J Natl Cancer Inst 1998;90:850–858.

19. Hughes TP, Kaeda J, Branford S, et al. Frequency of major molecular responses to imatinib or interferon alfa plus cytarabine in newly diagnosed chronic myeloid leukemia. N Engl J Med 2003;349:1423–1432.

20. White D, Saunders V, Lyons AB, et al. In-vitro sensitivity to imatinib-induced inhibition of ABL kinase activity is predictive of molecular response in de novo CML patients. Blood 2005;106: 2520–2526.

21. Hughes T, Deininger M, Hochhaus A, et al. Monitoring CML patients responding to treatment with tyrosine kinase inhibitors: review and recommendations for harmonizing current methodology for detecting BCR-ABL transcripts and kinase domain mutations and for expressing results. Blood 2006;108:28–37.

22. Cortes J, O'Brien S, Kantarjian H. Discontinuation of imatinib therapy after achieving a molecular response. Blood 2004;104:2204–2205.

23. Rousselot P, Huguet F, Rea D, et al. Imatinib mesylate discontinuation in patients with chronic myelogenous leukemia in complete molecular remission for more than 2 years. Blood 2007;109: 58–60.

24. Barrett J. Allogeneic stem cell transplantation for chronic myeloid leukemia. Semin Hematol 2003; 40:59–71.

25. Gratwohl A, Hermans J, Goldman JM, et al. Risk assessment for patients with chronic myeloid leukaemia before allogeneic blood or marrow transplantation. Chronic Leukemia Working Party of the European Group for Blood and Marrow Transplantation. Lancet 1998;352:1087–1092.

26. Hehlmann R, Berger U, Pfirrmann M, et al. Drug treatment is superior to allografting as first-line therapy in chronic myeloid leukemia. Blood 2007;109:4686–4692.

27. Wadhwa J, Szydlo RM, Apperley JF, et al. Factors affecting duration of survival after onset of blastic transformation of chronic myeloid leukemia. Blood 2002;99:2304–2309.

14

Chronic Lymphocytic Leukemia

Georg Aue and Adrian Wiestner

Chronic lymphocytic leukemia (CLL) is a neoplasm of small, mature B-lymphocytes in the peripheral blood, bone marrow, and lymphoid organs. CLL is the most common leukemia in Western countries but is rare in Hispanics and Asians. CLL accounts for about 25% of all leukemias. The incidence of CLL increases with age from $<1/100,000$ individuals at <40 years of age to $>20/100,000$ in persons over age 65, and the disease is almost twice as frequent in men as in women (1).

ETIOLOGY AND PATHOGENESIS

CLL has traditionally been viewed as an accumulative disease of clonal B cells that have a low proliferation rate and a defect in apoptosis. Molecular mechanisms in the pathogenesis likely include high expression of anti-apoptotic molecules such as Bcl-2 or defects in pro-apoptotic molecules. Recently, it has been shown that the CLL clone contains a considerable proliferative fraction that appears to locate primarily to the bone marrow and lymph nodes. The factors driving CLL cell proliferation and survival remain ill defined but likely include contact with antigens that can stimulate the leukemic cells through the B cell receptor and interactions with host stroma cells (2). No clear environmental etiologic factors have been identified, but a positive family history is one of the strongest risk factors for the development of CLL.

DIAGNOSIS

The World Health Organization (WHO) classification recognizes CLL and the closely related small lymphocytic lymphoma (SLL) as a neoplasm of small, round, CD5- and CD 23-expressing B lymphocytes that are present in the peripheral blood, bone marrow, and lymph nodes. The term SLL describes cases with the tissue morphology and immunophenotype of CLL but which are nonleukemic.

According to the National Cancer Institute-Working Group (NCI-WG)(3), the diagnosis of CLL is defined as:

1. Absolute lymphocytosis of $>5000/\mu l$, composed of morphologically mature appearing cells that is unexplained by other causes.
2. At least 30% lymphocytes in a normocellular or hypercellular marrow.
3. A monoclonal B-cell population with lymphocytes that express low levels of surface immunoglobulins and express CD5, CD19, CD20, and CD23.

CLINICAL MANIFESTATIONS

In current practice, the most common initial manifestation of CLL is the incidental detection of lymphocytosis on a routine blood test or the presence of asymptomatic lymphadenopathy. Abdominal fullness, fatigue, reduced exercise tolerance, or other constitutional symptoms can also be presenting complaints. Symptoms can precede the onset of anemia or clinically manifest organomegaly. With advanced stage, patients may have recurrent infections, weight loss, or symptoms related to anemia and thrombocytopenia.

CLL can cause most of the signs or symptoms of Non-Hodgkin's lymphoma. However, the pace of disease is typically slower than in the lymphomas, and the sudden onset of new symptoms, especially in previously untreated patients, should prompt to exclude other diagnoses. Lymphadenopathy in CLL is typically nontender but can become large enough to cause abdominal discomfort and fullness, and malaise. Even bulky lymphadenopathy does not generally cause obstruction or organ impairment. Splenomegaly is frequent, and hepatomegaly because of CLL infiltration of the liver can occur. Extranodal involvement is common, especially of the skin, but can also manifest as pulmonary nodules. Pleural infiltrations leading to effusions or gastrointestinal (GI) tract involvement leading to GI bleeding have been reported. Central nervous system involvement by CLL is unusual, and neurologic symptoms should be investigated to determine other etiologies, especially infections. While night sweats or low-grade fevers can be caused by CLL, it is important to also consider infection. Conversely, systemic infections may lead to a transient increase in lymph node size or in splenomegaly that may mimic transformation into high-grade lymphoma.

DIAGNOSTIC STUDIES AND LABORATORY FINDINGS

Complete Blood Count and Blood Smear

CLL cells are predominantly small, mature-appearing lymphocytes with round nuclei, clumped chromatin, and scant cytoplasm. Smudge cells, bare nuclei that appear squashed, are a classic feature. Prolymphocytes, medium-sized cells with prominent nucleoli, make up less than 10% of the lymphocytes in typical cases but may increase in rapidly progressive disease. Cases with more than 55% prolymphocytes are recognized as a distinct diagnostic entity called prolymphocytic leukemia (PLL). The absolute lymphocyte count in CLL is by definition greater than 5000/μl and can easily exceed $1\times10^5/\mu$l. In contrast, patients with SLL have a normal or only slightly increased lymphocyte count. Some circulating cells showing CLL features are also frequently observed in SLL. In advanced disease, anemia or thrombocytopenia are common, most often because of replacement of the bone marrow by tumor cells, with a possible contribution of hypersplenism. Autoimmune hematologic manifestations are also typical and more frequent in advanced disease or during treatment with purine analogs. Autoimmune hemolytic anemia (AIHA) and immune thrombocytopenia (ITP) are highly associated with CLL, while pure red cell aplasia (PRCA) is less seen and isolated neutropenia is rare.

Bone Marrow Biopsy

The bone marrow is always involved in CLL and in the vast majority of SLL cases. Distinct patterns of infiltration, which have some prognostic value, are recognized: nodular, interstitial, diffuse, or mixed. Advanced disease is often associated with a diffuse pattern of infiltration. Bone marrow biopsy, outside of clinical studies, may be reserved for cases presenting diagnostic difficulties or that have depressed peripheral blood counts.

Lymph Node Biopsy

A lymph node biopsy can distinguish between CLL and other lymphomas or may be necessary to exclude transformation in patients with rapidly enlarging nodes, especially if the growth preferentially affects a single nodal area. The lymph node architecture in CLL is effaced by an abundance of small lymphocytes with clumped chromatin. Mitotic activity is typically low.

Immunophenotyping and Flow Cytometry

Flow cytometry has become the single most helpful study to confirm a diagnosis of CLL, and immunophenotyping results may lead to additional tests of value in the differential diagnosis. CLL cells are B cells (CD19 positive) that express CD5 and CD23. These cells typically have weak expression of CD20, CD22, and surface immunoglobulin and are negative for FMC7, CD10, and CD103.

Cytogenetics

To fully evaluate cytogenetic abnormalities in CLL, it is necessary to use fluorescence in situ hybridization (FISH). FISH can identify abnormalities in approximately 80% of cases. In a pivotal study, chromosome 13q deletion was present in 55%, deletion of 11q in 18%, trisomy 12 in 16%, and deletion of 17p in 7%. No karyotypic abnormality was detected in 18%. Several other abnormalities were found less frequently, and 29% of patients had two or more aberrations (4). Because there is no CLL-specific chromosomal lesion, detection of these abnormalities is more pertinent for prognosis than diagnosis.

Imaging Studies

Computed tomography (CT) is the imaging method of choice to determine the extent of lymph node involvement in CLL and to evaluate response to treatment. CT can identify Rai stage 0 patients with visceral lymphadenopathy who have a clinical course similar to patients with Rai stage I (5). Positron emission tomography (PET) can be negative, and lymph nodes typically have only weak metabolic activity even in extensive disease. While PET is not helpful in the diagnosis of CLL, it can add valuable information in advanced stage or relapsed disease when transformation into high-grade lymphoma is a consideration.

Laboratory Studies

- Direct antiglobulin test (DAT) should be obtained in patients with anemia and pretreatment. Conversion of the DAT from negative to positive may herald the onset of AIHA.
- Serum immune globulins typically decrease with disease duration. Occasionally, a small M spike may be present.
- Beta-2-microglobulin (B2M) is typically elevated and increases with disease bulk. Low B2M levels (<3 mg/L) have been associated with better response to treatment (6).
- LDH is typically normal. Elevated LDH is seen with AIHA and may be modestly increased with rapidly progressive disease.
- A mild elevation of alkaline phosphatase is common. Elevated transaminases should trigger evaluation for viral hepatitis, especially if treatment with rituximab is considered.

DIFFERENTIAL DIAGNOSIS

The differential diagnosis of CLL includes the entire spectrum of lymphoproliferative diseases. Morphology, flow cytometry, immunohistochemistry, and cytogenetics are the tests with the best diagnostic yield. The main distinguishing features of closely related entities are briefly summarized in Table 14.1.

STAGING AND NATURAL HISTORY

The clinical course and the prognosis of CLL are extremely variable. Two staging systems have been used to risk-stratify CLL: the Rai classification (7) (Table 14.2), utilized in North America, and

TABLE 14.1. *Immunophemotype of B-cell Chronic Lymphocytic Leukemia and Lymphomas That Resemble It*

Entity	sIg	CD5	CD10	CD19	CD20	CD23	Karyotype/ Oncogenes
B-CLL	Weak	++	−	++	+	++	13q, 11q, trisomy 12, 17p
FL	++	−	++	++	++	+/−	t(14;18), BCL-2
MCL	++	++	−	++	++	−	t(11;14), Cyclin D1
MZL	+	−	−	++	++	−	No consistent anomaly
PLL	++	+/−	−	++	++	−	occ t(11;18)

B-CLL, B-cell chronic lymphocytic leukemia; FL, follicular lymphoma; MCL, mantle cell lymphoma; MZL, marginal zone lymphoma; PLL, prolymphocytic leukemia; sIg, surface immunoglobulin.

TABLE 14.2. *Rai Clinical Staging System*

Rai Stage	Modified Rai Staging Risk Group	Clinical Features	Median Survival (years)*
0	Low	Blood and marrow lymphocytosis	11.5
I	Intermediate	Lymphocytosis and adenopathy	11
II	Intermediate	Lymphocytosis and splenomegaly or hepatomegaly, with or without adenopathy	7.8
III	High	Anemia (Hb <11 g/dl)	5.3
IV	High	Thrombocytopenia (<100,000/μl)	7

*Based on 1674 patients from MD Anderson Cancer Center (7).

the Binet classification commonly used in Europe. Both are based on clinical and laboratory parameters and hold prognostic information.

The Binet classification distinguishes three stages: stage A, characterized by fewer than three areas of lymphoid involvement, where the spleen counts as one lymphoid area; stage B involves three or more lymphoid areas; stage C is characterized by anemia and/or thrombocytopenia, regardless of the extent of lymphoid involvement.

PROGNOSTIC FACTORS

In recent years, several molecular markers have been identified that hold important prognostic information independent of clinical stage and are therefore particularly valuable to assess early-stage patients. These markers primarily predict the pace of disease progression in untreated patients and overall survival. In contrast, response to treatment appears to be dominated by currently incompletely defined factors (8).

Immunoglobulin Variable Region Heavy Chain Gene Mutation

The immunoglobulin (Ig) expressed by B cells is composed of light and heavy chains encoded by distinct genes. The presence or absence of somatic mutations in the variable region of the heavy chain gene (VH) distinguishes between two disease subsets: patients whose CLL cells express unmutated IgVH genes (Ig-unmutated CLL) have a shorter survival than patients whose CLL cells express mutated IgVH genes (Ig-mutated CLL). Ig-mutated CLL can have a median survival of 20 or more years, typically a stable or slowly progressive course, and may never require treatment. In contrast, Ig-unmutated CLL is more rapidly progressive, requires treatment early, and is associated with a shorter median survival of 8 to 10 years (9).

ZAP-70

The tyrosine kinase ZAP-70 is essential for the T cell response to antigen. ZAP-70 is also expressed in several other cell types, including some B cell subsets. In CLL, high expression of ZAP-70 commonly is found in Ig-unmutated CLL and is rare in Ig-mutated CLL (10). ZAP-70 expression can be assessed by clinical flow cytometry and predicts the pace of disease progression as well as overall survival, even in early-stage patients. Median progression-free survival, measured as the time from diagnosis to treatment, is approximately 3 years in ZAP-70-positive CLL and reaches 9 years for ZAP-70-negative disease. Median overall survival in the two subtypes is about 9 years and can be as long as 25 years, respectively (11,12). ZAP-70 is a cytoplasmic protein that is expressed at lower levels in CLL B cells than in T cells, making the test technically challenging. Results close to threshold should therefore be interpreted with caution.

Cytogenetics

Deletions of chromosome 17p (p53 locus) or 11q (ATM locus) are associated with inferior outcome: median survival in these patients has been estimated at 32 months for 17p deletion and 79 months for

11q deletion. In contrast, the longest overall survival of 133 months has been associated with an isolated 13 q deletion (4,8). Because many patients may have more than one abnormality, a hierarchical model of genetic subgroups has been proposed, which assigns patients to the genetic subgroup of the prognostically dominant abnormality. For example, a combination of 13q deletion and 17p deletion is assigned to the prognostic group of 17p deletion. 17p deletions are relatively infrequent in newly diagnosed patients but are more common in relapsed or refractory disease. 17p also correlates with poor treatment response to chemotherapy (8).

Leukemia Cell-Surface Expression of CD38

Increased CD38 expression on the cell surface of CLL cells as measured by flow cytometry correlates with inferior outcome (13). CD38 expression is a partial surrogate for the Ig-gene mutation status and/or ZAP-70 expression in some studies but not others.

Lymphocyte Doubling Time

A lymphocyte doubling time of less than 12 months indicates more rapidly progressive disease and is stage-independent associated with decreased survival.

TREATMENT

When? The Paradigm of Watchful Waiting

Most patients with early-stage CLL are asymptomatic and have a relatively good long-term prognosis. Several randomized trials investigating immediate versus deferred chlorambucil-based treatment in early-stage patients showed a slightly inferior survival with immediate chemotherapy (14). Deferral of treatment or "watchful waiting" has therefore become the standard of care for patients with early-stage CLL. Periodical clinical evaluation including basic laboratory testing at 3- to 6-month intervals is a reasonable strategy for asymptomatic patients with relatively stable disease. Treatment is reserved for symptomatic or rapidly progressive disease (3,15). However, over the past decade patients increasingly are treated at earlier stages of disease, despite the absence of data that this approach is of long-term benefit.

Consensus treatment indications include (3):

- Constitutional symptoms due to CLL
- Symptomatic/massive (>10 cm) lymphadenopathy
- Symptomatic/massive splenomegaly (>6 cm below costal margin)
- Progressive marrow failure: worsening anemia and/or thrombocytopenia
- Rapidly progressive lymphocytosis (lymphocyte doubling time <6 months)
- Autoimmune cytopenias (ITP, AIHA, PRCA) poorly responsive to corticosteroid treatment

How to Treat Chronic Lymphocytic Leukemia? An Increasing Choice of Active Agents

Alkylating Agents

Prior to the introduction of purine analogs, oral chlorambucil was the drug of choice. Response rates between 40% and 80% were recorded. However, complete remissions are rare, and response duration is short. Combination regimens of cyclophosphamide, prednisone, and vincristine without (COP/CVP) or with addition of an anthracycline (CHOP) can induce more rapid responses and a higher response rate compared with single-agent chlorambucil, but these improvements did not translate into improved survival (14).

Purine Analogs

The purine analog fludarabine induced more complete responses and increased progression-free survival compared with chlorambucil in a randomized trial (16). There was no significant difference in overall survival, probably because of the crossover design of the study and the high response rate to fludarabine in patients who failed chlorambucil. Several other randomized protocols confirmed the superior activity of single-agent fludarabine compared with chlorambucil or with CAP (cylophosphamide, doxorubicin, prednisone) and found it equally as effective as CHOP (17). Myelosuppression, worse between days 12 and 16, lymphopenia, opportunistic infections, and the precipitation of autoimmune hematologic complications are among the main toxicities of fludarabine. Prolonged or repeat use of purine analogs can lead to severe suppression of hematopoiesis and protracted cytopenias. Other purine analogues, such as pentostatin and cladribine, are also effective in CLL, but these agents have been less studied.

Monoclonal Antibodies

Rituximab, a humanized anti-CD20 monoclonal antibody, is frequently used in CLL as part of combination regimens. As a single agent at 375 mg/m2 weekly for 4 weeks for initial therapy it can induce short-lived partial responses in up to 50% of patients (18). Rituximab has even more limited activity in refractory or relapsed disease. Dose escalation studies found only minor increases in responses that remain short lived. The first infusion of rituximab often induces a systemic cytokine release syndrome that can be life threatening because of severe hypotension and bronchospam. Premedication with antihistamines, slow infusion, and careful monitoring, especially during the first infusion, are recommended. Except for the infusional side effects, rituximab is very well tolerated and can be combined safely with chemotherapy.

Alemtuzumab, a humanized anti-CD52 monoclonal antibody, is FDA approved for fludarabine refractory CLL. The pivotal trial found a response rate of 33%, mainly partial responses (19). Importantly, alemtuzumab was equally effective in patients with or without 17p deletions. However, it appears to be less active in patients with bulky lymphadenopathy (>5 cm). Side effects include cytokine release syndrome, neutropenia, and pronounced lymphopenia, with an increased risk of opportunistic infections, making adequate antimicrobial prophylaxis necessary. Subcutaneous injection of alemtuzumab appears to be equally as effective and is associated with fewer side effects (20). Alemtuzumab is also being studied as a first-line treatment with promising activity, at least when compared with chlorambucil. Only recently has alemtuzumab been incorporated into combination regimens, but the added immunosuppression appears to lead to a significant increase in infectious complications.

Purine Analog Combination Regimens

The combination of fludarabine with rituximab induced more responses (84%), including more complete responses (CRs) (38%) than did fludarabine monotherapy in previously untreated patients (21). Two randomized trials have demonstrated that the combination of cyclophosphamide with fludarabine yields superior response rates and better progression-free survival (PFS) than did fludarabine as a single agent (22,23). A combination regimen of fludarabine, cyclophosphamide, and rituximab (FCR) achieved the highest reported complete response rate (70%) in a large phase II trial (6). However, more than one quarter of the patients experienced grade IV neutropenia, and 26% of patients were unable to complete all 6 cycles. Pentostatin, a purine analog with slightly different properties than fludarabine, in combination with cyclophosphamide and rituximab (PCR) also induced responses in 91% of previously untreated patients (24).

High-Dose Chemotherapy

While there have been promising results in studies of high-dose therapy followed by autologous stem cell rescue, the current consensus is that despite short-term effectiveness, chemotherapy does not alter CLL's natural history and is associated with considerable toxicity (15).

Allogeneic Stem Cell Transplantation

Allogeneic stem cell transplantation is a potentially curative treatment because of a potent graft-versus-leukemia effect. Nonmyeloablative conditioning regimens are increasingly preferred over myeloablative conditioning, mostly because the first approach has less acute toxicity and is better tolerated in the elderly. Most studies report a transplant-related mortality rate of about 20% at one year and a long-term, disease-free survival in the range of 50% (25). Allogeneic transplantation, especially for biologically fit patients with adverse disease features, should be considered and discussed early in the course of treatment and not just considered a last resort.

Treatment Considerations

Table 14.3 summarizes outcome for several treatment options in CLL. Comparisons between different studies are difficult because patient selection and disease stage affect outcome. Clearly treatment induces better responses in earlier-stage patients than in patients with advanced disease (6,23), and therefore lead time bias is an important confounder when comparing the efficacy of different treatment regimens outside of randomized studies. In addition, data on survival in many randomized trials is still too preliminary to allow firm conclusions—the effect of more intense treatment regimens on survival is therefore unproven. Commonly used first-line chemotherapy choices for CLL are 2 or 3 agent combinations of fludarabine, rituximab, and cyclophosphamide: FR, FC, and FCR are typically repeated every 28 days for up to 6 cycles (26). Patients relapsing after a successful treatment with a fludarabine-based regimen may respond well again to a similar regimen, but repeated exposure to purine analogs carries an increased risk of severe myelosuppression. Patients with relapsed or refractory disease may benefit from being referred to clinical trials.

Refractory disease has not yet been formally defined, but an increasingly accepted characterization includes lack of response to purine analog therapy or relapse within 6 months of achieving a response to such therapy (25). Such patients have poor survival prospects and often have adverse cytogenetic features (del 17p or del 11q) and/or have acquired p53 mutations. Purine analog-based combination chemotherapy can achieve response rates of up to 50% in fludarabine-refractory patients (27). Additional effective treatment options are limited but include alemtuzumab, allogeneic transplantation, high-dose methylprednisolone, and investigational agents such as flavopiridol or lenalidomide (25,28–30).

Supportive care in advanced-stage CLL will often focus on cytopenias and infections. IvIG replacement infusions are of modest benefit to reduce incidence and severity of bacterial infections. The protection conferred by vaccinations may be limited because of the immune defect in advanced disease, but nonlive vaccines can be administered safely and may be helpful. Anti-infective prophylaxis against pneumocystis and/or herpes infections is not typically necessary with single-agent fludarabine with or without rituximab but is part of many fludarabine and cyclophosphamide combination regimens (22,23). Alemtuzumab is associated with CMV reactivation, and monitoring for CMV is recommended.

COMPLICATIONS OF CHRONIC LYMPHOCYTIC LEUKEMIA AND THEIR TREATMENT

Autoimmune Manifestations

AIHA and ITP are common in CLL, and their incidence increases with advanced disease and purine analog treatment. These autoimmune complications as well as the less common PRCA often respond to prednisone or cyclosporine. Rituximab appears as a particularly useful and directed therapy in patients in whom autoimmune disease arises during purine analog treatment (31). Retreatment with purine analogs is generally not recommended because of the risk of the autoimmune manifestation recurrence and the potentially fatal outcome, especially with AIHA or ITP.

Infections

Infections from bacterial, viral, and fungal agents are the most important cause of morbidity and mortality in CLL. Immunosuppression secondary to chemotherapy and biologic agents, in particular alemtuzumab but also fludarabine, contribute to the increased incidence of infections. Prophylactic use of antibiotics in neutropenic or hypogammaglobulinemic patients is not recommended. Prophylaxis for

TABLE 14.3. Treatment Options in Chronic Lymphocytic Leukemia

Study	Regimen	N =	CR %	ORR %	PFS	OS	Treatment regimen (each cycle 28 days unless note differently):
First-line treatment							
Randomized phase III (16)	Flu vs. Cb	50 / 9	20 / 4	63 / 37	20 mo / 14 mo	66 mo / 56 mo	**fludarabine** 25 mg/m² iv day 1–5 compared with chlorambucil 40 mg/m² po day 1
Randomized phase III (23)	Flu vs. Flu + Cy	137 / 141	5 / 23	59 / 74	19 mo / 32 mo	N/A	**fludarabine** 25 mg/ m² iv days 1–5 and **cyclophosphamide** 600 mg/m² iv day 1
Randomized phase III (22)	Flu vs. Flu + Cy	182 / 180	7 / 24	83 / 95	20 mo / 48 mo	N/A	**fludarabine** 30 mg/m² iv day 1–3, **cyclophosphamide** 250 mg/m² iv day 1–3
Retrospective comparison (21)	Flu vs. Flu + R	178 / 104	20 / 38	63 / 84	45% at 2 y / 67% at 2 y	81% at 2 y / 93% at 2 y	**fludarabine** 25 mg/m² iv day 1–5, **rituximab** 375 mg/m² iv day 1
Phase II, single center (28)	Flu, followed by R	60	78	93	68% at 3 y	N/A	**fludarabine** 25 mg/m² iv day 1–5 for 6 cycles followed by 4 weekly doses of **rituximab** 375 mg/m² iv weekly
Phase II, single center (6)	Flu, Cy, R (FCR)	224	70	95	69% at 4 y	N/A	**rituximab** 375 mg/m² iv day 1 of course 1 and 500 mg/m² day 1 of courses 2–6; **fludarabine** 25 mg/m² iv day 2–4 of course 1 and days 1–3 of courses 2–6; and **cyclophosphamide** 250 mg/m² iv day 2–4 of course 1 and day 1–3 of courses 2–6
Phase II, 2 institutions (24)	Pen+Cy+R (PCR)	65	41	91	33 mo	N/A	**pentostatin** 2 mg/m² iv day 1, **cyclophosphamide** 600 mg/m² iv day 1, and **rituximab** 375 mg/m² iv day 1, repeated every 21 days
Relapsed/refractory patients							
Phase II, multicenter (19)	Alemtuzumab, 30 mg i.v.	93	3	33	5 mo (9.5 mo)*	16 mo	**alemtuzumab** 30 mg iv three times a week for 12 weeks
Phase II single center (29)	Flu+Cy+R	177	25	73	28 mo	42 mo	**rituximab** 375 mg/m² iv day 1 of course 1 and 500 mg/m² day 1 of courses 2–6; **fludarabine** 25 mg/m² iv day 2–4 of course 1 and days 1–3 of courses 2–6; and **cyclophosphamide** 250 mg/m² iv day 2–4 of course 1 and day 1–3 of courses 2–6
Phase II single center (20)	Alemtuzumab, 10 mg s.c.	16	50	25	N/A	N/A	**alemtuzumab** 10 mg sc three times a week for 18 weeks
Phase II, single center (27)	Lenalidomide	45	9	47	81% at 1y	N/A	**lenalidomide** 25 mg po day 1–21
Phase I, single center (30)	Flavopiridol	42	0	45	13 mo	N/A	See reference

Cb, chlorambucil; Cy, cyclophosphamide; Flu, fludarabine; mo, months; N/A, not applicable; OS, overall survival; median OS in months or projected OS with year of projection; Pen, pentostatin; PFS, progression free survival; median PFS in months or projected PFS with year of projection; R, rituximab; tiw, three times per week; y, years;
*PFS for responding patients.

pneumocystis and herpes infections is typically administered to patients receiving alemtuzumab or combination chemoimmunotherapies and may be especially beneficial in relapsed disease (17). However, younger patients receiving first-line treatment do not require this type of prophylaxis (22). Granulocyte-colony stimulating factor (G-CSF) maybe useful to reduce the duration of neutropenia associated with fludarabine combination regimens.

Richter's Transformation

Transformation to an aggressive, high-grade, large B-cell lymphoma or to a Hodgkin's lymphoma is called Richter's syndrome. Risk factors for the occurrence of Richters's syndrome remain incompletely defined, but its incidence does not seem to be increased as a result of prior treatment with fludarabine. Characteristic findings include systemic symptoms, rapid lymph node enlargement, LDH elevation, and paraproteinemia. Positron emission tomography can be helpful in the diagnosis of Richter's transformation. Treatment for Richter transformation is similar to high-grade lymphoma, but the response to treatment is usually short lived.

SELECT INTERNET RESOURCES

Ongoing clinical trials: http://www.clinicaltrials.gov
Education and patient information: http://www.clltopics.org
Research funding, education, and patient information: http://www.lymphoma.org

REFERENCES

1. American Cancer Society. Cancer Facts & Figures 2007. Atlanta: American Cancer Society: 2007. Available online at http://www.cancer.org/downloads/STT/CAFF2007PWSecured.pdf. Last accessed March 5, 2007.
2. Chiorazzi N, Rai KR, Ferrarini M. Chronic lymphocytic leukemia. N Engl J Med 2005;352: 804–815.
3. Cheson BD, Bennett JM, Grever M, et al. National Cancer Institute-sponsored Working Group guidelines for chronic lymphocytic leukemia: revised guidelines for diagnosis and treatment. Blood 1996;87:4990–4997.
4. Dohner H, Stilgenbauer S, Benner A, et al. Genomic aberrations and survival in chronic lymphocytic leukemia. N Engl J Med 2000;343:1910–1916.
5. Muntanola A, Bosch F, Arguis P, et al. Abdominal computed tomography predicts progression in patients with Rai stage 0 chronic lymphocytic leukemia. J Clin Oncol 2007;25:1576–1580.
6. Keating MJ, O'Brien S, Albitar M, et al. Early results of a chemoimmunotherapy regimen of fludarabine, cyclophosphamide, and rituximab as initial therapy for chronic lymphocytic leukemia. J Clin Oncol 2005;23:4079–4088.
7. Wierda WG, O'Brien S, Wang X, et al. Prognostic nomogram and index for overall survival in previously untreated patients with chronic lymphocytic leukemia. Blood 2007;109:4679–4685.
8. Grever MR, Lucas DM, Dewald GW, et al. Comprehensive assessment of genetic and molecular features predicting outcome in patients with chronic lymphocytic leukemia: results from the U.S. Intergroup Phase III Trial E2997. J Clin Oncol 2007;25:799–804.
9. Hamblin TJ, Davis Z, Gardiner A, et al. Unmutated Ig V(H) genes are associated with a more aggressive form of chronic lymphocytic leukemia. Blood 1999;94:1848–1854.
10. Wiestner A, Rosenwald A, Barry TS, et al. ZAP-70 expression identifies a chronic lymphocytic leukemia subtype with unmutated immunoglobulin genes, inferior clinical outcome, and distinct gene expression profile. Blood 2003;101:4944–4951.
11. Orchard JA, Ibbotson RE, Davis Z, et al. ZAP-70 expression and prognosis in chronic lymphocytic leukaemia. Lancet 2004;363:105–111.
12. Rassenti LZ, Huynh L, Toy TL, et al. ZAP-70 compared with immunoglobulin heavy-chain gene mutation status as a predictor of disease progression in chronic lymphocytic leukemia. N Engl J Med 2004;351:893–901.

13. Krober A, Seiler T, Benner A, et al. V(H) mutation status, CD38 expression level, genomic aberrations, and survival in chronic lymphocytic leukemia. Blood 2002;100:1410–1416.
14. Chemotherapeutic options in chronic lymphocytic leukemia: a meta-analysis of the randomized trials. CLL Trialists' Collaborative Group. J Natl Cancer Inst 1999;91:861–868.
15. Gribben JG. How I treat indolent lymphoma. Blood 2007;109:4617–4626.
16. Rai KR, Peterson BL, Appelbaum FR, et al. Fludarabine compared with chlorambucil as primary therapy for chronic lymphocytic leukemia. N Engl J Med 2000;343:1750–1757.
17. Oscier D, Fegan C, Hillmen P, et al. Guidelines on the diagnosis and management of chronic lymphocytic leukaemia. Br J Haematol 2004;125:294–317.
18. Hainsworth JD, Litchy S, Barton JH, et al. Single-agent rituximab as first-line and maintenance treatment for patients with chronic lymphocytic leukemia or small lymphocytic lymphoma: a phase II trial of the Minnie Pearl Cancer Research Network. J Clin Oncol 2003;21:1746–1751.
19. Keating MJ, Flinn I, Jain V, et al. Therapeutic role of alemtuzumab (Campath-1H) in patients who have failed fludarabine: results of a large international study. Blood 2002;99:3554–3561.
20. Cortelezzi A, Pasquini MC, Sarina B, et al. A pilot study of low-dose subcutaneous alemtuzumab therapy for patients with hemotherapy-refractory chronic lymphocytic leukemia. Haematologica 2005;90:410–412.
21. Byrd JC, Rai K, Peterson BL, et al. Addition of rituximab to fludarabine may prolong progression-free survival and overall survival in patients with previously untreated chronic lymphocytic leukemia: an updated retrospective comparative analysis of CALGB 9712 and CALGB 9011. Blood 2005;105:49–53.
22. Eichhorst BF, Busch R, Hopfinger G, et al. Fludarabine plus cyclophosphamide versus fludarabine alone in first-line therapy of younger patients with chronic lymphocytic leukemia. Blood 2006;107: 885–891.
23. Flinn IW, Neuberg DS, Grever MR, et al. Phase III trial of fludarabine plus cyclophosphamide compared with fludarabine for patients with previously untreated chronic lymphocytic leukemia: US Intergroup Trial E2997. J Clin Oncol 2007;25:793–798.
24. Kay NE, Geyer SM, Call TG, et al. Combination chemoimmunotherapy with pentostatin, cyclophosphamide, and rituximab shows significant clinical activity with low accompanying toxicity in previously untreated B chronic lymphocytic leukemia. Blood 2007;109:405–411.
25. Montserrat E, Moreno C, Esteve J, et al. How I treat refractory CLL. Blood 2006;107:1276–1283.
26. Del PG, Del Principe MI, Consalvo MA, et al. The addition of rituximab to fludarabine improves clinical outcome in untreated patients with ZAP-70-negative chronic lymphocytic leukemia. Cancer 2005;104:2743–2752.
27. Wierda W, O'Brien S, Wen S, et al. Chemoimmunotherapy with fludarabine, cyclophosphamide, and rituximab for relapsed and refractory chronic lymphocytic leukemia. J Clin Oncol 2005; 23:4070–4078.
28. Byrd JC, Shinn C, Waselenko JK, et al. Flavopiridol induces apoptosis in chronic lymphocytic leukemia cells via activation of caspase-3 without evidence of bcl-2 modulation or dependence on functional p53. Blood 1998;92:3804–3816.
29. Byrd JC, Lin TS, Dalton JT, et al. Flavopiridol administered using a pharmacologically derived schedule is associated with marked clinical efficacy in refractory, genetically high-risk chronic lymphocytic leukemia. Blood 2007;109:399–404.
30. Chanan-Khan A, Miller KC, Musial L, et al. Clinical efficacy of lenalidomide in patients with relapsed or refractory chronic lymphocytic leukemia: results of a phase II study. J Clin Oncol 2006; 24:5343–5349.
31. Hegde UP, Wilson WH, White T, et al. Rituximab treatment of refractory fludarabine-associated immune thrombocytopenia in chronic lymphocytic leukemia. Blood 2002;100:2260–2262.

15

Hodgkin's Lymphoma

Michael Craig, Jame Abraham, Wyndham H. Wilson,
and Elaine S. Jaffe

Classical Hodgkin's lymphoma (CHL) is a neoplastic disorder of the lymphoid system characterized by the presence of multinucleated giant cells of B-cell origin, known as Reed–Sternberg (RS) cells, in a background of numerous reactive lymphocytes. It is one of the few malignancies in which effective therapy has been developed, with over 75% of patients cured with chemotherapy and/or radiation. The steady decline in mortality because of CHL is primarily because of excellent results achieved with effective combination chemotherapy. It is considered a distinct disease entity from nodular lymphocyte predominant Hodgkin's lymphoma (NLPHL).

EPIDEMIOLOGY

Hodgkin's lymphoma is among the most common malignancies of young adults. It constitutes approximately 1% of all malignancies and 18% of all lymphomas. In the United States during 2007, about 8190 patients were diagnosed with CHL and 1070 patients died of CHL (1). In Europe and North America, there is a bimodal age distribution, with an increasing frequency between the second and third decades, and a second peak after the fifth decade.

PATHOLOGIC CLASSIFICATION

Table 15.1 lists the World Health Organization (WHO) Revised European American Lymphoma classifications, in comparison to older historical schemes (2).

- Classical HL.
  - Nodular sclerosis classical Hodgkin's lymphoma (NSCHL).
  - Mixed cellularity classical Hodgkin's lymphoma (MCCHL).
  - Lymphocyte depleted classical Hodgkin's lymphoma (LDCHL).
  - Lymphocyte-rich classical Hodgkin's lymphoma (LRCHL).
- Nodular lymphocyte-predominant Hodgkin's lymphoma (NLPHL).

NLPHL is a clinicopathologic entity of B-cell phenotype that is distinct from classic Hodgkin's lymphoma. The immunophenotypes for CHL and NLPHL are described in Table 15.2 (3).

PATHOLOGY

Hodgkin's lymphoma is somewhat unique among the malignant lymphomas in that the RS cells and variants, the malignant cells, constitute the minority of cells present in the tumor mass (Fig. 15.1). The neoplastic cells in classical Hodgkin's lymphoma are associated with a rich inflammatory background containing lymphocytes, eosinophils, neutrophils, histiocytes, and plasma cells in varying proportions. Molecular studies in recent years have provided evidence for the B-cell origin of the neoplastic cell in both classical HL and NLPHL, because the cells have undergone somatic mutations in

TABLE 15.1. *Historical Evolution of the Classification of Hodgkin's Lymphomas*

Jackson-Parker	Lukes-Butler	Rye	REAL/WHO
Paragranuloma	L&H, nodular LP	LPHL	NLPHL
	L&H, diffuse		LRCHL
Granuloma	NS	NS	NS
	MC*	MC*	MC
Sarcoma	LD, diff fibrosis	LD	LD
	LD, reticular		

*Defined as a category of exclusion, not with specific features.
L&H, lymphocytic and histiocytic; LD, lymphocyte depletion; LP, lymphocyte-predominant; LPHL, lymphocyte-predominant Hodgkin's lymphoma; LRCHL, lymphocyte-rich classic Hodgkin's lymphoma; MC, mixed-cellularity; NLPHL, nodular lymphocyte-predominant Hodgkin's lymphoma; NS, nodular-sclerosis.

the immunoglobulin variable region. However, the tumor cells down-regulate the B-cell program and are typically negative for most B-cell associated markers (4). They show constitutive activity of nuclear factor kappa B.

NSCHL requires the presence of a nodular growth pattern, broad bands of fibrosis, and a characteristic variant of the RS cell known as a lacunar cell. The lacunar cell has abundant clear cytoplasm with a sharply demarcated cell membrane. In formalin-fixed tissue a characteristic artifact often occurs; the cytoplasm of the cell retracts, leaving a clear space or lacunus. NSCHL is graded according to the proportion of neoplastic cells and the presence of necrosis, as well as depletion of normal lymphocytes. Two grades of NSCHL are identified in the WHO classification (2). This is the most common form of CHL, comprising 60% to 70% of cases, and has an equal distribution in males and females. NSCHL often involves mediastinal, supraclavicular, and cervical lymph nodes.

MCCHL is characterized by numerous classical RS cells in a rich inflammatory background, fine reticular fibrosis, and an absence of distinct fibrous bands. MCHD is more common in males than females and is the second most common type, affecting 15% to 25% of patients. It is frequently associated with disseminated disease at presentation, and B symptoms are also common. It is one of the variants of CHL, along with lymphocyte depletion, that is seen in association with human immunodeficiency virus (HIV) infection. MCCHL is the subtype most often positive for Epstein-Barr virus (EBV) sequences (2).

LDCHL is the rarest form of CHL, constituting approximately 1% of cases. Epidemiologically, it is seen in regions of the world of lower socioeconomic status and is also increased in frequency in HIV-infected individuals. It may be thought of as representing a further evolution of MCCHL, with more frequent malignant cells, a depletion of normal lymphocytes, and usually greater fibrosis, which is often diffuse and reticular in nature. Patients can also be elderly and present with B symptoms and advanced stage.

TABLE 15.2. *Immunophenotypic Criteria for the Classification of Hodgkin's Lymphoma*

Marker	NLPHL	Classic HL
CD30	−	+
CD15	−	+
CD20	+	−/+
EMA	+/−	−
LCA	+	−
BCL-6	+	−
Oct2, BOB.1	+	−(+)

HL, Hodgkin's lymphoma; NLPHL, nodular lymphocyte-predominant Hodgkin's lymphoma.

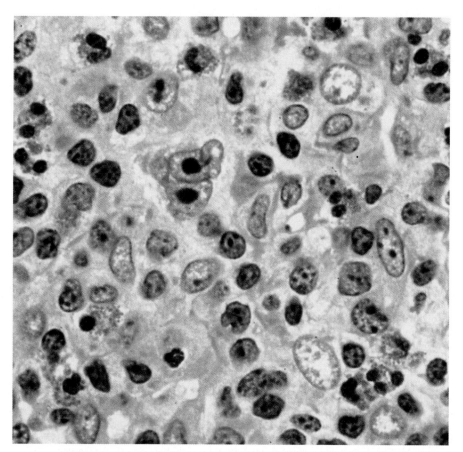

FIG. 15.1. Diagnostic Reed-Sternberg cell seen in classic types of Hodgkin's lymphomas (mixed cellularity, nodular sclerosis, lymphocyte depletion). Neoplastic cells in nodular lymphocyte-predominant Hodgkin's lymphomas are termed popcorn cells or L and H cells (lymphocytic or histiocytic predominance). Reed-Sternberg cells of the classic type generally are not seen in a nodular lymphocyte-predominant Hodgkin's lymphoma.

LRCHL is characterized by a cellular milieu rich in normal lymphocytes and a paucity of malignant cells that have the immunophenotype of classic RS cells. LRCHL may have a diffuse or nodular growth pattern and especially in its nodular form may be mistaken for nodular lymphocyte predominant HL. It tends to present in older individuals, often with isolated peripheral lymphadenopathy.

NLPHL differs from classical HL in its immunophenotypic profile, histologic characteristics, and clinical behavior (3). Classical RS cells are not seen. The neoplastic cells are referred to as lymphocytic and histiocytic (L & H) cells or popcorn cells. They have a lobulated nuclear contour, dispersed chromatin, and inconspicuous nucleoli. They generally cluster within nodules associated with lymphocytes and histiocytes. Initially, the background lymphocytes are predominantly of B-cell phenotype, but T cells may predominate in later stages. The neoplastic cells, the popcorn cells, are positive for CD20 and are generally negative for CD15 and negative or weakly positive for CD30. NLPHL affects patients of all ages and occurs more often in males than females. B symptoms are infrequent, but patients often have multiple relapses over time, similar to low-grade non-Hodgkin's lymphoma.

ETIOLOGY AND RISK FACTORS

The Epstein-Barr virus (EBV) has been linked to many cases of classical HL but is absent in NLPHL. EBV is most commonly found in MCCHL and LDCHL. Infectious mononucleosis appears to be a predisposing risk factor for subsequent EBV-positive CHL but not EBV-negative CHL (5). NSCHL is most common in North America and is more prevalent among individuals of higher socioeconomic status, whereas MCCHL and LDCHL are seen in underdeveloped regions of the world. The risk of classical HL is increased 5- to 10-fold in HIV-positive patients. Familial cases of CHL have been reported, and siblings of CHL patients are at slightly increased risk. There is a weak association with certain HLA types.

CLINICAL FEATURES

More than 80% of patients have cervical lymph node enlargement, and more than 50% will have mediastinal adenopathy. Lymph nodes are usually nontender, firm, and rubbery.

Constitutional symptoms ("B" symptoms):
• Unexplained fever (temperature, >38°C).
• Drenching night sweats.
• Unexplained weight loss (>10% of body weight, over 6 months before the diagnosis).

Other symptoms include fatigue, weakness, anorexia, alcohol-induced nodal pain, and pruritus. Staging (Ann Arbor/American Joint Committee on Cancer [AJCC] and Cotswold) is outlined in Table 15.3 (6–8).

PRETREATMENT EVALUATION

1. Excisional biopsy (and not needle biopsy) of a prominent node is highly recommended for diagnosis.
2. Detailed history with attention to unexplained fever, night sweats, and significant weight loss (constitutional symptoms).
3. Complete physical examination, including the lymh node examination and evaluation for hepatosplenomegaly.
4. Laboratory tests include
   • Complete blood count (CBC), erythrocyte sedimentation rate (ESR).
   • Biochemical tests of liver function, renal function, and serum uric acid.
5. Radiologic studies.
   • Chest radiograph and computed tomography (CT) scan of the chest, abdomen, and pelvis.
   • Positron emission tomography (PET) scan, often combined with CT, is helpful in some cases (9).

TABLE 15.3. *Staging*

Stage I—Involvement of single lymph node region or lymphoid structure (spleen, thymus, Waldeyer's ring) or involvement of a single extralymphatic site (IE).

Stage II—Involvement of two or more lymph node regions on the same side of the diaphragm (II), which may be accompanied by localized contiguous involvement of an extralymphatic organ or site (IIE). The number of anatomic sites may be indicated by numeric subscript.

Stage III—Involvement of lymph node regions on both sides of the diaphragm (III), which may also be accompanied by localized involvement of an associated extralymphatic organ or site (IIIE), by involvement of the spleen (IIIS), or both (IIIE+S).

Stage IV—Disseminated involvement of one or more extralymphatic organs, with or without associated lymph node involvement, or isolated extralymphatic organ involvement with distant (nonregional) nodal involvement.

Each stage is divided into A and B categories: B for those with defined systemic symptoms, and A for those without.
X, A mass >10 cm or a mediastinal mass larger than one third of the thoracic diameter; E, Involvement of a single extranodal site contiguous to a known nodal site; CS, Clinical staging; PS, Pathologic staging.

6. Bone marrow biopsy of the posterior iliac crest for those with abnormal CBC or clinical stage IIB, III, or IV.
7. Staging laparotomy and splenectomy for patients with early-stage disease above the diaphragm is no longer performed to assess occult disease because of more accurate radiologic staging and the equivalency of systemic treatment.

Prognostic Features

Favorable prognostic features include:

1. Sedimentation rate less than 50.
2. Patient age 50 years or younger.
3. Lymphocyte predominant or nodular sclerosing histology.
4. Absence of "B" symptoms (fever and loss of weight).
5. Fewer than three sites of involvement.
6. No bulky adenopathy, including mediastinal disease less than one third of the chest diameter on chest x-ray or tumor size <10 cm.

The International Prognostic Factors Project on Advanced Hodgkin's lymphoma prognostic score:

1. Albumin level of less than 4.0 g/dL.
2. Hemoglobin level of less than 10.5 g/dL.
3. Male sex.
4. Age of 45 years or older.
5. Stage IV disease.
6. White-cell count greater than 15,000/mm^3.
7. Absolute lymphocyte count of less than 600/mm^3 or a lymphocyte count that was less than 8% of the total white-cell count.

The 5-year progression-free survival according to the international prognostic factor score are as follows: 0 factors, 84%; 1 factor, 77%; 2 factors, 67%; 3 factors, 60%; 4 factors, 51%; and 5 or greater factors, 42% (10).

MANAGEMENT OF NEWLY DIAGNOSED CLASSICAL HODGKIN'S LYMPHOMA

The goal of therapy for CHL is cure. Advances in the systemic treatment of CHL have dramatically improved the response rate and survival. This is mainly because of careful staging, understanding of the pattern of spread, and advances in radiation and chemotherapy. In general, combined modality treatment incorporating chemotherapy with or without radiation is used for most patients with CHL (11). Therapy with radiation consists of treating regions of known disease (especially if bulky) plus adjacent nodal groups. Treatment selection is influenced by stage, prognostic factors, and short- and long-term toxicity. Response criteria for lymphoma, incorporating PET scan results, have been updated by consensus panel (9).

Radiation Treatment

Because of the availability of effective chemotherapy regimens, radiation as a single mode of treatment is used less commonly. In adult Hodgkin's lymphoma, the appropriate dose of radiation is 2500 cGy to 3000 cGy to clinically uninvolved sites and 3500 cGy to 4400 cGy to regions of initial nodal involvement. When these recommendations are individualized and modified with careful treatment technique; the risk of cardiac and pulmonary complications is reduced but not eliminated.

While considering radiation treatment, it is important to consider long-term complications such as breast cancer in young women and risk of lung cancer in patients with a history of smoking. Radiation

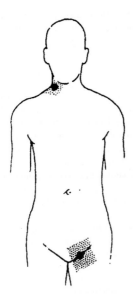

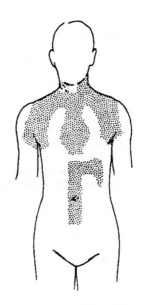

A Involved field irradiation

B Subtotal nodal irradiation
including mantle and spade fields

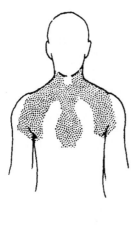

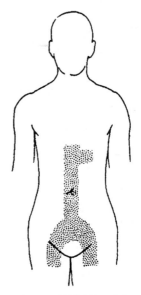

C Mantle field irradiation

D Inverted-Y field irradiation

FIG. 15.2. Radiation therapy fields used in treating Hodgkin's disease. When the fields shown in **(C)** and **(D)** are combined, this is commonly called total nodal irradiation (TNI). From Haskell CM. Cancer Treatment, 4th ed. Philadelphia: WB Saunders; 1995:965.

therapy is classically delivered to three major fields, known as the mantle, para-aortic, and pelvic or inverted-Y fields. Extended field (EF) radiation refers to the inclusion of adjacent clinically negative nodal sites (Fig. 15.2).

Chemotherapy

Aggressive chemotherapy produces long-term disease-free remissions, even in advanced CHL. The first "curative regimen" was mechlorethamine, Oncovin, procarbazine, prednisone (MOPP), which resulted in a 70% complete remission in stage III–IV patients. Subsequently, many regimens have been developed including ABVD (doxorubicin, bleomycin, vinblastine, and dacarbazine) and hybrids of MOPP and ABVD (12). Chemotherapy is usually administered for two cycles beyond complete response or stable disease, for a minimum of six cycles in advanced stages.

ABVD and MOPP contain different agents. Studies have shown that ABVD is less toxic and more effective than MOPP, with a higher freedom from progression and overall survival. At 10 years, the risk of developing treatment-related leukemia with the MOPP regimen is 2% to 3%, whereas it is 0.7% with ABVD (13).

Recently published data has shown that increased dose BEACOPP (bleomycin, etoposide, doxorubicin, cyclophosphamide, vincristine, procarbazine, and prednisone) for advanced CHL had an overall 5-year survival of 91% and freedom from treatment failure of 87% (14).

Commonly used regimens include:
1. ABVD: doxorubicin + bleomycin + vinblastine + dacarbazine (12).
2. BEACOPP: bleomycin + etoposide + doxorubicin + cyclophosphamide + vincristine + procarbazine + prednisone (14).
3. COPP/ABVD: cyclophosphamide + vincristine + procarbazine + prednisone/doxorubicin + bleomycin + vinblastine + dacarbazine.
4. MOPP: mechlorethamine + vincristine + procarbazine + prednisone.
5. MOPP/ABV hybrid: mechlorethamine + vincristine + procarbazine + prednisone/doxorubicin + bleomycin + vinblastine.
6. Stanford V: doxorubicin + vinblastine + mechlorethamine + etoposide + vincristine + bleomycin + prednisone. Radiation therapy is added to the involved field (15).

CHOOSING A REGIMEN

Historically, MOPP was considered the standard treatment for advanced CHL. Currently, ABVD is the standard treatment in North America. In a randomized study, the Cancer and Leukemia Group B (CALGB) compared leading regimens with an 8-year follow-up (Table 15.4). The results indicate that ABVD alone or MOPP/ABVD was superior to MOPP alone, in terms of remission, freedom from progression, and survival. A randomized study of ABVD versus MOPP-ABV showed equivalency but higher toxicity with MOPP-ABV.

The 12-week chemotherapy regimen, Stanford V, given in combination with radiation to sites of disease was introduced with objectives of maintaining or improving the rate of cure and minimizing the acute and long-term side effects. Stanford V is an abbreviated 12-week course of treatment in which myelosuppresive and nonmyelosuppressive treatments are alternated weekly. Clinical trials are ongoing to compare the efficacy of ABVD versus Stanford V.

A recent German study for patients with advanced-stage CHL using COPP/ABVD, BEACOPP, or increased dose BEACOPP, and consolidative radiation therapy to sites of initial bulky (5 cm or larger) or residual disease, showed a 5-year overall survival of 83% for COPP/ABVD, 88% for BEACOPP, and 91% for increased-dose BEACOPP. The actuarial rate of secondary acute leukemias 5 years after diagnosis of Hodgkin's lymphoma was 0.4% for COPP/ABVD, 0.6% for BEACOPP, and 2.5% for increased-dose BEACOPP ($p = 0.03$). Although this study suggests that dose intensity improves the survival of Hodgkin's lymphoma, this improvement must be balanced against the increased toxicity and risk of leukemia. BEACOPP is considered unsuitable for patients over age 65, associated with significant acute fatal toxicity.

TABLE 15.4. *Response and Survival from Different Regimens (CALGB study and German Lymphoma Group study)*

Regimen	Complete Response Rate	Survival Rate	Follow-up
MOPP	67%	64%	8 years
ABVD	82%	72%	8 years
MOPP/ABVD	83%	73%	8 years
BEACOPP (standard dose)	88%	88%	5 years
BEACOPP (increased dose)	96%	91%	5 years

ABVD, doxorubicin (adriamycin), bleomycin, vinblastin, and dacarbazine; BEACOPP, bleomycin, etoposide, doxorubicin, cyclophosphamide, vineristine, procarbazine; and prednisone; MOPP, merchlorethamine, oncovin, procarbazine, and prednisone.

Treatment Options

For treatment selection, patients can be divided into two major risk groups:

1. Stages I and II without B-symptoms or bulky disease are considered "favorable early stage" and at low risk for recurrence. Cure rate is >90%.
2. Stage IIB and stage I–II B with bulk are variably considered "early" or "advanced" by different study groups. Most U.S. groups treat them as "unfavorable early disease." Cure rate is >80%.
3. Stage III and IV are considered "advanced stage" and are at significant risk for recurrence. Cure rate is about 60% to 70%.

Treatment Recommendations for Classical Hodgkin's Lymphoma

In addition to the following information, Table 15.5 details commonly used treatment regimens (11).

1. Favorable early disease
   a. ABVD six cycles alone or ABVD two to four cycles with involved field radiation.
2. Unfavorable early disease
   a. ABVD six to eight cycles alone or ABVD four to six cycles with involved or EF radiation. One European randomized trial showed no difference in freedom from treatment failure or overall survival when EF radiation was replaced by involved field radiation (30 Gy to field, adding 10 Gy to bulk).
   b. Massive mediastinal disease (defined as a mediastinal mass width greater than one third of the maximum chest diameter or 10-cm mass) will receive combined modality therapy. Chemotherapy regimens such as ABVD plus radiation therapy to a mantle or modified mantle field should be considered. Patients with an early and a complete radiographic and PET response may not require radiation consolidation (pending results of clinical trials).
3. Advanced disease
   a. ABVD for six to eight cycles is the current standard. Treatment is usually continued two cycles after resolution of disease by imaging studies. Increased-dose BEACOPP for patients with or without radiation treatment for poor prognosis disease should be considered in younger patients.
   b. Addition of involved field radiation is usually considered, particularly for bulky disease. Recent evidence from a randomized trial suggests there may be no need to add radiation if a complete response can be achieved with combination chemotherapy.
   c. Stanford V is an effective regimen with shorter treatment duration (3 months) and is currently undergoing randomized comparison with ABVD-based treatment in intergroup trial E2496.

TABLE 15.5. *Commonly Used Treatment Regimen*

ABVD
Doxorubicin, 25 mg/m^2 per dose IV push for two doses, days 1 and 15 (total dose/cycle, 50 mg/m^2)
Bleomycin, 10 U/m^2 per dose IV push for two doses, days 1 and 15 (total dose/cycle, 20 U/m^2)
Vinblastine, 6 mg/m^2 per dose IV push for two doses, days 1 and 15 (total dose/cycle, 12 mg/m^2)
Dacarbazine, 375 mg/m^2 per dose IV infusion for two doses, days 1 and 15 (total dose/cycle,
    750 mg/m^2)
Treatment cycle repeats every 28 days.

MOPP
Mechlorethamine, 6 mg/m^2 per dose IV push for two doses, days 1 and 8 (total dose/cycle, 12 mg/m^2)
Vincristine, 1.4 mg/m^2 per dose IV push for two doses, days 1 and 8 (total dose/cycle, 2.8 mg/m^2)
Procarbazine, 100 mg/m^2 per day orally for 14 doses, days 1–14 (total dose/cycle, 1400 mg/m^2)
Prednisone, 40 mg/m^2 per day orally for 14 doses, days 1–14 (cycles 1 and 14 only)
    (total dose/cycle, 560 mg/m^2)
Treatment cycle repeats every 28 days.

Alternating MOPP/ABVD
Alternate MOPP and ABVD cycles by 28 days.

MOPP/ABV Hybrid
Mechlorethamine, 6 mg/m^2 IV push day 1 (total dose/cycle, 6 mg/m^2)
Vincristine, 1.4 mg/m^2 IV push day 1 (total dose/cycle, 1.4 mg/m^2; maximal dose, 2 mg)
Procarbazine, 100 mg/m^2 per day orally for 7 doses, days 1–7 (total dose/cycle, 700 mg/m^2)
Prednisone, 40 mg/m^2 per day orally for 14 doses, days 1–14 (total dose/cycle, 560 mg/m^2)
Doxorubicin, 25 mg/m^2 IV push day 8 (total dose/cycle, 25 mg/m^2)
Hydrocortisone, 100 mg IV day 8, before bleomycin (total dose/cycle, 100 mg)
Bleomycin, 10 U/m^2 IV push day 8 (total dose/cycle, 10 U/m^2)
Vinblastine, 6 mg/m^2 IV push day 8 (total dose/cycle, 6 mg/m^2)
Treatment cycle repeats every 28 days.

BEACOPP Standard Dose
Bleomycin, 10 mg/m^2 (day 8); *etoposide,* 100 mg/m^2 (days 1–3); *doxorubicin,* 25 mg/m^2 (day 1);
    cyclophosphamide, 650 mg/m^2 (day 1); *vincristine,* 1.4 mg/m^2 (day 8); *procarbazine,*
    100 mg/m^2 (days 1–7); and *prednisone* 40 mg/m^2 (days 1–14)
Regimen was repeated on day 22.
The maximum dose of vincristine is 2 mg.

Increased Dose BEACOPP
Bleomycin, 10 mg/m^2 (day 8); *etoposide,* 200 mg/m^2 (days 1–3); *doxorubicin,* 35 mg/m^2 (day 1);
    cyclophosphamide, 1250 mg/m^2 (day 1); *vincristine,* 1.4 mg/m^2 (day 8); *procarbazine,*
    100 mg/m^2 (days 1–7); and *prednisone* 40 mg/m^2 (days 1–14)
Regimen was repeated on day 22.
G-CSF starting on day 8 until count recovery.
The maximum dose of vincristine is 2 mg.

Stanford V
Mustard, 6 mg/m^2 IV weeks 1, 5, 9
Vincristine, 1.4 mg/m^2 IV weeks 2, 4, 6, 8, 10, 12 (maximal dose, 2 mg)
Prednisone, 40 mg/m^2 per day orally every other day weeks 1–9, taper
Doxorubicin, 25 mg/m^2 IV weeks 1, 3, 5, 7, 9, 11
Bleomycin, 5 U/m^2 IV weeks 2, 4, 6, 8, 10, 12
Vinblastine, 6 mg/m^2 IV weeks, 1, 3, 5, 7, 9, 11
Etoposide, 60 mg/m^2 IV daily for 2 days, weeks 3, 7, 11
—The maximum dose of vincristine is 2 mg.
—All drugs are administered on day 1, except for VP-16, which is given on days 1 and 2
—Taper prednisone by 10 mg of the total dose qod (every other day) on weeks 10 and 11
—Reduce the dose of vinblastine to 4 mg/m^2 on weeks 9 and 11 for patients over the age of
    50 years.
—Reduce the dose of vincristine to 1 mg on weeks 10 and 12 for patients over the age of 50 years.
—If mustard is unavailable, cyclophosphamide 650 mg/m^2 IV on weeks 1, 5, 9 may be substituted.

ABVD, doxorubicin (adriamycin), bleomycin, vinblastin, and dacarbazine; BEACOPP, bleomycin, etoposide, doxorubicin, cyclophosphamide, vincristine, procarbazine, and prednisone; G-CSF, granulocyte colony-stimulating factor; IV, intravenous; MOPP, merchlorethamine, oncovin, procarbazine, and prednisone.

Lymphocyte-Predominant Hodgkin Lymphoma

This subtype is associated with the propensity for multiple relapses even up to 15 years. Early stages of NLPHL without risk factors are treated with radiation alone or in some cases with observation following complete resection. Advanced stages are rare at diagnosis and may be associated with a poor prognosis. While such cases are usually treated like classical Hodgkin's lymphoma, the unique biology of NLPHL raises the question of whether it should be treated like an aggressive B-cell lymphoma (3). Indeed, phase II trials show high single-agent activity of rituximab in NLPHL, which is almost always CD20 positive. The use of rituximab combined with chemotherapy in the front-line setting is still considered investigational, and affected patients should be referred for trials because of the rarity of the disease.

COMPLICATIONS OF THERAPY

Radiation Therapy

Early Complications

Mantle field radiation may cause mouth dryness, pharyngitis, cough, and dermatitis. Subdiaphragmatic radiation may cause anorexia and nausea. Radiation can cause myelosuppression or thrombocytopenia.

Late Complications

Late complications of radiation therapy include hypothyroidism, pericarditis, and pneumonitis. Additionally, 15% of the patients receiving mantle radiation may experience electric shock sensation radiating down the back of the legs when the head is flexed, 6 to 12 weeks after the treatment. This may be because of transient demyelinization of the spinal cord, and it usually resolves spontaneously.

Patients who received cardiac radiation are at increased risk for coronary artery disease (CAD). Patients should be monitored and evaluated for other risk factors for CAD.

There is increased risk of secondary neoplasms (lung, breast, stomach, and thyroid). A twofold to eightfold increase in lung cancer is observed more than 5 years after the radiation treatment and persists through the second decade. The increased risk is greatest in inhaled tobacco users.

Breast cancer is inversely proportional to the age at radiation treatment. The relative risk (RR) is 136 if the patient is younger than 15 years, 19 for age group 15 to 24 years, and 7 for age group 24 to 29 years. The high risk is restricted to women irradiated before age 30 years. The average interval between radiation and diagnosis of breast cancer is 15 years. Breast examination should be part of follow-up for women at risk. Routine mammography should begin about 8 years after completion of the radiation.

CHEMOTHERAPY

Early Complications

Early complications of chemotherapy include nausea and vomiting, alopecia, myelosuppression, and infection.

Late Complications

Late complications of chemotherapy include sterility (primarily with MOPP-based regimens), neuropathy (primarily with vincristine), cardiomyopathy (doxorubicin), pulmonary fibrosis (bleomycin), and secondary leukemia (MOPP ± radiation).

TREATMENT OF HODGKIN'S LYMPHOMA IN RELAPSE

For successful management of patients with relapsed CHL, one should have a clear understanding of the sites of relapse, the time since the last treatment, and the details of the previous treatment. If the relapse is because of inadequate initial treatment, retreatment with chemotherapy or radiation is considered. Relapse after primary radiation is best managed with chemotherapy. Generally, relapse after primary combination chemotherapy should be consolidated with autologous stem cell transplant.

Salvage Chemotherapy Regimens

Nonanthracycline-containing regimens

1. ESHAP (etoposide, methylprednisolone, high-dose cytarabine, and cisplatin).
2. ICE (ifosfamide, carboplatin, and etoposide).
3. DHAP (dexamethasone, high-dose cytarabine, and cisplatin).
4. EIP (etoposide, ifosfamide, and cisplatin)

Anthracycline containing regimens

1. Dose-adjusted EPOCH (etoposide, prednisone, vincristine, cyclophosphamide, and doxorubicin).
2. EVA (etoposide, vincristine, and doxorubicin).
3. ASHAP (doxorubicin, cisplatin, high-dose cytarabine, and methylprednisolone).

POTENTIALLY CURATIVE TREATMENT APPROACH

Potentially curative treatment approach includes high-dose chemotherapy with autologous stem cell transplantation, combination chemotherapy, and EF radiation therapy.

PALLIATIVE TREATMENT

Palliative treatment includes investigational treatment, radiation treatment, and sequential single-agent chemotherapy (gemcitabine or vinblastine).

REFERENCES

1. Jemal A, Ward E, Murray T, et al. Cancer Statistics, 2007. CA Cancer J Clin 2007;57:43–56.
2. Jaffe ES, Harris, NL, Stein H, et al. (Eds). World Health Organization Classification of Tumours. Pathology and Genetics of Tumours of Haematopoietic and Lymphoid Tissues. Lyon, France: IARC Press; 2001:237–254.
3. Nogova L, Rudiger T, Engert A. Biology, clinical course and management of nodular lymphocyte-predominant Hodgkin lymphoma. Hematology Am Soc Hematol Educ Program 2006.266–272.
4. Mathas S. The pathogenesis of classical Hodgkin's lymphoma: a model for B-cell plasticity. Hematol Oncol Clin North Am 2007;21:787–804.
5. Hjalgrim H, Askling J, Rostgaard K, et al. Characteristics of Hodgkin's lymphoma after infectious mononucleosis. N Engl J Med 2003;349:1324–1332.
6. Lister TA, Crowther D, Suteliffe SB, et al. Report of a committee convened to discuss the evaluation and staging of patients with Hodgkin's disease: Cotswolds meeting. J Clin Oncol 1989; 7:1630–1636.
7. Mauch P, Larson D, Osteen R, et al. Prognostic factors for positive surgical staging in patients with Hodgkin's disease. J Clin Oncol 1990;8:257–265.
8. Urba WJ, Longo DL. Hodgkin's disease. N Engl J Med 1992;326:678–687.
9. Cheson B, Pfistner B, Juweid M, et al. Revised response criteria for malignant lymphoma. J Clin Oncol 2007;25:579–586.
10. Hasenclever D, Diehl V. A prognostic score for advanced Hodgkin's disease. N Eng J Med 1998;339:1506–1514.
11. Conners J. State-of-the-art therapeutics: Hodgkin's lymphoma. J Clin Oncol 2005;23:6400–6408.

12. Canellos GP, Anderson JR, Propert KJ, et al. Chemotherapy of advanced Hodgkin's disease with MOPP, ABVD, or MOPP alternating with ABVD. N Eng J Med 1992;327:1478–1484.
13. Swerdlow AJ, Douglas AJ, Hudson GV, et al. Risk of second primary cancers after Hodgkin's disease by type of treatment: analysis of 2846 patients in the British National Lymphoma Investigation. BMJ 1992;304:1137–1143.
14. Diehl V, Franklin J, Pfreundschuh M, et al. The German Hodgkin's Lymphoma Study Group Standard and Increased-dose BEACOPP chemotherapy compared with COPP–ABVD for advanced Hodgkin's disease. N Engl J Med 2003;348:2386–2395.
15. Horning SJ, Hoppe RT, Breslin S, et al. Stanford V and radiotherapy for locally extensive and advanced Hodgkin's disease: mature results of a prospective clinical trial. J Clin Oncol 2002; 20:630–637.

16

Non-Hodgkin's Lymphoma

Richard F. Little and Wyndham H. Wilson

The non-Hodgkin's lymphomas (NHL) are a heterogeneous group of lymphoid tumors that have distinctive clinical and biologic behaviors. NHL is thus not a single disease but a group of diseases. Accurate diagnosis of the specific NHL subtype is therefore critical to understanding management. Treatment approaches must take into account if the particular NHL is potentially curable. Even within a designated histopathologic classification, such as diffuse large B-cell lymphoma (DLBCL), there is considerable biological and clinical heterogeneity.

Refinement in diagnostic resolution is an evolving science and is dependent on morphologic, immunophenotypic, and genetic features. Recent advances have led to resolution of clinically relevant molecular-based distinctions among lymphomas through the identification of a tumor's histogenetic origins and gene transcription signatures.

EPIDEMIOLOGY

A steady increase in the age-adjusted incidence per 100,000 persons has been documented, with 11.1 cases in 1976 and 19.0 in 2000. Approximately one third of the increase may be attributed to a combination of iatrogenic immunosuppression and the acquired immune deficiency syndrome (AIDS) epidemic. Other potential causes include increased exposures to environmental carcinogens. NHL occurs more commonly in males, and Whites are affected more than African Americans.

In AIDS-related lymphomas (ARL), certain chemokine receptor variants are associated with different risks of B-cell NHL subtypes. These chemokine variants appear to be racially distributed, paralleling differences in ethnic incidence.

There are other differences in the epidemiology of lymphoma in human immunodeficiency virus (HIV)-infected and noninfected patients. For example, diffuse large B-cell lymphoma (DLBCL) comprises approximately 30% of lymphomas in HIV-noninfected and 70% to 80% of lymphomas in HIV-infected cases. The incidence of ARL has substantially decreased since the advent of highly active antiretroviral therapy (HAART) for HIV infection, but the risk remains substantially higher (100-fold) than in the HIV-noninfected population. Immunoblastic DLBCL subtypes mainly account for the decrease in incidence tumors, whereas the incidence of Burkitt lymphoma and the centroblastic variant of DLBCL appear to have been less affected by HAART. The median survival of patients with ARL has increased from approximately 4 to 11 months pre-HAART to almost 24 months since the advent of HAART. However, there has been no improvement in survival for AIDS-related Burkitt in the HAART era.

PATHOPHYSIOLOGY

A major known risk factor for NHL appears to be an abnormality of immune function (either immune deficiency or dysregulation) as in HIV infection, iatrogenic immune suppression, autoimmune diseases, congenital immune deficiencies, Wiskott-Aldrich, and X-linked lymphoproliferative disorder.

Infectious agents have been implicated. Gamma herpesviruses are linked to certain NHL subtypes, especially lymphomas associated with immune deficiency states. Epstein-Barr virus (EBV) is highly associated with African Burkitt lymphoma and AIDS-related DLBCL. The Kaposi's sarcoma–associated herpes virus (KSHV) (also known as human herpes virus-8 or HHV-8) is etiologically linked to primary effusion lymphomas that tend to occur specifically in AIDS and multicentric Castleman's disease, a rare lymphoproliferative disorder in which affected persons have markedly increased risk developing aggressive NHL.

Human retroviruses and RNA viruses are other risk factors. HTLV-1 is causative of adult T-cell leukemia/lymphoma. Hepatitis C virus is associated with splenic marginal zone lymphoma.

Other risk factors include environmental and occupational exposures, especially organic compounds such as organophosphate insecticides.

CLASSIFICATION

Lymphoma classification has evolved since Hodgkin's lymphoma was first described, and new technology has made it possible to move from purely histopathologic typing to the current World Health Organization (WHO) classification that includes immunophenotypic, molecular, genetic, and clinical elements to distinguish NHL subtypes (Tables 16.1 to 16.4).

NHLs are broadly classified as B-cell or T-cell lymphomas, depending on the lymphocyte lineage giving rise to the tumor. B lymphocytes give rise to B-cell NHL, 88% of all NHL. T lymphocytes give rise to T-cell NHL, 12% of NHL. Expression (or its lack thereof) of cell surface antigens and immunoglobulin proteins is dependent on the type of lymphocyte and its stage of differentiation. Analysis of these proteins in tumor cells is diagnostically useful as well as for determining tumor histogenesis.

TABLE 16.1. *Molecular Characteristics of B-Cell Lymphomas*

Histology	Cytogenetics	Oncogene/Protein	Immunoglobulin Gene Rearrangements	
			Heavy	κ λ
CLL/SLL*	t(14; 19)	Bcl-3	+	
	Trisomy 12, 13q			+
Lymphoplasmacytoid			+	+
Follicular center cell grade I, II, or III	t(14; 18)[†]	Bcl-2	+	
Marginal zone[‡]	Trisomy 3			
	t(11; 18)		+	
Mantle cell lymphoma	t(11; 14)	Bcl–1/Cyclin-D1	+	
Diffuse large B-cell[§]	t(3; 22)(q27;q11)	Bcl-6		+
		Bcl-2		
Primary mediastinal (thymic) large B-cell		MAL gene	+	+
Lymphoblastic lymphoma/leukemia			+	+/−
Burkitt's lymphoma	t(8; 14)(q24;q32)	c-myc	+	
	t(2; 8)(11p; q24)			λ+
	t(8; 22)(q24;q11)			κ+

*Trisomy 12 is seen in 30% of cases, and abnormalities in 13q are present in 25% of patients.
[†]t(14; 18) is present in 75% to 95% of follicular center cell non-Hodgkin's lymphoma.
[‡]Cytogenetic abnormalities have been seen in extranodal marginal zone non-Hodgkin's lymphoma.
[§]Bcl-2 rearrangements up to 30% and Bcl-6 up to 45% of cases of diffuse large B-cell lymphoma and 5. Bcl-2 is present in 30% of cases and c-myc is uncommon.
CLL/SLL, chronic lymphocytic leukemia/small lymphocytic lymphoma.

TABLE 16.2. *Molecular Characteristics of T-Cell Lymphomas*

Histology	Cytogenetics	Oncoprotein	TCR Gene Rearrangements
T-CLL/T-PLL	Inv14(q11; q32), Trisomy 8q	Bcl-3	+
Mycosis fungoides			+
Peripheral T-cell lymphoma, unspecified			+/−
Extranodal NK/T-cell	EBV +		−
Angioimmunoblastic* T-cell lymphoma	Trisomy 3 or 5, EVB +		+
ATLL	HTLV I integration +		+
Enteropathy T-cell	EVB −		β +
Hepatosplenic γ/δ T-cell lymphoma			δγ+
Systemic ALCL[†]	T(2; 5)	Alk+	+
Precursor T-lymphoblastic lymphoma/leukemia	Variable T(7; 9)	Tcl-4	Variable

*TCR gene rearrangement is present in 75% and IgH in 10%.
[†]TCR gene rearrangement in 90%.
ALCL, anaplastic large cell lymphoma; Alk, anaplastic lymphoma kinase gene; ATLL, adult T-cell lymphoma; NK, natural killer; T-CLL, T-cell chronic lymphocytic leukemia; T-PLL, T-cell prolymphocytic leukemia.

TABLE 16.3. *B-Cell Immunophenotype*

Histology	SIg	CIg	CD 5	10	11	15	20	23	30	34	43	45
CLL/SLL*	+/−	−/+	+	−	−/+		weak	+			+	
Lymphoplasmacytoid*	+	+	−	−	−/+		+	−			+/−	
Follicular center cell grade I–III*,[†]	+	−	−	+	−		+	−/+			−	
Marginal zone*,[‡]	+	+	−	−	+/−		+	−			−/+	
Mantle cell lymphoma*,[§]	+	−	+	−	−/(+ few)		+	−			+	
Diffuse large B-cell*	+/−	−/+	−/+	−/+			+	−				+/−
Primary mediastinal large cell*,[¶]	−	−	−/+	−/+		−	+	−	−/+			+/−
Precursor B lymphoblastic lymphoma/leukemia*,**	−	−/+		+/−			+			+/−		
Burkitt's lymphoma*	+		−	+			+	−				
Burkitt's-like lymphoma*	+/−	−/+	−	−/+			+					

*Positive B-Cell–associated antigens: CD19, CD20, CD22, and CD79
[†]SIg+: IgM +/−, IgD > IgG > IgA
[‡]SIg M > G > A and IgD−; CIg+ in 40%
[§]SIgM+ usually IgD+, κ > λ and CD11c−
[¶]M > G > A and IgD−; CIg+ in 40%
**TdT+, HLA − Dr+ and CD20−/+
CLL/SLL, chronic lymphocytic leukemia/small lymphocytic lymphoma.

TABLE 16.4. *T-cell Immunophenotype*

Histology	CD									
	1a	2	3	4	5	7	8	25	56	TdT
T-CLL/T-PLL		+	+	+	+	+	+	−		
Mycosis fungoides		+	+	+	+	−/+	−	−		
Peripheral T-cell lymphoma	+/−	+/−	+	+/−	−/+	+/−				
Angioimmunoblastic T-cell lymphoma		+	+	+	+					
Extranodal NK/T		+	−	−	+/−	+/−	−		+	
Enteropathy T-cell		+	−			+	+/−			
Adult T-cell lymphoma/leukemia		+	+	+	+	−	−	+		
Systemic anaplastic large-cell lymphoma*		−/+						+/−		
Hepatosplenic γ/δ		+	−				−		+	
Precursor T lymphoblastic lymphoma/leukemia	+/−	+/−	+	+	+/−	+	+			+

NK, natural killer; T-CLL, T-cell chronic lymphocytic leukemia; T-PLL, T-cell prolymphocytic leukemia.
*Cells CD30⁺.

There is an increasing appreciation of the relationship between tumor tissue origin and clinical behavior. DLBCL subtypes deriving from germinal center B cells have a better prognosis than those DLBCL of postgerminal center B-cell histigenic origin. In chronic lymphocytic leukemia/lymphoma (CLL), cases can be grouped according to whether the variable region of the immunoglobulin genes (IgV_H) shows sequence homology to germline IgV_H genes or evidence of somatic mutations. Prognosis is poorer in cases with unmutated IgV_H genes (pregerminal center histigenic origin) compared with cases with somatic mutations (postgerminal center B-cell histigenic origin).

WHO recognizes three major categories of lymphoid neoplasms: (i) B cell neoplasms, (ii) T and natural killer (NK) cell neoplasm, and (iii) Hodgkin's lymphoma.

Both lymphomas and lymphoid leukemias are included in the WHO classification. Solid and leukemic phases are present in many lymphoid neoplasms. The WHO classification stratifies these neoplasms primarily by lineage. Within each category, distinct diseases are defined according to a combination of morphology, immunophenotype, genetic features, and clinical syndromes.

A cell of origin is postulated for each neoplasm. For many, this cell of origin represents the state of differentiation of the tumor cells that are seen in the tissues, rather than the cell in which the initial transforming events occurs (not possible to know in many cases).

For further information regarding the WHO classification of tumors and to order the monograph for *Tumors of Haematopoietic and Lymphoid Tissues*, see http://www.iarc.fr/who-bluebooks/.

STAGING

Staging evaluation for systemic NHL includes:

I. Diagnostic confirmation by tissue biopsy
    A. Sufficient material is critical to conduct the studies needed to insure accurate diagnosis
    B. Needle biopsies generally yield inadequate tissue for these studies and should be avoided for primary diagnosis
    C. Important studies for diagnostic confirmation often include:
        1. Assessment of clonality
        2. Immunophenotypic, cytogenetic, and molecular studies
        3. Markers of histogenesis (B- versus T-cell origin and germinal center versus nongerminal center histogenesis)

4. Oncogene rearrangement can be diagnostically useful
   a. t(8;14) or MYC in Burkitt lymphoma
   b. t(14;18) or bcl-2 in follicular lymphoma
   c. t(2;5) or ALK in anaplastic large cell lymphoma
   d. t(11;14) or bcl-1 in mantle cell lymphoma
   e. Trisomy 3 or trisomy 18 (marginal zone lymphoma)

D. Some tumors (e.g., T-cell–rich B-cell lymphoma or lymphomatoid granulomatosis) have excess reactive T cells that may obscure the minority of diagnostic malignant B cells if inadequate tissue is obtained

II. History and physical examination

III. Viral testing if indicated by risk or lymphoma subtype
   A. HIV serology in all aggressive NHL
   B. HTLV-1 serology
   C. Hepatitis B and C serology

IV. Clinical and laboratory assessment of organ function
   A. Include CD4 cell count if HIV-positive
   B. In addition to routine blood tests:
      1. Lactate dehydrogenase (LDH; indirect measure of tumor burden and prognosis)
      2. Serum β_2 microglobulin
      3. Serum α-fetoprotein or β-human chorionic gonadotropin young males with an isolated mediastinal mass where the differential diagnosis includes mediastinal germ cell tumor

V. Chest radiograph, computed tomography scans of chest, abdomen, and pelvis

VI. Bone marrow biopsies

VII. Lumbar puncture with cytology should be performed in patients at risk of central nervous system (CNS) disease:
   A. DLBCL with elevated LDH and more than one extranodal site and/or lymphomatous involvement in the bone marrow
   B. All Burkitt lymphoma
   C. Some investigators recommend that all ARL cases (regardless of bone marrow and extranodal sites or histological subtype) be evaluated for CNS disease.

VIII. Positron emission tomography (PET) is useful for identifying sites of disease and for response assessment. Gallium scans are less sensitive and specific than PET, so of limited utility

IX. The Ann Arbor Staging System, initially developed for patients with Hodgkin's lymphoma, also is used in NHL. This system does not apply to lymphoblastic leukemia/lymphoma or to mycosis fungoides (Table 16.5)

RESTAGING FOR RESPONSE EVALUATION

At completion of therapy, repeat all restaging studies. Generally restaging after four cycles is indicated in aggressive lymphomas (repeat all abnormal tests). In indolent lymphomas, response to therapy may be slower; restaging can be performed less frequently.

TABLE 16.5. *Ann Arbor Staging System*

Stage	Description
I	Single lymph node region or single extralymphatic organ or site (IE)
II	Two or more lymph node regions on the same side of the diaphragm or single extranodal site with adjacent nodes (IIE)
III	Nodal regions on both sides of the diaphragm (III) or involving single extranodal site with adjacent nodes (IIIE), or spleen (IIIS), or both (IIISE)
IV	Diffuse or disseminated involvement of one or more extralymphatic organs; bone marrow, liver, brain involvement

Absence of associated symptoms is designated A; Presence of symptoms is designated B. "B" symptoms include unexplained fevers, unexplained >10% weight loss, sweats.

The rate of response to treatment may have prognostic value. Disease progression or no response implies extremely poor prognosis. Biopsy of residual masses after therapy may be required. PET scan may help to resolve whether a residual mass is malignant. Repeat staging procedures at regular intervals after treatment is completed.

PROGNOSTIC FEATURES

Prognostic features are related to disease and the individual patient.

Disease-related prognostic features include tumor bulk, stage, number of extranodal sites, histologic type, and tumor histogenesis. Indolent lymphomas are rarely curable but may have prolonged natural history. In DLBCL, there is a better prognosis with gene expression patterns similar to germinal center.

Other disease-related prognostic features include B cells (GCB) compared with those with gene expression patterns similar to activated B cells (postgerminal center histiogenic derivation),tumor proliferation as measured by immunohistochemistry (such as MIB-1) or molecular profiling, and high proliferation associated with cyclophosphamide, doxorubicin, vincristine and prednisone (CHOP) failure (may be overcome with infusional regimens such as dose-adjusted EPOCH [etoposide, prednisone, vincristine, cyclophosphamide, doxorubicin]), β_2-microglobulin.

Bcl-2 expression is associated with CHOP failure and may be partially overcome with rituximab. P53 mutation is associated with CHOP failure and may not be relevant in ARL. Bcl-6 expression is an independent predictor of improved disease-free survival in aggressive lymphomas.

Patient-related prognostic features include age and performance status.

Prognostic assessment and modeling have been developed to predict the outcome based on clinical presentation. The most commonly used model is International Prognostic Index (IPI) (Table 16.6). The IPI was initially developed for aggressive NHL but is applicable to other NHL subtypes. In the IPI, 1 point is assigned for each of the following:

1. Older than 60 years of age
2. Eastern Cooperative Oncology Group (ECOG) performance status 2 or more
3. LDH above normal
4. Two or more extranodal sites   *APLES*
5. Stage III or IV disease

In age-adjusted international index for patients younger than 60 years of age, 1 point each is assigned for:

1. Performance status 2 or more
2. LDH above normal
3. Stage III or IV disease

In ARL, the primary prognostic determinant is the CD4 cell count. Among those whose HIV is sensitive to HAART, the IPI and lymphoma-specific features appear to be of relatively greater prognostic.

TABLE 16.6. *International Prognostic Index for Diffuse Large B-Cell Lymphomas*

Risk Category	Score	Patients in Risk Group (%)	Complete Responses (%)	5-Year Disease-Free Survival (%)	5-Year Survival (%)
International Prognostic Index					
Low	0 or 1	35	87	70	73
Low-intermediate	2	27	67	50	51
High-intermediate	3	22	55	49	43
High	4 or 5	16	44	40	26

TREATMENT PRINCIPLES

Treatment of NHL is guided by clinical behavior. Approaches can been broadly classified by cell type and clinical behavior as indolent, aggressive, or highly aggressive. Conventional treatment has been chemotherapy, radiotherapy, or a combination of these modalities. Novel treatments, including monoclonal antibodies, are now in everyday practice. Ongoing clinical research will refine how newer treatments are used to augment or supplant current standards of care.

Indolent B-Cell and T-Cell Lymphomas

The natural history is one of a relatively slow-growing lymphoma with low potential for cure but with median survival measured in years to decades. Examples include grades I and II follicular lymphoma, B-chronic lymphocytic leukemia/small lymphocytic lymphoma, marginal zone B-cell lymphoma, and mycosis fungoides.

Indolent lymphomas transform into high-grade malignancies in approximately 40% of patients and lead to death; treatment for transformed lymphoma is similar to that of aggressive lymphomas, but outcomes are not as favorable (Table 16.7). Initial treatment depends on type of lymphoma, pace of the disease, and disease-associated morbidity. A slow-growing indolent lymphoma without associated symptoms may not require immediate treatment. Responses are not often durable, and early treatment of asymptomatic patients does not improve survival. An alternative approach to watchful waiting is to offer participation in research protocols.

Newer treatments may change the natural history (as with R-CHOP). Research treatments may be curative (as with active immunotherapy with tumor-specific idiotype vaccine or nonmyeloablative stem-cell transplantation). In all cases, stratify by prognostic features so that treatment can be directed more effectively toward those with the worst prognosis.

Most cases are disseminated at diagnosis and standard chemotherapy is not curative. Regimens include oral chlorambucil; cyclophosphamide, vincristine, and prednisone (CVP), fludarabine, and rituximab (monoclonal anti-CD20 antibody).

As a single agent in previously untreated follicular lymphoma, rituximab yields up to 75% response rates. Maintenance rituximab may prolong remission (at 3 years of median follow-up, duration of remission was 23 months versus 12 months, favoring rituximab maintenance group receiving 375 mg/m^2 every 2 months for 4 doses postinduction).

As a single agent in previously treated follicular lymphoma, rituximab can yield responses in 50% to 60% of cases, with a median response duration of 6 to 16 months. Rituximab with CHOP induces complete responses in up to 95% of previously untreated follicular lymphomas with a median response

TABLE 16.7. *Indolent Lymphoma Treatment*

Combination Chemotherapy	Treatment Description	Reference
CVP	**Cyclophosphamide** 400 mg/m^2 PO daily for 5 days, days 1–5 (total dose/cycle = 2000 mg/m^2) **Vincristine** 1.4 mg/m^2 IV on day 1 (maximum dose/cycle = 2 mg; total dose/cycle = 1.4 mg/m^2) **Prednisone** 100 mg/m^2 PO daily for 5 days, days 1–5 (total dose/cycle = 500 mg/m^2) Treatment is repeated every 21 days	(1)
Single Agents	Treatment Description	Reference
Fludarabine	**Fludarabine** 25 mg/m^2 per day IV for 5 days, days 1–5 (total dose/cycle = 125 mg/m^2) Treatment is repeated every 28 days	(2–4)
Rituximab	**Rituximab** 375 mg/m^2 IV weekly (total dose/week = 375 mg/m^2)	(5)

IV, intravenous; PO, orally.

duration not reached at 50 months of follow-up. Rituximab combined with fludarabine yields results similar to CHOP plus rituximab.

Radioimmunotherapy for Relapsed Disease

Yttrium 90-ibritumomab tiuxetan (Zevalin, Cell Therapeutics, Seattle, WA) is Food and Drug Administration (FDA)-approved and is well tolerated. In a randomized trial, Zevalin resulted in statistically and marginally clinically significant higher objective response rate (ORR) and complete response (CR) but not response duration compared with rituximab alone in relapsed or refractory low-grade, follicular, or transformed B-cell NHL.

Tositumomab and iodine-131 Tositumomab (Bexxar, GlaxoSmithKline, Research Triangle Park, NC) are approved by the FDA for the treatment of patients with CD20-positive, follicular, NHL, with and without transformation, when disease is refractory to rituximab and has relapsed after chemotherapy.

Indolent B-positive T-cell lymphomas at stage I disease may be curable with 10-year disease-free survival of approximately 50% with radiation alone. Because of the long natural history, this is a difficult disease to study. For example, a large phase 2 trial of more than 100 patients was initiated in 1984 but was not complete and published until 2003. A 10-year disease-free survival of 76% was reported, suggesting that combined radiation and chemotherapy may be superior to radiotherapy alone in stage I and II disease. Based on these results, a randomized trial has been initiated. There is interest in newer treatments (including immunotherapy) as potentially more effective. Large retrospective databases indicate that the observational strategy does not compromise survival compared with early intervention. Thus, combined modality therapy cannot be recommended as standard of care.

Stage II to IV disease treatment options include watchful waiting, autologous transplantation (associated with high risk of relapse), research approaches, vaccine immunotherapy, allogeneic transplantation, and conventional chemotherapy plus rituximab.

Data from a randomized phase II trial suggests chemotherapy followed by rituximab may yield superior results compared with concomitant administration. Randomized trial data suggests that in relapsed/resistant indolent lymphoma that maintenance rituximab improves progression-free survival regardless of whether rituximab was initially used (e.g., maintenance rituximab is used after either CHOP or R-CHOP induction).

For chronic lymphocytic leukemia/small lymphocytic lymphoma treatment options include fludarabine and rituximab, given concurrently or sequentially increase response rates. Alemtuzumab is approved for fludarabine-refractory disease, with response rates of approximately 30%. Cladribine may also be used.

For lymphoplasmacytoid lymphoma/Waldenström macroglobulinemia treatment options include conventional therapies including alkylating agents (especially chlorambucil), with or without corticosteroids. CHOP is sometimes used. Purine analogues such as fludarabine or cladribine are also active. Response rate (RR) to first-line therapy ranges from 38% to 85%. RR to fludarabine in previously treated patients ranges from 30% to 50%. Initial therapy with rituximab has produced overall response rates of 20% to 40%; there is a risk of IgM paraprotein flare. Preliminary data suggests a role for agents such as alemtuzumab and bortezomib. There is interest in thalidomide and analogs.

For marginal zone lymphoma associated with *Helicobacter pylori,* effective eradication of the infection can result in lymphoma regression and likely cure. For marginal zone lymphoma associated with autoimmune disease (such as Sjögren syndrome or Hashimoto's thyroiditis), chemotherapy with or without rituximab may be useful.

Local therapy such as surgery or regional irradiation may yield relatively long-term disease control. Splenectomy may be indicated for splenic marginal zone lymphoma. Cases associated with hepatitis C virus (HCV) infection may regress with effective HCV therapy.

Mycosis Fungoides

Mycosis fungoides is a cutaneous T-cell lymphoma that often has multiple skin plaques, nodules, and/or generalized erythroderma. Sézary syndrome is the late occurrence of nodal and leukemic disease. Prognosis depends on a number of features including disease extent. Median survival of approximately 10 years is seen in relatively indolent disease, but in those with poor prognostic features (older than 65 years of age, stage IVB), median survival may be only 1 year.

A variety of treatments have been reported for limited stage disease, but the extent to which outcomes are related to therapy or to the disease natural history is often not well documented.

Topical treatment should be used for local disease including topical gel formulation combining methotrexate and laurocapram, and topical nitrogen mustard; low-dose oral methotrexate, and topical bexarotene gel. Combined modality therapy including subcutaneous interferon-α and oral isotretinoin, followed by total-skin electron beam therapy and long-term maintenance therapy with topical nitrogen mustard and interferon-α has been reported as useful. Some reports suggest that interferon alone is just as effective.

Additionally, extracorporeal photopheresis with or without other modalities has been reported As well as denileukin diftitox (recombinant diphtheria toxin and interleukin [IL]-2) and alemtuzumab.

Primary Cutaneous Anaplastic Large Cell Lymphoma/Lymphomatoid Papulosis (CD30$^+$)

These are chronic recurrent skin diseases usually of a benign course. Lymphomatoid papulosis is considered to be an atypical lymphoproliferation rather than a true lymphoma but may develop into a lymphoma. Low-dose methotrexate and psoralen/ultraviolet A (UVA) therapy can reduce the skin lesions, but chronic therapy is required. The anaplastic lymphoma kinase (ALK) protein has been shown to identify a subgroup of patients with systemic anaplastic large cell lymphoma (ALCL) with an excellent prognosis, whereas ALK-negative ALCLs are more heterogeneous. ALK-positive cases are associated with younger age, more limited disease state, and better prognosis. ALK-negative cases are associated with older age, advanced disease stage, and poor prognosis.

AGGRESSIVE B-CELL LYMPHOMAS

Mantle Cell Lymphoma

Most patients present with advanced-stage disease. The median age is in the seventh decade, and the male to female ratio is high. Splenomegaly and gastrointestinal involvement is common. Unlike other aggressive lymphomas, it is incurable and has a short median survival of 3 to 5 years. The blastic variant may be more aggressive with a propensity for central nervous system (CNS) involvement (25%) and shorter survival. There may be a survival advantage in younger patients with stage IA or IIA treated with radiation therapy.

Diffuse Large B-Cell Lymphoma

Morphologic variants of DLBCL include centroblastic, immunoblastic, T-cell histiocyte rich, anaplastic, and plasmablastic variants.

A subtype of DLBCL, mediastinal (thymic) large B-cell lymphoma (Med-DLBCL), arises in the mediastinum and is of putative thymic B-cell origin. Med-DLBCL has distinctive clinical, immunophenotypic, and genotypic characteristics. Presenting features include localized disease and signs and symptoms related to a large anterior mediastinal mass. Dissemination to multiple organs can occur. CD19 and CD20 are present, while CD10 and CD5 are absent. Gains in chromosome 9p and REL gene support the concept of a subtype distinct from DLBCL arising in other sites.

Follicle center lymphoma grade III is an aggressive lymphoma with follicles present in the lymph node but having more than 15 centroblasts per high-power field. This tumor is potentially curable with aggressive therapy. Thus, care must be taken to distinguish this tumor from mantle cell and from grades I and II follicle center cell lymphoma.

Primary Effusion Lymphoma

All cases are associated with the KSHV, also known as human herpes virus-8 (HHV-8); more than 70% are coassociated with EBV. The tumor presents as effusions in the body cavities usually with an absence of nodal disease, giving rise to its alternative designation of body-cavity lymphoma. Primary effusion lymphoma (PEL) occurs most often in the setting of HIV infection. There is no defined effective standard of care, and median survival is generally 4 to 6 months with therapy.

TABLE 16.8. *Standard Therapy for Aggressive Non-Hodgkin's Lymphoma*

Combination Chemotherapy	Treatment Description	Reference
R-CHOP	**Rituximab** 375 mg/m^2 IV day 1	(6,7)
	Cyclophosphamide 750 mg/m2 IV day 1	
	(total dose/cycle = 750 mg/m^2)	
	Doxorubicin 50 mg/m^2 IV day 1	
	(total dose/cycle = 50 mg/m^2)	
	Vincristine 1.4 mg/m^2 IV day 1	
	(maximum dose/cycle = 2 mg; total dose/cycle = 1.4 mg/m^2)	
	Prednisone 50 mg/m^2 per day PO for 5 days, days 1–5	
	(total dose/cycle = 250 mg/m^2)	
	Treatment is repeated every 21 days	

Possible Alternatives include DA-EPOCH-R, ACVBP, CHOP every 14 days, CHOEP
See Table 16.9.
IV, intravenous; Po, orally.

Primary cutaneous large cell lymphoma often has an indolent course.

Lymphomatoid granulomatosis has a variable clinical course depending on its grade. Interferon may be useful in low-grade disease (grades I to II). Dose-adjusted EPOCH-R is useful in grade III disease.

TREATMENT PRINCIPLES

Rituximab with cyclophosphamide, doxorubicin, vincristine, and prednisone (R-CHOP) is the standard of care for curative intent in DLBCL (Table 16.8). Probability of cure can be estimated using prognostic models, such as the IPI. Addition of rituximab to CHOP appears to "equalize" various regimens to some extent. For example, the advantage of CHOEP (etoposide added to CHOP) over CHOP alone in young patients is no longer seen when rituximab is added to either regimen.

For stage I to II disease, three cycles of CHOP plus involved-field radiotherapy results in 5-year progression-free survival (PFS) of 77% and overall survival (OS) of 82%, better than with 8 cycles of CHOP alone (64% and 72%, respectively). However, R-CHOP now is commonly used in early-stage disease without radiation.

In advanced-stage disease, the OS and PFS are approximately 50% and 32%, respectively, at 5 years with CHOP.

Randomized trials show that addition of rituximab on day 1 of each CHOP cycle resulted in improved outcome in patients 60 to 80 years of age: complete response higher with rituximab (76% versus 63%), 2-year event-free survival (EFS) with rituximab (57% versus 38%), 2-year overall survival with rituximab (70% versus 57%), and rituximab appears to confer greater benefit in tumors with bcl-2 overexpression or lack of bcl-6 expression.

An intergroup phase 3 trial of R-CHOP versus CHOP with a second randomization to rituximab maintenance or not in older patients has shown that the greatest failure-free survival benefit is dependent on concomitant rituximab and CHOP, and that maintenance rituximab following R-CHOP confers no additional improvement.

Possible alternatives to R-CHOP as front-line therapy, or as salvage therapy (Table 16.9) include dose-adjusted-EPOCH-R, biweekly R-CHOP, and doxorubicin, cyclophosphamide, vindesine, bleomycin, and prednisone (ACVBP).

HIGHLY AGGRESSIVE B-CELL LYMPHOMA

Precursor B-Lymphoblastic Lymphoma/Leukemia

Most cases of precursor B-lymphoblastic lymphoma/leukemia (PBLL) (80%) present as leukemia. In lymphoma cases, nodal, cutaneous, and osseous involvement is common. PBLL should be distinguished from Ewing's sarcoma (ES) or primitive neuroectodermal tumor (PNET). PBLL may be negative for CD45 (leukocyte common antigen, a widely used marker for lymphoma) and may express

TABLE 16.9. *Alternative or Salvage Regimens for Aggressive Non-Hodgkin's Lymphoma*

Combination Chemotherapy	Treatment Description	Reference
EPOCH (dose adjusted)[*,†]	**Etoposide** 50 mg/m^2 per day by continuous IV infusion for 4 days, days 1–4 (total dose/cycle = 250 mg/m^2) **Doxorubicin** 10 mg/m^2 per day by continuous IV infusion for 4 days, days 1–4 (total dose/cycle = 40 mg/m^2) **Vincristine** 0.4 mg/m^2 per day by continuous IV infusion for 4 days, days 1–4 (total dose/cycle = 1.6 mg/m^2 [no cap]) **Prednisone** 60 mg/m^2 per dose PO every 12 h for 5 days, days 1–5 (total dose/cycle = 600 mg/m^2) **Cyclophosphamide** 750 mg/m^2 IV day 5 (total dose/cycle = 750 mg/m^2) **Filgrastim** 5 μg/kg per day SC starting day 6; continues until ANC >5000 cells/mm^3 Treatment is dose adjusted based on neutrophil nadirs and repeated every 21 days	(8, 9)
CHOEP	**CHOP with etoposide** 100 mg/m^2 IV days 1, 2, and 3	(10)
R-ICE	**Rituximab** 375 mg/m^2 IV 48 hours prior to cycle 1 and on day 1 of cycles 1–3 **Etoposide** 100 mg/m^2 IV days 3, 4, and 5 **Carboplatin** AUC 5: dose = 5 × [25 + Creatinine Clearance] capped at 800 mg IV on day 4 **Ifosfamide** 5000 mg/m^2 mixed with an equal amount of MESNA CIV for 24 hours on day 4	(11)
DHAP	**Cisplatin** 100 mg/m^2 by continuous IV infusion for 24 h on day 1 (total dose/cycle = 100 mg/m^2) **Cytarabine** 2000 mg/m^2 per dose IV over 3 h every 12 h for 2 doses on day 2 (total dose/cycle = 4000 mg/m^2) **Dexamethasone** 40 mg per day PO or IV for 4 days, days 1–4 (total dose/cycle = 160 mg/m^2) Treatment is repeated every 21–28 days	(12)
ESHAP	**Etoposide** 40 mg/m^2 per day over 1 h IV for 4 days, days 1–4 (total dose/cycle = 160 mg/m^2) **Methylprednisolone** 250–500 mg per day IV for 5 days, days 1–5 (total dose/cycle = 1250–2500 mg) **Cytarabine** 2000 mg/m^2 IV over 2 h on day 5 (total dose/cycle = 2000 mg/m^2) **Cisplatin** 25 mg/m^2 per day by continuous IV infusion for 4 days, days 1–4 (total dose/cycle = 100 mg/m^2) Treatment is repeated every 21–28 days	(13)
ACVBP	**Doxorubicin** 75 mg/m^2 IV day 1 **Cyclophosphamide** 1200 mg/m^2 per dose IV day 1 **Vindesine** 2 mg/m^2 IV days 1 and 5 **Bleomycin** 10 mg IV days 1 and 5 **Prednisone** 60 mg/m^2 per day PO days 1–5	(14)

*Etoposide, cyclophosphamide, and doxorubicin dosages may be increased by 20% from the previous cycle's dosage if there was no evidence of absolute neutropenia (ANC <500/mm^3) or thrombocytopenia (platelet count <25,000/mm^3).

†Increments in the doses of cyclophosphamide by 50 mg/m^2 and etoposide by 15 mg/m^2 each cycle is allowed if patient could tolerate without significant neutropenia.

ANC, absolute neutrophil count; AUC, area under the curve; civ, continuous intravenously; iv, intravenously; MESNA, 2-mercaptoethane sulfonate; PO, orally; SC, subcutaneously.

TABLE 16.10. *Outcome in Adults and Children with Burkitt's and Burkitt's-Like Lymphoma with CODOX-M/IVAC Regimen*

Number	Complete Response	Event-Free Survival at 2 Years
Children: 21	90%	85%
Adults: 20	100%	100%
Total: 41	95%	92%

From Magrath I, Adde M, Shaa A, et al. Adults and children with non-cleaved–cell lymphoma have a similar excellent outcome when treated with the same chemotherapy regimen. J Clin Oncol 1996;14:925–934, with permission.

CD99 (a marker for ES or PNET). PBLL accounts for approximately 2.5% of childhood NHL. ALL therapy strategy can yield 73% EFS at 10 years, superior to short-pulse B-NHL therapy.

Burkitt Lymphoma/B-Cell Acute Lymphocytic Leukemia

Immunophenotype, molecular, and cytogenetic analyses of the bone marrow or peripheral blood, or both, should be done. Surface immunoglobulin expression is characteristic. Cytogenetics shows t(8;14), t(2;8), or t(8;22).

Treatment may provoke tumor lysis syndrome, and prophylaxis should be used: alkalinize the urine with D5W plus 100 mEq sodium acetate at 100 to 150 mL/hr, add allopurinol, 600 mg, orally daily for 2 days, then 300 mg per day orally until resolution of the tumor lysis syndrome.

Aggressive chemotherapy includes cyclophosphamide, vincristine, doxorubicin, methotrexate/ifosfamide, mesna, etoposide, cytarabine (CODOX-M/IVAC) risk-stratified regimen (Tables 16.10–16.13). Three cycles of CODOX-M should be given for low risk (all of the following: normal LDH, WHO performance status 0 or 1, Ann Arbor stage I to II, and no tumor mass 10 cm or larger). Four cycles of alternating CODOX-M and IVAC should be administered for high risk (e.g., do not meet criteria for low risk above).

Other aggressive chemotherapy includes hyper-CVAD (cyclophosphamide, vincristine, Adriamycin, dexamethasone) regimen (Tables 16.14 and 16.15). The addition of rituximab may increase efficacy.

TABLE 16.11. *Estimate of 1-Year Event-Free Survival for Subgroups of High-Risk Patients Treated with CODOX-M/IVAC Regime for HIV-Unrelated Burkitt Lymphoma*

Variable	n	1-year Event-Free Survival (%)	(95% CI)	Log-rank p value
International Prognostic Index score				
0–1	6	83.3	(53.5–99.0)	
2	19	63.2	(41.5–84.9)	
3	14	57.1	(31.2–83.1)	0.8852

From Mead GM, Sydes MR, Walewski J, et al. An international evaluation of CODOX-M and CODOX-M alternating with IVAC in adult Burkitt's lymphoma: results of United Kingdom Lymphoma Group LYO6 study. Ann Oncol 2002; 13:1264–1274, with permission.
CI, confidence interval; CODOX-M/IVAC, cyclophosphamide, vincristine, doxorubicin, methotrexate/ifosfamide, mesna, etoposide, cytarabine; EFS, event-free survival; HIV, human immunodeficiency virus.

TABLE 16.12. *CODOX-M Regimen*

Day	Drug	Dose	Route	Time
1	Cyclophosphamide	800 mg/m^2	IV	
	Vincristine	1.5 mg/m^2 (max 2 mg)	IV	
	Doxorubicin	40 mg/m^2	IV	
	Cytarabine	70 mg	IT	
2–5	Cyclophosphamide	200 mg/m^2	IV	Daily
3	Cytarabine	70 mg	IT	
8	Vincristine	1.5 mg/m^2 (max 2 mg)	IV	
10	Methotrexate	1200 mg/m^2	IV	Over 1 hour
		240 mg/m^2	IV	Each hour over 23 h
11	Leucovorin	192 mg/m^2	IV	At hour 36
		12 mg/m^2	IV	Every 6 h until MTX level $<5 \times 10^{-8}$ M
13	G-CSF	5 μg/kg	SC	Daily until AGC $>10^9$/l
15	Methotrexate	12 mg	IT	
16	Leucovorin	15 mg	PO	24 h after IT methotrexate

From Mead GM, Sydes MR, Walewski J, et al. An international evaluation of CODOX-M and CODOX-M alternating with IVAC in adult Burkitt's lymphoma: results of United Kingdom Lymphoma Group LY06 study. Ann Oncol 2002;13:1264–1274.
Begin next cycle on the day that unsupported ANC is $>1.0 \times 10^9$/L, and unsupported platelet $>75 \times 10^9$/L.
AGC, absolute granulocyte count; ANC, absolute neutrophil count; CODOX-M, cyclophosphamide, vincristine, doxorubicin, methotrexate; G-CSF, granulocyte colony-stimulating factor; IT, intrathecally; IV, intravenously; MTX, methotrexate; PO, orally; SC, subcutaneously.

TABLE 16.13. *IVAC Regimen*

Day	Drug	Dose	Method	Time
1–5	Etoposide	60 mg/m^2	IV	Daily over 1 h
	Ifosfamide	1500 mg/m^2	IV	Daily over 1 h
	Mesna	360 mg/m^2 (mixed with ifosfamide) then 360 mg/m^2	IV	3 hourly (7 doses/24 h period)
1 and 2	Cytarabine	2 g/m^2	IV	Over 3 hours, 12 hourly (total of 4 doses)
5	Methotrexate	12 mg	IT	
6	Leucovorin	15 mg	PO	24 h after IT MTX
7	G-CSF	5 μ/kg	SC	Daily until AGC $>1.0 \times 10^9$/l

From Mead GM, Sydes MR, Walewski J, et al. An international evaluation of CODOX-M and CODOX-M alternating with IVAC in adult Burkitt's lymphoma: results of United Kingdom Lymphoma Group LY06 study. Ann Oncol 2002;13:1264–1274.
Begin next cycle CODOX-M) on the day the unsupported ANC is $>1.0 \times 10^9$/L, and unsupported platelet $>75 \times 10^9$/L
ANC, absolute neutrophil count; IT, intrathecally; IV, intravenously; IVAC, ifosfamide, mesna, etoposide, cytarabine; MESNA, 2-mercaptoethane sulfonate; MTX, methotrexate;. PO, orally; SC, subcutaneously.

TABLE 16.14. *Treatment Outcome with Hyper-CVAD Program by B-ALL Features: FAB, Immunophenotype, and Karyotype*

				Outcome				
				CR		Relapse		
Features	No.	%	% Age >60 Years	No.	%	No.	%	3-Year Survival (%)
Total	26		46	21	81	9	43	49
L3, t(8;14), t(2;8), or t(8;22)	7	31	14	7	100	1	14	86
L3, CALLA, t(8;14), t(2;8), or t(8;22)	2	8	50	1	50	None		50
L3, other, sIg+*	11	38	64	8	73	4	50	36
L3, CALLA, other, sIg+†	3	12	33	3	100	2	67	33
L2, t(8;14), sIg+ >90%	1	4	All	1	100	All		None
L1/L2, other, sIg+ >90†	2	8	50	1	50	All		None

From Thomas DA, Cortes J, O'Brien S, et al. Hyper-CVAD program in Burkitt's-type adult acute lymphoblastic leukemia. J Clin Oncol 1999;17:2461–2470, with permission.
B-ALL, B-cell acute lymphoblastic leukemia; CALLA, common acute lymphocytic anemia antigen; CR, complete remission; CVAD, cyclophosphamide, vincristine, Adriamycin, dexamethasone; FAB, French-American-British.

Preliminary data suggest R-EPOCH effective in Burkitt lymphoma. There is not yet sufficient data to recommend this treatment routinely outside of a research protocol, but favorable toxicity profile may confer rationale if a given patient cannot tolerate more established aggressive dose-intensive therapy.

TREATMENT OF RECURRENT AND REFRACTORY B-CELL LYMPHOMA

Many patients with NHL require additional therapy because of disease recurrence or refractoriness to therapy. Although grades I and II follicular lymphoma are not curable, high-dose chemotherapy followed by autologous transplant improves PFS. In aggressive NHL, approximately 40% to 50% of patients fail to achieve remission with conventional chemotherapy. Among those who do achieve a CR, 30% to 40% will relapse. These patients may benefit from salvage therapy (see Table 16.9).

Principles of Salvage Therapy

Conventional wisdom promotes the use of noncross-resistant chemotherapy such as DHAP (cisplatin, cytarabine, and dexamethasone), ESHAP (etoposide, methyl prednisolone, cytarabine, and cisplatin), and ICE (ifosfamide, carboplatin, etoposide). However, evolving understanding of cellular apoptotic response to chemotherapeutic stimuli suggests that true noncross-resistance drugs may not exist—as mechanisms for tumor resistance may not be entirely drug-specific—because of the intrinsic high apoptosis thresholds in refractory tumors. Both in vitro and empiric clinical data provide evidence that tumor resistance can be overcome by using drugs already administered but with different infusion schedules (e.g., by prolonged infusion regimens such as dose-adjusted EPOCH-R). In addition, other agents such as in ICE or ESHAP have also shown utility in the setting of relapsed and refractory NHL.

Rituximab added to conventional chemotherapy increases efficacy in CD20+ tumors.

TABLE 16.15. *Hyper-CVAD Alternating with High-Dose Methotrexate and Ara-C*

Cycle	Day	Drug	Dose	Route	Time
Odd numbers 1, 3, 5, and 7	1–3	Cyclophosphamide	300 mg/m² (total dose 1800 mg/m²)	IV	Each dose given over 2 hours every 12 hours for 6 doses
	1–3	Mesna	600 mg/m²	CIV	Infused over 24 hours daily for 3 days. Start 1 hour before cyclophosphamide and continue for 12 hours after last dose.
	4	Doxorubicin	50 mg/m²	IV	Over 2 hours
	4 and 11	Vincristine	2 mg	IV	
	4–11 and 11–14	Dexamethasone	40 mg/day	PO or IV	Daily starting 24 hours after the last dose of doxorubicin, until granulocytes are >30,000/μl or until day 21 (whichever comes first).
		G-CSF	10 μg/kg	SC	
Even 2, 4, 6, and 8	1	Methotrexate	1 g/m²	CIV	Infused over 24 hours
		Leucovorin	50 mg IV or PO is given	IV or PO	12 hours after the completion of methotrexate, followed by 15 mg IV or PO every 6 hours for 8 doses. At the end of the methotrexate infusion, 24 hours and 48 hours after completion, the methotrexate level is checked. If the level is >1 μM at 24 hours or >0.1 μM at 48 hours, the leucovorin dose is increased to 50 mg IV every 6 hours until the level is <0.1 μM.
	2–3	Ara-C	3 g/m²	IV	Given over 2 hours every 12 hours for 4 doses
		G-CSF	5 μg/kg	SC	Begin after chemotherapy completion until the ANC is >30,000/μL or until day 21 (whichever comes first). Then it is held for 1 day and the next cycle is started.

From Thomas DA, Cortes J, O'Brien S, et al. Hyper-CVAD program in Burkitt's-type adult acute lymphoblastic leukemia. J Clin Oncol 1999;17:2461–2470.
Central nervous system prophylaxis: MTX 12 mg IT on day 2 and ara-C 100 mg IT on day 8 of each cycle for 16 IT treatments in high-risk patients, four IT treatments in low-risk patients.
ANC, absolute neutrophil count; CIV, continuous intravenously; G-CSF, granulocyte colony-stimulating factor; IT, intrathecally; IV, intravenously; MTX, methotrexate; PO, orally; SC, subcutaneously.

High-dose chemotherapy and autologous stem cell transplantation (ASCT) may confer curative advantage in some patients whose disease is responsive to salvage chemotherapy. ASCT achieves long-term survival in up to 50% of patients with chemotherapy-sensitive relapsed DLBCL, and some prospective randomized studies have documented the superiority of ASCT over salvage chemotherapy for relapsed DLBCL. Patients with low-risk IPI are most likely to benefit. Patients with well-controlled HIV with relapsed NHL should not be routinely excluded from consideration for ASCT.

Allogeneic transplantation remains investigational. Nonmyeloablative or reduced intensity stem cell transplantation (RIST) attempts to exert immunologic effects against the tumor without the risk of high-dose chemotherapy. High-dose chemotherapy does not appear to overcome tumor resistance in the majority of cases. Graft engineering to enhance graft-versus lymphoma benefit and to decrease graft-versus-host complications remains an active area of investigation. Studies have not consistently shown strong graft-versus-lymphoma effects in the majority of patients.

ACQUIRED IMMUNE DEFICIENCY SYNDROME-RELATED LYMPHOMA (SYSTEMIC) TREATMENT CONSIDERATIONS

Many experts recommend CNS prophylaxis for all systemic ARL (Table 16.16). Standard-dose chemotherapy has supplanted low-dose therapy in the HAART era.

Randomized trial data indicates increased toxicity with CHOP, especially in those with fewer than 50 CD4 cells/mm^3. Preliminary analysis of a phase II randomized trial of dose-adjusted

TABLE 16.16. *Selected Regimens and Outcomes for Acquired Immune Deficiency Syndrome-Associated Non-Hodgkin's Lymphoma*

Regimen	Evaluable Patients	Median Baseline CD4 cells/mm^3	Complete Response Rate (%)	Median Progression-Free/ Overall Survival (mo)	Reference
Randomized R-CHOP	99	130	57.6	11.25/34.75	18
versus CHOP (+HAART)	51	147	47	9.5/27.5	
Infusional CDE	48	70	46	7.9*/12.8	19
Pooled results of 3 phase II trials of infusional CDE + rituximab (+ HAART)	74	161	70	Not yet reached (at 23 months FFS* is 59% and OS is 64%)	20
Dose-adjusted EPOCH (HAART deferment until chemotherapy completion)	39	198	74	Not yet reached (at 53 months, PFS is 73% and OS is 60%; OS is 87% if CD4 count over 100 cells/mm^3)	21
Phase II randomized R-dose-adjusted	38	190	65	FFS is 80% at 12 mo	22
EPOCH versus dose-adjusted EPOCH followed by rituximab maintenance	38	180	38	FFS is 72% at 12 mo	

CDE, cyclophosphamide, doxorubicin, and etoposide; CHOP, cyclophosphamide, doxorubicin, vincristine, and prednisone; EPOCH, etoposide, prednisone, vincristine, cycophosphamide, and doxorubicin; FFS, failure-free survival; HAART, highly active antiretroviral therapy; OS, overall survival; PFS, progression-free survival; R, rituximab.

EPOCH with rituximab given concurrently versus given as maintenance after completion of EPOCH reported no excess toxicity and a 1-year progression-free survival of 80%. Based on this data, rituximab with dose-adjusted EPOCH can be considered a reasonable choice for initial therapy in most cases of ARL.

There is no randomized data comparing the EPOCH and CHOP regimens in ARL. Investigators felt that given the initial data for EPOCH, inclusion of a CHOP arm in randomized trials would not be ethical, given the well-established short time to progression with CHOP (approximately 9 to 12 months). R-CHOP appears effective in small phase II trials in patients without adverse clinical features (e.g., CD4 cells <100 mm^3, prior AIDS, or performance status >1).

Some studies have suggested a role for dose-intense regimens for Burkitt lymphoma in AIDS (e.g., hyper-CVAD or CODOX-M), but toxicity is high. Combined with rituximab this is currently a research focus for this patient population. Limited data suggests that Burkitt lymphoma in AIDS responds to infusional chemotherapy and may be more effective when given with rituximab (e.g., dose-adjusted EPOCH, Table 16.17).

The use of concurrent HAART is unsettled. There are inadequate data to make evidence-based recommendations. A phase 2 trial of dose-adjusted EPOCH in ARL suggested that concurrent HAART is not necessary to achieve favorable results, provided effective antiretroviral therapy is initiated after treatment for lymphoma. Concerns to omit HAART during ARL therapy include overlapping toxicity, pharmacokinetic interactions, HAART adherence problems related to chemotherapy, and because chemotherapy will deplete CD4 cells regardless of HAART. Clinical trials that include HAART have not demonstrated clear clinically relevant problems with concurrent HAART. Many oncologists recommend continuing HAART if a patient is already on a stable well-tolerated regimen, but delaying HAART initiation until after lymphoma therapy in those who are not. However, pharmacokinetic interactions between chemotherapy and many HAART drugs have not been studied.

TABLE 16.17. *Dose-Adjusted EPOCH for AIDS-Related Lymphomas*

Etoposide	50 mg/m^2/day CIV days 1–4 (total dose/cycle = 250 mg/m^2)		
Doxorubicin	10 mg/m^2/day CIV days 1–4 (total dose/cycle = 40 mg/m^2)		
Vincristine	0.4 mg/m^2/day CIV days 1–4 (total dose/cycle = 1.6 mg/m^2 [no cap])		
Prednisone	60 mg/m^2 PO daily, days 1–5		
Cyclophosphamide	Cycle 1 dependent on CD4 cell count		
	CD4/mm^3	<100	187 mg/m^2 IV on day 5
		≥100	375 mg/m^2 IV on day 5
	Cycles 2 and beyond dependent on ANC nadir		
	ANC nadir	<500	Decrease dose by 187 mg/m^2
		≥500	Increase dose by 187 mg/m^2 (maximum dose is 750 mg/m^2)
Filgrastim	300 μg/ per day SC starting day 6; continues until ANC >5000 cells/mm^3		
	Treatment is repeated every 21 days		

Rituximab 375 mg/m^2 given on day 1 prior to EPOCH infusion may increase efficacy
HAART suspended until completion of all EPOCH cycles in original phase II trial; HAART continued in randomized multicenter phase II trial.
PCP prophylaxis for all patients and continued until CD4 >200 cells/mm^3
MAC prophylaxis for all patients with CD4 <100 cells /mm^3

From Sparano J, Lee J, et al. Randomized phase II trial of infusional EPOCH chemotherapy given either concurrently with or sequentially followed by rituximab in HIV-associated lymphoma: AIDS Malignancy Consortium Trial 034. Presented at: 10th International Conference on Malignancies in AIDS and Other Acquired Immunodeficiencies; October 16–17, 2006; Bethesda, MD.
ANC, absolute neutrophil count; CIV, continuous intravenously; EPOCH, etoposide, prednisone, vincristine, cycophosphamide, and doxorubicin; HAART, highly active antiretroviral therapy; IV, intravenously; MAC, mycobacterium avium complex; PCP, *Pneumocystis carinii* pneumonia; PO, orally; SC, subcutaneously.

ACQUIRED IMMUNE DEFICIENCY SYNDROME–RELATED PRIMARY BRAIN LYMPHOMA

For diagnosis, a major recent advance has been the ability to diagnose AIDS primary brain lymphoma (AIDS-PBL) more easily. Essentially 100% of AIDS-PBL are EBV associated. Combined EBV and PET or single photon emission computed tomography (SPECT) thallium can be used in a relatively noninvasive diagnostic approach, and brain biopsy can be avoided if the tests are concordant. If both EBV and PET/SPECT are positive, the positive predictive value for lymphoma is 100%. If both EBV and PET/SPECT are negative, the negative predictive value for lymphoma is 100%.

For treatment, the use of high-dose systemic methotrexate has not been adequately evaluated in HIV-infected patients. As AIDS-PBL virtually never occurs until CD4 cells are less than 50 per cubic millimeter, the importance of immune reconstitution with treatment should be considered a high priority in treatment to help prevent disease recurrence. Interest in high-dose chemotherapy with rituximab and HAART is a current research focus.

Standard of care remains radiotherapy. HAART, especially among those naïve to antiretroviral therapy, may result in substantial immune recovery and tumor control and thus should be initiated as soon as possible in patients with AIDS with focal brain lesions.

AGGRESSIVE T-CELL LYMPHOMA

Adult T-Cell Leukemia/Lymphoma

Rare in Western countries, this is the most common lymphoma in Asia and is caused by the human retrovirus, HTVL-1. Adult T-cell lymphoma (ATLL) may behave aggressively, but some clinical variants have a relatively indolent course. ATLL cannot be cured. Ameliorative treatments include interferon and doxorubicin-based combination chemotherapy.

Clinical Variants

Acute ATLL has a survival time ranging from a few weeks to more than 1 year. There is a leukemic phase with elevated white blood count, skin rash, generalized lymphadenopathy, organomegaly, constitutional symptoms, and high LDH. Hypercalcemia is common. Opportunistic infections occur as a result of an associated T-cell immunodeficiency.

For lymphomatous ATLL, survival also ranges from a few weeks to more than 1 year. The lymphoma is characterized by prominent lymphadenopathy without peripheral blood involvement. Hypercalcemia is less frequent than in the acute form, but generally patients have advanced-stage disease.

Chronic variant generally has a more protracted clinical course with longer survival, but it can transform into an acute phase with an aggressive course. There may be skin lesions and absolute lymphocytosis but without numerous atypical lymphocytes in the peripheral blood. Hypercalcemia is absent.

Smoldering ATLL is characterized by a more protracted clinical course and longer survival but can acutely transform into an aggressive tumor. More generally, the ATLL is indolent with normal white blood count and less than 5% circulating neoplastic cells. Skin or pulmonary lesions are common, but hypercalcemia is absent. Progression from chronic and smoldering to acute variants occurs in 25% of cases, usually after a long duration.

Enteropathy-Type T-Cell Lymphoma

Adult patients usually have a history of gluten-sensitive enteropathy. The geographic distribution is that of intestinal enteropathies, and hence the disease is rare in Western countries. Patients may present with abdominal pain and small bowel perforation. The prognosis is usually poor.

Extranodal Natural Killer/T-Cell Lymphoma, Nasal-Type

This is most prevalent in Asia, Mexico, and Central and South America, occurs most often in adults (men more than women), and is almost always EBV associated. The disease usually presents in the nasopharyngeal area with symptoms of obstruction, pain, or epistaxis. Tumors may cause extensive midfacial destructive lesions, termed lethal midline granuloma. Upper aerodigestive tract involvement may present with perforation. The skin is commonly involved. Treatment for localized disease is primarily radiation. Optimal outcome is dependent on careful planning of radiation fields and higher doses (50 to 60 Gy). The role of chemotherapy is unclear. At relapse (and less commonly at presentation), the disease may disseminate to extranodal sites such as the bone marrow and blood.

Angioimmunoblastic T-Cell Lymphoma

Angioimmunoblastic T-cell lymphoma or angioimmunoblastic lymphadenopathy with dysproteinemia (AILD) occurs most often in the middle aged and elderly with equal gender incidence, usually at an advanced stage with systemic symptoms. A pruritic skin rash is common. Laboratory findings include polyclonal hypergammaglobulinemia, circulating immune complexes, cold agglutinins with hemolytic anemia, positive rheumatoid factor, and antismooth muscle antibodies. The aggressive clinical course is responsive to steroids and chemotherapy, but most patients relapse and die from disease.

Peripheral T-Cell Lymphoma, Unspecified

Peripheral T-cell lymphoma (unspecified) accounts for nearly 50% of the peripheral T-cell lymphomas in Western countries and most commonly occurs in adults with equal gender incidence. Nodal involvement is the most common presentation, but bone marrow, liver, spleen, and extranodal involvement including skin is not uncommon. The clinical course is aggressive, and the disease responds poorly to therapy. The median survival at 5 years is poor at 20% to 30%.

Anaplastic Large Cell Lymphoma: Systemic and Primary Cutaneous Forms

The systemic form occurs in both children and adults and has either a T-cell or null phenotype; true anaplastic large-cell lymphomas with a B-cell phenotype are rare. It may involve lymph nodes or extranodal sites, including the skin, and half of patients have B symptoms and advanced states at presentation. It is highly responsive to chemotherapy and curable with OS and FFS of 75% and 60%, respectively, at 7 years.

The primary cutaneous form occurs mostly in adults and presents with isolated skin nodules. The clinical course is indolent. Skin lesions may spontaneously regress. Systemic disease is uncommon and occurs late in the disease course. This form may be incurable. Some cases appear to be within the spectrum of lymphomatoid papulosis type A.

Hepatosplenic γ/δ

Hepatosplenic γ/δ is a rare tumor that comprises fewer than 5% of T-cell neoplasms. Its peak incidence is in adolescents and young adults, and males are more often affected than females. The aggressive clinical course is associated with a median survival less than 2 years.

TREATMENT PRINCIPLES

T-cell lymphomas tend to have a poorer PFS and OS than aggressive B-cell lymphomas. Systemic ALCL is an exception and is among the most curable subtypes with doxorubicin-based treatment. Some T-cell subtypes have no potential for cure and should be approached palliatively, as in ATL and primary cutaneous anaplastic lymphoma. Other T-cell subtypes, including angioimmunoblastic and PTL, have low curative potential with conventional dose treatment and should be considered for trials targeting high-risk patients.

SUGGESTED READINGS

Bagley CM Jr, Devita VT Jr, Berard CW, et al. Advanced lymphosarcoma: intensive cyclical combination chemotherapy with cyclophosphamide, vincristine, and prednisone. Ann Intern Med 1972; 76:227–234.

Coiffier B, Lepage E, Briere J, et al. CHOP chemotherapy plus rituximab compared with CHOP alone in elderly patients with diffuse large B-cell lymphoma. N Engl J Med 2002;346:235–242.

Danhauser L, Plunkett W, Keating M, et al. 9-beta-D-arabinofuranosyl-2-fluoroadenine 5'-monophosphate pharmacokinetics in plasma and tumor cells of patients with relapsed leukemia and lymphoma. Cancer Chemother Pharmacol 1986;18:145–152.

Habermann TM, Weller EA, Morrison VA, et al. Phase III trial of rituximab-CHOP (R-CHOP) vs. CHOP with a second randomization to maintenance rituximab (MR) or observation in patients 60 years of age and older with diffuse large B-cell lymphoma (DLBCL). Presented at: 45th Annual Meeting of the American Society of Hematology; December 6–9, 2003; San Diego, CA.

Hersh MR, Kuhn JG, Phillips JL, et al. Pharmacokinetic study of fludarabine phosphate (NSC 312887). Cancer Chemother Pharmacol 1986;17:277–280.

Hutton JJ, Von Hoff DD, Kuhn J, et al. Phase I clinical investigation of 9-beta-D-arabinofuranosyl-2-fluoroadenine 5'-monophosphate (NSC 312887), a new purine antimetabolite. Cancer Res 1984; 44:4183–4186.

Kaiser U, Uebelacker I, Abel U, et al. Randomized study to evaluate the use of high-dose therapy as part of primary treatment for "aggressive" lymphoma. J Clin Oncol 2002;20:4413–4419.

Kaplan LD, Lee JY, et al. Rituximab does not improve clinical outcome in a randomized phase III trial of CHOP with or without rituximab in patients with HIV-associated non-Hodgkin's lymphoma: AIDS-malignancies consortium trial 010. Blood 2005;106:1538–1543.

Kewalramani T, Zelenetz AD, Nimer SD, et al. Rituximab and ICE (RICE) as second-line therapy prior to autologous stem cell transplantation for relapsed or primary refractory diffuse large B-cell lymphoma. Blood 2004;103:3684–3688.

Little RF, Pittaluga S, Grant N, et al. Highly effective treatment of acquired immunodeficiency syndrome-related lymphoma with dose-adjusted EPOCH: impact of antiretroviral therapy suspension and tumor biology. Blood 2003;101:4653–4659.

Magrath I, Adde M, Shad A, et al. Adults and children with small non-cleaved-cell lymphoma have a similar excellent outcome when treated with the same chemotherapy regimen. J Clin Oncol 1996; 14:925–934.

McLaughlin P, Grillo-Lopez AJ, Link BK, et al. Rituximab chimeric anti-CD20 monoclonal antibody therapy for relapsed indolent lymphoma: half of patients respond to a four-dose treatment program. J Clin Oncol 1998;16:2533–2833.

Mead GM, Sydes MR, Walewski J, et al. An international evaluation of CODOX-M and CODOX-M alternating with IVAC in adult Burkitt's lymphoma: results of United Kingdom Lymphoma Group LY06 study. Ann Oncol 2002;13:1264–1274.

Sparano J, Lee J, Kaplan LD, et al. Randomized phase II trial of infusional EPOCH chemotherapy given either concurrently with or sequentially followed by rituximab in HIV-associated lymphoma: AIDS Malignancy Consortium Trial 034. Presented at: 10th International Conference on Malignancies in AIDS and Other Acquired Immunodeficiencies; October 16–17, 2006; Bethesda, MD.

Sparano JA, Lee S, Chen MG, et al. Phase II trial of infusional cyclophosphamide, doxorubicin, and etoposide in patients with HIV-associated non-Hodgkin's lymphoma: an Eastern Cooperative Oncology Group Trial (E1494). J Clin Oncol 2004;22:1491–1500.

Spina M, Jaeger U, Sparano JA, et al. Rituximab plus infusional cyclophosphamide, doxorubicin, and etoposide in HIV-associated non-Hodgkin lymphoma: pooled results from 3 phase 2 trials. Blood 2005;105:1891–1897.

Thomas DA, Cortes J, O'Brien S, et al. Hyper-CVAD program in Burkitt's-type adult acute lymphoblastic leukemia. J Clin Oncol 1999;17:2461–2470.

Tilly H, Lepage E, Coiffier B, et al. Intensive conventional chemotherapy (ACVBP regimen) compared with standard CHOP for poor-prognosis aggressive non-Hodgkin lymphoma. Blood 2003; 102:4284–4289.

Velasquez WS, Cabanillas F, Salvador P, et al. Effective salvage therapy for lymphoma with cisplatin in combination with high-dose Ara-C and dexamethasone (DHAP). Blood 1988;71:117–122.

Velasquez WS, McLaughlin P, Tucker S, et al. ESHAP—an effective chemotherapy regimen in refractory and relapsing lymphoma: a 4-year follow-up study. J Clin Oncol 1994;12:1169–1176.

Wilson WH, Bryant G, Bates S, et al. EPOCH chemotherapy: toxicity and efficacy in relapsed and refractory non-Hodgkin's lymphoma. J Clin Oncol 1993;11:1573–1582.

Wilson WH, Grossbard ML, Pittaluga S, et al. Dose-adjusted EPOCH chemotherapy for untreated large B-cell lymphomas: a pharmacodynamic approach with high efficacy. Blood 2002;99:2685–2693.

17

Multiple Myeloma

Sandeep S. Dave and Cynthia E. Dunbar

EPIDEMIOLOGY AND RISK FACTORS

The annual incidence of multiple myeloma in the United States is approximately 4 per 100,000 (1,2). There is a slight male predominance. The incidence in African Americans is almost twice that in Caucasians. Median age at diagnosis is 66 years. The role of genetic factors is uncertain. There have been a few reported instances of familial clustering, but the vast majority of cases are sporadic (3). Exposure to radiation may play a role. An increased incidence has been noted in atomic bomb survivors exposed to more than 50 Gy as well in workers in nuclear power plants. There is little evidence to implicate other environmental causes.

PATHOPHYSIOLOGY

Multiple myeloma is characterized by the proliferation and accumulation of clonal plasma cells. The presence of somatic mutations in the complementarity determining regions (the antigen-binding portion) of the clonal immunoglobulin indicates the transforming event occurred in a postgerminal center B cell or a plasma cell itself.

The commonest chromosomal abnormality involves the heavy chain locus on chromosome 14, but there is no single cytogenetic abnormality that is characteristic of the disease. Chromosome 13 abnormalities are also common and are associated with poor prognosis.

At the gene-expression level, monoclonal gammopathy of unknown significance (MGUS) cannot be distinguished from multiple myeloma. However, normal plasma cells can be clearly distinguished from plasma cells of both MGUS and myeloma.

The clinical features of the disease result from bone marrow infiltration by the malignant clone, secretion of osteoclast-activating factors and cytokines, high levels of circulating immunoglobulin and/or free light chains, and depressed immunity.

DIAGNOSIS AND CLINICAL FEATURES

Clinical Features

The most common presenting symptom is bone pain, present in 60% of patients, especially in the back or chest. Weakness and fatigue are common and are often associated with a normochromic, normocytic anemia. Twenty-five percent of patients have renal insufficiency, and 20% of patients have hypercalcemia. Less than 5% of patients have clinically significant amyloidosis or hyperviscosity.

Diagnostic Criteria

The World Health Organization (WHO) major criteria for diagnosis includes:

1. Bone marrow plasmacytosis >30%
2. Plasmacytoma on biopsy

3. Presence of monoclonal protein (M protein) in serum or urine:
   a. Serum IgG >3.5 g/dL, or
   b. Serum IgA >2 g/dL, or
   c. Urine Bence-Jones protein >1 g/24hours.

The WHO minor criteria for diagnosis includes:

1. Bone marrow plasmacytosis 10% to 30%
2. M protein present, but less than major criteria concentration
3. Presence of lytic bone lesions
4. Reduced normal immunoglobulins to <50% of normal

The diagnosis of multiple myeloma requires a minimum of one major and one minor criterion, or three minor criteria including the presence of bone marrow plasmacytosis and the presence of M protein.

The distribution of monoclonal protein type in multiple myeloma patients is:

- IgG in 60% of patients
- Light chain only (Bence Jones proteinuria) in 20% of patients
- IgA in 17% of patients
- IgD in 2% of patients
- Biclonal in 1% of patients

Bone marrow involvement can be patchy; repeated marrow biopsies may be needed to make the diagnosis.

STAGING AND PROGNOSIS IN MULTIPLE MYELOMA

The Durie-Salmon Staging System (Table 17.1) is based on factors related to tumor burden. The system does not correlate well with prognosis and is being supplanted by the International Staging Sytem (Table 17.1), which is based upon β_2 microglobulin and serum albumin. Median survival ranges from 62 months for stage I compared with 29 months for stage III. Cytogenetic abnormalities have also been associated with survival with the presence of t(4;14) and t(14;16) and loss of 13q and 17p13 associated with a poor prognosis.

TABLE 17.1. *Staging Systems for Multiple Myeloma*

Durie Salmon System	
Stage I (myeloma mass, <0.6 × 10¹² cells/m²)	All of the following: Hgb, >10 g/dL; serum Ca, ≤12 mg/dL; ≤1 lesion on skeletal survey; IgG M protein, <50 g/L; IgA M protein, <30 g/L; urinary light chains, <4 g/24 h
Stage II (myeloma mass, 0.6–1.2 × 10¹² cells/m²)	Results fit neither stage I nor stage III
Stage III (myeloma mass, >1.2 × 10¹² cells/m²)	Any of the following: Hgb, ≤8.5 g/dL; serum Ca, >12 mg/dL; >1 lesion on skeletal survey; IgG M protein, >70 g/L; IgA M protein, >50 g/L; urinary light chain excretion, >12 g/24 h
Subclassification A	Serum creatinine, <2 mg/dL
Subclassification B	Serum creatinine, ≥2 mg/dL

International Staging System	
Stage I	β_2 microglobulin <3.5 mg/L and serum albumin >3.5 g/dL
Stage II	Neither stage I or stage II
Stage III	β_2 microglobulin >5.5 mg/L

Initial Evaluation

Suggested in the initial evaluation of multiple myeloma are:

- Complete history and physical examination
- Blood counts with differential and visual examination of the peripheral smear
- Serum electrolytes, blood urea nitrogen (BUN), and creatinine
- Calcium, magnesium, and phosphorus
- Uric acid
- β_2 microglobulin and serum albumin
- Serum lactate dehydrogenase (LDH)
- Serum protein electrophoresis (SPEP) with immunofixation and quantitation of immunoglobulins
- Serum free light chain (FLC) assay is more sensitive for the detection of monoclonal free light chains than urine immunofixation and is supplanting urine protein electrophoresis
- Urine protein electrophoresis (UPEP) and quantitation of light chains, if FLC is not available
- Radiographic skeletal survey
- Bone marrow biopsy and aspirate, with standard cytogenetics, and if possible fluorescent in situ hybridization (FISH) analysis for chromosome abnormalities. Standard cytogenetics are much less sensitive.
- Consider magnetic resonance imaging (MRI) of the spine, particularly if there are any spinal symptoms

An SPEP alone is inadequate because some forms of multiple myeloma secrete only light chains that are rapidly cleared to the urine.

A nuclear medicine bone scan is of no value because the disease produces osteolytic and not osteoblastic bone lesions.

DIFFERENTIAL DIAGNOSIS

Monoclonal gammopathy of unknown significance (MGUS) is characterized by M protein <3 g/dL, less than 10% plasma cells in the bone marrow, lack of symptoms, normal blood counts and renal function, and an absence of lytic lesions and evidence of end-organ involvement.

About 1% of patients/year experience progression to typical multiple myeloma. Smoldering multiple myeloma (SMM) is characterized by M protein >3 g/dL and/or greater than 10% plasma cells in the bone marrow, lack of symptoms, and an absence of lytic lesions and evidence of end-organ involvement.

About 3% of patients/year progress to typical multiple myeloma. Factors predicting progression include greater than 10% plasma cells in the bone marrow, detectable Bence-Jones proteinuria, and immunoglobulin IgA subtype.

Primary Amyloidosis

This disease is also a clonal expansion of plasma cells resulting in the overproduction of monoclonal light chains. Primary amyloidosis can be considered MGUS with clinical manifestations because of specific characteristics of the light chains that lead to their deposition as amyloid fibrils and multiorgan involvement. The proportion of bone marrow plasma cells may exceed 10%, but it is rarely greater than 20%. Lytic lesions are rare. The diagnosis is established by demonstrating the deposition of amyloid fibrils in a biopsy of affected tissue.

Metastatic Carcinoma

Malignant processes can produce lytic lesions and plasmacytosis. In the absence of significant M-protein in the blood or urine, the diagnosis of metastatic carcinoma must be actively excluded before the diagnosis of multiple myeloma is considered.

TREATMENT

Not all patients who fulfill the minimal criteria for the diagnosis of multiple myeloma require treatment. More specifically, patients with SMM or asymptomatic stage I multiple myeloma often remain stable for many years, and treatment has not been shown to prolong survival or to prevent progression in presymptomatic disease.

The main options include conventional chemotherapy (4,5), high-dose corticosteroids, dose-intensive chemotherapy with autologous hematopoietic cell rescue (6,7), allogeneic stem cell transplantation, as well as newer therapies such as thalidomide or its analogs and the proteosome inhibitor bortezomib. Bisphosphonate treatments can prevent or slow bone destruction and may also have antitumor activity.

No treatment modality with the possible exception of allogeneic stem cell transplantation is curative in multiple myeloma. However, event-free survival and overall survival are improved by approximately a year following autologous hematopoietic stem cell transplantation (HSCT) as compared with conventional chemotherapy, and newer agents such as thalidomide and bortezemib are effective in a significant percentage of patients with relapsed or refractory disease. The management of myeloma has become more complicated with this expanding set of therapeutic alternatives, but the lack of overlapping toxicities means that many patients even with advanced disease can be managed effectively as outpatients with reasonable quality of life. Survival from diagnosis has increased significantly over the past decade, particularly in patients under age 60, because of the activity of these new treatment modalities.

Treatment regimens are summarized in Table 17.2 (7–29). A flow chart outlining the treatment options for patients is shown in Figure 17.1.

Initial Therapy

All patients younger than 60 to 70 years of age should be considered for high-dose chemotherapy with autologous stem cell transplantation as consolidation therapy following initial treatment, although studies are ongoing to assess the upfront role of high-dose therapy and autologous transplantation versus combination therapy that includes new highly active agents. The most convincing data regarding survival advantage for autologous transplantation are in patients younger than 55 to 60, with somewhat conflicting data in the 60- to 70-year age group. Alkylating agents are damaging to hematopoietic stem cells. Hence, antilogous hematopoietic cells should be collected from the peripheral blood or bone marrow prior to any exposure to alkylators such as melphalan (4,5), and generally patients younger than 60 should not be treated with melphalan-containing regimens because of the adverse impact of even a few cycles of this agent on the ability to collect autologous peripheral blood stem cells.

Stem cell-sparing options for upfront therapy include dexamethasone in combination with thalidomide, bortezomib, or vincristine and adriamycin. The combination of thalidomide and dexamethasone is now Food and Drug Administration (FDA)-approved as first-line therapy and preserves stem cell collection options. Response rates approach 70%. VAD (Vincristine, Adriamycin, Dexamethasone) has been used as initial therapy in patients (6), often in the setting of preparation for autologous stem cell transplantation, with response rates comparable to melphalan plus prednisone. Typically three to four cycles of VAD are administered prior to transplantation. The combination of thalidomide and dexamethasone appears to yield equivalent results to VAD but is used much less frequently (7). Lenalidomide in combination with dexamethasone may have some adverse impact on collection of stem cells. High-dose dexamethasone alone is also useful for patients requiring concurrent radiation therapy or those with significant marrow involvement and cytopenias.

In symptomatic patients older than 70 and in younger patients who are not candidates for transplantation, the combination of oral melphalan with thalidomide and standard-dose prednisone (MPT) has shown high durable response rates and should be considered the current treatment of choice in the elderly. At a median follow-up of 18 months in a prospective randomized trial comparing MPT with MP, MPT was superior to MP, with an overall response rate of 76% versus 48%, and yielded better progression-free and overall survival. Toxicity was a serious problem, with 33% of patients discontinuing thalidomide because of deep vein thrombosis or neurotoxicity.

More aggressive regimens combining multiple cytotoxic agents such as VMBCP (Vincristine, Melphalan, BCNU/carmustine, Cyclophosphamide, Prednisone), VMCP (Vincristine, Melphalan, Cyclophosphamide, Prednisone), and VBAP (Vincristine, BCNU/carmustine, Adriamycin,

TABLE 17.2. *Treatment Regimens*

Regimen	Treatment description	Toxicities
Melphalan + Prednisone + Thalidomide (MPT)	Melphalan, 10 mg/m^2 per day PO for 4 days (d 1–4; total dose/cycle, 40 mg/m^2) + Prednisone, 60 mg/m^2 per day PO for 4 days (d 1–4; total dose/cycle, 40 mg/m^2) Thalidomide, 100 mg per day PO Cycle duration, 4–6 week. Start at low doses and increase if tolerated. Decrease doses if myelosuppression is prolonged.	Myelosuppression. Therapy-related myelodysplastic syndrome. Peripheral neuropathy, thromboembolism (up to 20% of patients). Strongly consider prophylaxis with enoxaparin or similar agent.
Melphalan + Prednisone + Thalidomide (MPT) Modified for Patients Age >75[28]	Melphalan, 0.2 mg/kg per day PO for 4 days (d 1–4) Prednisone, 2 mg/kg per day PO for 4 days (d 1–4; total dose/cycle, 40 mg/m^2) Thalidomide, 100 mg per day PO Cycle duration, 6 weeks.	Peripheral neuropathy (17% of patients). Thromboembolism (7% of patients).
Melphalan + Prednisone (MP)	Melphalan, 10 mg/m^2 per day PO for 4 days (d 1–4; total dose/cycle, 40 mg/m^2) + Prednisone, 60 mg/m^2 per day PO for 4 days (d 1–4; total dose/cycle, 40 mg/m^2) Cycle duration, 4–6 week. Start at low doses and increase if tolerated. Decrease doses if myelosuppression is prolonged.	Myelosuppression. Therapy-related myelodysplastic syndrome.
Thalidomide + Dexamethasone	Thalidomide, 200 mg per day PO Dexamethasone, 20 mg/m^2 per day PO for 4 days, repeated every 8 days (d 1–4, 9–12, and 17–20; total dose/cycle, 480 mg)	Thromboembolism (up to 20% of patients). Strongly consider prophylaxis with enoxaparin or similar agent.
Vincristine + Adriamycin + Dexamethasone (VAD)	Vincristine, 0.4 mg/day continuous IV infusion for 4 days (d 1–4; total dose/cycle, 1.6 mg) Doxorubicin, 9 mg/m^2 per day continuous IV infusion for 4 days (d 1–4; total dose/cycle, 36 mg/m^2) Dexamethasone, 40 mg per day PO for 4 days, repeated every 8 days (d 1–4, 9–12, and 17–20; total dose/cycle, 480 mg) Cycle repeats every 25 days	GI and myelotoxicity

(continued)

TABLE 17.2. *Treatment Regimens (continued)*

Regimen	Treatment description	Toxicities
High-Dose Chemotherapy and Autologous Stem Cell Transplantation	Conditioning regimen: Melphalan, 200 mg/m^2 IV as a single agent	Mucositis Up to 5% transplant-related mortality
Interferon-α	Interferon-α, 3 million units/m^2 SC, 3 doses/wk (total dose/wk, 9 million units/m^2)	CNS changes, cytopenias, fever, and myalgias
Thalidomide	Dosing is not thoroughly established. Doses ≥400 mg/day needed for relapsed/refractory disease. Smaller doses (<400 mg/day) may be sufficient for untreated disease.	Peripheral neuropathy (dose-limiting toxicity). Somnolence, constipation. Higher incidence of deep venous thrombosis, especially when used in combination with adriamycin-containing regimens. Consider placing such patients on prophylactic low-molecular-weight heparin.
Bortezomib	1.3 mg/m^2 as an IV bolus 2×/week for 2 wks, on days 1, 4, 8, and 11 in a 21-day cycle.	Thrombocytopenia, GI symptoms, fatigue, and sensory neuropathy.
Bortezomib + Liposomal Doxorubicin	1.3 mg/m^2 as an IV bolus 2×/week for 2 wks, on days 1, 4, 8, and 11 in a 21-day cycle. Liposomal doxorubicine 30 mg/m^2 should be administered as a 1-hr intravenous infusion on day 4 following bortezomib.	Thrombocytopenia, GI symptoms, fatigue, and sensory neuropathy, neutropenia, and anorexia.
Lenalidomide + Dexamethasone	Lenalidomide 25 mg qd po days 1–21 in a 28-day cycle Dexamethasone, 40 mg per day po for 4 days, repeated every 8 days (d 1–4, 9–12, and 17–20; total dose/cycle, 480 mg)	Thromboembolism (9%). Consider prophylaxis.
Pamidronate	Pamidronate, 90 mg IV infusion over 2–4 h, monthly	Fever, nausea, hypokalemia, hypocalcemia
Zolendronic acid	Zolendronic acid 4 mg IV infusion over 15 minutes, monthly	Renal toxicity has been reported with higher doses and shorter infusions. Fatigue, fever, hypophosphatemia, hypokalemia

CNS, central nervous system; d, day; GI, gastrointestinal; h, hours; IV, intravenously; po, orally; qd, every day; SC, subcutaneously.

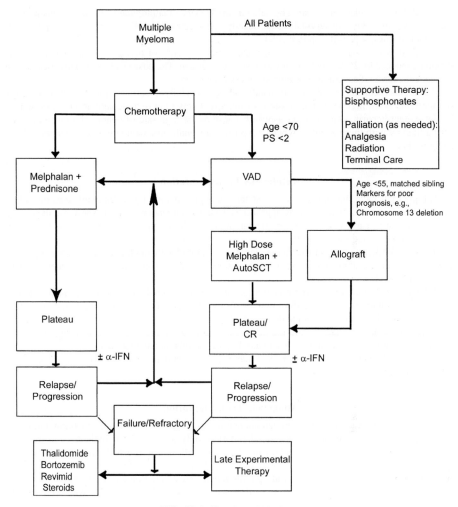

FIG. 17.1. Treatment strategy.

Prednisone) have failed to demonstrate consistent superiority to regimens containing melphalan as the only cytotoxic agent (5).

Chemotherapy should be administered for at least three cycles and, in responders, continued until the disease reaches a plateau phase. However, more than five to six cycles is generally not necessary and in the case of alkylating agents, is associated with a higher risk of secondary myelodysplastic syndrome/acute myeloid leukemia (MDS/AML). Two to three cycles must be administered before deeming a patient refractory to a regimen.

The plateau phase is defined as a stable M-protein in the serum and the lack of evidence of disease progression. Partial remission is defined at >50% reduction in serum paraprotein or >90% reduction in urine light chains. Complete remission (CR) is defined as no detectable serum or urine paraprotein and marrow plasma cells <5%. CR is extremely rare with conventional chemotherapy but can be reached in 20% to 50% of patients following a single or a double autograft, and the CR rate is higher with regimens incorporating novel agents such as thalidomide, lenalidomide, or bortezomib.

There is no evidence of additional efficacy of chemotherapy once patients enter a plateau phase, although the trials showing efficacy of thalidomide/prednisone/melphalan in elderly patients did continue with further cycles for 1 year. The value of maintenance thalidomide or pulse steroids remains under investigation. Overall survival is significantly impacted by the ability to achieve an objective response, even if it is a partial response (PR).

In patients with renal insufficiency (creatine clearance <50% of predicted), the melphalan dose should be reduced by 25% to prevent severe myelosuppression. The dose can be gradually escalated in subsequent courses if severe myelosuppression does not occur.

All patients receiving thalidomide or lenalidomide, especially in combination with chemotherapy and particularly during the first six months of therapy, likely require anticoagulation with low molecular weight heparin, coumadin, or aspirin because of the high rate of venous thromboembolism during therapy with these agents. (Whether aspirin is adequate anticoagulation is the subject of ongoing trials.)

Autologous Transplantation

Multiple trials have shown a survival advantage of approximately 1 year for autologous transplantation over conventional chemotherapy approaches. Data from a randomized trial show that there is no survival benefit to early versus late transplantation, although upfront autotransplantation resulted in longer progression-free survival (13).

There are conflicting data on whether tandem (two back-to-back) autologous transplantation is better than conventional single autologous transplantation, but a controlled trial showed a benefit for tandem transplants (11).

Melphalan at 200 mg/m^2 without radiation is considered the standard induction regimen. There is no proven benefit to purging the graft of tumor cells either by positive stem cell selection or antibody-mediated removal of tumor cells. In patients older than age 70 and in those with renal failure, melphalan is frequently dose-reduced to 140 mg/m^2 or 100 mg/m^2 to decrease toxicity. Thus, age and renal failure are not absolute contraindications to autologous transplantation approaches.

Treatment-related mortality should be less than 5%. Younger patients can receive transplants in the outpatient clinic.

Allogeneic Transplantation

After screening for the presence of a human leukocyte antigen (HLA)-matched sibling donor and assessment of cardiac, pulmonary and renal function, only about 10% of patients with multiple myeloma remain candidates for standard myeloablative allogeneic transplantation. Although the approach has the advantages of a tumor-free graft and the ability to produce a graft versus myeloma effect, the majority of patients who undergo allogeneic transplantation still relapse. In a series of 80 cases of newly diagnosed patients as well as patients with relapsed disease who were treated with allogeneic transplantation, only 5 patients were in continuous remission at 4 to 7 years after transplantation (16).

Myeloma patients have high treatment-related mortality from allogeneic transplantation, with high rates of serious infection presumed because of poor underlying immune function secondary to their disease. The development of nonmyeloablative regimens as well strategies that decrease the likelihood of graft-versus-host disease, such as T-cell depletion, may improve the outcomes in allogeneic transplantation. Current approaches focus on an initial autograft, and in high-risk patients proceeding immediately to a nonmyeloablative allograft.

Maintenance Therapy

Interferon Alpha

The data from the clinical trials are conflicting. Several but not all studies have shown a benefit from interferon alpha with increased freedom from progression for 6 to 12 months. Many patients are unable to tolerate the usual doses, and a majority need to either reduce the dose or discontinue the drug altogether. At present, interferon maintenance is rarely utilized.

Thalidomide

Thalidomide appears to improve event-free and overall survival in patients following autologous transplantation. Randomized clinical trials are currently in progress to evaluate whether the benefits routine thalidomide maintenance outweighs the risks of treatment-related toxicity.

Corticosteroids

Prednisone as a maintenance therapy has only been studied in patients responsive to VAD. In this setting, both progression-free survival and overall survival were higher in patients receiving maintenance therapy with prednisone at 50 mg every other day versus 10 mg every other day. The role of corticosteroids in patients undergoing autologous transplant is not known.

Relapsed or Refractory Disease Therapy

Patients who respond to their initial regimen eventually relapse. If postchemotherapy relapse occurs more than 6 months after the plateau state has been achieved, the original regimen can be reinstated. Most patients respond to the initial regimen, but the second response tends to be shorter in duration and more attenuated than the first. The highest rates of response in patients refractory to alkylating agents have been reported with VAD. At present, most relapsed patients receive thalidomide or lenalidomide with or without corticosteroids, or bortezomib.

Chemotherapy

VAD is the most frequently used conventional regimen. Patients with relapsed or refractory disease have a response rate of 60% and a median survival of 10 months. VMBCP and VBAP both have been used and produce response rates similar to those achieved with VAD.

Thalidomide

Thalidomide as a single agent produced a response in about 30% of patients who had relapsed or refractory disease. In combination with dexamethasone, the drug can induce a response in up to 60% of patients in this setting. Addition of melphalan increased the response rate to 75%, and the addition of liposomal doxorubicin yielded a response rate of 90%. However, higher response rates do not always correlate with better survival outcomes and are associated with more toxicity. Thus treatment should be tailored based on the aggressiveness of the disease as well as patient age and performance status.

Steroids

Dexamethasone and intravenous pulsed methylprednisolone in this setting have yielded response rates up to 40% (19).

Bortezomib

This proteosome inhibitor was shown to have an overall response rate of 35% in a group of patients who had been exposed to at least 2 prior therapies. A randomized phase 3 trial demonstrated superior event-free and overall survival compared with high-dose dexamethasone. Dose-limiting toxicity is thrombocytopenia.

Bortezomib in combination with liposomal doxorubicin improved event-freee survival compared with bortezomib alone in bortezomib-naive patients. This combination is now FDA approved in the United States for bortezomib-naive patients with relapsed multiple myeloma.

Lenalidomide

This thalidomide analog is FDA approved in the United States for use in combination with dexamethasone for patients with relapsed multiple myeloma. Overall response rate in a phase 3 trial was 59%.

Supportive Measures

Bisphosphonates

Bisphosphonates are widely used for the treatment and prevention of osteoporosis and in therapy of hypercalcemia. Bisphosphonates at appropriate doses can prevent the skeletal complications and improve quality of life in patients with advanced myeloma. There is also evidence for a survival benefit. Both intravenous pamidronate and zolendronic acid appear equally effective in preventing skeletal complication with similar rates of renal toxicity.

Oral bisphosphonates have failed to demonstrate similar efficacy in placebo-controlled trials. In the absence of significant toxicity or declining performance status, monthly treatment with intravenous bisphosophonates is recommended for all patients with multiple myeloma and bone disease. Treatment should be continued even if patients develop a skeletal event. Bisphosphonates are frequently used in patients without bone disease, although prospective clinical trial documenting efficacy in this setting are lacking. Multiple in vitro and biologic studies indicate the potential for an antimyeloma effect by stimulation of immune function or inhibition of interactions between myeloma cells and their microenvironment.

Radiation

Local radiation has a role for palliating symptomatic focal lesions, although if pain is the sole symptom and there is no impending fracture or cord compression, responses to chemotherapy, and in particular high-dose dexamethasone, can be equally rapid and effective.

Radiation to major bone-marrow regions should be avoided to collect adequate hematopoietic stem cells if needed. Systemic therapy with dexamethasone and/or thalidomide can occur simultaneously with local irradiation.

Surgical Options

Vertebroplasty and kyphoplasty are both commonly used and effective in alleviating symptoms from vertebral collapse.

Special Considerations

Renal Failure

Renal failure is usually multifactorial, secondary to light-chain nephrotoxicity, volume depletion, and hypercalcemia. Patients are treated with intravenous hydration, loop diuretics if hypercalcemia is present, and chemotherapy (typically high-dose pulse dexamethasone because of more rapid onset of action as compared with melphalan and prednisone) to decrease light chain production. Dialysis is used if necessary.

With the use of the above modalities, at least partial recovery of renal function is possible in the majority of patients, with the exception of those with significant amyloid deposition. Plasmapheresis may be used to decrease serum light chains (if detected on SPEP) but can only temporize until systemic therapy decreases production.

Hyperviscosity Syndrome

Hyperviscosity should be suspected in patients with unexplained mental status changes, worsening respiratory status, renal insufficiency, or bleeding. The syndrome is more common in the IgA and IgG3 subtypes. The diagnosis is made by measuring serum viscosity. Serum viscosity does not always correlate well with symptoms; thus, treatment should be initiated when the syndrome is suspected.

Plasmapheresis is effective for symptomatic hyperviscosity and should be continued until the serum viscosity has normalized. Therapy with a regimen containing high-dose dexamethasone results in the most rapid decrease in paraprotein production and should be used instead of melphalan and prednisone in patients with hyperviscosity.

Anemia

Erythropoietin has been shown to significantly decrease the frequency of transfusions and improve performance status and quality of life in anemic patients with multiple myeloma. Current guidelines for use of erythropoietin recommend Hgb <10 g/dL as the upper limit prior to the initiation of treatment. Treatment should be discontinued after the hemoglobin reaches 12 g/dL. The treatment should be discontinued if there is no evidence of a response (rise in Hgb >1 g/dL or decrease in transfusion requirements) in 6 to 8 weeks.

Follow-Up of Monoclonal Gammopathy of Unknown Significance and Smoldering Multiple Myeloma

Because both MGUS and SMM have a small but significant risk of progressing to multiple myeloma, it is important to periodically evaluate patients with these conditions. The frequency of periodic visits is based on the concentration of M-protein. If the serum M-protein is less than 2 g/dL with no other evidence of multiple myeloma, then the M-protein should be rechecked in 6 months, then annually if stable. If the serum M-protein is more than 2 g/dL with no other evidence of multiple myeloma, the M-protein should be rechecked in 3 months, then annually if stable.

Solitary Plasmacytoma

Plasmacytomas are tumors composed of plasma cells that are histologically identical to those seen in multiple myeloma. Overt multiple myeloma must always be excluded. Patients with soft-tissue plasmacytomas can be cured with local radiation. A majority of patients with solitary plasmacytomas of the bone develop systemic disease after receiving local radiation, suggesting that the presumed plasmacytoma was part of the systemic disease.

Plasma Cell Leukemia

Plasma cell leukemia is a very rare disease variant of multiple myeloma, occurring in about 2% to 4% of all cases. About 60% of cases present as primary disease. The diagnosis is made when the circulating plasma cell count is greater than 2000/mL, in addition to all the criteria for multiple myeloma. Prognosis is extremely poor, with median survival less than a year. Transplantation should be considered in all cases.

REFERENCES

1. Hallek M, Bergsagel PL, Anderson KC. Multiple myeloma: increasing evidence for a multistep transformation process. Blood 1998;91:3–21.
2. Riedel DA, Pottern LM. The epidemiology of multiple myeloma. Hematol Oncol Clin North Am 1992;6:225–247.
3. Lynch HT, Sanger WG, Pirruccello S, et al. Familial multiple myeloma: a family study and review of the literature. J Natl Cancer Inst 2001;93:1479–1483.
4. Case DC Jr, Lee DJ 3rd, Clarkson BD. Improved survival times in multiple myeloma treated with melphalan, prednisone, cyclophosphamide, vincristine, and BCNU: M-2 protocol. Am J Med 1977;63: 897–903.
5. Oken MM, Harrington DP, Abramson N, et al. Comparison of melphalan and prednisone with vincristine, carmustine, melphalan, cyclophosphamide, and prednisone in the treatment of multiple myeloma: results of Eastern Cooperative Oncology Group Study E2479. Cancer 1997; 79: 1561–1567.
6. Anderson H, Scarffe JH, Ranson M, et al. VAD chemotherapy as remission induction for multiple myeloma. Br J Cancer 1995;71: 326–330.
7. Weber D, Rankin K, Gavino M, et al. Thalidomide alone or with dexamethasone for previously untreated multiple myeloma. J Clin Oncol 2003;21:16–19.

8. Blade J, López-Guillermo A, Bosch F, et al. Impact of response to treatment on survival in multiple myeloma: results in a series of 243 patients. Br J Haematol 1994;88:117–121.
9. Child JA, Morgan GJ, Davies FE, et al. High-dose chemotherapy with hematopoietic stem-cell rescue for multiple myeloma. N Engl J Med 2003;348:1875–1883.
10. Zhan F, Hardin J, Kordsmeier B, et al. Global gene expression profiling of multiple myeloma, monoclonal gammopathy of undetermined significance, and normal bone marrow plasma cells. Blood 2002;99:1745–1757.
11. Attal M, Harousseau JL, Facon T, et al. Single versus double autologous stem-cell transplantation for multiple myeloma. N Engl J Med 2003;349:2495–2502.
12. Browman GP, Bergsagel D, Sicheri D, et al. Randomized trial of interferon maintenance in multiple myeloma: a study of the National Cancer Institute of Canada Clinical Trials Group. J Clin Oncol 1995;13:2354–2360.
13. Fermand JP, Ravaud P, Chevret S, et al. High-dose therapy and autologous peripheral blood stem cell transplantation in multiple myeloma: up-front or rescue treatment? Results of a multicenter sequential randomized clinical trial. Blood 1998;92:3131–3136.
14. Moreau P, Facon T, Attal M, et al. Comparison of 200 mg/m(2) melphalan and 8 Gy total body irradiation plus 140 mg/m(2) melphalan as conditioning regimens for peripheral blood stem cell transplantation in patients with newly diagnosed multiple myeloma: final analysis of the Intergroupe Francophone du Myelome 9502 randomized trial. Blood 2002;99:731–735.
15. Myeloma Trialists' Collaborative Group. Combination chemotherapy versus melphalan plus prednisone as treatment for multiple myeloma: an overview of 6,633 patients from 27 randomized trials. J Clin Oncol 1998;16:3832–3842.
16. Bensinger WI, Maloney D, Storb R. Allogeneic hematopoietic cell transplantation for multiple myeloma. Semin Hematol 2001;38:243–249.
17. Berenson JR, Crowley JJ, Grogan TM, et al. Maintenance therapy with alternate-day prednisone improves survival in multiple myeloma patients. Blood 2002;99:3163–3168.
18. UK myeloma forum. British Committee for Standards in Haematology. Diagnosis and management of multiple myeloma. Br J Haematol 2001;115:522–540.
19. Gertz MA, Garton JP, Greipp PR, et al. A phase II study of high-dose methylprednisolone in refractory or relapsed multiple myeloma. Leukemia 1995;9:2115–2118.
20. Singhal S, Mehta J, Desikan R, et al. Antitumor activity of thalidomide in refractory multiple myeloma. N Engl J Med 1999;341:1565–1571.
21. Richardson PG, Schlossman RL, Weller E, et al. Immunomodulatory drug CC-5013 overcomes drug resistance and is well tolerated in patients with relapsed multiple myeloma. Blood 2002;100:3063–3067.
22. Richardson PG, Barlogie B, Berenson J, et al. A phase 2 study of bortezomib in relapsed, refractory myeloma. N Engl J Med 2003;348:2609–2617.
23. Kyle RA, Gertz MA, Witzig TE, et al. Review of 1027 patients with newly diagnosed multiple myeloma. Mayo Clin Proc 2003;78:21–33.
24. Kyle RA. The role of bisphosphonates in multiple myeloma. Ann Intern Med 2000;132:734–736.
25. Barlogie B, Shaughnessy J, Tricot G, et al. Treatment of multiple myeloma. Blood 2004;103;20–32.
26. Palumbo A, Bringhen S, Caravita T, et al. Oral melphalan and prednisone chemotherapy plus thalidomide compared with melphalan and prednisone alone in elderly patients with multiple myeloma: randomized controlled trial. Lancet 2006;367:825–831.
27. Richardson PG, Sonneveld P, Schuster MW, et al. Bortezomib or high-dose dexamethasone for relapsed multiple myeloma. N Engl J Med 2005;352:2487–2498.
28. Hulin C, Virion J, Leleu X, et al. Comparison of melphalan-prednisone-thalidomide (MP-T) to melphalan-prednisone (MP) in patients 75 years of age or older with untreated multiple myeloma (MM). Preliminary results of the randomized, double-blind, placebo-controlled IFM 01–01 trial. J Clin Oncol ASCO Annual Meeting Proceedings 2007;25(18S):8001.
29. Nowrousian MR, Brandhorst D, Sammet C, et al. Serum free light chain analysis and urine immunofixation electrophoresis in patients with multiple myeloma. Clin Cancer Res 2005;11:8706–8714.

18

Hematopoietic Stem Cell Transplantation

Richard W. Childs and Ramaprasad Srinivasan

Hematopoietic stem cell transplantation (HSCT) is a potentially curative therapeutic modality widely used in the management of hematologic malignancies and a variety of nonmalignant disorders. Autologous HSCT typically involves administration of high-dose chemotherapy followed by infusion of hematopoietic stem cells procured from the recipient prior to myeloablative chemo/radiotherapy. In contrast, allogeneic HSCT involves infusion of hematopoietic stem cells collected from either a related or unrelated human leukocyte antigen (HLA)-compatible donor, following myeloablative or reduced-intensity conditioning of the recipient.

AUTOLOGOUS HEMATOPOIETIC STEM CELL TRANSPLANTATION

Autologous hematopoietic stem cell transplantation (auto-HSCT) was conceived as a means of overcoming lethal hematopoietic toxicity associated with high-dose chemotherapy in the treatment of dose-responsive malignancies (1,2). A role for auto-HSCT has been clearly established in the management of multiple myeloma and aggressive non-Hodgkin's lymphoma. Initial enthusiasm for this approach in solid tumors such as metastatic breast, ovarian, and lung cancer has been tempered by the failure of prospective randomized trials to demonstrate benefit over conventional treatments. The role of auto-HSCT continues to be explored in neuroblastoma and Ewing's sarcoma.

General Considerations

Most auto-HSCTs are performed using peripheral blood stem cells collected after mobilization with granulocyte colony-stimulating factor (G-CSF), with or without chemotherapy priming. The curative potential of auto-HSCT resides solely in the ability of high-dose chemotherapy to eradicate the underlying malignancy; no immune-mediated graft-versus tumor effects are generated. The high-dose chemotherapeutic regimen utilized is tailored to the malignancy based on its chemosensitivity profile; for instance, melphalan (200 mg/m^2) is the most widely used high-dose agent for multiple myeloma.

Infections related to chemotherapy-induced neutropenia and immunosuppression and extramedullary toxicities from high-dose chemotherapeutic agents account for the majority of complications occurring after auto-HSCT. There is a lower risk of treatment-related mortality (TRM) compared with allogeneic HSCT, typically less than 5% in most series.

Contamination of the stem cell product by malignant cells may limit the beneficial effects of high-dose chemotherapy. Efforts to purge tumor cells contaminating hematopoietic grafts by CD34$^+$ cell selection or by in vitro incubation of the stem cell graft with cytotoxic drugs remain investigational and have met with only moderate success.

Results of Autologous Hematopoietic Stem Cell Transplantation

Autologous Hematopoietic Cell Transplantation in Hematologic Malignancies

Multiple Myeloma

Large phase II trials have demonstrated high response rates (complete response 30% to 50%) and impressive disease-free survival (DFS) and overall survival (OS) rates (median, more than 5 years).

Randomized phase III trials in relatively young patients (less than 65 years of age) have shown superior response rates, DFS, and OS for auto-HSCT versus conventional chemotherapy (3).

Consecutive or tandem auto-HSCTs have been compared with single auto-HSCT in several randomized prospective studies. While some studies suggest improved DFS (but not OS) with the tandem approach, other large multicenter trials also indicated a survival benefit for tandem auto-HSCT. Subgroup analyses suggest that the survival benefit is most pronounced in patients who do not achieve a complete response (CR) or a very good partial response following the first auto-HSCT. Tandem auto-HSCT has also been compared with auto-HSCT followed by reduced-intensity or nonmyeloablative allogeneic HSCT, with at least one randomized study demonstrating superior overall survival and PFS with the latter approach.

Auto-HSCT is currently considered standard first-line therapy for relatively young patients (up to age 65) with myeloma and results in long-term CR rates of 5% to 10%. Melphalan (200 mg/m^2) is the most commonly used preparative regimen. The role of tandem auto-HSCT remains to be clearly defined, although some subgroups appear to benefit from this approach. Tandem auto/allo HSCT is a promising and potentially curative approach that requires further evaluation. The availability of newer, more effective and better tolerated antimyeloma agents such as bortezomib and lenolinamide is likely to lead to re-evaluation of the role auto-HSCT.

Lymphoma

Lymphomas are among the most common indications for auto-HSCT. The benefit of auto-HSCT has been most clearly observed in chemosensitive Hodgkin's disease and in intermediate- and high-grade non-Hodgkin's lymphoma (NHL). Auto-HSCT results in improved event-free and OS in patients with relapsed chemosensitive intermediate-/high-grade NHL, compared with conventional salvage therapy (4). Results from a randomized study suggest that initial treatment with auto-HSCT may benefit some patients with intermediate-/high-grade NHL, compared with standard treatment with cyclophosphamide, doxorubicin, vincristine, and prednisone (CHOP) chemotherapy.

For Hodgkin's disease, patients with chemosensitive disease in first relapse have improved event-free survival (EFS) with auto-HSCT compared with standard salvage chemotherapy. Patients with primary progressive disease (who progress despite first-line chemotherapy) may also benefit from auto-HSCT as part of a salvage regimen.

Incorporation of therapeutic antibodies such as rituximab (anti-CD20) in first-line treatment regimens has significantly improved the ability to treat several subsets of NHL. The benefit of auto-SCT in the era of B-cell targeted monoclonal antibodies remains to be determined.

Acute Myeloid Leukemia

Auto-HCT has been used both as postremission therapy in acute myeloid leukemia (AML) in first complete remission (CR1) and as therapy after relapse. Phase III studies in patients in CR1 suggest an improvement in DFS but not OS, compared with conventional postremission therapy. Further studies are required to clarify which, if any, prognostic subgroups are likely to benefit from auto-HSCT.

Autologous Hematopoietic Stem Cell Transplantation in Solid Tumors

The knowledge that some malignancies exhibit dose-dependent responses to chemotherapy led to the investigation of high-dose chemotherapy followed by auto-HCT in the treatment of solid tumors. Based on negative results from phase III trials, auto-HCT has been largely abandoned in the management of some malignancies (particularly metastatic breast cancer) but remains under investigation in several other solid tumor types.

Breast Cancer

While promising results from phase II studies in patients with metastatic breast cancer paved the way for randomized phase III studies of auto-HSCT, larger studies failed to demonstrate unequivocal benefit. At least seven large trials have compared auto-HSCT qurg standard chemotherapy in patients with metastatic breast cancer. Six demonstrated superior event-free survival with auto-HSCT, but none showed a survival advantage (5). Similar results were obtained in patients with high-risk breast cancer undergoing adjuvant auto-HSCT. Because of a lack of survival benefit and higher toxicity, there is little enthusiasm for further investigation of auto-HSCT in breast cancer.

Germ Cell Tumors

Phase II trials of auto-HSCT in relapsed or refractory germ cell tumors have yielded response rates of 40% to 65% and long-term survival rates of 15% to 40%. Patients with progressive disease or human chorionic gonadotropin levels greater than 1000 IU/L at transplantation, mediastinal primaries, and refractoriness to cisplatin-based therapy have a worse outcome and may not benefit from auto-HSCT.

An interim report from a European Group for Blood and Marrow Transplantation study suggested no advantage for auto-HSCT over standard salvage chemotherapy in patients failing cisplatin-based chemotherapy (6). Randomized studies are currently in progress to evaluate the role of auto-HSCT as initial therapy in germ cell tumors at high risk of relapse.

Other Tumors

Although still under study, available data do not suggest a clear benefit for auto-HSCT in ovarian and lung cancers.

When administered after an initial course of standard induction chemotherapy, auto-HSCT appears to improve short-term disease-free survival in neuroblastoma compared with conventional dose maintenance chemotherapy. However, a large randomized study was unable to demonstrate a survival advantage for patients undergoing auto-HSCT.

Some patients with Ewing's sarcoma/primordial neurectodermal tumor (PNET) and other soft-tissue sarcomas may benefit from high-dose chemotherapy. In the absence of evidence to support a survival benefit, patients should be treated with auto-HSCT only in a clinical trial.

ALLOGENEIC HEMATOPOIETIC STEM CELL TRANSPLANTATION

Allogeneic HSCT can cure patients with advanced chemotherapy-resistant hematologic malignancies (7–9). The first successful allogeneic HSCTs in humans were reported in 1968 (10–12). These transplants were performed in children with congenital immune deficiencies, with donor stem cells from HLA-compatible sibling donors. In the early years after the advent of allogeneic HSCT, immune deficiency syndromes and disorders of hematopoiesis constituted the major indications for the procedure; more recently, hematologic malignancies have become the usual reason for an allogeneic HSCT. Approximately 7000 allogeneic HCTs are performed annually in North America for a wide array of both malignant and nonmalignant disorders.

Indications for Allogeneic Hematopoietic Stem Cell Transplantation

Allogeneic HCT has been used as a potentially curative treatment modality in both malignant and nonmalignant diseases (Table 18.1). Currently, the most common indication for an allogeneic HSCT (approximately 75%) is an underlying hematologic malignancy (most often acute and chronic myelogenous leukemia, acute lymphocytic leukemia, and NHL). Nonmalignant conditions that are potentially curable by HSCT include disorders of hematopoiesis (such as aplastic anemia), immunodeficiency syndromes (such as Chediak-Higashi disease, severe combined immunodeficiency syndrome), congenital disorders of erythropoiesis (thalassemias), and inborn errors of metabolism (mucopolysaccharidoses). The advent of new treatment options for certain diseases (such as the tyrosine kinase inhibitor imatinib mesylate, which is effective in the treatment of chronic myelogenous leukemia) as well as improvements in the toxicity profile associated with HCT are likely to alter the indications for allogeneic transplantation.

TABLE 18.1. Indications for Hematopoietic Stem Cell Transplantation

Acute leukemias
Acute lymphoblastic leukemia (ALL)
Acute myelogenous leukemia (AML)

Chronic leukemias
Chronic myelogenous leukemia (CML)
Chronic lymphocytic leukemia (CLL)
Juvenile chronic myelogenous leukemia (JCML)
Juvenile myelomonocytic leukemia (JMML)

Myelodysplastic syndromes
Refractory anemia (RA)
Refractory anemia with ringed sideroblasts (RARS)
Refractory anemia with excess blasts (RAEB)
Refractory anemia with excess blasts
in transformation (RAEB-T)
Chronic myelomonocytic leukemia (CMML)
  deficiency

Stem cell disorders
Aplastic anemia (severe)
Fanconi anemia
Paroxysmal nocturnal hemoglobinuria
Pure red cell aplasia

Myeloproliferative disorders
Acute myelofibrosis
Agnogenic myeloid metaplasia (myelofibrosis)
Polycythemia vera
Essential thrombocythemia

Lymphoproliferative disorders
Non-Hodgkin's lymphoma
Hodgkin's disease

Phagocyte disorders
Chediak-Higashi syndrome
Chronic granulomatous disease
Neutrophil actin deficiency
Reticular dysgenesis

Inherited metabolic disorders
Mucopolysaccharidoses (MPS)
Hurler's syndrome (MPS-IH)
Scheie syndrome (MPS-IS)
Hunter's syndrome (MPS-II)
Sanfilippo syndrome (MPS-III)
Morquio syndrome (MPS-IV)
Maroteaux-Lamy syndrome (MPS-VI)
Sly Syndrome, β-C glucoronidase deficiency
  (MPS-VII)
Adrenoleukodystrophy
Mucolipidosis II (I-cell disease)
Krabbe disease
Gaucher's disease
Niemann-Pick disease
Wolman disease
Metachromatic leukodystrophy

Histiocytic disorders
Familial erythrophagocytic
  lymphohistiocytosis
Histiocytosis-X
Hemophagocytosis

Inherited erythrocyte abnormalities
β-Thalassemia major
Sickle cell disease

Inherited immune system disorders
Ataxia-telangiectasia
Kostmann syndrome
Leukocyte adhesion deficiency
DiGeorge syndrome
Bare lymphocyte syndrome
Omenn's syndrome
Severe combined immunodeficiency
  (SCID)
SCID with adenosine deaminase
Absence of T & B cells SCID
Absence of T cells, normal B cell SCID
Common variable immunodeficiency
Wiskott-Aldrich syndrome
X-linked lymphoproliferative disorder

Other inherited disorders
Lesch-Nyhan syndrome
Cartilage-hair hypoplasia
Glanzmann thrombasthenia
Osteopetrosis

Inherited platelet abnormalities
Amegakaryocytosis/congenital
  thrombocytopenia

Plasma cell disorders
Multiple myeloma
Plasma cell leukemia
Waldenstrom's macroglobulinemia

Other malignancies
Breast cancer
Ewing sarcoma
Neuroblastoma
Renal cell carcinoma

Adapted from list of transplant indications provided by the National Marrow Donor Program (NMDP).

**Antileukemic Potential of Allogeneic Hematopoietic Stem Cell Transplantation:
Underlying Principles**

In the 1960s and 1970s, allogeneic HSCT was largely viewed as a means of ensuring immunohematopoietic reconstitution or replacement after administration of high doses of chemotherapy with or without radiation. This premise still applies to the treatment of nonmalignant conditions where the major goal is to provide normal cellular components to replace or rectify an underlying deficiency. For hematologic malignancies, the dose-intensive preparative or conditioning regimen was initially considered to be critical for the eradication of the underlying malignancy, with HLA-matched donor stem cells used merely to reverse the accompanying fatal bone marrow ablation. However, over the last two decades, it has become increasingly evident that a donor immune-mediated antimalignancy effect, termed graft-versus-leukemia (GVL) or graft-versus-tumor (GVT), is central for the successful eradication of malignancies after allogeneic HCT. The following clinical observations have provided incontrovertible evidence for the existence of GVL and highlight the role of donor T lymphocytes in mediating this effect (7,8,13–15):

- Decreased risk of leukemia relapse in patients experiencing acute or chronic graft-versus-host-disease (GVHD).
- Increased risk of leukemia relapse in patients undergoing T-cell–depleted transplants.
- Increased risk of leukemia relapse in recipients of a syngeneic as opposed to nontwin sibling donor allografts.
- Ability of donor leukocyte infusions (DLI) to induce sustained remission in patients with chronic myeloid leukemia (CML) who relapse after transplantation.

Recognition of GVL has led to the development of low intensity or nonmyeloablative conditioning regimens, in which efficacy is largely dependent on the generation of donor immune-mediated antitumor responses.

Planning Allogeneic Hematopoietic Stem Cell Transplantation

Allogeneic HSCT is a complex procedure requiring careful planning and a multidisciplinary approach to patient management. Patient age, performance status, underlying disease, and donor availability must be factored into decisions regarding the type of transplantation (conventional myeloablative versus nonmyeloablative) and GVHD prophylaxis regimen.

Evaluation of Transplant Recipients

Donor-host HLA-compatibility is one of the most important factors affecting outcome after HSCT. Evaluation of the transplant recipient begins with HLA testing and a search for an appropriate donor. The initial donor search focuses on identifying a sibling matched at the allele level for HLA-A, B, and DR loci. If a suitable sibling donor is not available, a search for an HLA-compatible unrelated donor can be made through the National Marrow Donor Program (NMDP).

The evaluation also includes a thorough history and physical examination, with emphasis on the underlying diagnosis and its treatment, concomitant medical problems, performance status, transfusion history, and any history of opportunistic (particularly fungal) infections. An assessment is made of major organ function including pulmonary function testing and full cardiac evaluation. Serologic testing is performed to detect prior exposure to cytomegalovirus, herpesvirus, Epstein-Barr virus, hepatitis viruses, human immunodeficiency virus (HIV), toxoplasmosis, and varicella. Counseling is provided to focus on the potential benefits and risks of transplantation, need for a dedicated caregiver, and, when appropriate, fertility prospects.

Identification of a Suitable Donor

Matched Related Donor

Approximately one third of patients screened will have a suitable HLA-compatible sibling donor. While donors with a less than complete (6/6) HLA match can be used, greater HLA disparity increases the risk of both graft rejection and GVHD.

Syngeneic Donor

Identical twin transplants are rarely performed because high degrees of histocompatibility (including for minor histocompatibility antigens) minimize clinically meaningful GVL effects. Syngeneic donors may be used in the transplantation of nonmalignant diseases (such as severe aplastic anemia) where GVL is not required.

Matched Unrelated Donor

The NMPD search identifies a suitable donor for two thirds of Caucasians. Some minority groups are much harder to match. The matching process should be initiated as early as possible because the time to transplant, once a search is initiated, is 2 to 4 months. For a given degree of donor-host HLA-disparity, the risk of GVHD is higher with unrelated compared with related donors. Furthermore, the incidence of acute GVHD is higher with matched unrelated donors that are fully matched at a molecular level compared with HLA identical siblings.

Haplo-identical Donor

Most patients have a sibling, parent, or child with one matched HLA haplotype who could serve as donor. Transplants from haplo-identical donors are associated with a higher rate of GVHD, necessitating T-cell depletion in most circumstances to prevent life-threatening GVHD.

Umbilical Cord Cells

Blood collected from the placenta at the time of childbirth can be used as a source of hematopoietic stem cells. Most umbilical cord transplants are performed from unrelated donors that are mismatched at one or two HLA loci. While umbilical cord transplants are associated with a lower incidence of GVHD compared with mismatched related or unrelated transplants (even with HLA mismatching), their widespread use is limited by an increased risk of graft failure because of the small numbers of stem cells harvested. At first, umbilical cord transplants were typically limited to children and young adolescents. More recently, umbilical cord blood transplants, given as either a single unit or combined double cord units, have been used successfully in adults who lack an HLA identical sibling or matched unrelated donor.

Procurement of Hematopoietic Stem Cells

The majority of hematopoietic stem cells reside within the bone marrow, which traditionally served as the source of the allograft. However, the ability of G-CSF to mobilize hematopoietic stem cells into the circulation has led to the widespread use of peripheral blood stem cell allografts.

Obtaining stem cells from the bone marrow involves multiple aspirations from the iliac crests, a relatively safe procedure performed under general anesthesia. Mobilized stem cells are typically collected from the peripheral blood by apheresis after administration of G-CSF (10 to 15 μg/kg per day) for 4 to 6 days. G-CSF mobilized peripheral blood stem cell (PBSC) grafts usually contain higher numbers of $CD34^+$ progenitor cells as well as T cells ($CD3^+$ cells) compared with bone marrow grafts. Compared with bone marrow stem cells, transplants using PBSCs are associated with faster neutrophil and platelet engraftment, a reduction in transfusion requirements, a similar rate of acute GVHD, and a higher rate of chronic GVHD (16).

Given the ease of stem cell collection from both the practitioner and the donor perspectives, the higher progenitor cell yield, earlier engraftment, and some studies showing a possible survival advantage, the majority of allogeneic HCTs worldwide currently use mobilized peripheral blood as a source of hematopoietic stem cells.

Conditioning Regimen

A variety of conditioning regimens have been used in allogeneic HCT. The choice of conditioning regimen for a given patient is dictated by the underlying disease, the age of the patient, the presence

TABLE 18.2. *Preparative Regimens Commonly Used in Allogeneic Stem Cell Transplantation*

Myeloablative Regimens	
Cy/TBI	
Cyclophosphamide	120 mg/kg IV
TBI	1000–1575 cGy
Bu/Cy	
Busulfan	16 mg/kg PO or 12.8 mg/kg IV
Cyclophosphamide	120–200 mg/kg IV
Reduced-Intensity Regimens	
Flu/Low-dose TBI	
Fludarabine	90 mg/m^2 IV
TBI	200 cGy
Flu/Mel	
Fludarabine	125 mg/m^2 IV
Melphalan	180 mg/m^2 IV
Flu/Bu/ATG	
Fludarabine	180 mg/m^2 IV
Busulfan	8 mg/kg PO or 6.4 mg/kg IV
ATG	40 mg/kg IV
Cy/Flu	
Cyclophosphamide	120 mg/kg IV
Fludarabine	125 mg/m^2 IV

ATG, antithymocyte globulin; Bu, busulfan; Cy, cyclophosphamide; Flu, fludarabine; IV, intravenously; Mel, melphalan; PO, orally; TBI, total body irradiation.

of medical comorbidity, and donor characteristics (especially the degree of HLA compatibility). Table 18.2 lists some commonly used conditioning regimens.

Conventional or Myeloablative Conditioning

Myeloablative conditioning regimens serve a dual purpose:

- High doses of chemotherapy with or without radiation provide cytoreduction of the neoplasm, usually accompanied by eradication or ablation of host hematopoietic function.
- Conditioning suppresses the host's immune system, a prerequisite for preventing rejection of the transplant.

Tumor eradication in conventional transplants depends on both the transient cytoreductive properties of the conditioning agents and on more durable GVL effects mediated by donor immune cells. The two most commonly used regimens are cyclophosphamide in combination with either total body irradiation (TBI) or busulfan. TBI-based regimens have a higher incidence of secondary malignancies, growth retardation, and cataracts, while non-TBI regimens, particularly those containing busulfan, are associated with more veno-occlusive disease (VOD) and mucositis. The underlying condition often dictates the optimal conditioning regimen. For example, patients with acute lymphoblastic leukemia (ALL) appear to have a lower risk of relapse with TBI-based regimens.

Reduced-Intensity Conditioning

Reduced-intensity preparative regimens were devised in an effort to minimize conditioning-related morbidity associated with conventional transplants while retaining the immunosuppressive effects necessary to ensure engraftment. Reduced-intensity preparative regimens that do not eradicate host hematopoiesis are also referred to as nonmyeloablative conditioning regimens.

Tumor eradication in reduced-intensity transplants mainly depends on the donor immune-mediated GVL effect. These regimens are associated with a lower incidence of some conditioning-related toxicities

(VOD, mucositis, prolonged neutropenia, etc.). Reduced-intensity regimens are better tolerated by older patients (up to 70 years) and by those with medical comorbidities and have allowed allo-HSCT to be extended to these populations. Hematopoietic stem cell transplant registry data collected from the CIBMTR suggest that as of 2006, approximately 20% of all allogeneic transplants were performed using reduced-intensity conditioning.

Results of Allogeneic Hematopoietic Stem Cell Transplantation

Allogeneic HSCT is the only curative option for many patients with hematologic malignancies (2,7). In approximately 85% to 90% of all allogeneic transplants in the United States, an underlying hematologic malignancy serves as the indication.

Chronic Myeloid Leukemia

CML is a myeloproliferative disorder characterized by the presence of a characteristic t(9;22) (q34;q11) translocation, the Philadelphia chromosome. The natural history consists of a relatively indolent chronic phase with progression to the more aggressive accelerated phase and blast crisis. Although allogeneic HSCT is the only proven curative therapy for this condition, the introduction of targeted agents with remarkable efficacy (such as imatinib mesylate) has led to the acceptance of these drugs as standard first-line therapy for chronic phase CML. Consequently, allo-HSCT now is usually reserved for patients with accelerated phase or blast crises CML and for imatinib-resistant chronic phase patients.

In chronic phase CML, 65%–80% of patients undergoing transplantation from an HLA-compatible sibling, are cured; similar to slightly inferior results are now being reported in patients undergoing matched unrelated donor transplantation. Early results in patients receiving reduced-intensity conditioning are promising, but prospective studies are needed to determine if this approach is equivalent to conventional allo-HSCT. Transplantation is less effective in accelerated phase or blast crisis (where cure rates are 10% to 20%).

Younger patients and patients who undergo transplantation within a year of diagnosis have the best outcomes. Chronic phase CML is sensitive to GVL effects and a single DLI can reinduce remission in 70% of patients who relapse after transplantation. Patients with chronic phase CML who fail to achieve a cytogenetic remission with imatinib can be successfully salvaged with allo-HSCT.

Acute Myeloid Leukemia

The indication and timing for transplantation in AML and outcome after allogeneic HSCT depend on the risk category. Patients with intermediate or poor prognosis AML as determined by cytogenetics are at high risk for relapse after chemotherapy and should be evaluated for allogeneic HSCT in first remission (CR1) when an HLA-matched sibling donor is available. Patients transplanted in CR1 have a 45% to 60% probability of long-term DFS. Patients transplanted in first relapse or after induction of second complete remission (CR2) have only a 22% to 40% chance of long-term DFS. Outcomes after transplantation in first relapse or CR2 are comparable. Allogeneic HSCT in good prognosis AML is usually reserved for CR2 or first relapse, because the risk of TRM outweighs the benefits from early transplantation (CR1) in this group. Less than 20% of patients with primary induction failure or those beyond CR2 have durable leukemia remission after allogeneic HSCT.

Acute Lymphoblastic Leukemia

While a significant proportion of childhood ALL is curable with chemotherapy, the majority (60% to 70%) of adults with this disease relapse following initial chemotherapy. Patients older than 60 years of age, those with a leukocyte count higher than 30,000 per microliter, or with adverse cytogenetics [t(4;11), t(1;19), t(8;14) or t(9;22)] have a particularly poor prognosis. Allogeneic HSCT in CR1 is recommended for patients with poor prognostic features. Long-term DFS in this category approaches 40% to 60%. In patients without adverse factors, allogeneic transplantation is usually reserved for CR2. Patients undergoing transplantation in CR2 have long-term DFS of approximately 40%.

Myelodysplastic Syndrome

Allogeneic HSCT offers a 30% to 40% probability of long-term DFS in patients with myelodysplastic syndrome (MDS). The two most important factors predicting outcome after transplantation are blast percentage and cytogenetic risk group. Accordingly, patients with few blasts (refractory anemia or refractory anemia with ringed sideroblasts) enjoy a 50% to 75% long-term DFS, while more advanced stages (refractory anemia with excess blasts) are associated with a 30% DFS. Similarly, patients with good-risk cytogenetics have an approximately 50% probability of DFS compared with 10% or less for those with poor-risk cytogenetics. Nonetheless, allogeneic HSCT remains the only curative therapy for MDS and should be considered as a potential definitive therapy. Reduced-intensity HSCT is associated with a higher risk of relapse in patients with MDS than is conventional HSCT and should be reserved for patients who are not candidates for myeloablative HSCT or performed as part of well-designed trials.

Non-Hodgkin's Lymphoma

Low-Grade Non-Hodgkin's Lymphoma

Experience with allogeneic HSCT in low-grade lymphomas is largely restricted to patients undergoing the procedure late in the course of their disease after multiple chemotherapeutic options have been exhausted. In these circumstances, approximately 30% to 50% will achieve long-term DFS. The typically indolent disease course and profound susceptibility to GVL effects renders low-grade lymphomas amenable to management and cure using nonmyeloablative conditioning approaches.

Aggressive Non-Hodgkin's Lymphoma

The role of allogeneic HSCT in patients with intermediate- and high-grade lymphomas is unclear. Most studies have reported a high incidence of TRM with myeloablative transplantation in this group. As a consequence, allogeneic HSCT is generally reserved for those whom potentially curative autologous HSCT has failed or for those unlikely to benefit from an autologous transplant (patients with chemotherapy-resistant disease).

Multiple Myeloma

TRM rates of 50% have discouraged the use of conventional myeloablative transplantation for multiple myeloma. Nevertheless, there is evidence that donor immune-mediated graft-versus-myeloma effects can be curative. Recently, nonmyeloablative conditioning has been explored as a safer transplant approach to treat multiple myeloma. TRM has been significantly lower (less than 25%) compared with historical myeloma cohorts undergoing myeloablative conditioning; of importance, graft-versus-myeloma effects resulting in durable disease remission can be induced after reduced-intensity transplants. Autologous transplantation as myeloma cytoreduction followed by nonmyeloablative allogeneic transplantation as immunotherapy to eradicate minimal residual disease appears promising, with DFS of more than 50% in some studies.

Aplastic Anemia

Allogeneic HSCT can cure severe aplastic anemia (SAA). Early studies of allogeneic HSCT in patients with SAA were characterized by a high rate of graft rejection (up to 35% in some early series) and GVHD. Sensitization to histocompatibility antigens as a result of multiple transfusions and the use of cyclophosphamide alone as pretransplant conditioning accounted for these high rejection rates. Subsequent approaches added antithymocyte globulin (ATG) to cyclophosphamide to minimize graft rejection while preventing severe and potentially lethal GVHD. Additionally, the routine use of leukocyte-depleted and irradiated blood products has decreased the risk of graft rejection to less than 5%. A combination of cyclosporin A (CSA) and methotrexate is generally used as GVHD prophylaxis, with delayed and gradual withdrawal of immunosuppression to minimize the risk of GVHD. Patients under the age of 40 years receiving an allogeneic HSCT from an HLA-matched sibling have an excellent probability for cure, with long-term survival rates approaching 90% in children. Because of a lower incidence of chronic GVHD, bone marrow transplantation may result in superior outcome for SAA compared with peripheral blood stem cell transplantation.

Complications of Allogeneic Hematopoietic Stem Cell Transplantation

Complications of allogeneic HSCT are most commonly related to preparative regimen toxicities, infections occurring as a consequence of immunosuppression, or acute or chronic GVHD.

Conditioning-Related Toxicities

Conditioning-related toxicities vary depending on the type and doses of agents used in the preparative regimen. Nausea, vomiting, and mucositis occur commonly with myeloablative preparative regimens. Busulfan tends to be associated with more severe mucositis.

Hemorrhagic cystitis occurring early in the course of transplantation is usually associated with preparative regimens containing high-dose cyclophosphamide. In contrast, hemorrhagic cystitis more than 72 hours after conditioning is typically viral (polyomavirus BK or adenovirus). Attention to hydration and the routine use of 2-mercaptoethan sulfonate (MESNA) have virtually eliminated cyclophosphamide-associated hemorrhagic cystitis.

Opportunistic infections occur with conditioning-related neutropenia. Bacteria and fungi that are normally present in the skin, gastrointestinal tract, or respiratory tract cause the majority of these infections. Damage to gut mucosa and indwelling venous catheters serve as the portal of entry for most life-threatening gram negative or aerobic gram-positive organisms. The use of oral antibiotics such as quinolones for gut decontamination has decreased the incidence of gram-negative bacteremia.

Candida and aspergillus fungal infections occur commonly during conditioning-induced neutropenia. Prophylactic fluconazole appears to protect against sensitive candida. Trials comparing newer antifungal agents with improved safety profiles compared with amphotericin-B and with activity against aspergillus or resistant candida species are currently being conducted.

VOD is characterized by the triad of jaundice, tender hepatomegaly, and ascites occurring early posttransplant. Risk factors include:

- Advanced age.
- Conditioning with busulfan, with up to 30% of patients receiving oral busulfan developing this complication. This risk is decreased with the use of intravenous busulfan.
- Pre-existing liver disease.
- Development of acute GVHD.
- Transplants from matched unrelated and haploidentical donors.

Prophylaxis with oral ursodiol may be protective. VOD can be severe and life-threatening in approximately 25% of patients developing this complication. Treatment remains largely supportive, although defibrotide and recombinant tissue plasminogen activator have each been used with some success in severe VOD.

Graft-versus-Host Disease

GVHD is one of the most common complications of allogeneic HSCT. GVHD is a consequence of allogeneic donor T cells damaging normal recipient tissues. Based on the time of onset, clinical features, and pathophysiology, GVHD is classified as either acute or chronic (17).

Acute Graft-versus-Host Disease

Acute GVHD typically commences during the first 100 days after transplantation. Of HLA-matched sibling donor transplant recipients, 20% to 50% experience acute GVHD; the incidence is higher in transplants utilizing unrelated donors. The extent of donor-host HLA-disparity, recipient age, T-cell content of the graft, intensity of the conditioning regimen, and the type of GVHD prophylaxis regimen utilized influence the incidence and severity of GVHD.

The skin, gastrointestinal tract, and liver are the most common targets of alloreactive donor T cells. The following clinical and laboratory features should arouse suspicion of GVHD:

- Skin: erythematous maculopapular rash frequently involving the palms and soles. Severe cases can present with skin desquamation.
- Gastrointestinal: crampy abdominal pain and large volume watery diarrhea characterize GVHD of the colon and distal small bowel. In severe cases, bloody diarrhea or ileus may occur.
- Hepatic: elevated alkaline phosphatase and direct bilirubin accompanied by less pronounced increases in transaminases characterize acute GVHD of the liver.

Definitive diagnosis can be difficult because a variety of other conditions (drug-induced skin rash, viral colitis) can present with similar features. Biopsy and histopathologic examination of involved tissue is considered the criterion standard for diagnosing GVHD.

GVHD is a major contributor to TRM; strategies directed at preventing this complication are a critical aspect of transplant planning. Pharmacologic prophylaxis and graft T-cell depletion are established methods that effectively reduce the incidence and severity of GVHD. Cyclosporine or tacrolimus combined with methotrexate are usually used for GVHD prophylaxis. Effective T-cell depletion of the allograft can be achieved in vitro by $CD34^+$ cell selection or in vivo pharmacologically (as with Campath). However, T-depleted transplants are associated with a higher risk of graft failure, leukemia relapse, and opportunistic viral infections. Selective depletion of alloreactive T cells and T-depleted transplants with delayed T-cell add backs following transplantation are being explored as methods for reducing the incidence of GVHD without compromising GVL.

Treatment of established GVHD depends on the type and severity of involved organ (for grading of acute GVHD, see Table 18.3). While mild (grade I) skin GVHD can be managed effectively with topical steroids, visceral GVHD and more severe forms of cutaneous GVHD require systemic immunosuppressive therapy. Glucocorticoids (methylprednisone, typically at doses of 1 to 3 mg/kg per day) are the mainstay and are given in conjunction with cyclosporine or tacrolimus, with doses titrated to maintain therapeutic serum levels. Unfortunately, only about 50% of patients demonstrate durable responses to this form of therapy (for treatment of established acute GVHD, see Table 18.4).

Nonresponding or corticosteroid-refractory patients have a poor outcome, with mortality rates of more than 80%. The majority who develop steroid-refractory GVHD die from infectious complications or organ damage related to relentless immune attack. Comprehensive management strategies in patients with steroid-refractory GVHD with novel agents such as daclizumab and/or infliximab accompanied by

TABLE 18.3. *Grading of Acute Graft-versus-Host Disease*

	Organ involvement		
	Skin	Liver	GI
Stage			
1	Rash <25% of skin	Bilirubin 2–3 mg/dL	Diarrhea >500 mL/day *or* persistent nausea with histologic evidence of upper GI GVHD
2	Rash 25%–50% of skin	Bilirubin 3–6 mg/dL	Diarrhea >1000 mL/day
3	Rash >50% of skin	Bilirubin 6–15 mg/dL	Diarrhea >1500 mL/day
4	Generalized erythroderma	Bilirubin >15 mg/dL	Severe abdominal pain with or with bullae without ileus
Grade			
I	Stage 1–2	0	0
II	Stage 3 *or*	Stage 1 *or*	Stage 1
III	—	Stage 2–3 *or*	Stage 2–4
IV	Stage 4 *or*	Stage 4	—

From Przepiorka D, Weisdorf D, Martin P, et al. 1994 Consensus Conference on Acute GVHD Grading. Bone Marrow Transplant 1995;15:825–828, with permission.
GI, gastrointestinal; GVDH, graft-versus-host disease.

TABLE 18.4. *Treatment of Acute Graft-versus-Host Disease: The National Heart, Lung, and Blood Institute Approach*

Initial management

Grade I GVHD (stage 1–2 skin)
Topical corticosteroid therapy

Grade II–IV GVHD
• High-dose methylprednisolone 1–10 mg/kg per day up to a maximum of 500 mg/day IV 3–6 days *and*
• IV cyclosporine or IV tacrolimus
• Steroids tapered once response is evident over 10–14 days
• All patients receiving ≥1 mg/kg of methylprednisolone undergo routine surveillance blood cultures every 3 days
• All patients with ≥grade III GI GVHD receive prophylactic antibiotic therapy against enteric organisms (e.g., ampicillin-sulbactam)

Management of steroid-refractory GVHD
(GVHD not responsive to 6 or more days of continuous therapy with ≥1 mg/kg methyl-prednisolone)
A) Treatment
• Rapid taper of methylprednisolone to ≤1 mg/kg
• Daclizumab (monoclonal antibody to interleukin-2 receptor-α) 1 mg/kg on days 1, 4, 8, 15, 22
• Infliximab (monoclonal antibody to tumor necrosis factor-α) 10 mg/kg on days 1, 8, 15, 22
B) Supportive care
• All patients with GI GVHD are maintained NPO
• All patients with ≥grade III GI GVHD receive prophylactic antibiotic therapy against enteric organisms (e.g., ampicillin-sulbactam)
• All patients with steroid-refractory GVHD and those patients who receive ≥1 mg/kg methylprednisolone for more than 6 days receive prophylaxis against aspergillus (e.g., liposomal amphotericin, 5 mg/kg per day, or voriconazole)
• All patients receiving ≥1 mg/kg of methylprednisolone undergo routine surveillance blood cultures every 3 days

GI, gastrointestinal; GVHD, graft-versus-host disease; IV, intravenously; NPO, nothing by mouth.

targeted infectious prophylaxis against enteric bacteria and aspergillus appears to be a promising strategy (Table 18.4) (18).

Chronic Graft-versus-Host Disease

The onset of chronic GVHD is usually between 100 days and 2 years after transplantation. It affects 20% to 50% of recipients of allogeneic bone marrow transplants and up to 80% receiving an allogeneic peripheral blood stem cell transplant. Risk is increased by a prior history of acute GVHD, older patient age, the use of HLA-mismatched or unrelated donors, DLI, and/or the use of peripheral blood stem cell allografts. Patients may present with a myriad of clinical features including lichenoid or sclerodermatous skin changes, elevated liver function tests, xerostomia, dry eyes, diarrhea, bronchiolitis obliterans, and thrombocytopenia with or without pancytopenia.

Most clinicians use a two-stage staging system: limited GVHD, representing localized skin involvement and extensive GVHD, which includes patients with more diffuse skin involvement or involvement of other target organs. Investigators at the National Institutes of Health (NIH) have recently proposed a system for the diagnosis and classification of chronic GVHD based on a combination of histopathologic, clinical, laboratory, and radiologic features (19).

Therapy typically consists of cyclosporine or tacrolimus given in conjunction with low-dose corticosteroids. Alternative agents include mycophenolate mofetil, thalidomide, photochemotherapy with oral methoxypsoralen therapy followed by ultraviolet-A photophoresis (PUVA), and monoclonal antibodies directed against T or B lymphocytes or cytokines implicated in pathogenesis (daclizumab, rituximab, etc). A high risk of bacterial infections in patients with chronic GVHD warrants routine use antibiotic prophylaxis against encapsulated bacteria and opportunistic pathogens.

Pulmonary Complications

Pulmonary complications may occur both early and late after transplantation, and they may be infectious or noninfectious in etiology.

Pulmonary Complications Attributable to Infections

Fungi (aspergillus and other agents) as well as viruses (cytomegalovirus, respiratory syncytial virus, influenza, parainfluenza, etc.) can cause life-threatening pneumonia in the posttransplant setting. Early diagnosis, prophylactic or preemptive therapy (such as using ganciclovir or foscarnet for cytomegalovirus [CMV] antigenemia), and prompt institution of definitive therapy when available are the major principles guiding management of these complications. The risk of *Pneumocystis carinii* pneumonia is greatest in the first 6 months after transplantation, particularly in patients receiving T-depleted grafts or those suffering from chronic GVHD; prophylaxis with sulfa/trimethoprim or inhaled pentamidine virtually eliminates this complication.

Idiopathic interstitial pneumonitis usually occurs early after transplantation and is characterized by fever, hypoxia, and diffuse pulmonary infiltrates. Total body irradiation or drugs with pulmonary toxicity (like busulfan) in the preparative regimen increase the risk of this complication.

Diffuse alveolar hemorrhage is a relatively infrequent but frequently fatal complication of allogeneic HSCT. It is characterized by the rapid onset of dyspnea, cough, and hypoxia with diffuse bilateral infiltrates on radiography. High-dose corticosteroids and more recently recombinant factor VIIa may be of therapeutic benefit, but the condition is lethal in 40% to 50% of cases.

Infectious Complications

Recipients of allogeneic HSCT continue to be at risk for infections beyond the period of conditioning-related neutropenia, with viral and fungal pathogens and encapsulated bacteria posing the greatest hazards (20). Factors influencing infectious risk include the presence of acute or chronic GVHD, the extent of immunosuppressive pharmacotherapy in the posttransplant period, T-cell depletion of the graft, and the use of partially HLA-mismatched or unrelated donors.

Bacterial Infections

Gram-negative bacteremia associated with gastrointestinal GVHD and venous catheter-related infections (predominantly gram positive pathogens) occur with greatest frequency in the first 3 to 4 months after transplantation.

Recurrent sinus and pulmonary infections are associated with chronic GVHD. Antibiotic prophylaxis against encapsulated organisms, using penicillin or an appropriate alternative, reduces the risk of these infections.

Patients with recurrent infections and low serum immunoglobulin levels may benefit from prophylactic intravenous immunoglobulin (IVIg) infusions.

Fungal Infections

Fungal infections constitute a major cause of mortality after allogeneic HSCT: 60% to 70% of patients developing invasive fungal infections die despite antifungal therapy. Yeast (candida species) and molds (aspergillus) account for the majority of opportunistic fungal infections in the posttransplant period.

Candida infections typically occur early in the course of transplantation, often near the end of the neutropenic phase. Candidal infections can manifest as mucocutaneous candidiasis, candidemia, or with visceral involvement (the liver and spleen are most commonly involved). Routine prophylaxis with fluconazole offers protection against sensitive strains of candida.

Invasive aspergillus infections usually involve the lungs, paranasal sinuses, and the central nervous system, although dissemination to other visceral organs has been described. Predisposing factors are corticosteroids, severe GVHD, non-HLA identical and unrelated stem cell donors, and/or transplantation in rooms lacking laminar air flow.

Invasive fungal infections are difficult to eradicate. Fluconazole may be effective against sensitive candida strains (such as *Candida albicans*). Amphotericin B, lipid formulation amphotericin, and newer agents such as the echinocandins (caspofungin) and voriconazole have demonstrated efficacy against aspergillus and a wide spectrum of candida species.

The diligent application of preventive measures such as avoiding the indiscriminate use of corticosteroids remains the most effective strategy for minimizing mortality related to invasive fungal infections.

Viral Infections

Cytomegalovirus

While advances in screening and preventive therapy have reduced CMV-related mortality, CMV infection continues to be a major contributor to posttransplant morbidity. CMV is a DNA virus belonging to the herpesvirus family. Posttransplant CMV infection is most often a consequence of viral reactivation in patients with prior exposure to CMV and is observed in 50% to 70% of CMV seropositive recipients. Reactivation typically occurs in the first 100 days after transplantation. Primary infection in CMV-seronegative recipients can follow transplantation from a seropositive donor. Acquisition of primary infection from CMV-positive transfusion products has been all but eliminated with routine use of leukocyte-depleted or CMV-negative blood products. GVHD, the use of T-cell–depleted allografts, and corticosteroid/CSA/tacrolimus use increase the risk of CMV reactivation.

Interstitial pneumonitis is the most common and serious manifestation of CMV disease, followed by enteritis/colitis. Other manifestations include febrile episodes and marrow suppression resulting in thrombocytopenia with or without neutropenia. Mortality rates with CMV pneumonitis range from 65% to 85%.

Ganciclovir or foscarnet given in conjunction with IVIg improves the outcome associated with CMV disease (Table 18.5). Early detection methods including polymerase chain reaction (PCR) for viral DNA and immunofluorescence for detecting viral antigen in leucocytes predict the subsequent development of CMV disease. Preemptive therapy with ganciclovir or foscarnet (Table 18.5) begun when CMV reactivation is first detected (either PCR or immunofluorescence assay) has dramatically reduced the incidence of CMV pneumonitis/enteritis and consequently CMV-related mortality. Newer approaches for treatment of or prophylaxis against CMV disease include adoptive transfer of ex vivo expanded CMV-specific cytotoxic T lymphocytes.

TABLE 18.5. *Surveillance and Management of Cytomegalovirus: The National Heart, Lung, and Blood Institute Approach*

Surveillance
(CMV PCR)
• Weekly posttransplant until day 100
• Continue surveillance beyond day 100 in the event of late CMV reactivation, continued immunosuppressive therapy, or if clinically indicated

Management of CMV antigenemia*
Induction: Ganciclovir 5 mg/kg IV q12h or foscarnet 90 mg/kg IV q12h or valganciclovir 900 mg PO twice daily × 7 days,* followed by
Maintenance: Ganciclovir 5 mg/kg IV every day 5 times per week (M–F) or Foscarnet 90 mk/kg IV every day 5 times per week (M–F) or daily valganciclovir 900 mg PO every day × 7 days

Management of CMV Disease†
Induction: Ganciclovir or foscarnet IV (at induction doses) q12h × 14 days and IVIg 500 mg/kg IV QOD × 14–21 days
Maintenance: Ganciclovir 5 mg/kg IV every day × 30 days

*If PCR shows two consecutive increases in copy number, continue induction and consider other treatment options (e.g., switching from ganciclovir to foscarnet) until PCR turns negative.
†Foscarnet may be the drug of choice in patients who have cytopenias and CMV reactivation or CMV disease.
CMV, cytomegalovirus; IV, intravenously; IVIg, intravenous immunoglobulin; PCR, polymerase chain reaction; PO, orally.

Epstein-Barr Virus–Associated Lymphoproliferative Disorder

Epstein-Barr virus (EBV)-related lymphoproliferative disorder is a B-cell malignancy arising as a consequence of impaired T-cell immunity against EBV. EBV lymphoproliferation is a relatively rare complication, affecting approximately 1% of all allogeneic transplant recipients, but certain types of transplants (especially T-cell depleted) are associated with a significantly higher risk. The natural course of untreated EBV-lymphoproliferative disorder is rapid progression culminating in death. Allograft T-cell depletion, transplants from HLA-mismatched and unrelated donors, and the use of immunosuppressive agents predispose to the development of this malignancy.

Treatment with a monoclonal antibody to CD20 (rituximab), DLI, or adoptive infusion of EBV-specific cytotoxic T cells are all effective in eradicating this disease, particularly when combined with withdrawal of immunosuppression. Monitoring for EBV reaction by PCR should be considered in patients at high risk for EBV-related lymphoproliferative disorder.

Other Viral Infections

Patients undergoing allogeneic HSCT are at risk for infectious complications associated with the herpesviruses, varicella zoster, and various respiratory viruses (respiratory syncytial virus, influenza, parainfluenza). Adenoviruses or polyoma virus BK may appear clinically as hemorrhagic cystitis. Because cellular immunity is impaired in the posttransplant setting, normally self-limiting viral infections can have fatal sequelae.

Graft Failure

Graft failure is the inability to achieve (primary) or maintain (secondary) persistent donor hematopoiesis. Graft failure mediated by the recipient immune system is referred to as graft rejection. Graft failure is relatively uncommon in patients undergoing transplantation from an HLA-identical sibling donor (less than 2%). T-cell depletion, the use of HLA-mismatched or unrelated donor grafts, and alloimmunization caused by repeated transfusions are factors that increase the risk of graft rejection.

In myeloablative HSCT, primary graft failure presents as persistent pancytopenia (more than 3 to 4 weeks) after conditioning and is associated with a high mortality rate. Secondary graft failure is characterized by initial recovery of blood counts followed by a later loss of donor hematopoiesis.

Up to 50% of patients with graft rejection can be salvaged by repeat conditioning or immunosuppression (as with OKT3 antibody plus corticosteroids) followed by reinfusion of a T-cell–replete allograft. Graft failure can also result from infections, drugs, or chronic GVHD. In these settings, patients can often be salvaged with hematopoietic growth factors (such as G-CSF) with or without additional stem cells.

Late Sequelae of Transplantation

Secondary Malignancies

In addition to EBV-related lymphomas discussed above, leukemias and solid tumors can complicate allogeneic HSCT. The risk of solid tumors in transplant survivors at 10 years is increased eightfold compared with age-matched controls. Melanomas, tumors of the bone, liver, central nervous system (CNS), and thyroid are commonly encountered secondary malignancies. Younger patient age at transplantation and TBI-based conditioning regimens predispose to the development of secondary solid tumors.

Other Late Complications

Growth retardation, infertility, restrictive pulmonary disease, cataracts, endocrine dysfunction, avascular necrosis of bones, osteopenia, and neurocognitive defects are other delayed sequelae of allogeneic HSCT.

Reduced-Intensity and Nonmyeloablative Hematopoietic Stem Cell Transplantation

The high risk of transplant-related mortality with conventional transplants and the appreciation that GVL effects can cure some hematologic malignancies provided the impetus for the development of reduced-intensity and nonmyeloablative conditioning regimens (21,22). The basic principles underlying these regimens include reduced-intensity conditioning to induce adequate host immunosuppression for donor allograft "take" while minimizing toxicities related to dose-intensive conditioning, manipulation of posttransplant immunosuppression and administration of DLIs to promote rapid transition to complete donor immunohematopoiesis, and reliance on the GVL effect for eradication of the underlying malignancy.

A variety of different conditioning regimens have been used, and the cumulative experience from various transplant centers has led to the following observations. (i) Several conditioning-related toxicities such as VOD and mucositis are absent or mild compared with myeloablative transplants. (ii) Transplant-related mortality is substantially lower (7% to 20%) than that associated with standard or myeloablative transplants (25% to 40%). (iii) The improved toxicity profile has expanded the eligibility of allogeneic transplantation to older patients (to 70 years of age) and patients with comorbid medical conditions.

GVL effects against several hematologic malignancies including acute and chronic myelogenous leukemia, acute lymphocytic leukemia, chronic lymphocytic leukemia, NHL, and multiple myeloma have been observed. However, at least in some malignancies (notably MDS), the risk of relapse following reduced-intensity conditioning appears to be higher than that following myeloablative transplantation. Prospective randomized comparisons are required to determine if relapse risk and outcome in individual malignancies can be adversely affected by using reduced-intensity conditioning.

Pilot trials of nonmyeloablative HCT in solid tumors have shown for the first time the ability of the GVT effect to induce disease regression in treatment-refractory metastatic solid tumors. Renal cell carcinoma provides the best example of a tumor that may be susceptible to GVT effects (23); GVT effects have also been described in other solid tumors including breast, pancreatic, colon, and ovarian carcinoma (24).

Alternative Donor Transplantation

Transplantation from Matched Unrelated Donors

A 6/6 HLA matched sibling donor can be identified in less than one third of patients evaluated for an allogeneic HSCT. Suitable volunteer donors registered with the National Marrow Donor Program can be identified for many patients who do not have a matched sibling donor, but would otherwise be considered a candidate for an allogeneic HSCT. As many as 70% of Caucasians are estimated to have at least one HLA-matched donor available, but it is more difficult to find appropriately matched donors for patients belonging to some racial/ethnic subgroups.

Outcome following matched unrelated HSCT has improved significantly with the introduction of routine molecular typing of HLA loci (as opposed to serologic typing) to identify donor-host compatibility. Transplantation using donors who are HLA-identical at the HLA-A, -B, -C, -DR, and -DQ loci by high resolution molecular typing (10/10 match) leads to outcomes approaching that following matched sibling transplants; however, GVHD remains higher with unrelated donors, even when they are complete 10/10 HLA matches at a molecular level.

Transplantation from Mismatched Related Donors

Siblings with mismatches at one or more HLA loci can be used as donors for allogeneic HSCT. However, the incidence of both graft failure and GVHD is higher in recipients of partially matched sibling transplants.

Haploidentical transplants utilize parents, siblings, children, or other family members who share one haplotype with the recipient as donors. The high risk of lethal GVHD accompanying haploidentical transplantation mandates extensive T-cell depletion of grafts. In addition, strategies including the use of high CD34+ cell dose and nonmyeloablative conditioning have been utilized in a bid to improve outcome in transplants using mismatched related donors. Donor-host killer immunoglobulin-like receptor (KIR) incompatibility may affect outcome following haploidentical transplantation; transplants in which recipient cells do not express HLA molecules that can inhibit donor KIR are associated with a lower risk of GVHD and disease relapse, notably in patients with myeloid malignancies (25). Current evidence suggests that natural killer cell alloreactivity may mediate both the heightened GVL effects and reduced GVHD incidence in KIR-incompatible haploidentical transplants. It may be possible to select donors who are KIR-mismatched to maximize NK alloreactivity.

Umbilical Cord Transplants

Cord blood, collected from peripartum placenta, contains stem cells with remarkable proliferative capability. Cord blood is increasingly used as an alternative source of stem cells for allogeneic HSCT. Most cord blood transplants are performed using a cord unit that is mismatched at 1 or 2 HLA loci (5/6 or 4/6 HLA match). Most studies have reported the incidence of acute GVHD is similar and the incidence of chronic GVHD is lower with mismatched cord blood transplants compared with matched unrelated transplant. Both their proliferative potential and their relatively immature lymphocyte content (which lead to a lower incidence of GVHD) are viewed as advantages over other alternative stem cell sources such as haploidentical and unrelated donors. Furthermore, because umbilical cord allografts are derived from previously collected and stored cord blood, they are more immediately available than are unrelated donor grafts, which require donor preparation and then the collection of stem cells once a suitable donor is identified. The major limitation of cord blood as a source of hematopoietic stem cells (particularly in adults) is the relatively small number of cells that can be obtained from single cord blood units. A minimum of 1.5×10^7 nucleated cells/kg and/or $\geq 1.2 \times 10^5$ CD34+ cells/kg are required to obtain acceptable engraftment rates.

Early studies of cord blood transplants in children established the feasibility of this procedure, which was associated with acceptable engraftment rates (85% in one study) and low rates of acute GVHD (<10% in matched cord blood transplants) (26). Several retrospective analyses comparing cord blood transplants to unrelated donor marrow transplants (27,28) indicate that cord blood transplants are typically associated with delayed hematopoietic recovery (median neutrophil recovery time of 22 to 27 days and median platelet recovery time of 60 days in one study), leading to a higher risk of infectious complications. Despite HLA mismatching, the incidence of acute GVHD is similar and the rate of chronic GVHD is lower with cord blood transplants than with fully matched unrelated donors. TRM, disease relapse rates, and DFS following cord blood transplants are comparable with those seen in transplants using unrelated donor marrow.

The simultaneous use of multiple cord blood units from different donors and ex vivo expansion of cord blood stem cells are being explored in efforts to overcome the limitations imposed by low stem cell dose. Several recent studies have shown that umbilical cord blood transplants are a feasible transplant approach for adults, with results only slightly inferior to those observed with transplants using matched unrelated donors.

REFERENCES

1. Blume KG, Thomas ED. A review of autologous hematopoietic cell transplantation. Biol Blood Marrow Transplant 2000;6:1–12.
2. Thomas ED. Bone marrow transplantation: a review. Semin Hematol 1999;36(4 Suppl 7):95–103.
3. Attal M, Harousseau JL, Stoppa AM, et al. A prospective, randomized trial of autologous bone marrow transplantation and chemotherapy in multiple myeloma. Intergroupe Francais du Myelome. N Engl J Med 1996;335:91–97.
4. Philip T, Guglielmi C, Hagenbeek A, et al. Autologous bone marrow transplantation as compared with salvage chemotherapy in relapses of chemotherapy-sensitive non-Hodgkin's lymphoma. N Engl J Med 1995;333:1540–1545.
5. Antman KH. Randomized trials of high dose chemotherapy for breast cancer. Biochim Biophys Acta 2001;1471:M89–M98.
6. Pico JL, Rosti G, Kramar A, et al. A randomised trial of high-dose chemotherapy in the salvage treatment of patients mailing first-line platinum chemotherapy for advanced germ cell tumors. Ann Oncol 2005;16(7):1152–1159.
7. Childs RW. Allogeneic hematopoietic cell transplantation. In: De Vita VT Jr, Hellman, S, Rosenberg SA, eds. Principles and Practice of Oncology. 7th ed. London: Lippincott Williams & Wilkins, 2004.

8. Storb R. Allogeneic hematopoietic stem cell transplantation—yesterday, today, and tomorrow. Exp Hematol 2003;31:1–10.
9. Mathe G, Amiel JL, Schwarzenberg L, et al. Adoptive immunotherapy of acute leukemia: experimental and clinical results. Cancer Res 1965;25:1525–1531.
10. Gatti RA, Meuwissen HJ, Allen HD, et al. Immunologic reconstitution of sex-linked lymphopenic immunological deficiency. Lancet 1968;ii:1366-1369.
11. Bach FH, Albetini RJ, Joo P, et al. Bone-marrow transplantation in a patient with the Wiskott-Aldrich syndrome. Lancet 1968;2:1363–1366.
12. deKoning J, van Bekkum DW, Dicke KA, et al. Transplantation of bone marrow cells and fetal thymus in an infant with lymphopenic immunological deficiency. Lancet 1969;i:1223-1227.
13. Antin JH. Stem cell transplantation-harnessing of graft-versus-malignancy. Curr Opin Hematol 2003;10:440–444.
14. Riddell SR, Berger C, Murata M, et al. The graft versus leukemia response after allogeneic hematopoietic stem cell transplantation. Blood Rev 2003;17:153–162.
15. Horowitz MM, Gale RP, Sondel PM, et al. Graft-versus-leukemia reactions after bone marrow transplantation. Blood 1990;75:555–562.
16. Bensinger WI, Martin PJ, Storer B, et al. Transplantation of bone marrow as compared with peripheral-blood cells from HLA-identical relatives in patients with hematologic cancers. N Engl J Med 2001;344:175–181.
17. Vogelsang GB, Lee L, Bensen-Kennedy DM. Pathogenesis and treatment of graft-versus-host disease after bone marrow transplant. Annu Rev Med 2003;54:29–52.
18. Srinivasan R, Chakrabarti S, Walsh T, et al. Improved survival in steroid-refractory acute graft-versus-host disease after nonmyeloablative allogeneic transplantation using a daclizumab-based strategy with comprehensive infection prophylaxis. Br J Hematol 2004;124:777–786.
19. Shulman HM, Kleiner D, Lee SJ, et al. Histopathologic diagnosis of chronic graft-versus-host disease: National Institutes of Health Consensus Development Project on Criteria for Clinical Trials in Chronic Graft-versus-Host Disease: II. Pathology Working Group Report. Biol Blood Marrow Transplant 2006;12:31–47.
20. Leather HL, Wingard JR. Infections following hematopoietic stem cell transplantation. Infect Dis Clin North Am 2001;15:483–520.
21. Storb RF, Champlin R, Riddell SR, et al. Non-myeloablative transplants for malignant disease. Hematology (Am Soc Hematol Educ Program) 2001;375–391.
22. Anagnostopoulos A, Giralt S. Critical review on non-myeloablative stem cell transplantation (NST). Crit Rev Oncol Hematol 2002;44:175–190.
23. Childs R, Chernoff A, Contentin N, et al. Regression of metastatic renal-cell carcinoma after non-myeloablative allogeneic peripheral-blood stem-cell transplantation. N Engl J Med 2000;343: 750–758.
24. Childs RW, Srinivasan R. Allogeneic hematopoietic cell transplantation for solid tumors. In: Blume KG, Forman SJ, Appelbaum FR, eds. Thomas' Hematopoitic Cell Transplantation. 3rd ed. Malden, MA: Blackwell Science, 2004:1177–1187.
25. Ruggeri L, Capanni M, Urbani E, et al. Effectiveness of donor natural killer cell alloreactivity in mismatched hematopoietic transplants. Science 2002;295:2097–2100.
26. Wagner JE, Kernan NA, Steinbuch M, et al. Allogeneic sibling umbilical-cord-blood transplantation in children with malignant and non-malignant disease. Lancet 1995;346:214–219.
27. Rocha V, Labopin M, Sanz G, et al. Transplants of umbilical-cord blood or bone marrow from unrelated donors in adults with acute leukemia. N Engl J Med 2004;351:2276–2285.
28. Laughlin MJ EM, Rubinstein P, Wagner JE, et al. Outcomes after transplantation of cord blood or bone marrow from unrelated donors in adults with leukemia. N Engl J Med 2004;351:2265–2275.

19

Thrombocytopenia

Patrick F. Fogarty and Cynthia E. Dunbar

PLATELET BIOLOGY

Platelets are anucleate blood cells that participate in *primary hemostasis*, the formation of a platelet plug at sites of vascular injury. Platelets are produced from *megakaryocytes*, multinucleate hematopoietic cells located in the bone marrow. Cytokines such as thrombopoietin are necessary for normal platelet maturation and release. Once released into the circulation, the average life span of a platelet is 7 to 10 days. Platelets are removed from the circulation when they are activated and utilized at sites of vascular injury or as they become senescent. At any given time, up to one third of the platelet mass is stored in the spleen, providing a reserve of platelets that may be released during periods of physiologic stress. The normal platelet concentration in the blood is 150,000 to 350,000/uL as measured in most hospital laboratories.

ETIOLOGY AND CLINICAL FEATURES OF THROMBOCYTOPENIA

Thrombocytopenia may occur because of decreased production of platelets, increased consumption of platelets, increased sequestration of platelets, or any combination of these mechanisms (Table 19.1).

Regardless of the cause of thrombocytopenia, "platelet-type" bleeding is typically mucocutaneous and is characterized by petechiae, ecchymoses, epistaxis, and gingival and conjunctival hemorrhages. Less commonly, severe thrombocytopenia may lead to gastrointestinal, genitourinary, or central nervous system bleeding.

Spontaneous bleeding or bruising normally does not occur until the platelet count has fallen below 10,000 to 20,000/uL. The rate of decline of the platelet count may also influence the likelihood of unprovoked bleeding, presumably because of compensatory processes that may occur over time in the setting of persistent thrombocytopenia. Patients with dysfunctional platelets may bleed with higher platelet counts. Patients with thrombocytopenia and platelet counts greater than 20,000 to 30,000/uL without bleeding usually do not require immediate treatment to increase the platelet count. A platelet count of 80,000 to 100,000/uL is generally regarded as adequate for hemostasis during most invasive procedures, including surgery (Table 19.2).

DISORDERS CHARACTERIZED BY DECREASED PRODUCTION OF PLATELETS

Bone Marrow Failure

Congenital disorders, such as *Fanconi's anemia or dyskeratosis congenita*, typically present early in life; these syndromes often cause depression of other blood cell lineages (i.e., white cells and red cells) in addition to the platelet count, but in a significant minority of cases isolated thrombocytopenia can be the presenting abnormality.

Other disorders such as *congenital amegakaryocytic thrombocytopenia* and the *Thrombocytopenia with absent radius (TAR) syndrome* are characterized by isolated thrombocytopenia.

TABLE 19.1. *Causes of Thrombocytopenia*

Disorders Characterized by Decreased Production of Platelets

Bone marrow failure syndromes
  Congenital (amegakaryocytic thrombocytopenia, Fanconi's anemia, dyskeratosis congenita, Shwachman-Diamond syndrome, thrombocytopenia-absent radii syndrome, Wiskott-Aldrich Syndrome)
  Acquired (aplastic anemia, amegakaryocytic thrombocytopenia)
Myelodysplasia
Marrow infiltration (neoplastic, infectious)
Chemotherapy-induced
Irradiation-induced
Cyclic thrombocytopenia
Folate, B_{12} or iron (advanced cases) deficiency
Ethanolism

Disorders Characterized by Increased Clearance of Platelets

Immune thrombocytopenic purpura
Heparin-induced thrombocytopenia
Thrombotic thrombocytopenic purpura/Hemolytic-uremic syndrome
Disseminated intravascular coagulation (HELLP syndrome)
Posttransfusion purpura
Neonatal alloimmune thrombocytopenia
Von Willebrand disease, type IIB
Antiphospholipid antibody syndrome
Mechanical destruction (aortic valvular dysfunction; extracorporeal bypass)

Disorders Characterized by Increased Sequestration of Platelets

---

Hypersplenism*
Other conditions
Artifactual (pseudothrombocytopenia)
Drug-induced[†]
Gestational thrombocytopenia
HIV-associated thrombocytopenia
Infection- and sepsis-related thrombocytopenia
Hemophagocytosis
Qualitative platelet disorder-related (Bernard Soulier disease, grey platelet syndrome, May-Hegglin anomaly)

---

*See Table 19.5.
[†]See Table 19.6.

TABLE 19.2. *Target Platelet Count Values for Commonly Encountered Clinical Scenarios**

Goal or Intervention	Desired platelet count (/uL)
Prevention of spontaneous intracranial bleeding	>5000–10,000
Prevention of spontaneous mucocutaneous bleeding	>10,000–30,000
Placement of central vascular catheters	>20,000–30,000 (compressible site)
	>40,000–50,000 (noncompressible site or tunneled catheter)
Use of anticoagulant medications in therapeutic doses	>40,000–50,000
Invasive procedures	
Endoscopy with biopsy	>60,000
Liver biopsy	>80,000
Major surgery	>80,000–100,000

*Values are approximate and reflect target ranges for patients with otherwise intact hemostasis. Patients with thrombocytopenia and bleeding may benefit from augmentation of the platelet count (e.g., by platelet transfusion) irrespective of the platelet value.

Wiskott-Aldrich syndrome (WAS) is an X-linked recessive disorder that comprises a triad of thrombocytopenia, eczema, and immunodeficiency. Thrombocytopenia occurs because of decreased megakaryocytopoiesis along with increased destruction of abnormal platelets. Thrombocytopenia may improve with splenectomy, but allogeneic hematopoietic stem cell transplantation alone is potentially curative for the disorder.

Adults patients with *acquired amegakaryocytic thrombocytopenia* initially may appear to have immune thrombocytopenic purpura (see below), but the bone marrow reveals markedly reduced or absent megakaryocytes instead of normal or increased numbers; the disorder may progress to aplastic anemia. Patients with acquired aplastic anemia rarely can present with isolated thrombocytopenia. Marked bone marrow hypocellularity with decreased megakaryocytes would suggest this diagnosis. (For more discussion of the treatment of these entities, please see Chapter 6.)

Myelodysplasia

Thrombocytopenia is a common feature of myelodysplasia (MDS). Mild thrombocytopenia with macrocytosis, with or without anemia or neutropenia, in an older individual is a typical presentation. In contrast, an isolated very low platelet count (less than 20,000/ul) without any other blood count abnormalities is not typical for MDS.

Examination of the bone marrow aspirate and blood smear may suggest MDS if megakaryocytic dysplasia (including small and mononuclear "micromegakaryocyte" forms) and maturation abnormalities of erythrocytic and granulocytic precursor cells are present. Cytogenetic abnormalities (especially deletion of chromosome 5q or monosomy 7), if present, also indicate MDS as the underlying diagnosis (see Chapter 7).

Treatment of thrombocytopenia because of MDS can be difficult. Hematopoietic cytokines such as G-CSF or IL-11 are not effective, and newer therapies such as the immunomodulatory agent lenalidomide lead to platelet count responses in only a minority of individuals (see Chapter 7). Thrombopoietic stimulants in clinical trials are showing promise. Chronic transfusion of platelets may be indicated if the thrombocytopenia is severe and accompanied by bleeding. Because MDS platelets mature abnormally and may be defective, bleeding can occur at counts that would otherwise be hemostatic; thus, a higher threshold for prophylactic transfusion may be necessary.

Marrow Infiltration

Infiltration of the bone marrow by malignant cells may cause thrombocytopenia but usually only after massive replacement of the marrow space by tumor cells or immature hematologic precursor cells has occurred. In these scenarios, however, thrombocytopenia is rarely the sole blood count abnormality. Examination of the bone marrow biopsy and aspirate is required to diagnose marrow infiltration-related thrombocytopenia.

The acute and chronic leukemias, myeloma, and lymphoma are the most common tumors resulting in cytopenias because of neoplastic marrow infiltration. Certain *infections* (such as tuberculosis and ehrlichiosis) can result in formation of granulomas in the bone marrow that supplant the normal marrow architecture and lead to decreased production of blood cells, including platelets. Effective treatment of the underlying condition should be expected to restore a low platelet count to the normal range, but platelet transfusions may be required initially if bleeding is present or invasive procedures are planned (see Table 19.2).

Irradiation and Chemotherapy

Irradiation and/or myelotoxic chemotherapy induce thrombocytopenia via direct toxicity to megakaryocytes or more immature hematopoietic stem and progenitor cells. The degree and duration of thrombocytopenia depends on the intensity and the type of the myelotoxic regimen. Chemotherapy-induced thrombocytopenia typically resolves more slowly than neutropenia and/or anemia, especially following repetitive cycles of treatment.

A recombinant IL-11-like cytokine (Neumega, Wyeth, Madison, NJ) has been approved for the prevention of chemotherapy-induced severe thrombocytopenia, but its use is limited by significant side effects such as allergic reactions, fluid retention, and cardiovascular phenomena. Trials of novel platelet growth factors for chemotherapy-induced thrombocytopenia are underway (1).

Cyclic Thrombocytopenia

This exceedingly rare disorder is characterized by episodes of thrombocytopenia that occur cyclically, typically every 3 to 6 weeks. The thrombocytopenia is frequently severe and may be associated with significant bleeding. Treatment with oral contraceptives (female patients), androgens, immunosuppressive agents (such as azathioprine), or thrombopoietic growth factor has lead to responses in some cases.

Nutritional Deficiencies

Folate deficiency (commonly associated with alcoholism) and vitamin B_{12} deficiency may cause decreased megakaryocytopoiesis and thrombocytopenia, typically in conjunction with anemia. In contrast, thrombocytosis is typical in cases of significant iron deficiency; in very severe iron deficiency, however, thrombocytopenia may also occur. In any of these situations, replacement of the deficient vitamin or mineral should correct the thrombocytopenia.

DISORDERS CHARACTERIZED BY INCREASED CLEARANCE OF PLATELETS

Immune Thrombocytopenic Purpura

Immune thrombocytopenic purpura (ITP) is an acquired autoimmune disorder in which the production of antiplatelet antibodies results in platelet destruction, causing thrombocytopenia that may lead to bleeding. Patients typically present with markedly reduced platelet counts and mucocutaneous bleeding or may have only a mildly or moderately depressed platelet count that is discovered on a routine blood count. Because most of the available treatments have considerable toxicity, therapy should be offered only to symptomatic patients or to those felt to be at high risk for serious bleeding.

Epidemiology

The annual incidence of ITP in adults has been estimated to be about 2 cases per 100,000 persons and increases with age (2).

Pathophysiology

Pathogenic antiplatelet antibodies can be identified in approximately 75% of patients with ITP. These autoantibodies are commonly directed against the platelet glycoprotein complexes IIb/IIIa and/or Ib/IX, but other platelet protein targets have been identified. The antibody-coated platelets are then cleared by reticuloendothelial macrophages in the liver and/or spleen, resulting in a reduced life span of platelets from approximately 7 days to less than 2 days. Adult-onset ITP is generally idiopathic and becomes chronic but may occur in association with disorders of lymphoproliferation (lymphoma or chronic lymphocytic leukemia [CLL]) or immune dysregulation (systemic lupus erythematosus, human immunodeficiency virus [HIV] infection). In contrast, ITP in children typically follows a viral infection and frequently resolves spontaneously without specific therapy (3).

Presentation

Typically, new-onset severe ITP (platelets <30,000/uL) manifests with petechial bruising and bleeding from mucous membranes, including conjunctival hemorrhages, gingival bleeding, and epistaxis.

Milder disease (platelet count >50,000/uL) often presents as an asymptomatically low platelet count on a routine blood count.

Diagnosis

Because no single test or group of tests is diagnostic for ITP, the diagnosis is primarily one of exclusion. New-onset, isolated thrombocytopenia with no other readily apparent cause (including medication-related) in an otherwise asymptomatic adult generally may be regarded as sufficient grounds for the diagnosis of ITP and subsequent initiation of medical therapies (if appropriate based on the degree of thrombocytopenia).

The presence of other cytopenias, age greater than 60 years, or failure of primary therapy (corticosteroids for a trial of one week), however, should prompt bone marrow examination before consideration of other therapies. The presence of abnormal or decreased numbers of megakaryocytes or abnormal marrow cellularity should redirect the diagnostic evaluation away from ITP as a cause of the thrombocytopenia.

All patients should be screened for hepatitis B and C and HIV infection (see below).

Treatment

Individuals with mild or moderate thrombocytopenia (platelets >30,000/ul) who do not require a higher platelet count for surgery or active bleeding should not receive treatment. Rather, they may be observed at regular intervals for disease progression. Adults with platelet counts of <20,000 to 30,000/ul or those with significant bleeding generally should be treated (3,4).

Initial Management

Initial management generally consists of a short course of *corticosteroids* (prednisone 1 mg/kg/day for 7 to 10 days with subsequent rapid tapering or "pulse" dexamethasone 40 mg daily for 4 days). A significant increase in the platelet count should be seen within 3 to 7 days. In the event of a platelet response, prednisone may be tapered rapidly until a dose of 20 mg/day is reached; thereafter, tapering should proceed more slowly (e.g., by dose decrements of no more than 5 mg per adjustment, occurring no more frequently than once every 2 to 3 weeks). Patients who initially respond to dexamethasone typically receive pulse treatments monthly for at least 6 months.

For patients with serious active bleeding and/or very severe thrombocytopenia (<5000 to 10,000/ul), *intravenous immune globulin* (IVIg; 1 gm/kg/day for 2 days) or *anti-D* (WinRho [Baxter Healthcare Corporation, Deerfield, IL] 75 ug/kg/dose; appropriate for nonsplenectomized, Rh blood type-positive, nonanemic patients only) can be given in addition to corticosteroids to decrease clearance of antibody-coated platelets. Responses are generally seen within 3 to 5 days of IVIg or anti-D administration.

Platelet transfusions may be administered if the presentation is complicated by serious (e.g., intracranial) bleeding. Transfused platelets are expected to be cleared very rapidly in the presence of antiplatelet antibodies but may improve hemostasis temporarily.

Chronic Treatment

Unfortunately, despite a high initial response rate (60% to 75%), the majority of adults with ITP experience relapse once initial treatments are reduced or discontinued. The decision to administer second- or third-line agents for the treatment of refractory ITP must take into consideration the risk of thrombocytopenic bleeding as well as the significant toxicites of most of these treatments. Treatment is appropriate for patients with platelet counts <30,000/ul or clinically significant bleeding.

IVIg and *anti-D* (see above) may be used to decrease clearance of antibody-coated platelets by reticuloendothelial cells. *Anti-D* should be considered in Rh+ patients only. Both IVIg and anti-D produce rapid increases in the platelet count in a majority of patients; however, the effect is transient and the agents must be readministered every 2 to 3 weeks in most instances. They can be particularly useful for patients that require intermittent elevation of the platelet count for surgical procedures or other periods of increased bleeding risk.

The monoclonal anti-B cell antibody *rituximab* (anti-cd20), given at a dose of 375 mg/m^2 weekly for 4 weeks, induces initial and long-term responses in about 50% and 25%, respectively, of adults with severe, chronic ITP (5).

Other treatments for steroid and/or splenectomy-refractory ITP include *very high-dose pulse dexamethasone*, single-agent *vincristine, cyclosporine, danazol, mycophenolate mofetil, dapsone*, Helicobacter pylori *treatment, azathioprine, vitamin C, interferon, plasma exchange*, and *immunoadsorption over staphylococcal protein A columns* (3,4). Most of these therapies have response rates of 30% or less and can be associated with significant side effects. *Combination chemotherapy or high-dose chemotherapy with autologous stem cell support* has resulted in durable complete remissions in a subset of patients with severe, refractory ITP (6).

Splenectomy traditionally was performed after the platelet count failed to respond durably to corticosteroids but at the present time is usually reserved for cases of severe thrombocytopenia that has failed to respond to second- or third-line treatments, especially when complicated by clinically significant bleeding. A 65% to 75% response rate immediately postprocedure and durable response rates of 60% to 70% are typical (7). All patients must receive immunization against encapsulated bacterial organisms (pneumococcus, *H. influenzae*, meningococcus) several weeks prior to splenectomy if possible. Laparoscopic splenectomy results in decreased morbidity and shorter hospitalizations than open procedures.

Results of early trials of *novel thrombopoietin receptor agonists* in patients with severe, chronic ITP are encouraging, showing a clinically significant rise in the platelet count in a majority of patients and good tolerability (8,9).

Pregnancy-Associated Immune Thrombocytopenic Purpura

Pregnant women with platelet counts <30,000/uL during the second or third trimester, or with platelet counts <10,000/uL or bleeding in any trimester, should be treated. Intermittent infusions of *IVIg* or moderate-dose oral prednisone (commonly given on an every-other-daily schedule) are standard. *Splenectomy* during the first or second trimester may be considered for women whose ITP has failed treatment with IVIg and steroids and who have platelet counts <10,000/uL with associated bleeding. *Platelets* may be administered prophylactically prior to cesarean section in women who have platelet counts <10,000/uL or mucocutaneous bleeding near the time of delivery. A platelet count of >50,000/uL generally is regarded as adequate prior to cesarean section or vaginal delivery.

Heparin-Induced Thrombocytopenia

Heparin-induced thrombocytopenia (HIT) is an antibody-mediated disorder that results in platelet activation and clearance. Although the disorder produces thrombocytopenia, patients with HIT paradoxically are at high risk for thrombosis. If HIT is suspected, heparin should be discontinued immediately, and, if appropriate, alternative anticoagulation administered.

Epidemiology

HIT occurs in approximately 3% of patients who are treated with unfractionated heparin (10); as many as half of these individuals will develop thrombosis.

Pathophysiology

The pathogenesis of HIT begins with binding of the heparin molecule to platelet factor 4 (PF4), a platelet alpha granule protein that becomes antigenic when bound to heparin. The heparin-PF4 complex stimulates formation of an IgG antibody (HIT antibody) that binds both to the heparin-PF4 complex (via its Fab portion) and to platelet Fc receptors (via its Fc portion). Binding of the HIT antibody to platelets activates them, resulting in release of procoagulant microparticles, platelet clearance, and subsequent thrombocytopenia. PF4 also binds to polysaccharides (e.g., heparan sulfate) on the endothelial surface;

recognition of these PF4-polysaccharide complexes by HIT antibodies may lead to endothelial damage, expression of tissue factor, and further hypercoagulability.

Presentation

The typical presentation of HIT involves a hospitalized patient who develops thrombocytopenia within 5 to 10 days of receiving heparin. Other presentations, however, are possible.

The presenting platelet count may be in the normal range, but a decline of 50% or more from the baseline value in a heparin-treated patient may signify HIT. Platelet counts generally do not fall below 30,000/uL.

Spontaneous bleeding (including petechiae) is not typical, even in patients who have markedly decreased platelet counts. Bleeding, elevated coagulation tests, or severe thrombocytopenia generally should point the investigation away from HIT.

Venous (upper or lower limb, dural sinus) or arterial (lower limb, cerebrovascular accident, myocardial infarction, other locations) thromboses frequently occur in patients with HIT. The risk of HIT-related thrombosis persists for at least 30 days after the discontinuation of heparin (11).

In a minority of patients with HIT, thrombosis is the presenting clinical sign; in these cases, an unrecognized decline in the platelet count almost always has preceded the thrombosis.

Delayed-onset HIT describes *new* thrombocytopenia and venous or arterial thrombosis that occurs up to 14 days after completion of an uneventful course of heparin therapy. Thrombocytopenia and thrombosis typically worsen if heparin is administered.

Amanestic Response

HIT may occur within 1 to 4 days of re-exposure to heparin in patients who have received heparin within the prior 100 days because of prior formation and persistence of HIT antibodies. Sometimes the amanestic response is heralded by an acute systemic reaction characterized by fever, chills, hypotension, and/or cardiovascular compromise immediately after exposure to heparin; an abrupt fall in the platelet count is always observed.

Diagnosis

Strictly, the diagnosis of HIT requires both an appropriate clinical context and confirmatory laboratory testing (e.g., demonstration of HIT antibodies). Because of the limited availability of HIT-specific laboratory assays, however, *any patient in whom the clinical suspicion for the disorder is high should be managed as though he or she has HIT, even if the results of diagnostic tests are pending or unavailable.*

Clinical Factors

Thrombocytopenia (or >50% decline from the baseline platelet count) or thrombosis in a patient who has recently been exposed to heparin may indicate HIT; see *Presentation*. The timing of the decline in platelet count or appearance of thrombosis should be compared with the timing of the onset of exposure to heparin. An appropriate increase in the platelet count after discontinuation of heparin plus the absence of any other plausible explanation for thrombocytopenia may be regarded as diagnostic for HIT in the absence of confirmatory laboratory testing. A careful review of the hospital chart (including nursing notes) may be necessary to document administration of heparin, especially if its use was transient (heparin flushes) or its form covert (heparin-impregnated catheters).

Laboratory Diagnosis

Laboratory diagnosis is achieved by one or both of two types of assays. Both tests have a sensitivity of approximately 90%. The **ELISA** (enzyme-linked immunosorbent assay) **for PF4-heparin associated IgG** measures binding of HIT antibodies in the patient's serum to a PF4-heparin complex that has been used to coat wells of a microtiter plate; an anti-IgG antibody with a label is applied and the binding quantified. **Platelet activation assays** (less commonly available) measure activation of donor platelets in the presence of the patient's serum and a high and low concentration of heparin; increased release of adenosine triphosphate (ATP) (chemiluminescence method) or ^{14}C-serotonin (12) in the presence of therapeutic concentrations of heparin (0.05–0.3 U/mL) indicates HIT. Some heparin-treated patients who have not demonstrated a decline in the platelet count (and thus do not have HIT) nonetheless demonstrate HIT antibodies by ELISA; in these cases, platelet activation assays (which have a higher specificity than ELISA) are likely to be negative.

Treatment

All forms of *heparin must be discontinued* immediately. (In patients in whom laboratory testing for HIT eventually proves negative or in whom an alternative explanation for thrombocytopenia has been found, heparin may be subsequently restarted.) *Doppler ultrasound of the lower extremities* should be performed to rule out subclinical deep vein thrombosis. Because (i) HIT patients rarely bleed and (ii) transfused platelets may worsen the already increased thrombotic risk by providing substrate for HIT antibodies, platelet transfusions are rarely indicated.

Warfarin is contraindicated as initial treatment of clinically proven or suspected HIT because of its propensity to exacerbate hypercoagulability by reduction of plasma levels of proteins C and S.

Because of the high rate of serious thrombosis among patients with HIT, an *alternative anticoagulant* (Table 19.3) should be administered in all cases of suspected or proven HIT.

- Up to 50% of patients with HIT develop thrombosis within 30 days of recognition of the thrombocytopenia.
- The thrombocytopenia of HIT generally is *not* considered to be a contraindication to the use of anticoagulants, due to the underlying prothrombotic state.
- Some patients with HIT require anticoagulation for additional reasons (e.g., after interventional cardiac procedures, concurrent thrombosis).

The alternative anticoagulant should be continued at least until significant recovery of the platelet count has occurred or (patients with thrombosis) until the platelet count has recovered substantially and adequate anticoagulation with warfarin has been achieved (see *Longer-Term Anticoagulation*, below). If an alterative anticoagulant is not used, the patient should be followed closely until the platelet count has recovered for signs or symptoms of thrombosis.

Longer-Term Anticoagulation

Patients with HIT who develop thrombosis should receive anticoagulation with warfarin for a total duration of 3 to 6 months at an international normalized ratio of 2.0–3.0. Warfarin should not be initiated, however, until *both* therapeutic anticoagulation with an alternative anticoagulant has been achieved *and* the platelet count has recovered substantially. (Note: Synergy between warfarin and argatroban requires a special approach to interpretation of the INR.)

Thrombolysis/Thromboembolectomy

Low-dose or very low-dose thrombolytic agents may be indicated in acute limb ischemia or life-threatening pulmonary embolism caused by HIT-associated thrombi. Surgical removal of large-vessel, arterial thrombi may be indicated if the limb is threatened and other treatments have failed. Patients managed by either chemical or surgical means require concomitant use of an alternative anticoagulant, regardless of the degree of thrombocytopenia.

Intravenous Hemoglobin, Plasma Exchange, and Aspirin

IVIg, plasma exchange, and aspirin usually are not used unless thrombocytopenia and/or life-threatening thromboses are worsening or persistent despite initiation of an alternative anticoagulant.

TABLE 19.3. *Alternative Anticoagulants in the Treatment of Heparin-Induced Thrombocytopenia*

Agent	Description	Indication	Dosing	Comment
Argatroban	Synthetic direct thrombin inhibitor	Prophylaxis or treatment of HIT, including postpercutaneous coronary intervention	Obtain baseline PTT. Start continuous infusion at 0.5–1.2 μg/kg/min. Titrate to achieve PTT of 1.5 to 3 times the baseline value. Do not allow PTT to exceed 100 seconds nor the infusion rate to exceed 10 μg/kg/min.	• Patients with hepatic insufficiency: initial infusion rate = 0.5 μg/kg/min. • Increases the INR in warfarin-treated patients; interpret INR accordingly.
Lepirudin (*Refludan*®)	Recombinant hirudin; direct thrombin inhibitor	Treatment of HIT with associated thrombosis	Obtain baseline PTT. Give slow bolus of 0.4 mg/kg then continuous infusion of 0.15 mg/kg/hr. Titrate to achieve PTT of 1.5 to 2.5 times baseline value. PTTs should be obtained 4 hours after starting the infusion and at least daily during treatment.	• Patients with renal insufficiency: initial bolus = 0.2 mg/kg. = 0.2 mg/kg. • 50% of patients develop antidrug antibodies that increase half life; may necessitate a decrease in dose
Bivalirudin (*Hirulog*®)*	Semi synthetic derivative of hirudin	N/A	N/A	N/A
Danaparoid sodium (*Orgaran*®)*	Mixture of negatively charged glycosaminoglycans (heparin sulfate, dermatan sulfate, chondroitin sulfate)	N/A	N/A	• Monitoring difficult (requires anti-Xa levels and dana paroid calibration curve) • 10% cross-reactivity with HI antibodies

*Not available in the United States (Refludan, CSL Behring, Marburg, Germany; Hirulog, Biogen, Cambridge, MA; Orgaran, Schering-Plough, Kenilworth, NJ).
HIT, heparin-induced thrombocytopenia; INR, international normalized ratio; N/A, not applicable; PTT, partial thromboplastin time.

Retreatment with Heparin

HIT antibodies probably do not persist beyond 100 days from the initial episode of HIT (13), in which case very transient use of heparin subsequent to this time period may be safe. If possible, however, heparin should be avoided in all patients with a prior history of HIT, and an alternative anticoagulant should be used. If heparin is essential (such as in cardiopulmonary bypass), it should not be given until absence of HIT antibodies has been confirmed by ELISA or platelet activation methods, and its use should be limited to the procedure.

Low-Molecular-Weight Heparins The prevalence of HIT among patients treated with low-molecular-weight heparins (LMWHs) is much lower than that observed with unfractionated heparin, principally because of the smaller molecular size of the LMWHs, which decreases their binding to PF4 and their immunogenicity. However, a small but reproducible rate of cross-reactivity of HIT antibodies with LMWHs indicates that they should not be used in the treatment of acute HIT.

Nonimmune Heparin-induced Thrombocytopenia Nonimmune HIT describes a small decrease in the platelet count observed after the initiation of heparin; the phenomenon is not immune-mediated and presumably is caused by heparin-induced, PF4-independent platelet aggregation. The decrease in platelets generally is <10,000 to 30,000/uL and normally is not significant enough to result in thrombocytopenia. Heparin does not need to be discontinued in this scenario.

Thrombotic Thrombocytopenic Purpura

Thrombotic thrombocytopenic purpura (TTP) and the related disorder, the *hemolytic-uremic syndrome* (HUS), are characterized by microangiopathic hemolytic anemia and the formation of platelet-rich thrombi in the arterial and capillary microvasculature; hence, they also are known as *thrombotic microangiopathies* (TMA). As platelets are consumed, thrombocytopenia develops; anemia results from hemolysis and bleeding. Early aggressive intervention with plasma exchange is crucial in most cases because of the extremely high mortality rate for the disorder.

Epidemiology

The incidence of sporadic TTP is approximately 3 to 4 cases/100,000 persons (14); there is a slight female predominance. Most cases of endemic HUS occur in children, are related to infection with enteropathogenic bacteria, and are more prevalent in summer or warm climates. TMA occurs at an increased rate during pregnancy and in the peripartum period.

Pathophysiology

The TMAs are thought to arise from factors that directly or indirectly cause platelet aggregation and/or endothelial cell damage, leading to the formation of microvascular thrombi and ischemia in involved organs. These factors include toxins, cytokines, drugs, or deficiencies in the function of the von Willebrand factor cleaving protease (VWFCP, or ADAMTS-13). Red cells are sheared as they negotiate thrombotic obstructions and fibrin strands in the microvasculature, leading to hemolytic anemia. Consumption of platelets results in thrombocytopenia and bleeding.

Patients with **congenital TTP** have decreased activity of the VWFCP (15), which is a metalloproteinase whose normal function is to cleave newly synthesized, ultra-large VWF (ULVWF) multimers released in the plasma into multimers of smaller size. ULVWF multimers bind to platelets more avidly than smaller VWF molecules; thus, ULVWF in the plasma may incite platelet aggregation.

In **sporadic TTP**, an acquired deficiency of VWFCP results from production of an autoantibody against the VWFCP (16), leading to an accumulation of ULVWF in the plasma and excessive platelet aggregation.

Pregnancy-associated TTP-HUS may stem from decreased levels of the VWFCP that naturally occur in the second and third trimesters; in some cases an antibody to VWFCP is present (17).

In many cases of **endemic HUS**, Shiga toxin from *E. coli* (especially type 0157:H7) is thought to promote platelet aggregation by damaging endothelial cells or by other mechanisms.

Drugs such as *cyclosporine, quinine, ticlopidine, clopidogrel, mitomycin C, and bleomycin* may cause TMA by endothelial cell injury and/or proaggregatory effects on platelets. Antibodies inhibiting the VWFCP have been described in patients who received some of these medications (18,19).

TMA in the setting of **cancer, hematopoietic stem cell transplantation,** or **HIV infection** has not been linked to abnormalities of VWFCP, but effects on endothelial cells or platelets may be responsible.

Presentation

All patients with TMA have microangiopathic hemolytic anemia (MAHA). Varying degrees of bleeding and neurologic impairment (more typical of TTP) or symptoms related to renal failure (predominant in HUS) may also be present (Table 19.4). Microangiopathic hemolytic anemia, thrombocytopenia, fever, renal insufficiency, and neurologic system abnormalities (the classic pentad) occur in less than half of patients with TTP (20). Most patients with HUS have a recent or current diarrheal illness.

Children with diarrhea-associated TMA usually are said to have HUS (hemolytic *uremic* syndrome) because of the degree of renal impairment. In adults, TTP and HUS are often difficult to distinguish because of the overlap of symptoms, but if renal dysfunction predominates, the syndrome usually is classified as HUS.

Manifestations of renal insufficiency may include elevated creatinine, azotemia, proteinuria, hematuria, and/or oliguria.

Neurologic impairment (from microthrombi in the cerebral vasculature) occurs in about 75% and 30% of patients with TTP and HUS, respectively, and includes headache, somnolence, confusion, seizures, and (less commonly) paresis and coma.

Diagnosis

TMA is a clinical diagnosis; the presence of new-onset MAHA and thrombocytopenia (and/or renal failure) in the absence of any other plausible explanation suffice for the diagnosis. MAHA is *essential* to the diagnosis of TTP-HUS and is defined by anemia with positive markers of intravascular hemolysis (elevated lactate dehydrogenase [LDH], elevated indirect bilirubin, decreased haptoglobin, and reticulocytosis) and negative direct antiglobulin (Coombs) test (DAT). The blood smear shows >3 schistocytes per high-power microscopic field.

Clinical features such as an antecedent bloody diarrheal illness and/or renal insufficiency (more typically associated with HUS), or neurologic abnormalities with or without fever (more typically associated with TTP), or recent or current pregnancy, or treatment with associated drugs, or cancer, or recent hematopoietic stem cell transplantation are diagnostically corroborative. **Stool culture for *E. coli* 0157:H7** or assays for antibody against Shiga or Shiga-like toxins, or against specific bacterial lipopolysaccharide, may be positive in patients with endemic HUS. **Assays for the VWFCP** may be abnormal in congenital or sporadic (acquired) TTP; these specialized tests are not available widely and most require substantial processing time, so treatment decisions must be made on clinical grounds. The PT, aPTT and fibrinogen are typically within the normal range in TMA.

Treatment

Without plasma exchange, the mortality rate of sporadic TTP exceeds 90% (14). For this reason, the diagnosis of TMA should be made promptly and treatment with plasma exchange instituted expeditiously. An important exception is children or adults with endemic (*E. coli* diarrhea-associated) HUS, who generally recover with supportive care within 3 weeks, without plasma exchange.

Plasma exchange should be initiated as soon as appropriate vascular access has been obtained. It should be performed once daily until the LDH and platelet count are normal for 2 to 3 days; up to 3 weeks of treatment may be required. Failure to respond to once-daily therapy requires twice-daily treatments; once the LDH and platelet count indicate response, once-daily treatments can be resumed until these parameters have normalized for 2 to 3 days, then the treatments can be discontinued. Alternatively, treatments may be continued every other day, then weekly, for a short period of time, if the TMA was associated with severe clinical symptoms.

bleeding is present; in this case, human leukocyte antigen (HLA) antigen-matched platelets are preferred. Future transfusions should be administered judiciously, with washed or Pl^{A1}-negative blood products.

Neonatal Alloimmune Thrombocytopenia

Neonatal alloimmune thrombocytopenia (NAIT) is a cause of severe thrombocytopenia in neonates. It occurs when fetal platelet antigens cross the placenta and trigger formation of maternal alloantibodies that can then enter the fetal circulation, bind platelets, and induce thrombocytopenia. Antibodies commonly have specificity for human platelet antigen [HPA]-1a, also known as Pl^{A1}. The presence of certain maternal platelet phenotypes (such as the homozygous HPA-1b state) appears to influence the risk of the disorder, especially if the fetus inherits a different, paternal platelet phenotype.

The thrombocytopenia is typically severe, and a high prevalence of intracranial hemorrhage (ICH) during or following delivery is observed, resulting in neonatal death in 5% of cases of NAIT. Thrombocytopenia typically resolves by 2 to 3 weeks of age (25).

IVIg, with or without *corticosteroids*, is recommended for any neonate with platelet counts <20,000 to 25,000/uL. Random donor or (ideally) irradiated maternally antigen-matched platelets are often administered in cases of ICH. Subsequent pregnancies are regarded as high risk for recurrent NAIT.

Von Willebrand Disease, Type 2B

This type of von Willebrand Disease (VWD) is characterized by an abnormal von Willebrand Factor (VWF) that has increased affinity for its platelet receptor, glycoprotein Ib. Becasue of the bridging action of VWF, platelets aggregate in vivo and are cleared, typically resulting in a mild thrombocytopenia. VWD is discussed in detail in Chapter 21.

Extracorporeal Circulation-Related Thrombocytopenia

Passage of the blood for prolonged periods outside the body in an artificial circuit (such as used for cardiac bypass surgery) typically results in platelet activation and clearance. Thrombocytopenia generally is not severe. Other common causes of thrombocytopenia in the postsurgical patient (such as HIT, DIC, and sepsis-related and drug-induced thrombocytopenia) concomitantly must be considered.

DISORDERS CHARACTERIZED BY INCREASED SEQUESTRATION OF PLATELETS

Hypersplenism results in sequestration of blood cells (including platelets) in an enlarged or abnormal spleen. Mild to moderate thrombocytopenia is most commonly observed, but if the bulk of the platelet mass is contained within a massively enlarged spleen, thrombocytopenia can be severe.

TABLE 19.5. *Selected Causes of Splenomegaly*

Lymphoproliferation	**Congestion**
Lymphoma	Cirrhosis
Chronic lymphocytic leukemia	Heart failure
Collagen vascular disease (Felty syndrome, lupus)	
Autoimmune lymphoproliferative disorder	**Hemolysis**
	Hereditary spherocytosis
Myeloproliferation	Paroxysmal nocturnal hemoglobinuria
Myeloid leukemia	Thalassemia
Polycythema vera	
Essential thrombocythemia	**Infection**
	Viral (CMV, EBV, hepatitis)
Inborn Errors of Metabolism	Parasitic (malaria, babesiosis)
Gaucher disease	
Niemann-Pick disease	**Immunodeficiency**
	Common variable immunodeficiency

CMV, cytomegalovirus; EBV, Epstein-Barr virus.

Splenomegaly with hypersplenism is almost always an acquired condition, resulting from many different underlying disorders (Table 19.5). If adequate production of platelets can be documented and significant splenomegaly with thrombocytopenia is present, *splenectomy* may be considered in some cases. *Splenic embolization* and *splenic irradiation* are alternatives to removal of the spleen that generally do not result in maximal platelet responses. They may be considered, however, in patients with significant hypersplenism and disorders such as CLL or lymphoma who cannot tolerate surgery.

OTHER CAUSES OF THROMBOCYTOPENIA

Pseudothrombocytopenia

For reasons that are unclear, the calcium chelation induced by the anticoagulant ethylenediaminetetraacetic acid (EDTA) (present in blood-collecting tubes) causes changes on the platelet membranes of certain patients that expose cryptic antigens to which preformed, otherwise nonpathogenic agglutinating antibodies may bind, causing platelet clumping. Typically, automated cell counters (such as those that are present in most hospital laboratories) will report a falsely low platelet count; examination of the blood smear reveals platelet clumps. Normalization of the platelet count upon automated determination from a blood specimen collected in *citrate* anticoagulant and/or disappearance of platelet clumps on a blood smear obtained from a *fingerstick* source yields a correct assessment of platelet number and confirms the presence of this benign phenomenon.

Drug-Induced Thrombocytopenia

By definition, drug-induced thrombocytopenia develops after initiation of a given drug, resolves when the offending medication is discontinued, and may recur if the agent is reintroduced (26). The mechanisms by which many drugs may lead to a low platelet count, however, have not been elucidated.

Chemotherapeutic agents are clearly linked to decreased platelet production. **Quinine purpura** is a type of *drug-induced immune thrombocytopenia (DITP)*, in which antibody-mediated destruction of platelets after exposure to a given drug. Quinine is thought to induce a conformational change in the platelet membrane allowing exposure of an otherwise cryptic antigen; circulating antibodies then bind the antigen, but only in the presence of the drug. Patients with DITP present with severe thrombocytopenia (<20,000/uL) and mucocutaneous bleeding, including purpura and ecchymoses. Thrombocytopenia should resolve within days to weeks of discontinuing the agent. In cases of severe bleeding, *IVIg* and *platelet transfusions* appear to be more effective than steroids in inducing responses.

Other medications frequently associated with thrombocytopenia are listed in Table 19.6.

Gestational Thrombocytopenia

The blood volume increases by as much as 40% to 45% over baseline during pregnancy, causing a progressive hemodilution. Cytopenias result, although production of blood cells is normal or increased. Approximately 10% and less than 1% of pregnant women experience platelet counts <100,000/uL and <50,000/uL by the third trimester, respectively; the incidence of ITP is thought to be even lower. Severe thrombocytopenia in pregnancy (<50,000/uL) should prompt investigation to rule out a pre-existing condition, pre-eclampsia or a pregnancy-related thrombotic microangiopathy; if negative, the etiology may be presumed to be ITP and treated accordingly (see ***Immune Thrombocytopenic Purpura***, above).

Human Immunodeficiency Virus–Related Thrombocytopenia

Thrombocytopenia in HIV infection may result both from immune-mediated phenomena leading to increased clearance of platelets and ineffective platelet production, possibly because of direct infection of megakaryocytes with HIV. Improvement or resolution of thrombocytopenia after initiation of *antiretroviral therapy* in newly diagnosed patients is commonly observed; if possible, *zidovudine (AZT)* (27) should be included in the antiretroviral regimen because data on the efficacy of other antiretroviral agents in the correction of thrombocytopenia is limited. If the thrombocytopenia proves

TABLE 19.6. *Drugs Associated with Thrombocytopenia*

Antimicrobials	**Cardiovascular Agents**
Amphotericin	Amiodarone
Ampicillin	Captopril
Isoniazid	Digoxin
Rifampin	Hydrochlorothiazide
Methcillin	Procainamide
Piperacillin	Quinidine
Sulfisoxazole	
Trimethoprim-sulfimethsoxazole	**Neuropsychiatric Agents**
	Carbemazepine
Antiplatelet agents	Chlorpromazine
Anagrelide	Diazepam
Abciximab	Haldoperidol
Eptifibatide	Lithium
Ticlopidine	Methyldopa
Tirofiban	
	Other
Analgesics/Anti-inflammatory Agents	Gold
Acetominophen	Heparin
Diclofenac	Mycophenolate mofetil
Ibuprofen	Interferon-α
Sulindac	Quinine
	Most chemotherapeutic drugs
H$_2$ Blockers	
Cimetidine	
Ranitidine	

Adapted from DeLoughery T. Hemorrhagic and thrombotic disorders in the intensive care setting. In: Kitchens C, Alving BM, Kessler C, eds. Consultative Hemostasis and Thrombosis. Philadelphia: W.B. Saunders Company; 2002:493–513; George JN, Raskob GE, Shah SR, et al. Drug-induced thrombocytopenia: A systematic review of published case reports. Ann Intern Med 1998;129:886.

refractory, therapies commonly used in the treatment of ITP (*IVIg, anti-D*, steroids, splenectomy, others) are used, but the potentially immunosuppressive effects of some of these approaches need to be taken into consideration.

Infection- and Sepsis–Related Thrombocytopenia

Thrombocytopenia in the setting of infection or sepsis is common. DIC is often implicated in critically ill patients, but other causes, such as megakaryocyte-specific effects or increased clearance because of fever or splenic enlargement, may be responsible.

Transient thrombocytopenia is commonly observed in the setting of many viral infections; certain bacterial infections, such as ehrlichiosis, rickettsial disease, and dengue characteristically produce thrombocytopenia. A corroborative travel history and directed microbiologic testing are usually necessary to make the diagnosis. If the platelet count does not return to baseline with effective antimicrobial treatment or after resolution of the infection, an alternative etiology should be sought.

Hemophagocytosis

Hemophagocytosis is a process in which bone marrow macrophages (histiocytes) engulf cellular components of the marrow. The phenomenon is considered to be nonspecific if it is found only sporadically within an aspirate smear, but the observation of abundant histiocytes with intracytoplasmic white cells, red cells, or platelets in the setting of peripheral cytopenias indicates a pathogenic process.

In adults, sepsis (28) or Epstein Barr virus (EBV)–related infection or malignancy (29) can drive T cells to produce cytokines that mediate hemophagocytosis, leading to thrombocytopenia. In these cases, the treatment is principally immunosuppressive, but the disorder often is aggressive and unresponsive to treatment.

Familial Hemophagocytic lymphohistiocytosis is a rare, autosomal recessively-inherited disorder featuring hemophagocytosis, fever, organomegaly, and hypertriglyceridemia or hypofibrinogenemia; it presents at a young age. The only curative treatment is allogeneic hematopoietic stem cell transplantation.

Qualitative Disorders

Several heritable platelet anomalies of structure or function (including the *May-Hegglin anomaly* and the *Bernard-Soulier syndrome*) are typically associated with a mild thrombocytopenia. These are discussed in more detail in Chapter 21.

REFERENCES

1. Rice L. Drug evaluation: AMG-531 for the treatment of thrombocytopenias. Curr Opin Invest Drugs 2006;7:834–841.
2. Frederiksen H, Schmidt K. The incidence of idiopathic thrombocytopenia in adults increases with age. Blood 1999;94:909–913.
3. Cines DB, Blanchette VS. Immune thrombocytopenic purpura. N Engl J Med 2002;346:995–1008.
4. Cines DB, Bussel JB. How I treat idiopathic thrombocytopenic purpura. Blood 2005;106:2244–2251.
5. Cooper N, Stasi R, Cunningham-Rundles S, et al. The efficacy and safety of B-cell depletion with anti-CD20 monoclonal antibody in adults with chronic immune thrombocytopenic purpura. Br J Haematol 2004;125:232–239.
6. Huhn RD, Fogarty PF, Nakamura R, et al. High-dose cyclophosphamide with autologous lymphocyte-depleted peripheral blood stem cell (PBSC) support for treatment of refractory chronic autoimmune thrombocytopenia. Blood 2003;101:71–77.
7. Schwartz J, Leber MD, Gillis S, et al. Long-term follow-up after splenectomy performed for immune thrombocytopenic purpura (ITP). Am J Hematol 2003;72:94–98.
8. Bussel JB, Kuter DJ, George JN, et al. AMG 531, a thrombopoiesis-stimulating protein, for chronic ITP. N Engl J Med 2006;355:1672–1681.
9. Jenkins JM, Williams D, Deng Y, et al. Phase 1 clinical study of eltrombopag, an oral, nonpeptide thrombopoietin receptor agonist. Blood 2007;109:4739–4741.
10. Warkentin TE, Levine MN, Hirsh J, et al. Heparin-induced thrombocytopenia in patients treated with low-molecular-weight heparin or unfractionated heparin. N Engl J Med 1995;332:1330–1335.
11. Warkentin TE, Kelton JG. A 14-year study of heparin-induced thrombocytopenia. Am J Med 1996;101:502–507.
12. Sheridan D, Carter C, Kelton JG. A diagnostic test for heparin-induced thrombocytopenia. Blood 1986;67:27–30.
13. Warkentin TE, Kelton JG. Temporal aspects of heparin-induced thrombocytopenia. N Engl J Med 2001;344:1286–1292.
14. Torok TJ, Holman RC, Chorba TL. Increasing mortality from thrombotic thrombocytopenic purpura in the United States—analysis of national mortality data, 1968–1991. Am J Hematol 1995;50:84.
15. Furlan M, Robles R, Galbusera M, et al. von Willebrand factor-cleaving protease in thrombotic thrombocytopenic purpura and the hemolytic-uremic syndrome. N Engl J Med 1998;339:1578–1584.
16. Tsai HM, Lian EC. Antibodies to von Willebrand factor-cleaving protease in acute thrombotic thrombocytopenic purpura. N Engl J Med 1998;339:1585–1594.
17. Lattuada A, Rossi E, Calzarossa C, et al. Mild to moderate reduction of a von Willebrand factor cleaving protease (ADAMTS-13) in pregnant women with HELLP microangiopathic syndrome. Haematologica 2003;88:1029–1034.
18. Moake JL. Thrombotic thrombocytopenic purpura and the hemolytic uremic syndrome. Arch Pathol Lab Med 2002;126:1430–1433.
19. Tsai HM, Rice L, Sarode R, et al. Antibody inhibitors to von Willebrand factor metalloproteinase and increased binding of von Willebrand factor to platelets in ticlopidine-associated thrombotic thrombocytopenic purpura. Ann Int Med 2000;132:794–805.

20. Ridolfi RL, Bell WR. Thrombotic thrombocytopenic purpura: report of 25 cases and a review of the literature. Medicine 1981;60:413.
21. Bell WR, Braine HG, Ness PM, et al. Improved survival in thrombotic thrombocuytopenic purpura-hemolytic-uremic syndrome. N Engl J Med 1991;325:398–403.
22. De la Rubia J, Plume G, Arriaga F, et al. Platelet transfusion and thrombotic thrombocytopenic purpura. Transfusion 2002;42:1384–1385.
23. Chemnitz J, Draube A, Scheid C, et al. Successful treatment of severe thrombotic thrombocytopenic purpura with the monoclonal antibody rituximab. Am J Hematol 2002;71:105–108.
24. Shulman NR, Aster RH, Leitner A, et al. Immunoreactions involving platelets. V. Posttransfusion purpura due to a complement-fixing antibody against a genetically controlled platelet antigen. A proposed mechanism for thrombocytopenia and its relevance to "autoimmunity." J Clin Invest 1961;40:1597.
25. Mueller-Eckhardt C, Grubert A, Weisheit M, et al. 348 cases of suspected neonatal allo-immune thrombocytopenia. Lancet 1989;1:363.
26. George JN, Raskob GE, Shah SR, et al. Drug-induced thrombocytopenia: a systematic review of published case reports. Ann Intern Med 1998;129:886.
27. Hymes KB, Greene JB, Karpatkin S. The effect of azidothymidine on HIV-related thrombocytopenia. N Engl J Med 1988;318:516.
28. Stephan F, Thioliere B, Verdy E, et al. Role of hemophagocytic histiocytosis in the etiology of thrombocytopenia in patients with sepsis syndrome or septic shock. Clin Infect Dis 1997;25: 1159–1164.
29. Watson HG, Goulden NJ, Manson LM, et al. Virus-associated hemophagocytic syndrome: further evidence for a T-cell mediated disorder. Br J Haematol 1994;86:213.

20

Disorders of Hemostasis, I: Coagulation

Patrick F. Fogarty

INTRODUCTION: APPROACH TO THE BLEEDING PATIENT

Abnormalities of the activity of coagulation proteins and related molecules, decreased platelet function, or disruption of the vasculature (e.g., by surgery or trauma) can lead to bleeding. Careful assessment of both the clinical history and laboratory testing are necessary to establish the reason for bleeding.

Initial laboratory studies in a patient with new-onset or recent bleeding include a platelet count, activated partial thromboplastin time (aPTT), prothrombin time (PT), and fibrinogen. If the bleeding is moderate to severe, a hemoglobin level and specimen for red cell cross-matching should also be sent.

The *character, timing, and location* of the bleeding should be considered. Is the bleeding spontaneous or associated only with invasive procedures or trauma? If periprocedural, is the bleeding immediate or delayed? Mucocutaneous bleeding (epistaxis, gingival hemorrhage, petechiae/ecchymoses, gastrointestinal and urinary tract bleeding) are more characteristic of a defect in the activity of platelets, whereas soft-tissue bleeding or hemarthrosis suggests a deficiency in the activity of coagulation factors.

The *clinical context* is very important in determining the reason for bleeding. Hemorrhage in a patient who has been receiving heparin or warfarin may indicate excess anticoagulation or presence of a previously undetected lesion. Bleeding after allogeneic transplantation or treatment with certain drugs may occur because of thrombotic microangiopathy (TMA). Bleeding in an individual who is in septic shock may point to disseminated intravascular coagulation (DIC). New-onset, diffuse bleeding in a patient who is pregnant or postpartum may signify the hemolysis, elevated liver enzyme levels, and low platelet count (HELLP) syndrome or other entities. Postsurgical bleeding may stem from a number of causes, but an initial consideration should be deficient hemostasis because of a traumatized, bleeding vessel as well as a coagulation factor defect or deficits.

A positive *family history* of bleeding raises the clinical suspicion for heritable disorders such as hemophilia A or B (X-linked recessive inheritance) or von Willebrand disease (autosomal-dominant inheritance).

Importantly, bleeding does not necessarily indicate an intrinsic abnormality of hemostasis. Individuals with perfectly normal coagulation and platelet function will bleed given a sufficient hemostatic challenge (trauma, surgery, invasive malignancy, etc).

THE COAGULATION SYSTEM

Coagulation Factors: Background

Coagulation factors (clotting factors) are synthesized in the liver. Factors II, VII, IX, X, XI, and XII are *serine proteases* that are inactive as synthesized and acquire enzymatic capability when cleaved (activated) by other proteins. Tissue factor and factors V and VIII are not enzymes but serve as *cofactors* for coagulation reactions. A postsynthetic step in the production of factors II, VII, IX, and X and the natural anticoagulant proteins C and S requires the activity of a *vitamin K-dependent carboxylase* that modifies the aminoterminus of each factor, enabling it to function.

The activity of all clotting factors culminates in a principal event: the generation of thrombin at sites of vascular injury. Thrombin activates platelets and cleaves fibrinogen to form fibrin; therefore, it assists in both primary hemostasis (formation of an occlusive platelet plug) and secondary hemostasis (clot formation) at sites of blood vessel compromise.

The normal *laboratory range* of factor activity levels is ~50% to 150% and is derived from plasma activity as observed in a reference pool of normal donors. The *hemostatic level* of a given clotting factor (i.e., the level of factor necessary to maintain normal hemostasis) typically is much lower. For instance, 5% activity of factor VIII is well below the laboratory reference range but usually is sufficient to prevent spontaneous bleeding.

The Coagulation Cascade

The *coagulation cascade* illustrates the activation of coagulation factors in the formation of a fibrin clot. It comprises the *tissue injury* (also known as *extrinsic*), *contact* (also known as *intrinsic),* and *common pathways of coagulation* (Fig. 20.1). The arrangement of these pathways within the coagulation cascade probably best reflects the activity of clotting factors in vitro, whereas in vivo, the pathways not only interact at multiple points but also function in concert with the activation and aggregation of platelets to achieve hemostasis.

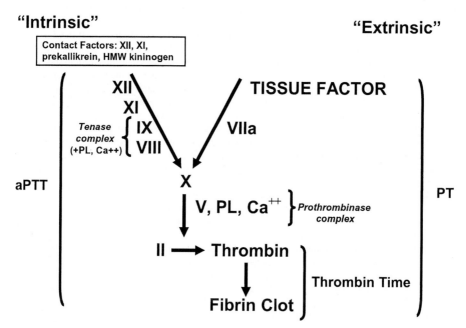

FIG. 20.1. The coagulation cascade. The **tissue injury pathway** of coagulation begins with the binding of activated factor VII (VIIa) to tissue factor (TF), which is provided by cell membranes. VIIa converts X to Xa. The *prothrombinase complex*, formed by the binding of Xa to Va in the presence of phospholipid and Ca^{2+}, converts II (prothrombin) to IIa (thrombin). The **contact pathway** of coagulation begins with the activation of factor XII to XIIa by kallikrein. XIIa cleaves XI to XIa; XIa cleaves IX to IXa. IXa forms a complex with VIIIa in the presence of phospholipid and Ca^{2+} (*tenase complex*) and converts X to Xa. Xa, in the presence of Va, PL, and Ca^{2+}, then cleaves II (prothrombin) to IIa (thrombin). The **common pathway** involves the cleavage of II by prothrombinase to yield thrombin, and thrombin cleavage of fibrinogen to form fibrin, which is then cross-linked via the action of XIIIa. Activation of coagulation usually begins with the tissue injury system, which provides feedback to the contact system by IIa-mediated activation of factor XI. There are additional points of interaction between the pathways (not indicated).

Tissue Injury Pathway

The tissue injury pathway of coagulation begins with the binding of activated factor VII (VIIa) to tissue factor (TF). The TF-VIIa complex mediates the conversion of X to Xa. The *prothrombinase complex*, formed by the binding of Xa to Va on a phospholipid (PL) surface (usually platelet membranes) in the presence of Ca^{2+}, converts II (prothrombin) to IIa (thrombin).

Contact Pathway

Activation of contact factors at the site of vascular injury leads to the conversion of factor XII to XIIa, and the sequential conversion of XI to XIa and IX to IXa. IXa complexes with VIIIa, PL, and Ca^{2+}, forming the *tenase complex*, which converts X to Xa. Xa, in a complex with Va, PL, and Ca^{2+} then cleaves II (prothrombin) to IIa (thrombin). The TF-VIIa complex can also activate IX leading to the subsequent formation of the tenase complex.

Common Pathway

The tissue injury and contact pathways converge in the common pathway, where X is converted to Xa and prothrombin (II) is cleaved to form thrombin. Thrombin then cleaves fibrinogen to form fibrin, which is then cross-linked via the action of XIII.

Common Coagulation Tests

An understanding of the basic laboratory tests for coagulation assists in the evaluation of bleeding disorders.

The *prothrombin time (PT)* is performed by adding thromboplastin (TP), composed of crude or recombinant tissue factor (TF) plus Ca^{2+}, to plasma that has been anticoagulated with citrate, and the time to formation of a fibrin clot is measured. Because the PT comprises reactions of coagulation that occur in the tissue injury and common pathways of coagulation, deficiencies in the activity of II, V, VII, X, or fibrinogen may prolong the PT.

The *International Normalized Ratio (INR)* was developed to standardize the reporting of PT values in warfarin-anticoagulated patients. Standardization is necessary because commercially available TP reagents have varying potencies that directly impact the PT; one TP may yield a different PT result than another when the same sample is tested. The potency of a given TP is expressed in terms of the *International Sensitivity Index (ISI)*.

Because the INR was developed to report factors measured by the PT that are decreased by warfarin impairment of vitamin K-mediated synthesis (i.e., it is not standardized for abnormalities of factor V and fibrinogen), the INR should be used only to describe anticoagulation in patients who are receiving warfarin. In all other patients (e.g., patients with liver disease), the PT should be referenced. The formula for the INR is $(PT_{patient}/PT_{mean\ normal})^{ISI}$.

The *activated partial thromboplastin time (aPTT)* begins with the addition of a contact activating agent to citrate-anticoagulated plasma. PL and Ca^{2+} are added, and the time to formation of a fibrin clot is measured. Because the aPTT reflects reactions of coagulation that occur in the contact and common pathways of coagulation, deficiencies in the activity of factors II, V, VIII, IX, X, XI, or XII may prolong the aPTT. A deficiency of other contact factors, such as prekallikrein or high molecular weight kininogen (HMWK), may also prolong the aPTT. Abnormalities of fibrinogen rarely impact the aPTT.

The *long-incubation aPTT* is performed by incubating the patient sample with activating agents for 10 minutes prior to the addition of PL and Ca^{2+}. If the contact factor prekallikrein is deficient, this extra incubation time allows activation of factor XII and correction of the aPTT.

Mixing studies are performed using a mixture of 50% patient plasma and 50% normal control plasma; the PT or aPTT is then performed as usual. Correction of a prolonged PT or aPTT with mixing generally implies a qualitative or quantitative abnormality of one or more clotting factors in the patient plasma. In contrast, failure of the PT or aPTT to correct completely upon mixing suggests the presence of an inhibitor in the patient plasma that neutralizes a component of the patient *and* normal plasma. Both lupus anticoagulants (LAs) and inhibitors to specific clotting factors can result in a prolonged aPTT or PT that does not correct upon mixing.

When evaluating a prolonged aPTT, an aPTT is performed on the mixture, then the mixture is allowed to incubate for an hour and the aPTT is repeated; some inhibitors of factor VIII are maximally inhibitory at 1 hour or more postmix. For instance, the aPTT on a 1:1 mixture of normal and patient plasma containing a factor VIII inhibitor may show correction initially but demonstrate a prolongation at 1 hour. Occasionally, a weak lupus anticoagulant (LA) may produce a prolonged aPTT or PT that *corrects* on mixing (1).

The *bleeding time (BT)* involves making a controlled incision in soft tissue (usually at a site on the forearm) and measuring the time to cessation of bleeding. Anemia and abnormalities of coagulation factors, platelets, or the vasculature may prolong the BT. The BT does *not* correlate with risk of surgical bleeding in most patients (2). The PFA-100 (Siemens Healthcare Diagnostics, Deerfield, IL) (3) has been used in place of the BT as a global assessment of platelet function (see Chapter 21).

The *thrombin time (TT)* involves the addition of exogenous thrombin to patient plasma, inducing cleavage of fibrinogen to fibrin and the formation of a fibrin clot. The most common cause of a prolonged TT is the presence of heparin in the sample, which can be confirmed by documentation of a normalization of the TT when the test is repeated using a heparin-binding agent such as protamine or Heparsorb (Organon Teknika, Durham, NC). Abnormalities of fibrinogen and circulating heparin-like anticoagulants also cause a prolonged TT. The *reptilase time* is also used to assess abnormalities of fibrinogen (reptilase cleaves fibrinogen to fibrin). Unlike thrombin, however, reptilase is not inhibited by the presence of heparin. Thus, a prolonged thrombin time in conjunction with a normal reptilase time usually indicates heparin contamination, whereas prolongation of both tests indicates a qualitative abnormality of fibrinogen.

The *functional fibrinogen assay* assesses fibrinogen concentration by addition of an excess of thrombin to a sample of diluted plasma.

Specialized Coagulation Tests

The *anti-Xa assay* provides information about the degree of anticoagulation that has occurred in the patient plasma because of the effect of heparin (unfractionated or low molecular weight) on factor Xa in the sample. By convention, samples should be drawn 4 to 6 hours after LMWH administration to estimate anticoagulation.

Two common tests for lupus anticoagulants include the *Dilute Russell's viper venom time* (DRVVT) and the *Staclot* (Diagnostica Stago, Parsippany, NJ) *assay*. These tests are used to identify an LA and distinguish an inhibitor of a clotting factor from an LA as the cause of a prolongation in the aPTT that does not correct with mixing. Other systems for the diagnosis of LAs are available (1).

Russell's viper venom in the DRVVT directly activates X in the patient sample, ultimately leading to the conversion of fibrinogen to fibrin. LAs inhibit the DRVVT, leading to a prolonged reaction time. If the DRVVT is prolonged, the presence of a LA is confirmed by repeating the test in a system that contains excess phospholipid (DRVVConfirm®), which neutralizes the LA and prevents it from interfering in the reaction, resulting in normalization the DRVVT. The Staclot assay involves performance of an aPTT with or without hexagonal phase phospholipids (HPE). If a LA is present, the aPTT will be shorter in the HPE-containing sample because of neutralization of the LA by HPE.

The *Bethesda Assay* is a special type of mixing study that involves incubation of dilutions of patient plasma with normal (control) plasma to assess the potency of an inhibitor (generally to factor VIII) in the patient plasma. After a 2-hour incubation phase, a factor VIII assay (or other appropriate factor assay, as indicated) is performed on each dilution (and on samples used to create a control curve); as the proportion of patient plasma in the mixture decreases, the effect of the inhibitor decreases, and the factor assay clotting time shortens.

The potency of the inhibitor is expressed in *Bethesda units (BU)*. The reciprocal of the dilution of the mixture of patient and normal control plasma that contains ~50% of normal factor VIII activity is the inhibitor titer in BU. For instance, if 50% inhibition of normal FVIII activity occurred at a 1:40 dilution, the inhibitor titer would be said to be 40 BU. The Nijmegen modification to the Bethesda assay includes slightly different buffers to stabilize the proteins during the incubation period (4).

Assays for Specific Clotting Factors

Factor activity levels can be assessed by clot-based reactions (that use modifications of the aPTT or PT), and some factors by chromogenic systems. Factor activity levels are generally reported as percentages (of "normal" activity) or in units per milliliter (U/mL), with 1 U/mL corresponding to 100% of the factor found in 1 mL of normal plasma. Usually, levels of 25% to 40% are necessary to prolong the PT or aPTT. Mild or moderate deficiencies of a given clotting factor may lead to an elevated PT or aPTT, but may be adequate for hemostasis.

The *euglobulin clot lysis time (ECLT)* measures time to dissolution of a fibrin clot; a shortened ECLT indicates activation of the fibrinolytic system. The most common cause of a shortened ECLT is DIC, in which fibrinolysis is activated in response to an activation of coagulation. Deficiencies in the activity of plasminogen activator inhibitor or alpha-2-antiplasmin also shorten the ECLT (see below).

DIFFERENTIAL DIAGNOSIS OF ABNORMAL COAGULATION TESTS

Conditions that predispose to bleeding or produce abnormal coagulation test results can be divided into those entities that prolong the aPTT, PT, or both (Table 20.1 and Figs. 20.2 to 20.4).

Conditions Associated with a Prolonged Activated Partial Thromboplastin Time

LAs are a very common cause of a prolongation in the aPTT that does not correct completely on mixing. LAs were so named because of their frequent presence in patients with systemic lupus erythematosus and tendency to prolong coagulation tests by interacting with phospholipid in the test sample. In contradistinction to their name, however, LAs are *not* physiologic anticoagulants; additionally, over one half of patients with LAs do not have connective tissue disease (see Chapter 22). LAs are diagnosed using the methods described above.

Hemophilia A and B

More frequently than with any other factor essential to the aPTT reaction, a deficiency of factor VIII causes a prolongation in the aPTT that corrects completely on mixing. Congenital factor VIII deficiency is referred to as hemophilia A. (Factor VIII is also decreased in moderate and severe von Willebrand disease; see below.) Congenital deficiency of factor IX is referred to as hemophilia B.

TABLE 20.1. *Common Causes of Abnormal Coagulation Studies*

Prolonged aPTT	Prolonged PT and PT	Prolonged aPTT	Prolonged BT
Lupus anticoagulant	Lupus anticoagulant	Lupus anticoagulant	Thrombocytopenia
Heparin in sample (at clinically relevant concentrations)	Liver disease	Liver disease	Disorders of platelet function
Deficiency of, or inhibitor to, factors VIII, IX, XI, XII	Warfarin use	Warfarin use	Von Willebrand disease
	Vitamin K deficiency	Vitamin K deficiency	
Deficiency of, or inhibitor to, prekallikrein or HMWK	Deficiency of, or inhibitor to, factors II,VII, X	Deficiency of, or inhibitor to, factors II, V, or X	Disorders of vasculature (e.g., Ehlers-Danlos)
Hypo- or dysfibrinogenemia	Hypo- or dysfibrinogenemia	DIC	Anemia
Traumatic venipuncture	Heparin in sample (at high concentration only)	Heparin in sample (PT prolonged at high concentration only)	

aPTT, activated partial thromboplastin time; BT, bleeding time; DIC, disseminated intravascular coagulation; HMWK, high-molecular-weight kininogen; PT, prothrombin time.

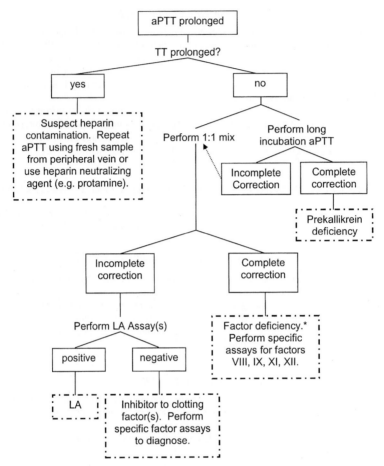

FIG. 20.2. Laboratory diagnostic algorithm for a prolonged aPTT and normal PT. aPTT, activated partial thromboplastin time; LA, lupus anticoagulant. *Occasionally, weak LAs can cause a prolongation in the aPTT that corrects completely on mixing. In this scenario, factor assays may be indicated in addition to LA testing, especially if demonstration of hemostatic factor levels is regarded as important (e.g., in a preoperative patient).

Hemophilia A is estimated to occur in one per 5000 to 10,000 live male births; hemophilia B is about one fifth as common. The disorders are inherited in an X-linked recessive fashion: males are affected, whereas females are carriers and are generally not affected unless significant lyonization has occurred favoring the X chromosome bearing the abnormal copy of the FVIII gene. There is no race predilection (5).

The presentation of the disease relates to the level of residual factor activity in the plasma. Severe hemophilia (<1% factor activity) typically presents in infancy with bleeding at circumcision or in early childhood with spontaneous bleeding into soft tissues (muscles) or joints and intracranial, gastrointestinal, or urinary bleeding. Moderate hemophilia (1% to 5% factor activity) is typified by less severe bleeding than that observed in severe disease, whereas individuals with mild hemophilia (>5% activity) usually do not experience spontaneous bleeding but may bleed upon significant hemostatic challenges such as trauma or surgery.

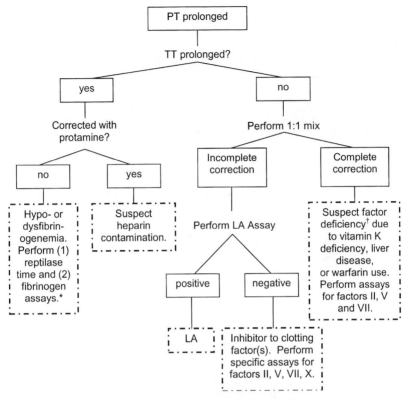

FIG. 20.3. Laboratory diagnostic algorithm for a prolonged PT and normal aPTT. LA, lupus anticoagulant; PT, prothrombin time; TT, thrombin time.
*Decreased functional fibrinogen in conjunction with a normal immunologic fibrinogen indicates an abnormal fibrinogen (dysfibrinogenemia), whereas decreased functional and immunologic assays are typical of hypofibrinogenemia.
[†]Occasionally, LAs can cause a prolongation in the PT that corrects on mixing.

Factor concentrates are the mainstay of treatment; both plasma-derived and recombinant products are commercially available. For acute major bleeding (e.g., intracranial) or prophylaxis prior to major surgery, doses of 50 U/kg (FVIII) or 100 U/kg (FIX) are administered by intravenous bolus infusion every 8 to 12 hours for 1 to 14 days, depending on the anatomic location and severity of the bleeding. Less severe bleeding (hemarthrosis) or prophylaxis prior to moderately invasive procedures (such as endoscopy with biopsy) may be addressed with lower doses of factor. Patients with mild hemophilia A may respond to infusion of DDAVP (0.3 mcg/kg/dose), but a trial should be done in the nonbleeding state to document a rise of the FVIII activity level into the hemostatic range. The oral antifibrinolytic agent *aminocaproic acid* (Amicar, Wyeth-Ayerst, Philadelphia, PA), given at a dose of 1 to 2 g every 4 to 6 hours, may be useful for patients with mucosal or oral bleeding, or bleeding associated with dental procedures.

Gene therapy (delivery of normal factor VIII or IX genes to patients with hemophilia) is in the initial phases of clinical investigation (5). Prophylactic factor replacement therapy (twice or thrice weekly infusions) is routinely used as a means of preventing the morbidity incurred from recurrent joint bleeding. It is more common among children than adults; generally, the practice is begun by the age of four years (6).

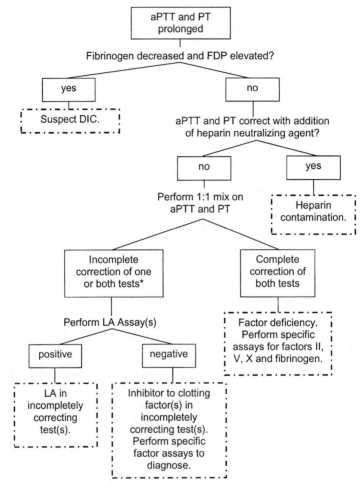

FIG. 20.4. Laboratory diagnostic algorithm for a prolonged aPTT and PT. aPTT, activated partial thromboplastin time; DIC, disseminated intravascular coagulation; FDP, fibrin degradation products; LA, lupus anticoagulant; PT, prothrombin time.
*Co-existing conditions, such as vitamin K deficiency (leading to a prolonged PT) and a concomitant LA (leading to an elevated aPTT), are possible.

Inhibitors

Hemophiliacs (usually with severe disease) who have received factor concentrates as treatment for bleeding are at risk for inhibitor formation. Over 25% of patients with hemophilia A and less than 5% of patients with hemophilia B will develop inhibitors to factor VIII or IX, respectively. The potency of the inhibitor is expressed in Bethesda Units (BU). Low-titer inhibitors (<5 BU) often may be overcome by increasing the dose or frequency of infused factor concentrate. It is usually not possible to overcome high-titer inhibitors (>5 BU) using this approach, however, and administration of prothrombin complex concentrates and/or recombinant factor VIIa is necessary.

Von Willebrand Disease

Von Willebrand disease (VWD), because of the lack of adequate VWF to bind and protect circulating factor VIII from clearance, can lead to low VIII levels and a prolongation in the aPTT (see Chapter 21). The prolongation in the aPTT corrects on mixing.

Factor XI Deficiency

Factor XI deficiency (hemophilia C) typically results in a prolonged aPTT that corrects on mixing. It is inherited in an autosomal-recessive manner and is most prevalent in the Ashkenazi Jewish population, where the frequency of heterozygotes is approximately 12% (7). It typically causes a mild bleeding tendency that is worsened by trauma or surgery. Levels of factor XI do not correlate well with bleeding symptoms. Fresh frozen plasma (FFP) may be used prophylactically or for treatment of bleeding, and adjunctive *aminocaproic acid* decreases unmitigated fibrinolysis, making it useful for chronic prophylaxis, oral bleeding, dental work, or minor surgical procedures.

Although *Factor XII deficiency and deficiencies of prekallikrein and HMWK* may lead to a prolonged aPTT, these conditions do *not* cause bleeding.

Acquired Inhibitors to Coagulation Proteins

Occasionally, adults without a prior history of hemophilia develop high-titer inhibitors to factor VIII; not infrequently, a concomitant lymphoproliferative or immune disorder is present. Immunosuppressive treatment with steroids or chemotherapy usually is effective (8).

Heparin Contamination

The presence of heparin in the sample used for the aPTT determination may be verified by documenting normalization of the aPTT after the test is repeated using a heparin-binding agent.

Other Factors

Warfarin may mildly prolong the aPTT because of depletion of factors II, XI, or X.

Occasionally, *traumatic venipuncture* may cause the aPTT to be prolonged because of the direct activation of coagulation at the site of venipuncture, leading to depletion of crucial coagulation proteins in the collected specimen. The blood should be redrawn with careful technique during phlebotomy and the aPTT repeated to document normalization. (Traumatic venipuncture may also lead to a *shortening* of the aPTT because of small amounts of thrombin generation.)

Conditions Associated with a Prolonged Prothrombin Time

Vitamin K Deficiency

Vitamin K deficiency can cause an elevated PT that typically corrects completely on mixing. The vitamin K-dependent factors that are measured by the PT are II, VII, and X.

Malabsorption or deficient dietary intake of vitamin K (from green leafy vegetables such as cabbage, cauliflower, and spinach, cereals, soybeans, and other foods) or decreased production by intestinal bacteria (which may be destroyed by antibiotics) may lead to vitamin K deficiency.

For treatment, *vitamin K* (phytonadione) may be administered via parenteral, oral, or subcutaneous routes (9). Intravenous administration (1 mg/day) results in faster normalization of a prolonged PT than subcutaneous dosing but occasionally has been associated with anaphylaxis; therefore, intravenous doses should be administered slowly (over 30 minutes) while the patient is monitored.

At least partial correction of the PT is expected within 24 hours after parenteral administration of vitamin K if vitamin K deficiency is the only reason for the prolongation in the PT.

Coagulopathy of Liver Disease

Hepatic insufficiency leads to decreased synthesis of clotting factors, such as the vitamin K-dependent factors and, with more severe disease, factors V, VIII, XI, XII, and fibrinogen, resulting in a prolonged PT (and with severe disease, aPTT) that correct(s) on mixing.

In contradistinction to coagulopathy because of isolated vitamin K deficiency, liver disease may feature a reduced factor V level in addition to decreased levels of factors II, VII, IX, and X.

Warfarin Ingestion

Warfarin inhibits the vitamin K-dependent carboxylase that is important for the synthesis of factors II, VII, IX, and X. Decreased functional levels of factors II, VI,I and X may prolong the PT and produce an elevated INR.

Supratherapeutic INRs that are not associated with bleeding generally are managed by temporarily withholding warfarin to allow the INR to descend into the desired range and restarting the warfarin at a lower dose.

Critically elevated INRs (>9) may be addressed with temporary discontinuation of warfarin, plus administration of vitamin K or FFP if the patient is felt to be at very high risk of bleeding.

For treatment of warfarin-associated major bleeding, the warfarin should be discontinued and FFP (4 units), prothrombin complex concentrate (such as *Bebulin* [Baxter International, Deerfield, IL), 35 units/kg/dose), or rhVIIa (*NovoSeven* [NovoNordisk, Princeton, NJ], 15–90 ug/kg/dose [10]) should be administered along with intravenous or oral vitamin K.

Lupus Anticoagulants

Lupus anticoagulants can cause a mild prolongation in the PT (see above).

Hypo/Dysfibrinogenemia

Quantitative or qualitative abnormalities of fibrinogen typically produce a long TT and reptilase time (see above), but the PT also may be prolonged (Fig. 20.3). The PT is much more sensitive to hypo/dysfibrinogenemia than is the aPTT.

Defects in the function of fibrinogen are more commonly acquired (e.g., cirrhosis or active liver disease) than congenital. For instance, DIC characteristically produces a consumptive hypofibrinogenemia.

Replacement of fibrinogen in a bleeding patient with hypo/dysfibrinogenemia is best accomplished by administration of *cryoprecipitate*, using a target plasma fibrinogen level of 80 to 100 mg/dL.

Deficiencies of Individual Clotting Factors

Congenital deficiencies of isolated coagulation factors (for example, VII) leading to a prolonged PT are extremely rare and typically are inherited in autosomal recessive pattern.

Antibodies to Bovine Factor V

Topical bovine thrombin (used in orthopedic, neurologic, and vascular surgery) contains bovine factor V, which is antigenic in some individuals. The resulting antibovine factor V antibody cross-reacts with human factor V, resulting in an acquired factor V deficiency and prolongation of the PT. Bleeding has been reported in some of these patients (11). Patients also may develop antibodies to bovine thrombin that can prolong the TT if bovine thrombin is used in the assay. The TT normalizes when a human thrombin is used instead because the bovine and human antibodies usually do not cross-react.

Conditions Associated with a Prolonged Activated Partial Thromboplastin Time and Prothrombin Time

Coagulopathy of Liver Disease

If hepatic insufficiency is extreme, multiple factor deficiencies can result in a prolonged PT and aPTT.

Deficiencies of Individual Clotting Factors

Isolated deficiencies of factors II, V or X are rare but may prolong both the PT and aPTT.

Disseminated Intravascular Coagulation

Depletion of coagulation factors via diffuse activation of coagulation may cause a prolongation in both the PT and aPTT (see Chapter 21).

Lupus Anticoagulants

Lupus anticoagulants can prolong both the aPTT and PT (see above).

Conditions Associated with Bleeding and Normal Coagulation Tests

Factor XIII Deficiency

Activated factor XIII cross-links fibrin strands, stabilizing the fibrin clot. Individuals with a deficiency of factor XIII characteristically develop delayed bleeding several hours to days following surgery or trauma. Traumatic soft-tissue and joint bleeds, recurrent pregnancy loss, and spontaneous intracranial hemorrhages also have been described (12).

Clot lysis or enzymatic assays and sequencing of either of the two genes that encode the molecule may be diagnostic.

Treatment of bleeding consists of infusion of *cryoprecipitate* or *FFP*.

Alpha-2-Antiplasmin Deficiency

In the normal scenario, alpha-2-antiplasmin inhibits plasmin, thus limiting fibrinolysis. Patients with alpha-2-antiplasmin deficiency experience accelerated digestion of fibrinogen and fibrin clots and have increased bleeding (13). Infusion of *FFP* replaces antiplasmin (note: SDP plasma does *not* contain antiplasmin).

Plasminogen Activator I (PAI-1) Deficiency

This extremely rare disorder causes a mild to moderate bleeding tendency because of an accelerated rate of lysis of fibrin clots (14).

Congenital and Acquired Abnormalities of the Vasculature and Integument

Congenital and acquired abnormalities of the vasculature and integument can cause increased fragility of blood vessels and bruising or bleeding despite normal coagulation, fibrinolysis, and platelet function. Such conditions include hereditary hemorrhagic telangiectasia (Osler-Weber-Rendu disease), heritable defects of collagen (Ehlers-Danlos syndrome, osteogenesis imperfecta), acquired collagen-associated conditions (scurvy, prolonged glucocorticoid administration, the normal aging skin), and other anomalies (Marfan syndrome, amyloidosis, vasculitis). There is no effective treatment for bruising associated with the congenital disorders; preventative measures to reduce the risk of trauma should be followed. Repletion of vitamin C (scurvy) and reduction of corticosteroids (glucocorticoid excess) ameliorate bruising associated with those acquired processes (15).

REFERENCES

1. Brandt JT, Tripplett DA, Alving B, et al. Criteria for the diagnosis of lupus anticoagulants: an update. Thromb Haemost 1995;74:1185–1190.
2. Lind SE. The bleeding time does not predict surgical bleeding. Blood 1991;77:2547.

3. Carcao MD, Blanchette VS, Dean JA, et al. The platelet function analyzer (PFA-100): a novel in-vitro system for evaluation of primary hemostasis in children. Br J Haematol 1998;101:70.

4. Verbruggen B, Novakova I, Wessels H, et al. The Nijmegen modification of the Bethesda assay for factor VIII: C inhibitors. Improved specificity and reliability. Thromb Haemost 1995;73:247.

5. Bolton-Maggs PH, Pasi J. Haemophilias A and B. Lancet 2003;361:1801–1809.

6. Schramm W. Experience with prophylaxis in Germany. Semin Hematol 1993;30(Suppl 2):12–15.

7. Seligsohn U. High gene frequency of factor XI (PTA) deficiency in Ashkenazi Jews. Blood 1978;51:1223.

8. Ludlam CA, Morrison AE, Kessler C. Treatment of acquired hemophilia. Semin Hematol 1994;31:16.

9. Raj G, Kumar R, McKinney WP. Time course of reversal of anticoagulant effect of warfarin by intravenous and subcutaneous phytonadione. Arch Intern Med 1999;159:2721–2724.

10. Deveras RA, Kessler CM. Reversal of warfarin-induced excessive anticoagulation with recombinant human VIIa concentrate. Ann Intern Med 2002;137:884–888.

11. Ortel TL, Charles LA, Keller FG, et al. Topical thrombin and acquired coagulation factor inhibitors: clinical spectrum and laboratory diagnosis. Am J Hematol 1994;45:128–135.

12. Mikkola H, Palotie A. Gene defects in congenital factor XIII deficiency. Thromb Hemost 1996;22:393–398.

13. Saito H. Alpha 2-plasmin inhibitor and its deficiency states. J Lab Clin Med 1988;112:671–678.

14. Lee MH, Vosburgh E, Anderson K, et al. Deficiency of plasma plasminogen activator inhibitor 1 results in hyperfibrinolytic bleeding. Blood 1993;81:2357–2362.

15. Goodnight S. Primary vascular disorders. In: Colman R, Hirsch J, Marder VJ, et al, eds. Hemostasis and thrombosis: basic principles and practice, 4th Ed. Philadelphia: Lippincott Williams and Wilkins; 2001:945–953.

21

Disorders of Hemostasis, II

Patrick F. Fogarty

In addition to thrombocytopenia (Chapter 19) and primary deficiencies in the activity of coagulation proteins (Chapter 20), disseminated intravascular coagulation, von Willebrand disease, and qualitative abnormalities of platelets can also result in bleeding.

DISSEMINATED INTRAVASCULAR COAGULATION

Although it frequently manifests as bleeding, disseminated intravascular coagulation (DIC) begins as a result of an uncontrolled local or systemic *activation* of coagulation because of an underlying disorder. DIC may be acute or chronic, limited or diffuse, and accompanied by thrombosis or hemorrhage. Disorders that are associated with DIC are listed in Table 21.1.

Pathophysiology

The normal mechanisms that regulate clot formation and dissolution are imbalanced in DIC, allowing intravascular coagulation to proceed preferentially (1). The inciting events are numerous but generally involve either overwhelming release of tissue factor (see Chapter 20) by cellular, vascular, or hypoxemic injury; or the presence of endogenously or exogenously-derived procoagulant molecules (e.g., bacterial lipopolysaccharide, proteins produced by neoplastic cells, or snake venom). As the acute primary process continues to drive coagulation, clotting factors and platelets are consumed, leading to bleeding commensurate with the degree of consumption. If activation of coagulation is chronic and low grade, however, clotting factors and platelets may be replenished sufficiently so as to avert bleeding; in these patients, hypercoagulability predominates, manifest as thrombosis (e.g., Trousseau syndrome).

Presentation

The appearance of DIC always indicates a serious underlying because of another disorder (Table 21.1) when unexplained bleeding and/or abnormalities in routine coagulation are observed.

The hemorrhage of DIC is typically diffuse and may involve bleeding at sites of surgical incisions or vascular access catheters, as well as urinary, gastrointestinal, pulmonary, central nervous system, or cutaneous hemorrhage. Acral cyanosis and petechial and ecchymotic lesions may also occur. Widespread DIC-associated truncal and extremity bruising (*purpura fulminans*) usually is limited to children or follows a viral infection.

Any degree of thrombocytopenia, hypofibrinogenemia, and prolongation of the activated partial thromboplastin time (aPTT) and prothrombin time (PT) is possible, but DIC rarely produces a platelet count less than 20,000/uL. Occasionally the DIC will be manifest by only moderately abnormal laboratory tests, without clinically significant thrombosis or bleeding. Patients with thrombosis and chronic DIC because of malignancy may have a normal or even elevated platelet counts.

Severe systemic DIC may lead to widespread tissue hypoxia and multiorgan dysfunction; hepatic, neurologic, cardiac, and renal impairment may occur. The development of multiorgan dysfunction is associated with a high mortality rate.

TABLE 21.1. *Conditions Associated with Disseminated Intravascular Coagulation*

Condition	Example
Tissue damage	Trauma, burns
Sepsis	Gram-negative or -positive bacterial infection; rickettsial or viral infection
Shock	Cardiogenic, septic
Pregnancy-related	Toxemia, placental abnormalities (abruption or previa), amniotic fluid embolism, retained uterine placental or fetal tissue (HELLP syndrome)
Vascular stasis	Cavernous hemangiomas (Kasabach-Merritt syndrome), abdominal aortic aneurysm
Fat embolism	Fracture of long bones, sickle cell crisis
Malignancy	Acute promyelocytic leukemia, adenocarcinoma (Trousseau syndrome)
Injection of toxic procoagulant molecules	Snake bites

Diagnosis

Typically, acute DIC is suspected when a patient with a predisposing condition (Table 21.1) develops bleeding or thrombosis and/or a perturbation in laboratory tests indicative of DIC. DIC is a dynamic condition, especially in the acutely ill patient; considerable variation in laboratory markers from timepoint to timepoint is possible, making analysis of trends rather than isolated values of greatest relevance to management. Laboratory parameters may show:

- Increased (prolonged) aPTT, PT, or thrombin time (TT) because of consumption of clotting factors and/or fibrinogen (most patients)
- Decreased fibrinogen (compared with baseline)* because of consumption of fibrinogen
- Increased products of fibrinogen and fibrin degradation (FDPs; D-dimer assay) because of plasmin-mediated cleavage of fibrinogen and fibrin. The D-dimer assay measures fibrin products that have been cross-linked by activated factor XIII
- Decreased platelet count (compared with baseline)* because of clearance resulting from activation and aggregation at the sites of local prothrombotic reactions (most patients)
- Fragmented red cells (schistocytes) on peripheral blood smear because of microvascular hemolysis (10% to 20% of patients with DIC)

Treatment

The clinical and laboratory manifestations of DIC are expected to resolve with correction of the inciting disorder. This might entail effective administration of antimicrobials to a patient with sepsis, treatment of malignancy, surgery to repair an aneurysmal dilatation, removal of conceptus and placenta, or another intervention as dictated by the clinical scenario. If the DIC is severe enough to have eventuated in multiorgan dysfunction, management in an intensive care unit is usually required.

Blood products should not be administered to patients with acute DIC unless clinically significant bleeding is present or if the risk of bleeding is felt to be high (e.g., thrombocytopenia in patient who has sustained major trauma); there is, however, no reason to withhold blood products for fear of "fueling the fire." If bleeding is present, *platelet transfusions* may be administered to stop clinical bleeding; a target platelet count of 20,000 to 30,000/uL (most cases) or >50,000/uL (intracranial or life-threatening hemorrhage) is reasonable. Higher target ranges may be desired for patients who are to undergo invasive procedures such as major surgery, but the consumptive process may make achieving the goal difficult.

---

* Especially in early DIC, the platelet count and fibrinogen may be reduced from the baseline value but still remain within the normal laboratory reference range.

Cryoprecipitate may be administered for bleeding in the setting of fibrinogen levels that are consistently less than 80 to 100 mg/dl. *Fresh frozen plasma (FFP)* should be given only to patients with significant bleeding and a prolonged PT and aPTT.

Because of its potential to exacerbate hemorrhage, *heparin* should be considered in acute DIC only in cases of bleeding when DIC is ongoing despite appropriate treatment. It should not be given unless the platelet count can be supported to 50,000/uL or higher and there is no central nervous system or diffuse gastrointestinal bleeding. If heparin is to be used, a low-dose infusion (6 to 10 U/kg/hr) with no bolus dose is recommended. An improving platelet count and fibrinogen concentration signifies that the treatment is effective. Heparin is contraindicated in patients with placental abruption or other obstetrical conditions that will require surgical management, because the anticoagulation is likely to complicate the curative treatment.

The use of *fibrinolysis inhibitors* and *antithrombin concentrates* in acute DIC is controversial. Fibrinolysis inhibitors may have a role in patients with profuse bleeding who have failed to respond to other management, in whom FDPs are felt to be inhibiting platelets.

Laboratory parameters (PT, PTT, fibrinogen. and platelet count) should be monitored at least every 6 hours in the acutely ill patient with DIC, and clinical bleeding should be followed to assess efficacy of therapeutic measures.

HELLP syndrome (*h*emolysis, *e*levated *l*iver enzymes, and *l*ow *p*latelets) is a severe form of DIC affecting women in the peripartum period that produces clinically significant hemolytic anemia and hepatocellular injury. It may be difficult initially to distinguish the disorder from thrombotic thrombocytopenic purpura (TTP) (see Chapter 19), but the presence of hepatic dysfunction (leading to elevated transaminases) may sway the diagnosis toward HELLP. Introduction of placental proteins into the maternal circulation has been thought to be etiologic. Gross hemoglobinuria with renal dysfunction and hypotension are common; the mortality rate is high. As with other forms of DIC, management is principally supportive, but in HELLP it also must include evacuation of the uterus, either by delivery of a term or near-term infant, or by dilatation and curettage to remove retained placental or fetal fragments.

Acute promyelocytic leukemia (APL) is frequently associated with DIC, potentially because of procoagulant molecules (tissue factor and others) contained within circulating promyelocytes. Bleeding in a patient with APL who presents with laboratory parameters consistent with DIC should be treated emergently; in addition to the appropriate use of platelets and cryoprecipitate, initiation of chemotherapy within 24 hours of diagnosis is recommended (see Chapter 11).

Trousseau syndrome is a form of chronic DIC in which recurrent episodes of venous thromboembolism (VTE) complicate an underlying malignancy, especially adenocarcinomas. Experience in the management of the disorder has suggested that anticoagulation with warfarin in not effective in preventing further VTE; instead, subcutaneous low-molecular-weight heparin in therapeutic doses is usually necessary to prevent recurrence of thromboembolism (see Chapter 23).

VON WILLEBRAND DISEASE

Epidemiology

Von Willebrand disease (VWD) is the most common inherited bleeding disorder; up to 1% of the population has levels of von Willebrand factor (VWF) that are below the laboratory reference range, although not all of these individuals experience excessive bleeding (2).

Pathophysiology and Classification

VWF is an unusual extremely large multimeric glycoprotein that is synthesized in endothelial cells and megakaryocytes. Binding of VWF to its receptor, platelet glycoprotein Ib (GPIb), tethers platelets to one another and to the subendothelial collagen matrix, localizing them to the site of injury. This interaction is especially important in vessels such as arterioles, where a "high shear" state is present. VWF also binds to factor VIII (FVIII) in the circulation, protecting it from clearance. Types 1 and 3 VWD involve quantitative decreases in VWF, while type 2 disease is characterized by qualitative (i.e., functional) abnormalities in the VWF molecule (Fig. 21.1).

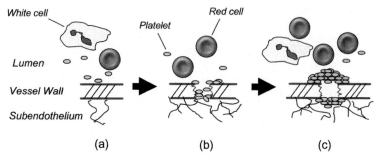

FIG. 21.1. *Primary hemostasis.* **(A) Normal conditions.** Under physiologic conditions, platelets do not interact with the endothelium. **(B) Adhesion.** Upon disruption of the blood vessel wall, subendothelial collagen and fibronectin are exposed, leading to platelet adhesion. In the arterial/arteriolar circulation, subendothelial von Willebrand factor (VWF) assists in the adherence of platelets to the site of injury via binding to the platelet glycoprotein (GP) Ib receptor. **(C) Aggregation.** Tissue factor interacts with factor VIIa, present locally, to catalyze the formation of thrombin. Thrombin, collagen, and other molecules bind to receptors on the platelet membrane, leading to platelet activation. Fibrinogen crosslinks platelets via their GPIIb/IIIa receptors, promoting formation of an occlusive plug that prevents additional blood loss through the break in the vessel wall. VWF also bridges between platelets via their GPIb and GPIIb/IIIa receptors.

Type 1 includes approximately 75% to 80% of patients, the majority of which do not have an identified causal mutation in the VWF gene, which is located on chromosome 12. Patients usually have mild or moderate bleeding.

Type 2 includes 4 subtypes; patients usually have moderate to severe bleeding symptoms and present before adulthood. *Type 2A* (10% to 15% of VWD) involves mutations in VWF that cause either a defect in intracellular transport (2A, type 1) or render the molecule more susceptible to proteolysis (2A, type 2). Laboratory testing (Table 21.2) typically shows a more marked decrease in VWF activity assays compared with antigen. *Type 2B* (5% of VWD) mutations result in an abnormal structure in the binding site for platelet GPIb (A1 domain, Fig. 21.1) and are responsible for a "gain-of-function" defect that allows spontaneous binding of the abnormal VWF to platelets in the circulation. Patients typically have thrombocytopenia because of removal of VWF-bound platelet aggregates. The ristocetin-induced platelet aggregation (RIPA) (Table 21.2) shows an increase in platelet aggregation to low concentrations of ristocetin.[1] *Type 2N* (uncommon) features mutations in VWF that decrease its ability to bind and protect FVIII from clearance, resulting in decreased FVIII levels in the plasma and a phenotype similar to hemophilia A. Soft-tissue and joint bleeding are common. The presence of affected females in the family is an important clue to consider this diagnosis. Laboratory studies show decreased FVIII (2% to 10%), and normal VWF function and antigen. *Type 2M* (very uncommon) results from mutations affecting the A1 domain in a different area from those mutations in type 2B. These result in decreased binding of platelets to VWF.

Type 3 VWD (rare) is caused by a variety of mutations of the VWF molecule, including larger deletions; patients may be homozygous for a given mutation or double heterozygotes. Severe bleeding manifests in childhood. FVIII is usually about 5%, and VWF levels usually are too low to detect.

Presentation

Bleeding symptoms usually involve mucous membranes. Epistaxis, oral bleeding, menorrhagia, and gastrointestinal bleeding are common. Individuals with marked abnormalities of VWF usually present

---

[1]*Pseudo* or *platelet type VWD* is caused by a defect in the platelet GPIb molecule, allowing it to bind to the patient's normal VWF with increased avidity and leading to a type 2B clinical phenotype. Mixing studies using a modified RIPA (patient's platelets and control plasma) distinguish it from type 2B VWD.

TABLE 21.2. *Laboratory Evaluation of Von Willebrand Disease*

Laboratory Test	Method or Premise	Indication
VWF antigen (ELISA)	Binding to an anti-VWF antibody quantitatively measures VWF in plasma	Initial workup
VWF activity (ristocetin cofactor assay)	Ristocetin promotes binding of patient plasma VWF to normal platelets (via GPIb); decreased platelet aggregation indicates abnormal or reduced VWF in patient's plasma	Initial workup
Factor VIII activity level	FVIII levels are reduced in moderate or severe VWD	Initial workup
Ristocetin-induced platelet aggregation (RIPA)	Type 2B mutation results in increased aggregation of patient PRP with low concentrations of ristocetin	Diagnosis of VWD type 2B
VWF multimer assay	Assess distribution of VWF multimers by electrophoresis	Diagnosis of VWD type 2
Platelet-associated VWF activity or antigen	Patient's platelets are lysed to assess amount and activity of intraplatelet (i.e., α-granule) VWF	Rarely indicated, but might be helpful if bleeding diathesis is present and other testing is negative

GPIb, platelet membrane receptor glycoprotein Ib; PRP, platelet-rich plasma; VWD, von Willebrand disease; VWF, von Willebrand factor.

earlier in life with bleeding at the time of mucous membrane-related procedures (tooth extractions, tonsillectomy), or at menarche.

Diagnosis

The diagnosis of VWD is based on a typical history of bleeding (i.e., mucous membrane-related) and confirmatory laboratory testing. Because many individuals with laboratory values of VWF that are below the reference range do not have bleeding, low VWF levels in a patient with bleeding may not necessarily be indicative of VWD. Hence, other causes (e.g., structural anomalies in nasal vessels in an individual with epistaxis) should be sought concomitantly. The *personal and family history* of bleeding should be carefully documented.

Initial Testing for Von Willebrand Disease

A *VWF antigen level* (by ELISA) and a *VWF activity* (by ristocetin cofactor assay) should be performed. The latter involves addition of ristocetin at 1.2 mg/mL to a mixture of patient plasma (the VWF source) and washed normal platelets. Ristocetin binds to VWF, allowing it to bind GPIb on the platelet membrane, causing platelet aggregation. The *factor VIII activity* may be abnormal. A *VWF multimer study* detecting the distribution of multimers and a *RIPA* is performed once a diagnosis of VWD has been made, to assess for types 2A or 2B VWD (Table 21.2). Testing of family members should be done, if possible, which aids in the diagnosis of patients with borderline results.

Treatment

The patient's type of VWD, past response to bleeding challenges, current medications, and general medical condition should be considered (Table 21.3) (2).

DDAVP (desmopressin acetate) indirectly causes release of VWF and factor VIII from storage sites (primarily the endothelium). After intravenous administration, levels of both factors are increased two- to five-fold for about 6 to 12 hours. Prior to use of DDAVP for clinically significant

TABLE 21.3. *Treatment of Von Willebrand Disease*

Type	Treatment	Comment
1	DDAVP; VWF replacement concentrates	DDAVP effective in most patients
2A	DDAVP; VWF replacement concentrates	Response may not be as marked to DDAVP as in type I
2B	Possibly DDAVP; VWF replacement concentrates	DDAVP may worsen thrombocytopenia; perform therapeutic trial with measurement of post-DDAVP platelet count
2N	DDAVP; VWF replacement concentrates	FVIII half-life may be shortened because of lack of binding by abnormal VWF
2M	DDAVP; VWF replacement concentrates	
3	DDAVP; VWF replacement concentrates; platelet transfusions if inadequate response to VWF replacement	Increase initial dose of VWF replacement concentrate to 50 IU/kg

DDAVP dose is 0.3 μg/kg IV in 50 mL saline over 20 minutes, or nasal spray 150 μg in each nostril (total, 300 μg) for weight >50 kg or 150 μg in one nostril for <50 kg, every 8 to 12 hours, maximum of 2 to 3 doses in a 48-hour period; monitor for hyponatremia. Nasal spray may be particularly helpful for home use in women with excessive menstrual bleeding because of VWD.
Replacement VWF concentrates are indicated for major bleeding or severe VWD; dose is 20 to 30 IU/kg q12h (give for 3 to 10 days for major bleeding or following surgery). Intermediate purity plasma-derived factor VIII concentrates contain VWF; recombinant or monoclonally purified factor VIII concentrates do not. Monitor clinical status and VWF antigen or activity to determine efficacy and need for dose modifications; patients may require an increase in dose despite an "adequate" VWF level.
Antifibrinolytic agents (such as epsilon aminocaproic acid, 50 mg/kg 4 × daily for 3 to 5 days; maximum 20 gm/d) are often used in conjunction with other therapies; they are especially useful for mucosal bleeding (e.g., dental procedures).
DDAVP, Desmopressin acetate; IV, intravenously; VWD, von Willebrand disease; VWF, von Willebrand factor.

bleeding or as prophylaxis prior to invasive procedures, patients should undergo a therapeutic trial to document responsiveness to the medication (as assessed by increased VWF levels into the hemostatic range and lack of worsening thrombocytopenia [type 2B patients]). More than 2 doses, given 12 to 24 hours apart, generally should be avoided in a 24- to 48-hour period, as tachyphylaxis and serious hyponatremia (because of fluid retention) can occur after repeated doses. Nonsteroidal antiinflammatory agents may aggravate this latter effect (3).

VWF concentrates are used when bleeding is not controlled with DDAVP, or as prophylaxis prior to an invasive procedure or for clinically significant bleeding, in patients who are less likely to be responsive to DDAVP (most type 3 and some type 2 patients). Humate-P (CSL Behring, King of Prussia, PA) is an intermediate-purity antihemophilic factor that contains VWF and is labeled with VWF ristocetin cofactor units. Cryoprecipitate generally is not recommended because of its lack of viral inactivation.

Antifibrinolytic agents such as epsilon aminocaproic acid (Amicar, Wyeth-Ayerst, Philadelphia, PA) and topical agents (including topical thrombin, Gelfoam, and fibrin sealant) are used adjunctively; epsilon aminocaproic acid may be particularly helpful for dental procedures.

Pregnancy and Von Willebrand disease

VWF levels increase two- to threefold during the last two trimesters of pregnancy; type I VWD patients whose VWF levels have reached the normal range during the third trimester may not require treatment during delivery. In more severely affected patients, DDAVP can be administered prophylactically, beginning usually after the onset of labor. (Patients with type 2B VWD who have experienced worsening thrombocytopenia during pregnancy should receive VWF replacement therapy and platelets, not DDAVP.) Because VWF levels fall rapidly within the 24 hours after delivery, DDAVP may be helpful for patients with VWD who have peripartum bleeding. If DDAVP is not effective, VWF replacement concentrates should be given (2).

QUALITATIVE PLATELET DISORDERS

Most disorders of platelet function are acquired; heritable qualitative platelet disorders are rare. When critical pathways of platelet biochemistry are perturbed, bleeding typically occurs, but because of redundancy of biochemical and receptor pathways that mediate the function of platelets, other defects may be detectable only on laboratory testing and do not produce clinically significant bleeding. In most cases, transfusion of platelets or other therapies will (temporarily) augment hemostasis in a patient with a congenital or acquired qualitative platelet disorder who has bleeding or who is to undergo an invasive procedure.

Platelet Biochemistry

Primary hemostasis describes the formation of a platelet plug at the site of vascular injury (Fig. 21.1). In a variety of reactions that are not entirely sequence-specific, individual circulating platelets must adhere to the denuded endothelial surface, undergo activation through receptor-ligand interactions, release the contents of their granules (i.e., platelet secretion), and aggregate to form a physical barrier to continued blood loss. Additionally, phospholipid in the platelet membrane participates in localizing and promoting the activity of coagulation factors.

Adhesion

Subendothelial molecules such as VWF, collagen, and fibronectin mediate adhesion of platelets to the exposed subendothelial matrix at sites of vessel wall compromise. In "high-shear" states such as arterioles, VWF is especially important, because it tethers the platelet to the endothelial surface via interaction with its receptor, platelet glycoprotein (GP) Ib (GPIb).

Activation

Subendothelial collagen activates platelets; thrombin, which has been generated locally in reactions following the interaction of factor VIIa and tissue factor (provided by the membranes of cells), also activates platelets by binding to receptors on the platelet surface and initiating a series of signal transduction events.

Secretion

Agonists such as collagen, thrombin, adenosine triphosphate (ADP), and epinephrine bind to their receptors on the platelet membrane and induce a series of biochemical events that cause platelets to release the contents of their granules (Table 21.4), which act to promote further activation and aggregation.

Aggregation

Binding of agonists also promotes a conformational change in the platelet GP IIb/IIIa receptor, exposing its binding sites for fibrinogen and VWF; these molecules can then bridge between individual platelets at the site of vascular injury, promoting the formation and stability of the platelet plug.

TABLE 21.4. *Characteristics of Platelet Granules*

	Alpha Granules	Delta (dense) Granules
Number per platelet	30–50	3–7
Visualization	Light microscopy (Wright's stain), electron microscopy	Electron microscopy
Contents	VWF, PDGF, PF4, TSP, FV, FXI, protein S, fibronectin; fibrinogen, IgG, P-selectin	ADP, ATP, serotonin, calcium

FIX, factor IX; FV, factor V; IgG, immunoglobulin G; PDGF, platelet-derived growth factor; PF4, platelet factor 4; VWF, von Willebrand factor.

Participation in Coagulation Reactions

The platelet membrane is rich in phospholipid, which is a required component for reactions involving clotting factor complexes.

Platelet Function Testing

Platelet Aggregation Studies (Platelet-Rich Plasma System)

The premise of **platelet aggregation** testing is that the cellular component (i.e., platelets) in a suspension of platelet-rich plasma (PRP) impedes transmission of light through the suspension. When any of a variety of agonists (collagen, thrombin, ADP, epinephrine) is added, aggregation occurs, consolidating the cellular component to the bottom of the reaction tube and allowing the passage of light through the plasma component. The increase in light transmission as aggregation occurs is plotted as a function of time (Fig. 21.2). Ideally, the waveform shows two physiologic processes: a *primary wave* represents initial aggregation as platelet receptors are activated and become available to bind proaggregatory molecules such as fibrinogen, and a *secondary wave* indicates further aggregation that is stimulated by the release of platelet granule contents. Routinely, **secretion of platelet granule contents** (Table 21.4) is assessed in tandem with platelet aggregation; after stimulation of platelets with an agonist, release of ATP into solution is measured through a chemiluminescence procedure and plotted as a function of time.

Platelet Function Analyzer

The platelet function analyzer (PFA) device, PFA-100 (Dade Behring, Newark, DE), assesses the formation of a platelet plug. Citrated whole blood is aspirated through a capillary leading to an aperture in a collagen-impregnated membrane; either ADP or collagen is added as an agonist. Platelets are activated and aggregate, progressively occluding the aperture. The time to complete occlusion is measured and compared with a normal range. Though less sensitive, an advantage of the PFA is that it is less time consuming and laborious than standard platelet aggregation studies (4).

Measurement of Granule Contents (Rarely Indicated)

Centrifugation of PRP produces a platelet pellet; the platelet membranes are then disrupted, liberating intracellular/intragranular proteins into the lysate. The molecule of interest is then assessed (e.g., VWF, by ristocetin cofactor assay, for intragranular VWF).

Acquired Disorders

Drugs

The most common acquired qualitative platelet disorders are caused by the use of medications that directly or indirectly impair platelet function (Table 21.5); of these, aspirin and the nonsteroidal anti-inflammatory drugs (NSAIDs) are most frequently responsible. Patients who present with bruising or platelet-type bleeding and whose platelet function testing shows abnormal aggregation or secretion should be questioned regarding current medications, especially recently initiated drugs and including over-the-counter, naturopathic, and herbal agents. Treatment of clinically significant drug-induced platelet dysfunction first involves discontinuation of the offending agent and may require additional measures (Table 21.6).

Aspirin irreversibly inhibits the platelet cyclooxygenase enzyme, which is responsible for the conversion of membrane-associated arachidonic acid to thromboxane A_2 (TxA_2); the inhibition is constant for the entire life span of the platelet ($\sim$7 days). Once liberated from the platelet, TxA_2 binds to receptors on adjacent platelets, initiating secretion of platelet granule contents and further promoting aggregation. Platelet aggregation studies (Fig. 21.2) show decreased reactivity to most agonists, including low concentration of thrombin and collagen, but normal aggregation with high concentrations of thrombin and collagen. Using the PFA-100 system, aspirin-induced platelet dysfunction is evident in an increased time to aperture occlusion with the epinephrine/collagen reagent, while that of the ADP/collagen reagent is unaffected.

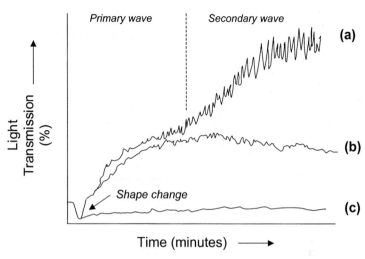

FIG. 21.2. *Platelet aggregation studies.* Platelet aggregation studies involve the addition of agonists (collagen, thrombin, ADP, arachidonic acid, or epinephrine) to a suspension of platelet-rich plasma (PRP); the agonist induces aggregation of platelets and allows transmission of light through the plasma component of the PRP. **(A)** In the **normal scenario**, the binding of an agonist to its platelet receptor initiates a *shape change* that temporarily decreases light transmission; subsequently, a *primary wave of platelet aggregation* is recorded (as increased light transmission) as fibrinogen binds its receptor, GPIIb/IIIa, and begins to cross-link platelets. Unlike the other agonists, collagen does not induce a primary wave. A *secondary wave* occurs as signal transduction events (resulting from platelet activation) eventuate in augmented binding of GPIIb/IIIa by fibrinogen and release of platelet granules, whose contents are able to induce further aggregation. **(B)** In **storage pool disease (SPD)**, platelet aggregation to ADP and other agonists typically shows an initial wave of aggregation, but the aggregates subsequently dissociate because of reduced or absent release of platelet granule contents. Because release of granules is largely dependent on thromboxane, the **aspirin effect** produces a similar platelet aggregation profile to that of SPD when ADP or epinephrine is used, but stronger agonists such as thrombin and collagen can circumvent the thromboxane pathway and produce a normal aggregation curve. **(C)** Because of a lack of GP IIb/IIIa expression on the platelet surface, platelets from patients with **Glanzmann's thrombasthenia** show absent aggregation to all agonists except ristocetin.

NSAIDs reversibly inhibit platelet cyclooxygenase; their inhibitory effect persists only as long as the drug is present in the circulation. *Selective inhibitors of cyclooxygenase-2* (COX-2) do not bind or impair platelet cyclooxygenase (COX-1).

Platelet glycoprotein IIb/IIIa inhibitors are used in the management of patients with acute coronary syndromes or before or following percutaneous coronary intervention (PCI), frequently in conjunction with heparin. *Eptifibatide* is a small molecule that binds the GP IIb/IIIa receptor, inhibiting the binding of its ligands, fibrinogen, VWF, and others, hindering platelet aggregation. The usual dose in patients with normal renal function is bolus of 180 μg/kg, followed by a continuous infusion of 2.0 μg/kg/min. *Abciximab* is a monoclonal antibody against GP IIb/IIIa that also inhibits binding of these proaggregatory ligands; the usual dose is a 0.25 mg/kg intravenous bolus followed by a 12- to 24-hour intravenous infusion of 10 μg/min. Abciximab-bound platelets can be cleared at an accelerated rate because of interaction between the Fc portion of the antibody and Fc receptors on reticuloendothelial macrophages in the liver and spleen, producing thrombocytopenia that in some cases (<1.0%) is severe.

TABLE 21.5. *Substances Associated with Platelet Dysfunction**

Platelet-directed agents	Chemotherapeutic drugs
Aspirin	BCNU
NSAIDS (except COX-2 inhibitors)	Daunorubicin
Dipyridamole (Aggrenox, Boehringer Ingelheim Pharmaceuticals, Ridgefield, CT)	Mithramycin
Clopidogrel (Plavix, Bristol-Myers Squibb/Sanofi Pharmaceuticals Partnership Bridgewater, NJ)	**Psychiatric medications**
	Selective serotonin reuptake inhibitors
Ticlopidine (Ticlid, Roche Pharmaceuticals, Nutley, NJ)	(e.g., fluoxetine, paroxetine, sertraline)
Abciximab (ReoPro, Eli Lilly, Indianapolis, IN)	Tricyclic antidepressants (e.g., imipramine,
Eptifibatide (Integrilin, Schering Corporation, Kenilworth, NJ)	amitriptyline, nortriptyline)
Tirofiban (Aggrastat, Medicure Pharma, Somerset, NJ)	**Other agents**
	Nitrates
Anesthetics	Antihistamines (diphenhydramine,
Dibucaine	chlorpheniramine)
Procaine	Ethanol
Halothane	Omega-3 fatty acids (eicosapentaenoic acid)
	"Wood ear" mushrooms
Antibiotics	Radiographic contrast dye
Penicillins (penicillin G, ticarcillin, nafcillin, piperacillin, methicillin, ampicillin)	
Cephalosporins (cefazolin, cefotaxime)	
Nitrofurantoin	

*Most of these agents have been reported to cause abnormalities in platelet aggregation or the bleeding time, rather than bleeding.
Adapted from George JN, Shattil SJ. Acquired disorders of platelet function. In Hoffman R, Benz EJ, Shattil SJ, et al, eds. Hematology: basic principles and practice, 3rd ed. New York: Churchill Livingstone; 2000:2174.
BCNU, bischloroethylnitrosourea; COX-2, cyclooxygenase-2; NSAIDS, nonsteroidal anti-inflammatory drugs.

Ticlopidine and *clopidogrel* irreversibly inhibit the binding of ADP to its receptor on the platelet membrane, impairing the ADP-dependent binding of fibrinogen to GPIIb/IIa, decreasing platelet aggregation. Neutropenia and aplastic anemia have been reported with increased frequency in patients taking ticlopidine (5); TTP has been described with use of ticlopidine and less frequently with clopidogrel (6,7).

Dipyridamole is used to prevent recurrent stroke or transient ischemic attack, usually in conjunction with aspirin. It inhibits ADP- and collagen-induced platelet aggregation via an effect on intracellular cyclic AMP.

Other Substances

Serotonin reuptake inhibitors (SSRIs) may impair the function of platelets by reducing the serotonin content of platelet dense granules. *Omega-3 fatty acids* may disrupt the phospholipid membrane of the platelet and interfere with reactions of coagulation that normally take place on the platelet surface.

Myelodysplasia/Myeloproliferation

The platelets that are produced in myelodysplasia (MDS) and the myeloproliferative disorders (chronic myeloid leukemia, essential thrombocythemia, polycythemia vera, and idiopathic myelofibrosis) may show abnormal receptor-ligand interactions, ineffective signal transduction, or decreased secretion of platelet granule contents; in a minority of patients these abnormalities lead to bleeding (8).

Renal Failure/Uremia

Platelets from individuals with impaired kidney function frequently show abnormalities upon aggregation testing. Although plasma urea itself may not be causative, other factors, such as increased lev-

TABLE 21.6. *Treatment of Qualitative Platelet Disorders*

Nature of Defect in Platelet Function	Prophylaxis Prior to Invasive Procedures	Treatment of Bleeding
Acquired		
Drug-induced	If possible, discontinue drug at least 7 days prior to procedure (ASA, ticlopidine, clopidogrel), or at least 6 to 12 hours (eptifibatide) or 24 to 48 hours (abciximab) prior to procedure	Discontinue drug; platelet transfusion until drug has been cleared and/or hemostasis is achieved.
MDS/MPD	Platelet transfusion only if significant thrombocytopenia or prior history of bleeding	Platelet transfusion
Renal failure	DDAVP,* platelets; hemodialysis prior to procedure	Platelets, DDAVP, cryo, high-dose estrogens (see text); possibly, hemodialysis. Keep Hct >30%.
Cardiac bypass-related	Not applicable	Platelet transfusions if clinically significant bleeding
Congenital		
Bernard-Soulier syndrome	Platelets, possibly DDAVP*	Platelets, possibly DDAVP. Menses suppression may be required, rhVIIa
Glanzmann's thrombasthenia	DDAVP*, platelets. Pregnancy: platelets at delivery and 3 to 7 days postpartum	Platelets, DDAVP, Amicar, rhVIIa
Storage pool disease (alpha granule, delta granule, or combined deficiency)	Platelets, DDAVP*	Platelets, DDAVP; possibly rhVIIa
Disorders of signal transduction	Platelets; possibly DDAVP*	Platelets, possibly DDAVP

*If DDAVP is to be used as prophylaxis prior to invasive procedures, a therapeutic trial confirming correction of a prolonged bleeding time after administration of DDAVP is recommended.
Amicar, aminocaproic acid; ASA, aspirin; cryo, cryoprecipitate; DDAVP, desmopressin acetate; Hct, hematocrit; MDS/MPD, myelodysplasia/myeloproliferative disorders; rhVIIa, recombinant human factor VIIa.

els of nitric oxide (9) or other products can cause decreased binding of fibrinogen to platelet GP IIb/IIIa or impaired release of platelet granules. Some of these patients experience clinically important bleeding, especially gastrointestinal (9). DDAVP (standard doses) (3), cryoprecipitate, and high-dose estrogens (Premarin [Wyeth Pharmaceuticals, Philadelphia, PA], 50-mg single dose) (10) have been suggested to be of benefit in uremia-related bleeding. Because the presence of adequate numbers of intravascular red cells may facilitate interaction of platelets with the vessel wall, red cell transfusions are recommended in patients with anemia related to renal failure who are bleeding, to keep the hematocrit above 30% (11). Platelet transfusion may be beneficial temporarily if other measures fail and bleeding persists. If a dialyzable substance in the uremic plasma is responsible for the defect in platelet function, hemodialysis also may be beneficial, albeit temporarily.

Cardiac Bypass

Cardiac bypass causes defects in both platelet number and function. As platelets pass through the extracorporeal oxygenating circuit, they contact the artificial surfaces of the system and are activated; they also are fragmented by distortional trauma. Both phenomena lead to their accelerated clearance. Following bypass, a decrease in the platelet count, abnormalities in platelet morphology on the blood smear, and impaired in vitro platelet aggregation are observed in most patients (12), but these effects typically persist for 24 to 48 hours following bypass. Platelet transfusion may be given for serious bleeding.

Congenital Disorders

Inherited disorders of platelet function are rare and produce varying degrees of platelet-type bleeding, usually beginning within the first decade of life. Heritable disorders of platelet function may also remain clinically silent until unmasked by a significant hemostatic challenge. Prophylaxis prior to invasive procedures and treatment of significant hemorrhage may require transfusion of normal platelets or use of DDAVP (3), antifibrinolytic agents, or (refractory bleeding) recombinant human factor VIIa (3,13,14) (Table 21.6).

Bernard-Soulier Syndrome

Bernard-Soulier syndrome (BSS) comprises a triad including large platelets, moderate thrombocytopenia, and a prolonged bleeding time; individuals with this disorder have reduced or abnormal expression of platelet glycoprotein Ib/IX (the receptor for VWF) on the surface of their platelets. BSS is autosomal recessively inherited. Platelet aggregation studies are normal with all agonists except ristocetin. BSS is distinguished from VWD in that the reduced ristocetin-induced platelet aggregation in BSS is corrected by the addition of normal platelets, whereas in VWD, it is corrected by the addition of normal plasma (which contains adequate VWF). The diagnosis can be confirmed by platelet flow cytometry.

Glanzmann's Thrombasthenia

Glanzmann's thrombasthenia is a recessively inherited qualitative or quantitative abnormality in GP IIb/IIIa expression on the platelet surface. Without adequate functional IIb/IIIa to bind fibrinogen and VWF (both of which cross-link platelets), platelet aggregation is markedly impaired (Fig. 21.2). Patients may present with mucocutaneous bleeding in infancy. Interestingly, the severity of clinical bleeding does not correlate well with the degree of deficiency of IIb/IIIa (15). Allogeneic HSCT has been used in the management of severe cases (16).

Storage Pool Disease

Storage pool disease (SPD) is characterized by abnormalities in number or content of platelet granules. Defects in alpha-granules, dense granules, or both (Table 21.4) may be present. Platelet aggregation to ADP (Fig. 21.2) typically shows an initial wave of aggregation, but the aggregates subsequently dissociate because of reduced or absent release of granule contents, which reinforce the aggregatory response. Most patients have a prolonged bleeding time. A variable bleeding diathesis results. More commonly, patients may have *release defects* wherein granules are present, but signaling necessary for release of granule contents is defective.

Albinism-Associated Storage Pool Disease

Albinism-associated SPD occurs in the context of disorders characterized by oculocutaneous albinism, such as the Hermansky-Pudlak and Chediak-Higashi syndromes. Impaired biogenesis of dense granules, lysosomes, and melanosomes may be responsible for the reduced number of dense granules in these patients (17).

Nonalbinism-Associated Storage Pool Disease

Nonalbinism-associated SPD occurs in a variety of other conditions (thrombocytopenia with absent radius [TAR] syndrome, Ehlers-Danlos syndrome, Wiskott-Aldrich syndrome, Osteogenesis imperfecta). Defects in dense granules may relate more to granular content rather than number (18) and may occur in conjunction with alpha-granule abnormalities (alpha-delta SPD). Decreased or empty dense granules can be visualized on electron microscopy.

Gray Platelet Syndrome

The *gray platelet syndrome* (19) is a rare, inherited disorder characterized by abnormalities of platelet alpha granules, thrombocytopenia, and fibrosis in the bone marrow; consanguinity is common. A lifelong history of mild to moderate mucocutaneous bleeding usually is present. Review of the blood smear typically shows agranular platelets that appear "gray" on Wright's staining because of a lack of azurophilic granules. In contrast to dense granule deficiency, platelet aggregation to epinephrine, ADP, and arachidonic acid is often normal, while thrombin and collagen produce variable results. The diagnosis is confirmed with electron microscopy.

Quebec Platelet Disorder

The *Quebec platelet disorder* (20) is an extremely rare disorder that is characterized by abnormal platelet factor V, mild thrombocytopenia, and prolonged bleeding time (BT), leading to a moderate bleeding diathesis. Bleeding is unresponsive to platelet transfusion.

Scott Syndrome

Scott syndrome (21) is an extremely rare disorder characterized by spontaneous bleeding because of a platelet membrane defect that does not support the binding of coagulation factors. Patients have a normal bleeding time and platelet aggregation studies.

Congenital Disorders of Signal Transduction

Congenital disorders of signal transduction include defects in receptor-agonist interactions, G-protein activation, platelet enzymatic activity, and phosphorylation of signaling proteins (22).

Isolated Laboratory-Specific Defects

Individuals with phenotypically normal hemostasis occasionally demonstrate reduced or (less frequently) absent aggregation to one or more agonists on platelet aggregation testing. These abnormalities, which may be genetically determined, probably reflect interindividual differences in the reactivity of platelets to certain ligands and do not necessarily indicate an increased risk for spontaneous or trauma-induced hemorrhage, unless a tendency to bleed has been previously demonstrated.

Other Conditions

The *May-Hegglin anomaly* features mild to moderate thrombocytopenia, large platelets, and characteristic leukocyte azurophilic inclusions (Dohle bodies). While the large size of the platelets implies a qualitative abnormality, patients generally do not bleed excessively and aggregation studies are normal. An autosomal dominantly inherited disorder, it is a manifestation of mutated nonmuscle myosin heavy chain IIA, which has been implicated in the related disorders Sebastian syndrome, Fechtner syndrome, and Epstein syndrome; these feature varying degrees of sensorineural hearing loss, nephritis, cataracts, and leukocyte inclusions (23).

REFERENCES

1. Bick RL. Disseminated intravascular coagulation current concepts of etiology, pathophysiology, diagnosis, and treatment. Hematol Oncol Clin North Am 2003;17:149–176.
2. Rick ME. Treatment of von Willebrand disease. In Rose BD, ed. UpToDate (online textbook of medicine). Wellesley, MA: UpToDate; 2003.

3. Mannucci PM. Desmopressin (DDAVP) in the treatment of bleeding disorders: the first 20 years. Blood 1997;90:2515–2521.

4. Carcao MD, Blanchette VS, Dean JA, et al. The platelet function analyzer (PFA-100): a novel in-vitro system for evaluation of primary hemostasis in children. Br J Haematol 1998;101:70–73.

5. Symeonidis A, Kouraklis-Symeonidis A, Seimeni U, et al. Ticlopidine-induced aplastic anemia: two new case reports, review, and meta-analysis of 55 additional cases. Am J Hematol 2002;71: 24–32.

6. Moake JL. Thrombotic thrombocytopenic purpura and the hemolytic uremic syndrome. Arch Pathol Lab Med 2002;126:1430–1433.

7. Bennett CL, Connors JM, Carwile JM. Thrombotic thrombocytopenic purpura associated with clopidogrel. N Engl J Med 2000;342:1773–1777.

8. Landolfi R, Marchioli R, Patrono C. Mechanisms of bleeding and thrombosis in myeloprolifera-tive disorders. Thromb Haemost 1997;78:617–621.

9. Zuckerman GR, Cornette GL, Clouse RE, et al. Upper gastrointestinal bleeding in patients with chronic renal failure. Ann Int Med 1985;102:588–592.

10. Boyd GL, Diethelm AG, Gelman S, et al. Correcting prolonged bleeding during renal transplan-tation with estrogen or plasma. Arch Surg 1996;131:160–165.

11. Turrito VT, Weiss HJ. Red blood cells: their dual role in thrombus formation. Science 1980; 207:541–543.

12. Kestin AG, Valeri CR, Khuri SF, et al. The platelet function defect of cardiopulmonary bypass. Blood 1993;82:107–117.

13. Bellucci S, Caen J. Molecular basis of Glanzmann's Thrombasthenia and current strategies in treatment. Blood Rev 2002 Sep;16:193–202.

14. Buchanan GR. Quantitative and qualitative platelet disorders. Clin Lab Med 1999;19:71–86.

15. George JN, Caen JP, Nurden AT. Glanzmann's thrombasthenia: the spectrum of clinical disease. Blood 1990;75:1383–1395.

16. Bellucci S, Devergie A, Gluckman E, et al. Complete correction of Glanzmann's thrombasthenia by allogeneic bone-marrow transplantation. Br J Haem 1985;59:635–641.

17. Shalev A, Michaud G, Israels SJ, et al. Quantification of a novel dense granule protein (granulo-physin) in platelets of patients with dense granule storage pool deficiency. Blood 1992;80: 1231–1237.

18. Weiss HJ, Lages B, Vicic W, et al. Heterogenous abnormalities of platelet dense granule ultra-structure in 20 patients with congenital storage pool deficiency. Br J Haematol 1993;83:282–295.

19. Raccuglia G. Gray platelet syndrome: a variety of qualitative platelet disorder. Am J Med 1971; 51:818–828.

20. Hayward CPM, Rivard GE, Kane WH. An autosomal dominant, qualitative platelet disorder associated with multimeric deficiency, abnormalities in platelet factor V, thrombospondin, von Willebrand factor, and fibrinogen, and an epinephrine aggregation defect. Blood 1996;87: 4967–4978.

21. Sims PJ, Wiedmer T, Esmon CT, et al. Assembly of the platelet prothrombinase complex is linked to vessiculation of the platelet plasma membrane: studies in Scott syndrome, an isolated defect in platelet procoagulant activity. J Biol Chem 1989;264:17049–17057.

22. Rao K, Gabbeta J. Congenital disorders of platelet signal transduction. Arterioscler thromb Vasc Biol 2000;20:285–289.

23. Seri M, Pecci A, Di Bari F, et al. MYH9-related disease: May-Hegglin anomaly, Sebastian syndrome, Fechtner syndrome, and Epstein syndrome are not distinct entities but represent a variable expression of a single illness. Medicine 2003;82:203–215.

22

Venous Thromboembolism

Steven J. Lemery* and Craig M. Kessler

Venous thromboembolism (VTE) occurs in an estimated 100 individuals per 100,000 population each year in the United States; however, the incidence of VTE in people over 80 years of age is approximately 500 events per 100,000 population per year (1). Pulmonary embolism (PE) occurs at about half the rate of VTE; however, this may underestimate the incidence because autopsy data were not included in these estimates (1). Pulmonary emboli frequently cause death in hospitalized patients because the diagnosis is often missed; many of these events are potentially preventable. Furthermore, chronic VTE-induced pulmonary hypertension complicates PE in about 4% of cases after 2 years of follow-up (2). Deep venous thrombosis (DVT) most commonly occurs in the lower extremities, but virtually any venous vascular bed can be involved. The frequency of upper extremity DVTs, particularly those associated with the use of long-term indwelling central venous access devices, is somewhat unclear and the need to prevent them somewhat controversial. When upper extremity DVTs arise, the potential for subsequent pulmonary embolization is substantial, estimated to be as high as 25% in some trials.

Clinicians continue to recognize Virchow's triad of vascular stasis, endothelial injury, and hypercoagulability as the major factors contributing to thrombosis. With modern laboratory techniques, many of the biochemical, autoimmune, and heritable variables that lead to a hypercoagulable state can be detected and explained.

DEEP VENOUS THROMBOSIS AND PULMONARY EMBOLISM

Thrombosis of the deep veins of an extremity often is the initial manifestation of the more devastating entity of PE. Symptoms and signs associated with DVT include calf or leg swelling (88%), pain (56%), tenderness (55%), warmth (42%), erythema (34%), Homan's sign (13%), and palpable cord (6%) (3).

Alternatively, a DVT may remain asymptomatic and not discovered until a patient experiences symptoms of a PE. A patient who develops a pulmonary embolus may experience dyspnea (77%), chest pain (55%), hemoptysis (13%), syncope (10%), and sudden death (3).

The signs that accompany PE are tachypnea (70%), tachycardia (43%), hypoxia/cyanosis (18%), and hypotension (10%) (3).

DVT causes long-term morbidity because of chronic leg pain, cyanosis, venous dilatation and congestion, swelling, cutaneous ulceration, and decreased mobility, the so-called postthrombotic syndrome (PTS). Within 6 years of initial DVT treatment with heparin alone, postthrombotic syndrome develops in up to 80% of involved extremities; approximately 20% of contralateral extremities may also develop postthrombotic manifestations despite no evidence of prior overt DVT (4). Gradient compression stockings (typically 20 to 30 mm pressure) should be applied to the affected lower extremity shortly after the DVT has been diagnosed so that the development of severe postthrombotic signs and symptoms can be mitigated. Compression stockings are not substitutes for an adequate anticoagulation regimen but are useful adjuncts for rehabilitative exercise programs. Thromboembolic deterrent (TED) stockings do not provide equivalent benefits. The initiation of gravity-based exercise regimens (e.g., walking, jogging, and so forth, rather than swimming) is also extremely important in the prevention

*The views expressed are the result of independent work and do not necessarily represent the views or findings of the U.S. Food and Drug Administration of the United States.

and mitigation of PTS. Unfortunately, compression stockings or sleeves for upper extremity DVTs are not as beneficial or convenient.

A distinction is made between distal DVT in the lower extremity below the popliteal vein trifurcation in the calf and those designated as proximal DVT, which involve the popliteal and more proximal venous system. Calf vein DVTs are considered lower risk for PE in contrast to the higher risks of PE associated with proximal DVT. Approximately 25% of distal DVTs will propagate proximally within 1 to 2 weeks if left untreated, increasing the risks of subsequent PE and development of postthrombotic syndrome. Furthermore, the finding of distal DVT by duplex Doppler ultrasound may simply represent the residual DVT after a portion of the source clot has embolized to the lung.

RADIOGRAPHIC DIAGNOSIS OF DEEP VENOUS THROMBOSIS

Because of its general availability, noninvasive nature, and sensitivity and specificity, ultrasonography is the first diagnostic test typically used when DVT is suspected. Venography, the criterion standard for the diagnosis of DVT, requires iodine-based contrast dyes to diagnose DVT through the presence of an intraluminal-filling defect. The invasive nature of the procedure, the difficulty in ascertaining adequate venous access in a swollen extremity, the potential allergic reactions, and the renal insufficiency that can develop because of viscosity of the dye load all limit the practicality and usefulness of venography for most situations. That being said, venography is used frequently in clinical research studies to provide a more sensitive indication of the antithrombotic efficacy of new anticoagulant medications. Venography may also be useful in instances where ultrasound is not feasible or is equivocal and a diagnosis of DVT must be known. Ultrasonography is considerably more sensitive for the detection of proximal DVT than for distal DVT. Venography often detects asymptomatic DVT, usually located distally in the venous vasculature of the lower extremities. The clinical relevance of distal DVT is uncertain because they embolize less frequently; however, if a distal DVT propagates proximally, significant PE may develop.

Compression ultrasound with venous imaging enhances the diagnosis of DVT by direct visualization of an occlusive or partially occlusive thrombus, noncompression of a vein, and/or lack of blood flow observed with Doppler. Sensitivity ranges from 89% to 100%, and specificity ranges from 86% to 100% (5). Unfortunately, sensitivity may be lower in patients with asymptomatic DVT (5). Serial evaluations with ultrasound improve sensitivity, because an undiagnosed distal DVT can be discovered when it propagates proximally. Furthermore, an ultrasound can accurately diagnose a Baker's cyst, which occasionally mimics DVT. One limitation of ultrasound is the difficulty in differentiating between a new recurrent DVT in the ipsilateral extremity of a patient who has previously carried the diagnosis, especially if the previous DVT has not resolved. Impedance plethysmography may be useful in this instance. Bilateral ultrasound of lower extremities should be considered because "clot burden" may influence the decision on duration of anticoagulation.

DVT can be diagnosed using magnetic resonance venography (MRV). One prospective blinded study reported sensitivity greater than 94% and specificity greater than 90% for the diagnosis of DVT (6). MRV directly visualizes thrombi in a noninvasive manner, and MRV can image proximal veins in the pelvis. Major disadvantages include cost, availability, and lack of uniform expertise in reading images.

PULMONARY EMBOLISM DIAGNOSIS: ECHOCARDIOGRAPHY, ELECTROCARDIOGRAPHY AND RADIOGRAPHY

PE generally occurs through the embolization of distal lower extremity thrombi; however, PE also can complicate upper extremity DVT and occur after removing an indwelling central venous access device. Less commonly, PE may originate in the inferior vena cava (particularly in association with renal cell carcinoma) or the heart via a patent foramen ovale or mural thrombus in the right ventricle. In addition, the diagnosis of PE may be delayed when the PE is accompanied by concurrent arterial thromboembolic events such as a cerebrovascular accident, where there is paradoxical embolization of DVT through a patent foramen ovale.

Diagnostic methods with low specificity for the diagnosis of PE include electrocardiography (ECG), echocardiography, and chest radiography. Suggestive ECG findings of PE include new right atrial or ventricular enlargement; new right bundle branch block, or the classic S1Q3T3 pattern; and supraventricular arrhythmias.

Suggestive findings of PE on echocardiogram include right ventricular dilatation, often with myocardial hypokinesis (most common); pulmonary artery dilatation; right ventricular mural thrombi; tricuspid regurgitation; and loss of inspiratory collapse of the inferior vena cava.

Transthoracic or transesophageal echocardiogram confirmation of right ventricular hypertension can assist in the decision regarding thrombolysis with right heart failure. Both echocardiography and spiral computed tomography (CT) have a low sensitivity for PE located in peripheral pulmonary vessels. Chest radiographic findings suggestive of a pulmonary embolus include a Hampton's hump or a focal paucity of blood vessel perfusion.

PULMONARY EMBOLISM DIAGNOSIS

Angiography

The criterion standard for the diagnosis of PE remains pulmonary angiography; an intraluminal-filling defect confirms the presence of an embolus. Angiography is not the initial diagnostic test of choice because it requires an invasive procedure and is associated with risks of stroke, renal failure caused by contrast dye osmotic load, hematoma at the venous access site, anaphylaxis caused by iodine contrast dye, and even death, usually secondary to induced arrhythmias. Nevertheless, when making a diagnosis is necessary, the potential risks are usually outweighed by the benefits of obtaining an accurate diagnosis and facilitating the implementation of thrombolytic therapy or anticoagulation. Initiating extended oral or parenteral anticoagulation without a firm diagnosis of PE confers a considerable and potentially unwarranted risk of hemorrhagic complications.

Computed Tomography and Ventilation/Perfusion Scanning

The two most commonly ordered tests to diagnose PE are the ventilation/perfusion lung scan (V/Q) and a helical or spiral CT scan of the chest. CT is widely available and can diagnose other potential pathologic causes of dyspnea. The advantages of V/Q scanning over CT include the lack of need for contrast dye and ability to diagnose distal vascular PE, which the spiral CT frequently cannot detect. The initial test of choice depends on local availability, radiologic expertise, and patient factors. Patient factors to consider include history of contrast dye for CT and the ability to perform ventilation maneuvers required for a V/Q scan.

The V/Q scan evaluates mismatches in pulmonary perfusion compared with that of ventilation. The test was prospectively evaluated as part of the PIOPED I study in 1990 (7). The clinical pretest probability of PE was combined with V/Q scan results to determine posttest probability for PE in 755 patients who underwent both pulmonary angiography and a V/Q scan. The PIOPED I study investigators defined a high pretest clinical probability as conveying an 80% to 100% chance of having a PE, while a low pretest clinical probability was associated with a 0% to 19% chance of having a PE (7). V/Q scan results are most informative when the results match the clinical pretest probability. The following study results demonstrate why additional testing is often necessary after obtaining V/Q scan results:

• Forty percent of patients with a low-probability V/Q scan but a high pretest clinical probability of PE actually had a PE (7),
• Fifty-six percent of patients with a high-probability V/Q scan but a low pretest clinical probability of PE had a PE (7).

Based on the PIOPED I results, pulmonary angiography is often performed in high-risk patients despite a low- or intermediate-probability V/Q scan. Serial Doppler examinations of the lower extremities are another diagnostic option for patients at lower risk, such as a patient with an intermediate pretest probability for PE and a low- or intermediate-probability V/Q scan (16% and 28% chances of having a PE, respectively) (7).

The diagnostic characteristics of computed tomographic angiography (CTA) or CTA with venous-phase imaging (CTA-CTV) has been assessed in a large trial (PIOPED II, n = 824) (8). The PIOPED II investigators used the Wells score to determine the clinical probability of PE. Similar to the characteristics of the V/Q scan, the predictive values for CTA varied based on the clinical assessment. The positive predictive values of a positive CTA finding in a patient with high, intermediate, or low pretest probability of PE were 96%, 92%, and 58%, respectively (8). Negative predictive values of a positive CTA finding were 60%, 89%, and 96% in the three groups, respectively (8). CTA-CTV displayed very similar findings compared with CTA; the only predictive value difference greater than 5% using the two different methods was in the negative predictive value for a patient with high clinical probability of PE (60% CTA versus 82% CTA-CTV) (8). Caution should be used in interpreting this difference because of the small number of subjects studied in this subgroup. The authors of PIOPED II concluded that additional testing for PE is necessary when the clinical probability is inconsistent with the imaging results (8). Furthermore, caution should be exercised in extrapolating this study's findings to all centers that have different levels of expertise in both the acquisition and interpretation of CTA and CTA-CTV.

LABORATORY DIAGNOSIS OF VENOUS THROMBOEMBOLISM

The D-dimer assay has been used as an adjunct to exclude DVT and PE. When a cross-linked fibrin clot is degraded by plasmin, D-dimers are formed. A sensitive enzyme-linked immunosorbent assay (ELISA) test for D-dimers, if negative in a patient with a low pretest probability of VTE, essentially excludes VTE. The ELISA's low specificity for VTE requires that further diagnostic testing be conducted. Elevated levels of D-dimers are produced by many conditions including cancer, pregnancy, sepsis, sickle cell crisis, and surgery. The D-dimer assay may be a useful adjunct in predicting the risk of future VTE in patients who experienced VTE. The PROLONG Study indicated that patients with positive D-dimers 1 month after the completion of at least 3 months anticoagulation for idiopathic VTE had a significantly higher risk for recurrent VTE, which was mitigated by continued anticoagulation. In this study, patients with abnormal D-dimers who did not reinitiate anticoagulation manifested a 15% incidence of rethrombosis over the 18-month observation period compared with a bleeding or thrombosis rate of 2.9% if anticoagulation were continued. Additionally, the adjusted hazard comparing the rates of recurrent thromboembosim among those patients with an abnormal D-dimer level compared to patients with a normal D-dimer level was 2.27 (95% CI, 1.15–4.46) (9).

DEEP VENOUS THROMBOSIS IN SITES OTHER THAN THE DISTAL VEINS OF THE LOWER EXTREMITIES

DVT can have devastating consequences when it occurs in unusual sites. DVT of the subclavian and axillary veins are most commonly associated with the presence of indwelling venous access devices. Malignancies involving the superior sulcus (so-called Pancoast tumors) and mediastinum may cause DVT in the superior vena cava and subclavian veins. Bilateral upper extremity DVTs are uncommon and should prompt a search for malignancy. More worrisome are DVT that involve the hepatic (and splanchnic), retinal, and renal veins, or the cerebral venous structures. DVT of the hepatic (the Budd-Chiari syndrome [BCS]) and splanchnic veins results in abdominal pain caused by an engorged liver (hepatic vein clot), ascites, portal hypertension, and bowel ischemia. BCS is usually an acute clinical complication of cirrhosis and acquired hypercoagulable states including pregnancy; myeloproliferative disorders; hereditary hypercoagulable states, including deficiencies of proteins C and S; and paroxysmal nocturnal hemoglobinuria. The clonal V671F point mutation in the Janus 2 kinase (JAK2V617F) tyrosine kinase, which occurs in a large proportion of myeloproliferative disorders (MPD) (particularly polycythemia rubra vera), should be assessed in patients with BCS or portal vein thrombosis to rule out MPD. Treatment options for splanchnic vein thrombosis include anticoagulation, thrombolysis, and consideration of orthotopic liver transplantation in a patient with liver failure. In addition, acute reduction of red blood cell mass and/or platelet count should be considered if the splanchnic vein thrombosis is because of an underlying MPD.

ACQUIRED THROMBOPHILIC STATES

Heparin-Induced Thrombocytopenia and Heparin-Induced Thrombocytopenia with Thrombosis

Heparin-induced thrombocytopenia (HIT) is a thrombogenic state caused by antibodies formed after exposure predominantly to unfractionated heparin. These antibodies bind to the heparin-platelet factor 4 (PF4) complex and secondarily promote thrombosis in vivo in both venous and arterial sites by aggregating platelets. In general, platelet counts begin to decrease 5 to 9 days after the initiation of heparin. Thrombocytopenia may occur earlier in patients previously administered heparin in the past 100 days. A diagnosis of HIT is supported by an ELISA assay that detects PF4-heparin antibodies and/or by platelet aggregation assays, which detect spontaneous aggregation of platelets induced by the addition of heparin to the patient's platelet-rich plasma. Sensitivity of platelet aggregation assays can be increased when patient's platelets are "loaded" with radioactive serotonin; serotonin release from platelets is detected as a marker of platelet activation in vitro, after the addition of heparin. The most sensitive test is the serotonin-loaded platelet aggregation assay; however, false-positive platelet aggregation assays and ELISA for PF4-heparin antibodies are not uncommon (10). Small exposures to unfractionated heparin, including flushing of intravenous lines, may precipitate HIT. Low-molecular-weight heparins (LMWH) uncommonly precipitate HIT but can exacerbate HIT once it occurs in association with unfractionated heparin.

Multiple agents are available for the treatment of HIT when anticoagulation is undertaken in the presence of thrombocytopenia. Traditional low-molecular-weight heparin preparations such as enoxaparin, dalteparin, and tinzaparin can cross-react with the PF4-heparin antibodies produced by unfractionated heparin and are not recommended for anticoagulation in HIT/heparin-induced thrombocytopenia with thrombosis (HITTS). Lepirudin (a recombinant form of hirudin), bivalirudin (a small synthetic molecule [molecular weight (MW) = 2180 D] with homology to the two amino acids of hirudin), and argatroban (a small, synthetically derived compound [MW = 527] that binds to thrombin in a reversible manner) are direct thrombin inhibitors that have proven effective for anticoagulation during the thrombocytopenia of HIT and for treatment of thrombosis in HITTS. Lepirudin is antigenic, and antibody formation results in excessive anticoagulation. Lepirudin is contraindicated in the presence of renal insufficiency. Bivalirudin (approved in HIT only for patients undergoing percutaneous coronary intervention) and argatroban are both hepatic-excreted, nonantigenic, and short-acting and should be used with caution in patients with liver disease. None of these agents have specific antidotes if excessive bleeding occurs in association with their use. Clinicians should refer to the drug's labels to guide dosing and conversion to oral anticoagulant therapy. Finally, the synthetic pentasaccharide fondaparinux does not appear to cross-react with heparin and is being investigated as an alternative anticoagulant for the treatment of HITTS.

Nephrotic Syndrome

The nephrotic syndrome confers an elevated risk of both renal vein thrombosis and DVT/PE. Membranous glomerulonephritis confers the highest risk of renal vein thrombosis (20% to 30%) (11). Predisposition toward hypercoagulability is because of reductions of modulators of coagulation; antithrombin III and protein S are lost in the urine (11). Increased levels of procoagulant factors are also observed, including factors V, VIII, and fibrinogen (11). The routine use of prophylactic anticoagulation for patients with nephrotic syndrome has not been established by randomized controlled trials; however, some experts advocate prophylactic anticoagulation for patients with nephrotic syndrome caused by membranous glomerulonephritis or with the antiphospholipid syndrome who have additional risk factors including extreme albuminuria (11). Low-molecular-weight heparin anticoagulation is contraindicated in renal insufficiency.

Antiphospholipid Antibody Syndrome

Proposed mechanisms to explain how antiphospholipid antibodies (APA) mediate the development of thrombosis include binding of APA to β_2-glycoprotein I (β_2-GPI) complexed to phospholipid exposed on the surface of injured or activated endothelial cells, oxidant based injury to endothelin, and interference with regulatory proteins such as annexin V and protein C (12).

Antiphospholipid antibodies are associated with infections such as syphilis, but these APA are less thrombogenic and often transient.

Testing for APA is accomplished directly by using specific assays to quantitate levels by ELISA or indirectly through the detection of antiβ_2-GPI antibodies. The functional expression of APA is designated as the lupus anticoagulant (LAC), which prolongs phospholipid-dependent clotting assays. Assays include the dilute Russell viper-venom time, the dilute prothrombin or tissue thromboplastin inhibition test, and the kaolin clotting time. Because the APA is directed against phospholipid, a useful confirmatory test for the LAC is the platelet neutralization assay, in which the prolonged activated partial thromboplastin test, characteristic of the LAC, is shortened or normalized after incubating patient plasma with normal platelets; these platelets will provide enough phospholipid to adsorb the LAC and allow the coagulation test to proceed normally.

Two positive tests for APA, obtained at least 6 weeks apart, are required to fulfill the laboratory criteria for the APA syndrome. Clinical criteria for the diagnosis of the APA syndrome include detection of venous and/or arterial thrombotic events, autoimmune thrombocytopenic purpura, marantic endocarditis, multiple spontaneous abortions before the tenth week of gestation, or unexplained death of a morphologically normal fetus after the tenth week of gestation. Thrombosis can occur in virtually any vascular bed, and patients may present with a catastrophic syndrome with thrombosis in multiple vascular sites, including cerebrovascular accidents and DVT.

Treatment strategies should focus on modification and elimination of risk factors, such as smoking and oral estrogen contraceptives. For a thrombotic complication, systemic anticoagulation should be initiated. To prevent VTE recurrence, a randomized, double-blind, prospective study showed that dosing warfarin to an international normalized ratio (INR) of 2.0 to 3.0 was equally effective as higher intensity warfarin regimens to achieve an INR of 2.5 to 3.5 (13). In general, anticoagulation after a thrombotic event should be long term; future studies may delineate if certain subgroups may safely discontinue anticoagulation (12).

Hypercoagulability of Malignancy

VTE frequently complicates malignancy and results in significant morbidity and mortality. The estimated prevalence of VTE in patients with cancer is 10% to 15% and as high as 28% in pancreatic cancer (14). Cancer promotes thromboses through a variety of mechanisms: release of tissue factor, activation of factor X by a cancer procoagulant, endothelial-tumor cell interactions, and platelet activation. Hypercoagulability associated with malignancies is designated as the Trousseau syndrome and manifests as disseminated intravascular coagulation, nonbacterial thrombotic endocarditis, PE, DVT, and arterial thromboses. Occasionally, chemotherapy agents promote thrombosis, possibly through direct injury to the vascular endothelium. Of equal importance is the observation that adjuvant therapy with SERMS (selective estrogen receptor modulators), such as tamoxifen, or antiangiogenic medications, such as thalidomide and lenalidomide for the treatment of multiple myeloma and bevacizumab for the treatment of breast, colon, or lung malignancies, can all increase the potential thrombogenicity beyond what is usually observed in the chemotherapy treatment of those cancers in the absence of those agents. Central venous indwelling catheters often complicate cancer care because of thrombus formation in the catheter itself and the vessel into which it has been inserted (15).

Treatment of the hypercoagulability of cancer can be challenging and should be individualized. Rethrombosis often occurs despite adequate treatment with warfarin; furthermore, patients with cancer are at a high risk for bleeding secondary to surgeries, local tumor factors, and thrombocytopenia associated with chemotherapy. The U.S. Food and Drug Administration (FDA) recently approved dalteparin for the extended treatment of symptomatic venous thromboembolism in patients with cancer based on the large clinical CLOT trial that showed a reduction in objectively confirmed, symptomatic DVT and/or PE during the 6-month study period when compared with oral anticoagulation (15.7% versus 8%) (16,17). Dalteparin appeared to reduce the incidence of rethrombosis most significantly in the first month of treatment compared with warfarin. It has not been established whether this reduction in recurrent VTE is similar for all low-molecular-weight heparin (LMWH) preparations.

Paroxysmal Nocturnal Hemoglobinuria

Paroxysmal nocturnal hemoglobinuria (PNH) causes intravascular hemolysis, bone marrow failure, and thrombotic events. Diagnosis can be made rapidly by flow cytometric detection of deficient CD55 and CD59 on peripheral blood erythrocytes and neutrophils. Patients with large clones (greater than 50%) carry a high risk of thrombotic events, which include unusual sites such as the hepatic or mesenteric veins. Hypercoagulability is the most common cause of death in this disease. The etiology of the thrombogenicity has not been elucidated, and treatment of thrombosis with anticoagulation can be difficult. One nonrandomized study showed decreased risks of thrombosis in patients who were prophylaxed with warfarin (18), but it is not unusual for PNH patients to continue to experience venous and/or arterial thrombotic complications during anticoagulation treatment.

SURGERY AS AN ACQUIRED RISK FOR THROMBOSIS

Surgery imparts a significant predisposing risk for thrombosis. Surgery and trauma induce hypercoagulability through multiple mechanisms: direct endothelial injury, activation of the coagulation cascade (through the release of tissue factor), and platelet activation. Risk varies with the indications for surgery, anesthesia time, patient age, and the presence of underlying heritable or acquired hypercoagulable states. VTEs most frequently occur with hip or knee arthroplasty, hip fracture surgery, spinal cord injury, major trauma, and any surgery performed in the context of malignancy. Patients undergoing these procedures should receive prophylaxis against the formation of thrombosis; options include graduated pneumatic compression stockings plus LMWH, adjusted dose heparin, fondaparinux, and oral anticoagulation with warfarin to achieve an INR goal of 2 to 3 (19). DVT prophylaxis should be individualized depending on bleeding risk, history of previous thrombosis, history of heparin-induced thrombocytopenia, presence of renal insufficiency, and type of surgery; refer to published guidelines to assist in management (19). Outpatient surgical procedures performed in patients younger than 40 who can be made readily ambulatory do not require prophylactic anticoagulation. Prolonged prophylactic anticoagulation postsurgery may be indicated for patients undergoing total hip replacement (at least until the patient is mobile) and for those in whom a malignancy persists.

MICROANGIOPATHIC HEMOLYTIC STATES

Microangiopathic hemolytic anemias are commonly associated with thrombosis. Thrombotic thrombocytopenic purpura (TTP) is the paradigm. TTP is characterized by thrombocytopenia, microangiopathy, renal insufficiency, fever, and central nervous system abnormalities.

Clinicians should suspect TTP when thrombocytopenia and microangiopathic hemolysis coexist. Thrombosis causes the secondary manifestations of renal insufficiency and central nervous system alterations. TTP may be precipitated by an acquired quantitative or qualitative deficiency of von Willebrand factor (VWF) protease, resulting in abnormally large, unprocessed circulating VWF multimers that have potent platelet-activating properties. Initial treatment for TTP involves immediate administration of corticosteroids combined with aggressive plasmapheresis and exchange of the patient's total plasma volume with normal plasma. TTP is a readily treatable disease but has a mortality rate of approximately 20% (compared with almost 100% mortality untreated) (20).

Disseminated intravascular coagulation (DIC) is characterized by systemic thrombosis, mediated by pathologic overproduction of thrombin. DIC is the consequence of other concurrent disease processes, especially evident in patients with active malignancy, obstetrical catastrophes, or trauma. Treatment for DIC is challenging, with primary therapy targeted toward eradicating the underlying precipitant and secondary therapy intended to ameliorate the bleeding and/or thrombotic consequences of the consumptive coagulopathy. If unrelenting bleeding ensues in the context of hypofibrinogenemia (fibrinogen consumption and degradation) and thrombocytopenia, supportive care in the form of cryoprecipitate, fresh frozen plasma, and platelet transfusions may be considered but should be implemented concurrently with heparin at subtherapeutic VTE doses. DIC caused by acute promyelocytic leukemia is best approached with all-*trans*-retinoic acid for the underlying leukemia.

MYELOPROLIFERATIVE DISORDERS

Myeloproliferative disorders (MPD) have been associated with thrombosis, especially true of polycythemia rubra vera and essential thrombocythemia. MPDs, paradoxically, are also associated with an increased risk of hemorrhage, but thrombotic complications are the most common cause of death in MPD. The thrombotic risk of polycythemia is often exacerbated by the hyperviscosity produced by a markedly increased red cell mass. Treatments for polycythemia vera include repeated phlebotomy to decrease red cell volume/hyperviscosity and cytotoxic agents such as hydroxyurea to reduce erythrocyte, leukocyte, and platelet production, with the ultimate goal to minimize the risk of thrombosis. Polycythemia vera associated erythromelalgia is usually treated with low-dose aspirin 81 mg daily.

Therapy to prevent thrombosis is usually considered for patients with essential thrombocythemia who are older than 60 or have a prior history of thrombosis. Guidance is provided by a randomized trial evaluating low-dose aspirin plus anagrelide versus hydroxyurea (HU) (21). Hydroxyurea plus aspirin was associated with a lower risk of arterial thrombosis, serious hemorrhage, and transformation to myelofibrosis than anagrelide, a specific platelet lowering noncytotoxic and nonchemotherapy agent. VTE incidence was higher in the HU group; however, the totality of the data when statistically analyzed for composite endpoints favored treatment with HU (21). Blood counts should be followed closely during HU therapy, and HU is contraindicated in pregnant women or for women who desire to become pregnant.

Other acquired risk factors for thrombosis include increased age, immobility, prior VTE, myocardial infarction, certain drugs and biological therapies, pregnancy, and hormone therapy (22). Table 22.1 lists acquired and heritable hypercoagulable states.

HERITABLE HYPERCOAGULABLE STATES

Inherited hypercoagulable states associated with an increased risk of VTE include activated protein C resistance (factor V Leiden gene polymorphism); prothrombin gene mutation; deficiencies of protein C, protein S, and antithrombin III; and hyperhomocysteinemia.

TABLE 22.1. *Hypercoagulable States*

Acquired hypercoagulable states
   Heparin-induced thrombocytopenia
   Nephrotic syndrome
   Antiphospholipid antibody syndrome
   Malignancy
   Paroxysmal nocturnal hemoglobinuria
   Surgery
   Microangiopathic hemolytic anemia (TTP/HUS/DIC)
   Myeloproliferative disorders
   Increased age
   Immobility
   Trauma
   Prior venous thromboembolism
   Myocardial infarction
   Pregnancy
   Hormone therapy
   Presence of a venous access device
Heritable hypercoagulable states
   Activated protein C resistance
   Prothrombin gene mutation (G20210A)
   Protein C deficiency
   Protein S deficiency
Antithrombin III deficiency
Hyperhomocyteinemia

DIC, disseminated intravascular coagulation; HUS, hemolytic-uremic syndrome; TTP, thrombotic thrombocytopenic purpura.

There may also be heritable hypercoagulable states precipitated by persistent elevations of coagulation factors VIII, IX, and XI. More uncommon inherited hypercoagulable states include dysfibrinogenemias or other deficiencies of the fibrinolytic system (plasminogen deficiency). Clinicians should base decisions on whom to screen on how the results will affect clinical management and/or how the results will affect the patient and his or her family; for example, oral estrogen contraception use is not recommended for hypercoagulable women. Screening for a thrombophilic hypercoagulable state should be considered for a young patient with a positive family history of thrombosis, unprovoked thrombosis, or recurrent thrombosis. Appropriate genetic counseling should be performed before these tests are administered, and testing should be timed appropriately. For example, protein C, protein S, and antithrombin III levels may be reduced during an active thrombosis, which can create a false-positive test result. Furthermore, warfarin will reduce the activities of the vitamin K-dependent modulators of clotting factors, protein C and protein S. Heparin and warfarin may affect test results for the lupus anticoagulant, and this diagnosis is best established after anticoagulation is discontinued.

ACTIVATED PROTEIN C RESISTANCE (FACTOR V LEIDEN)

A mutation in coagulation factor V (Arg506Gln; factor V Leiden gene polymorphism) results in a protein that is no longer susceptible to inactivation by activated protein C proteolysis. Factor V Leiden, occurring in about 5% of the Caucasian population, is the most common known inheritable risk factor for VTE but has little effect on arterial thrombotic potential (23). Most patients who carry the mutation do not develop thrombosis; however, additive risk factors, including estrogen use and the coexistence of the prothrombin mutation, greatly increase the risk of VTE. Laboratory testing includes direct detection of an abnormal but characteristic gene mutation in factor V, accomplished by polymerase chain reaction (PCR), and indirectly by evaluating the effects of factor V Leiden in an in vitro laboratory test for activated protein C resistance (this latter assay should not be performed while the patient is receiving warfarin).

PROTHROMBIN MUTATION (G20210A)

The second most common gene mutation responsible for congenital hypercoagulability is the prothrombin G20210A polymorphism. As with factor V Leiden, VTE predominates in patients with the prothrombin gene mutation, with arterial thrombosis being unusual. This mutation is associated with elevated prothrombin levels, mainly in Caucasians, and was found to have a crude 2.8 odds ratio for the development of thrombosis (24). G20210A can be indirectly assayed by measuring a prothrombin level, but direct genetic testing with PCR is more frequently performed.

DEFICIENCIES OF PROTEINS S, C, AND ANTITHROMBIN III

These three proteins are synthesized in the liver and have a modulatory function in homeostasis of the coagulation cascade. Protein S is a cofactor of activated protein C that serves to inactivate factors Va and VIIIa. Antithrombin III inhibits factors II, Xa, XIa, IXa, and XIIa (25). Heparin complexes to antithrombin III, greatly potentiating the serine protease inhibitory activity of antithrombin III. These enzymes can be quantitatively or qualitatively abnormal in hypercoagulable individuals. Severe deficiencies of these enzymes may result in VTE at a young age, including newborns. Arterial thrombotic complications are unusual. These deficiencies are uncommonly detected in the general population, but they are responsible for 5% to 9% of idiopathic VTE (22).

HYPERHOMOCYSTEINEMIA

Controversy exists regarding the contribution of hyperhomocysteinemia to the development of VTE. The HOPE-2 placebo-controlled randomized trial (n = 5522) studied homocysteine-lowering therapy as a means to decrease the risk of VTE (a secondary endpoint). Despite the lower homocysteine levels in the treated group, the incidence of VTE was the same in both study arms (26). Vitamin B_{12}, folate, and vitamin B6 lower homocysteine levels; however, it is unknown whether vitamin therapy will reduce the risk of recurrent VTE in a patient with high homocysteine levels below that of treatment with anticoagulation alone.

INITIAL TREATMENT FOR ACUTE VENOUS THROMBOEMBOLISM

Anticoagulation is the primary prophylaxis and first therapy for thrombosis and for prevention of recurrent VTE. In certain situations, treatment may include additional modalities, such as fibrinolytic therapy or insertion of an inferior vena cava filter.

DVT or PE should be treated initially with systemic anticoagulation in the form of unfractionated heparin (UFH), LMWH, or fondaparinux. The goal is to prevent the propagation or embolism of a clot while the endogenous fibrinolytic system dissolves the clot locally. Oral anticoagulation with warfarin should not be used as a single agent for the initial treatment of thrombosis; warfarin causes a transient hypercoagulable state, and its use without systemic anticoagulation can result in severe skin necrosis.

The choice of the initial treatment for VTE depends on several factors. The American College of Physicians and the American Academy of Family Physicians offers guidelines that recommend that the initial treatment of DVT and PE should proceed with either UFH or LMWH (27). Oral anticoagulation with warfarin can be initiated concurrently with at least a 5-day overlap with LMWH or UFH, and the heparin can be discontinued when the INR is in the therapeutic range of 2 to 3. Warfarin as a single "unopposed" anticoagulation agent should be avoided in the context of VTE because underlying hypercoagulability can be exacerbated as the vitamin K-dependent modulators of coagulation (e.g., proteins S and C) will be reduced rapidly. LMWH and fondaparinux are more expensive than UFH; however, overall hospitalization and laboratory monitoring expenses are less with LMWH and fondaparinux. Unfractionated heparin requires more frequent monitoring because it complexes with acute phase reactant proteins, resulting in unpredictable plasma levels of anticoagulation. LMWH requires monitoring only in special situations, including renal failure, pregnancy, and at both extremes of body mass index. LMWH should be followed with antifactor Xa levels whenever laboratory monitoring is required. LMWH and fondaparinux are contraindicated in renal failure and should be used with extreme caution and with dose reduction in patients with mild renal insufficiency, as the kidneys excrete LMWH. UFH may be preferred in a patient at risk for bleeding, because its half-life is shorter, and its action can be reversed with protamine. In contrast, there is no specific antidote for LMWH (or fondaparinux) if untoward hemorrhage occurs. Protamine sulfate's ability to reverse LMWH is unpredictable. LMWH and fondaparinux are less likely than UFH to cause HIT.

EXTENDED TREATMENT TO PREVENT RECURRENT VENOUS THROMBOEMBOLISM

When a patient is receiving appropriate anticoagulation with UFH or LMWH for acute VTE, warfarin therapy can be initiated concurrently. Heparin overlap therapy as bridging for long-term anticoagulation with warfarin should continue for a minimum of 5 days and not be terminated until a therapeutic INR of 2 to 3 is reached. Standard practice is to initiate warfarin at 5 mg daily because of possible overanticoagulation at higher doses. A double-blinded randomized study, however, showed that warfarin at 10 mg for 2 days followed by dose adjustment determined by a nomogram (28) was not associated with an increased bleeding risk. Caution should be used in patients with potential vitamin K deficiency, because this strategy may increase the risk of overanticoagulation. Vitamin K-deficient patients may have a mildly elevated prothrombin time prior to warfarin treatment. Common examples of patients who are at increased risk for vitamin K deficiency include those who are elderly, malnourished, postsurgical, or on antibiotics.

The FDA has recently recommended that initial warfarin dosing be optimized by individualized genetic testing for CYP2C9 and vitamin K epoxide reductase polymorphisms to predict how the patient will respond to the initial warfarin dose. Because the CYP2C9*2,*3 and the VKORC1 variant alleles are associated with increased warfarin sensitivity, it is hypothesized that foreknowledge of these important polymorphisms will allow for more efficient and timely anticoagulation and will avoid risks of bleeding because of excessive dosing. The generalized adoption of pharmacogenomic, individualized dosing for initial oral warfarin has lagged because of (i) ethnic variability of the most significant alleles; (ii) the fact that genetic variability may be less important to the success of warfarin dosing than are food interactions and drug-drug interactions; (iii) the increased cost associated with genetic screening without guarantee of reimbursement; and (iv) the lack of availability of timely testing. Whether this approach will be more cost effective and more favorable from the risk-benefit perspective remains to be determined by adequately powered prospective clinical studies.

Warfarin is the favored standard treatment for long-term anticoagulation because of its lower cost and established risk-benefit profile. Dalteparin sodium is FDA approved for the extended treatment and subsequent prevention of recurrent symptomatic venous thromboembolism in patients with cancer. Unique risks of long-term LMWH use include osteopenia and heparin-induced thrombocytopenia (the latter risk is uncommon in this setting).

The ideal intensity of the INR for warfarin anticoagulation to prevent recurrent idiopathic VTE has been studied in two large prospective, randomized trials, which have yielded conflicting results. In the placebo-controlled PREVENT trial, low-intensity anticoagulation with the target INR of 1.5 to 2.0 reduced the recurrent VTE rate by two thirds (29). In a randomized, two-arm study of standard warfarin anticoagulation in Canada to achieve an INR between 2 and 3 versus a low-intensity INR arm with target INR between 1.5 and 2.0, the standard dosing regimen was over 60% more effective ($p = 0.03$) than low-intensity warfarin anticoagulation in reducing the cumulative probability of recurrent thromboembolism (30). There was no difference in bleeding complications between the two dosing intensities. The differences between the two studies may be related to trial design. For instance, the Canadian trial, in contrast to the PREVENT study, included cancer patients, who more likely would experience warfarin resistance.

In general, for an unprovoked idiopathic DVT, at least 3 to 6 months of anticoagulation are recommended (27). A massive life-threatening PE requires indefinite anticoagulation, similar to the recommendations for recurrent idiopathic VTE (unless the risk of life-threatening bleeding on anticoagulation exceeds the risk of a fatal PE—an IVC filter may be indicated in this uncommon instance). The PREVENT trial corroborated that patients with idiopathic VTE have a high incidence of recurrent VTE and benefit from long-term anticoagulation (29). As previously discussed, the antiphospholipid antibody syndrome requires prolonged warfarin therapy. Individuals with cancer may be hypercoagulable and anticoagulation should probably be continued as long as the malignancy is present. Patients with transient risk factors (i.e., trauma) usually require anticoagulation for 3 to 6 months (27). Patients with increased D-dimers, elevated FVIII activities, or evidence of significant residual DVT at 1 month after discontinuing anticoagulation appear to be at increased risk for rethrombosis and should be considered for reinstatement and indefinite continuation of their anticoagulation regimen.

INFERIOR VENA CAVA FILTERS IN THE TREATMENT OF DEEP VENOUS THROMBOSIS OR PULMONARY EMBOLUS

Inferior vena cava (IVC) filters are inserted to prevent thrombi originating in the venous vasculature of the lower extremities from embolizing to the pulmonary circulation. The IVC filter is placed by an interventional radiologist. Major reasons for the placement of an IVC filter include strong contraindications to the use of anticoagulants, intolerance to or noncompliance with anticoagulants, and recurrent PE despite adequate systemic anticoagulation. A randomized study revealed that, in the short term, an IVC filter decreases the incidence of pulmonary embolus, but at 2 years the difference was not statistically significant (30). In addition, there were more DVT in the IVC filter group, with the potential of greater morbidity from postphlebitic syndrome (31). Individuals with permanent IVC filters probably benefit from lifelong anticoagulation. The use of retrievable IVC filters should be considered in most clinical situations because they provide flexibility for either future removal or maintenance as a permanent intervention against PE.

FIBRINOLYTIC THERAPY

Fibrinolytic therapy has been generally reserved for patients with massive PE associated with right ventricular dilatation and overload with hemodynamic compromise. That subcohort of patients with systolic blood pressure <90 mm Hg, or a blood pressure drop >40 mm Hg for >15 minutes, not caused by cardiac arrhythmias, sepsis, or hypovolemia, may benefit from thrombolytic therapy with improved survival (32).

Nevertheless, no clinical study has confirmed a survival advantage when using thrombolytic agents. Some practitioners consider thrombolytic therapy for patients with new right heart failure or moderate to severe pulmonary hypertension in the setting of PE. Fibrinolysis is investigational in selected patients with massive ileofemoral DVT to decrease development of postthrombotic complications. Systemic thrombolytic therapy with massive ileofemoral DVT is likely to fail because of venous hypertension and the inability to perfuse the thrombus with the fibrinolytic agent. Rather, catheter-directed intrathrombus delivery of the thrombolytic agent is indicated. Careful patient selection and informed consent are critical to avoidance of the morbidity and mortality associated with thrombolysis: elderly individuals with systemic hypertension are at greatest risk. Patients frequently bleed at the venotomy site if the venipuncture is not performed flawlessly. Because of an intracerebral bleed rate approaching 0.6%, and approximately 2% major bleeds elsewhere, thorough discussion with a patient regarding potential risks and benefits is important.

Surgical and mechanical thrombectomy procedures may be indicated for the small number of patients with massive PE and DVT who are not candidates for fibrinolytic therapy. There is a lower potential risk of bleeding complications using mechanical approaches compared with systemic or catheter-directed thrombolytic therapy. Stent placement after thrombolysis or mechanical thrombectomy should be considered for venous stenosis or short-segment residual thrombus at the site of original DVT.

REFERENCES

1. White H. The epidemiology of venous thromboembolism. Circulation 2003;107:I–4.
2. Pengo V, Lensing AWA, Prins MH, et al. Incidence of chronic thromboembolic pulmonary hypertension after pulmonary embolism. N Engl J Med 2004;350:2257–2264.
3. Anderson FA, Wheeler HB, Goldberg RJ, et al. A population-based perspective of the hospital incidence and case-fatality rates of deep vein thrombosis and pulmonary embolism. The Worchester DVT Study. Arch Intern Med 1991;151:933–938.
4. Elliot MS, Immelman EJ, Jeffery P, et al. A comparative randomized trial of heparin versus streptokinase in the treatment of acute proximal venous thrombosis: an interim report of a prospective trial. Br J Surg 1979;66:838–843.
5. Tapson VF, Carroll BA, Davidson BL, et al. The diagnostic approach to acute venous thromboembolism. Clinical practice guideline. American Thoracic Society. Am J Resp Crit Care Med 1999;160:1043–1066.
6. Fraser DGW, Moody AR, Morgan PS, et al. Diagnosis of lower-limb deep venous thrombosis: a prospective blinded study of magnetic resonance direct thrombus imaging. Ann Intern Med 2002; 136:89–98.
7. Saltzman HA, Alavi A, Greenspan RH, et al. Value of the ventilation/perfusion in acute pulmonary embolism: results of the Prospective Investigation of Pulmonary Embolism Diagnosis (PIOPED). JAMA 1990;263:2753–2759.
8. Stein PD, Fowler SE, Goodman LR, et al. Multidetector computed tomography for acute pulmonary embolism. N Engl J Med 2006;354:2317–2327.
9. Palareti G, Cosmi B, Legnani C, et al. D-Dimer testing to determine the duration of anticoagulation therapy. N Engl J Med 2006;355:1780–1790.
10. Warkentin TE. Heparin-induced thrombocytopenia: pathogenesis and management. Br J Haematol 2003;121:535–555.
11. Orth SR, Ritz E. The nephrotic syndrome. N Engl J Med 1998;338:1202–1211.
12. Levine JS, Branch DW, Rauch J. The antiphospholipid syndrome. N Engl J Med 2002;346: 752–763.
13. Crowther MA, Ginsberg JS, Julian J, et al. A comparison of two intensities of warfarin for the prevention of recurrent thrombosis in patients with the antiphospholipid antibody syndrome. N Engl J Med 2003;349:1133–1138.

14. Caine GJ, Stonelake PS, Lip GYH, et al. The hypercoagulable state of malignancy: pathogenesis and current debate. Neoplasia 2002;4:465–473.

15. Bick RL. Cancer-associated thrombosis. N Engl J Med 2003;349:109–111.

16. Lee AY, Levine MN, Baker RI, et al. Low-molecular-weight heparin versus a coumarin for the prevention of recurrent venous thromboembolism in patients with cancer. N Engl J Med 2003; 349:146–153.

17. Food and Drug Administration. Fragmin (dalteparin) injection label, 2007. Center for Drug Evaluation and Research Web site. Available at http://www.fda.gov/cder/foi/label/2007/020287s035lbl.pdf. Accessed December 18, 2008.

18. Hall C, Richards S, Hillmen P. Primary prophylaxis with warfarin prevents thrombosis in paroxysmal nocturnal hemoglobinuria (PNH). Blood 2003;102:3587–3591.

19. Geerts WH, Pineo GF, Heit JA, et al. Prevention of venous thromboembolism. Chest 2004;126: 338S–400S.

20. George JN. Evaluation and management of patients with thrombotic thrombocytopenic purpura. J Intensive Care Med 2007;22:82–91.

21. Harrison CN, Campbell PJ, Buck G, et al. Hydroxyurea compared with anagrelide in high-risk essential thrombocythemia. N Engl J Med 2005;353:33–45.

22. Anderson FA, Spencer FA. Risk factors for venous thromboembolism. Circulation 2003;107(23 Suppl 1):I9–I16.

23. Ridker PM, Miletich JP, Hennekens CH, et al. Ethnic distribution of factor V Leiden in 4047 men and women. Implications for venous thromboembolism screening. JAMA 1997;277:1305–1307.

24. Poort SR, Rosendaal FR, Reitsma PH, et al. A common genetic variation in the 3N-untranslated region of the prothrombin gene is associated with elevated plasma prothrombin levels and an increase in venous thrombosis. Blood 1996;88:3698–3703.

25. Zwicker J, Bauer KA. Thrombophilia. In Kitchens CS, Alving BM, Kessler CM, eds. Consultative Thrombosis and Hemostasis. Philadelphia: W.B. Saunders Company; 2002:181–196.

26. Ray JG, Kearon C, Yi Qilong, et al. Homocysteine-lowering therapy and risk for venous thromboembolism: a randomized trial. Ann Intern Med 2007;146:761–767.

27. Snow V, Qaseem A, Barry P, et al. Management of venous thromboembolism: A clinical practice guideline from the American College of Physicians and the American Academy of Family Physicians. Ann Intern Med 2007;146:204–210.

28. Kovacs MJ, Roger M, Anderson DR, et al. Comparison of 10-mg and 5-mg warfarin initiation nomograms together with low-molecular-weight-heparin for outpatient treatment of acute venous thromboembolism. A randomized, double-blind, controlled trial. Ann Intern Med 2003;138: 714–719.

29. Ridker PM, Goldhaber SZ, Danielson E, et al. Long-term, low-intensity warfarin for the prevention of recurrent venous thromboembolism. N Engl J Med 2003;348:1425–1434.

30. Kearon C, Ginsberg JS, Kovacs MJ, et al. Comparison of low-intensity warfarin therapy with conventional-intensity warfarin therapy for long-term prevention of recurrent venous thromboembolism. N Engl J Med 2003;349:631–639.

31. Decousus H, Leizorovicz A, Parent F, et al. A clinical trial of vena caval filters in the prevention of pulmonary embolism in patients with proximal deep-vein thrombosis. N Engl J Med 1998;338: 409–415.

32. Task Force on Pulmonary Embolism, European Society of Cardiology. Guidelines on the diagnosis and management of acute pulmonary embolism. Eur Heart J 2000;21:1301–1336.

23

Consultations in Anticoagulation

Pallavi P. Kumar and Barbara M. Alving

This chapter provides guidelines for the treatment of venous thromboembolism (VTE) in patients who require special consideration, such as those who have underlying cancer or who are pregnant. The chapter also discusses the prevention and treatment of postphlebitic syndrome and peripheral vascular disease (PAD), two chronic vascular problems that can coexist as patients age.

PROPHYLAXIS AND TREATMENT OF VENOUS THROMBOEMBOLISM IN THE PATIENT WITH CANCER IN SPECIFIC CLINICAL SETTINGS

Patients with malignancy have an increased risk for VTE because of multiple factors: hypercoagulability resulting from increased production and release of procoagulant factors such as tissue factor; prolonged immobilization; narrowing of vascular flow caused by tumor obstruction; vascular damage induced by chemotherapy, hormonal therapy, or antiangiogenic agents; and long-term indwelling devices, such as central venous catheters. As long as the cancer is active, the increased risk for VTE is present; the cancers most commonly associated with VTE are those of the lung, gastrointestinal tract, breast, and prostate gland.

Recommendations for anticoagulation are based primarily on clinical trial data or small studies in which patients with malignancy were only a minor subset (fewer than 20% of participants). In general, unfractionated heparin (UFH), low-molecular-weight heparin (LMWH), and oral anticoagulants have been the mainstay of therapy. Because LMWH undergoes renal excretion, patients with kidney impairment who receive LMWH should be monitored by measurement of the antifactor Xa activity. The creatinine clearance should be calculated before initiation of LMWH in elderly patients, because they may have renal dysfunction despite having normal creatinine values. Monitoring should also be used in severely obese patients (body mass index [BMI]$\geq$40) who are to receive therapeutic doses of LMWH and should be considered for those who are obese (BMI $\geq$30), especially if the patient has moderate to severe renal insufficiency (creatinine clearance less than 60 mL/min) (1).

The target antifactor Xa levels (based on measurements 4 hours after LMWH injection) for patients who are on treatment doses of LMWH are 0.5 to 1.2 U/mL for twice daily dosing. For once daily dosing, the target is between 1 and 2 U/mL. (The levels are measured in plasma derived from blood drawn into tubes containing sodium citrate.)

Primary Prophylaxis in Cancer Patients Undergoing Surgical Intervention

In studies published between 1969 and 1984, the rate of VTE in general surgical patients who did not receive prophylaxis was between 15% and 30%, with fatal PE between 0.2% and 0.9% (2). Prophylaxis is now routinely provided to postoperative surgical patients and is especially indicated for those with underlying cancer. Once-daily LMWH appears to be as safe and effective as injections of UFH given two or three times each day and provides convenience as well as a better quality of life for the patient (3,4). In the Clinical Center at the National Institutes of Health, enoxaparin is the LMWH utilized. However, other LMWH, such as nadroparin calcium, dalteparin, ardeparin, tinzaparin, and reviparin, may be considered (5–12) (Table 23.1).

TABLE 23.1. *Primary Prophylaxis in Patients with Cancer in the Perioperative Period*

Surgical Intervention	Drug of Choice	Dose	Initiation of Dose	Other	Duration of Treatment
Abdominal/ Pelvis	Enoxaparin (LMWH)	40 mg SQ daily	10–14 hours preoperatively	Recommend use of compression stockings with anticoagulant	28 days
Orthopedic	Enoxaparin (LMWH)	30 mg SQ q12hr OR 40 mg SQ daily	12–24 hours postoperatively 10–12 hours preoperatively	Recommend use of compression stockings or intermittent pneumatic compression with LMWH	Under debate: 30–35 days showed significant reduction of VTE
Neurosurgery	Enoxaparin	40 mg SQ daily	Started 12–24 hours postoperatively	Use compression stockings and/ or intermittent pneumatic compression with LMWH	Until hospital discharge

LMWH, low-molecular-weight heparin; SQ, subcutaneous; VTE, venous thromboembolism.

Primary Prophylaxis in Cancer Patients Receiving Chemotherapy, Hormonal, and/or Antiangiogenic Treatment

Patients with cancer who are undergoing treatment should be considered for prophylaxis if they have one or more of the following: a history of VTE, a large mass compressing a major vessel, or treatment that includes tamoxifen or an antiangiogenic agent, such as thalidomide. Treatment in these patients should be individualized; if prophylaxis is chosen, LMWH (i.e., enoxaparin 40 mg/day or UFH [low dose]) should be considered, because these regimens have been effective in other clinical settings (2). The administration of warfarin at a fixed dose of 1 mg/day is not recommended.

Primary Prophylaxis in Cancer Patients Who Are Immobilized/Hospitalized

Acutely ill hospitalized medical patients undergo a threefold reduction in VTE when treated with LMWH (enoxaparin at a daily dose of 40 mg) compared with controls receiving no treatment. This conclusion is derived from the MEDENOX trial, a double-blind randomized study of 1102 patients with acute medical illnesses who received prophylaxis against VTE (14.9% of these patients had cancer or a history of cancer) (Table 23.2) (13). Patients were randomized to 1 of 3 groups that would re-

TABLE 23.2. *Primary Prophylaxis in Patients with Cancer Hospitalized for Acute Medical Conditions: The MEDENOX Trials*

Recommended Prophylaxis for Venous Thromboembolism	Dose	Duration of Treatment	Incidence of Venous Thromboembolism	Other
Enoxaparin versus Placebo	40 mg SQ daily	6–14 days (days of hospitalization)	5.5% versus 14.9% $p < 0.001$	The significant reduction in VTE with enoxaparin was maintained at 3 months

LMWH, low-molecular-weight heparin; SQ, subcutaneous; VTE, venous thromboembolism.

ceive for 6 to 14 days the subcutaneous daily administration of 40 mg of enoxaparin, 20 mg of enoxaparin, or placebo. The primary outcome was VTE during the ensuing 3 months. The outcome favored prophylactic treatment with subcutaneous enoxaparin at a dose of 40 mg daily. Adverse events, which included hemorrhage, local reaction, thrombocytopenia, and death from any cause, were not different between the groups receiving enoxaparin and placebo. The weakness of this study was that a more appropriate control group should have been one receiving UFH.

Primary Prophylaxis in Patients with Brain Metastases and Primary Brain Tumors

The causes of VTE in patients with primary and metastatic brain tumors are multifactorial and include hypercoagulability, venous stasis, tumor burden, and treatments that may induce a low-grade disseminated intravascular coagulation (DIC). The challenge in using anticoagulation is balancing the risk of thrombosis with the risk of precipitating intracranial hemorrhage. Studies have shown both increased risk as well as benefit with the use of LMWH prophylaxis in the nonsurgical setting (14).

For patients undergoing surgery, the recommended prophylaxis is to initiate LMWH 24 hours postoperatively; this is associated with minimal risk (Table 23.3) (10). In one study of patients with brain tumors, prophylaxis was initiated before surgery; this study was terminated early because of the increased incidence of intracranial bleeding (15).

Treatment of Venous Thromboembolism in Patients with Primary Brain Tumors or Brain Metastases

Treatment doses of UFH or LMWH can be administered safely to patients with primary brain tumors or brain metastases who develop VTE (14). However, the patients should undergo careful monitoring; the risk for hemorrhagic complications may be increased in patients with vascular metastatic tumors and for those who have certain tumors, such as metastatic melanoma. An option to anticoagulation is placement of an inferior vena cava filter, which also is associated with risks as well as benefits.

Treatment of Patients with Trousseau's Syndrome

Trousseau's syndrome is a spectrum of venous and arterial thromboembolic disorders predating or associated with a malignancy (3,16). Patients with this syndrome, even if adequately anticoagulated with warfarin according to the international normalized ratio (INR), may have recurrent thrombi. UFH and LMWH are efficacious, but dosing depends on the clinical setting. For example, a patient with an acute deep vein thrombosis (DVT) may require enoxaparin at therapeutic doses, whereas DIC may be controlled with lower doses. LMWH reduces the rate of recurrent thrombi without increasing bleeding and may also improve quality of life (Table 23.4) (3,16).

TABLE 23.3. *Evidence for Favorable Benefit/Risk Ratio with Anticoagulation after Neurosurgery*

Associated with High Risk of Venous Thromboembolism	Recommended Treatment	Duration of Treatment	Outcome
Patients after surgery for brain tumors	40 mg enoxaparin subcutaneously daily with compressive stockings OR compressive stockings alone	Begin within 24 hours after neurosurgery and continue for more than 7 days	Rate of VTE: 17% with LMWH + stockings versus 32% with stockings alone $p = 0.004$ 3% in each group had major bleeding

LMWH, low-molecular-weight heparin; VTE, venous thromboembolism.

TABLE 23.4. *Treatment of Patients with Trousseau's Syndrome*

Clinical Manifestations of Trousseau's	Recommended Treatment for Trousseau's Syndrome	Dose	Length of Treatment	Other Comment
Spontaneous recurrent or migratory venous thrombosis Arterial thrombosis Microangiopathy Marantic endocarditis Acute/chronic DIC–thrombotic versus bleeding state	LMWH for Trousseau's syndrome	Variable; 30 mg SQ twice a day has been used	Requires treatment as long as tumor persists	Further studies are needed to compare efficacy, safety, and costs of LMWH with other anticoagulants

DIC, disseminated intravascular coagulation; LMWH, low molecular weight heparin; SQ, subcutaneous.

General Approach in Treating Venous Thromboembolism in Cancer Patients

In general, treatment of VTE in patients with cancer consists of LMWH or UFH followed by warfarin for at least 3 months (9,17). However, for patients who may be bedridden, critically ill, and/or malnourished, continued indefinite long-term treatment with LMWH may be preferable to warfarin. Most institutions have a nomogram that guides the dosing and monitoring of UFH. General guidelines are provided in Table 23.5 (9,17).

TABLE 23.5. *General Approaches in Treating Patients with Cancer Who Develop Venous Thromboembolism*

Treatment for Venous Thromboembolism	Recommended Dose	Duration of Treatment	Other Comments
LMWH (enoxaparin) + warfarin	1 mg/kg twice daily + 5–10 mg oral warfarin daily (dose adjust to maintain INR goal of 2.0–3.0)	LMWH for at least 5 days, start warfarin on the second day. Concurrently INR goal maintained for 2 days before stopping LMWH	Continue for at least 3 months or longer depending on clinical setting; long-term LMWH can also be used
UFH + warfarin	Initial bolus 5000 units IV followed by approximately 1280 U/hr + 5–10 mg oral warfarin daily (dose adjust to maintain INR goal of 2.0–3.0)	UFH for at least 5 days, start warfarin on the second day Concurrently INR goal maintained for 2 days before stopping UFH	UFH adjusted to maintain an aPTT of 60–85 seconds (the targeted APTT should be equivalent to antifactor Xa activity level of 0.3 to 0.7 U/ml)
			Warfarin continued for at least 3 months

aPTT, activated partial thromboplastin time; INR, international normalized ratio; IV, intravenously; LMWH, low-molecular-weight heparin; UFH, unfractionated heparin; VTE, venous thromboembolism.

Anticoagulation Options

For patients who develop recurrent VTE despite adequate anticoagulation with warfarin (INR, 2–3), long-term treatment with LMWH may prove efficacious. This approach was validated in a study of patients with cancer and acute VTE who were randomized to receive either LMWH (dalteparin, 200 IU/kg body weight) once daily for 5 to 7 days followed by a coumarin derivative for 6 months or LMWH alone (dalteparin, 200 IU/kg) daily for 1 month followed by a daily dose of 150 IU/kg for 5 months (18). In the 6-month period, 27 of 336 patients in the LMWH group had recurrent VTE events compared with 53 of 336 patients in the oral anticoagulant group. This finding was statistically significant ($p = 0.002$). There was no significant difference between the two groups with respect to the incidence of bleeding.

If thrombocytopenia occurs during anticoagulation, the following differential should be considered: chemotherapy-induced thrombocytopenia, DIC, heparin-induced thrombocytopenia (HIT), thrombotic thrombocytopenic purpura, immune thrombocytopenic purpura, bone marrow failure, and folate or vitamin B12 deficiency.

Patients with HIT usually have a reduction in platelet count that begins 5 or more days after starting heparin therapy, although patients with prior heparin exposures may develop a low platelet count more rapidly. HIT can also become apparent 1 to 2 weeks after heparin has been discontinued. If HIT is a consideration, heparin must be discontinued and other anticoagulation initiated; choices include a direct thrombin inhibitor, such as argatroban or hirudin. An alternative that can be administered subcutaneously is fondaparinux, a synthetic pentasaccharide capable of inhibiting factor Xa through its interaction with antithrombin; it does not have activity against thrombin. The fondaparinux-platelet factor 4 complex is not recognized by antibodies and therefore has been used successfully as an alternative agent in patients with HIT; however, it has not yet been approved by the Food and Drug Administration (FDA) for use in such patients (19).

Thrombosis and Venous Access Devices

One complication of long-term central venous catheters is thrombosis, which can involve the tip of the catheter alone, the length of the catheter forming a fibrin sheath, or the veins of the upper extremities, neck, and mediastinum (20). One current approach to prophylaxis against catheter-related DVT at the Clinical Center is to reserve anticoagulation for those patients who have had a catheter-related thrombosis or who are at very high risk for thrombosis; these patients would receive warfarin at a dose to achieve an INR of 1.5 to 2 or a daily injection of enoxaparin (1 mg/kg) with the knowledge that either of these treatments places the patients at some increased risk for bleeding (20).

For those patients who have developed a catheter-related DVT, treatment can be initiated with LMWH for 5 to 7 days, followed by warfarin (INR, 2–3) or enoxaparin at a dose of 1 mg/kg/day for the lifetime of the catheter. Thrombolytic therapy has also been used successfully to clear the venous occlusion and thus maintain patency of the vessel (20). Thrombolytic therapy is also used to lyse thrombi that are within catheters; the occlusion can be reversed according to the protocol described in Table 23.6 (20).

Indications for Inferior Vena Cava Filters in a Cancer Patient

The use of inferior vena cava (IVC) filters should be based on the contraindications to anticoagulation and/or failure of adequate anticoagulation. Patients who receive IVC filters are initially protected against PE; however, they are at increased risk for recurrent DVT, IVC thrombosis, and thrombosis at the insertion site. Filters that can be retrieved are now available and can help reduce the morbidity associated with permanent IVC filters. If the retrievable filter is not removed within the time frame indicated by the manufacturer, then it can become technically difficult to retrieve, and the vascular surgeon or interventional radiologist may recommend that it remain permanently in place.

Two examples of retrievable filters that have been approved by the FDA are the Gunther Tulip Retrievable Vena Cava Filter (Cook, Inc, Bloomington, IN) and the OptEase Retrievable Vena Cava Filter (Cordis Endovascular, Miami Lakes, FL). The retrievable vena cava filters made by both of these manufacturers also can remain in place permanently. The Gunther Tulip retrievable filter is generally

TABLE 23.6. *Thrombolysis of Catheter Occlusion*

Event	Treatment	Recommended Dose	Duration of Treatment	Other Comments
Thrombus at the tip of the catheter (ball-valve clot) or fibrin sheath	tPA (or Urokinase)	2 mg (5000 to 10,000 U)	Instill for 30–120 minutes into the catheter	Success defined by withdrawing 3 cc of blood and infusion of 5 cc of saline through the catheter—successful 70% to 90% of the time; repeat if not successful.
Thrombus occlusion despite tissue plasminogen activator (tPA)	tPA OR Urokinase	1 mg/hr	Infusion for 6 hours	Requires 10–15 cc (1 mg/cc) be made to prime the intravenous tubing. Then run in 1–2 cc to fill the catheter and then start the infusion*
		40,000 U/hr	Infusion for 6–12 hours into the catheter	

recovered after 7 to 10 days but in some cases recovery has been extended to 3 to 4 weeks. The OptEase retrievable filter can be recovered after being in place for as long as 23 days. Data on the duration of dwelling time prior to recovery is still being obtained and has been reported mainly for trauma patients who have received the retrievable filter in the acute care setting (21).

PREVENTION AND TREATMENT OF VENOUS THROMBOEMBOLISM IN PREGNANCY

Although maternal mortality is rare in pregnant women who live in developed countries, pregnancy-associated PE remains one of the most frequent causes of death. The evaluation and management of VTE in pregnancy are complicated by difficulty in interpreting symptoms, concern about performing imaging that may be hazardous to the fetus, and the need to consider possible complications of anticoagulation in both the mother and the fetus.

Diagnosis of Venous Thromboembolism During Pregnancy

In pregnant women, symptoms of lower extremity edema, back pain, and/or chest pain are often attributed to pregnancy rather than to a possible VTE. D-dimer assays are not helpful in establishing a diagnosis of VTE in late pregnancy because of the high rate of false-positive test results due to increasing levels of D-dimer during the last trimester. Radiologic studies have to be assessed carefully in terms of potential risks of ionizing radiation on the fetus. Compression ultrasonography of the proximal veins is recommended as the initial test for suspected DVT. If results are equivocal or an iliac vein thrombosis is possible, then magnetic resonance venography should be considered, because it does not carry radiation risks and is reliable. Finally, evaluation of a pregnant woman for PE would include a ventilation/perfusion (V/Q) lung scan. The perfusion scan should be completed first, and if it is abnormal, then a ventilation scan does not need to be performed. The diagnostic role of the spiral computed tomography (CT) scan in pregnant women has not been established.

TABLE 23.7. *Single Episode of Prior Venous Thromboembolism Associated with a Transient Risk Factor*

Treatment During Pregnancy	Treatment During Postpartum Period
Surveillance	Begin anticoagulation with UFH or LMWH and then overlap with warfarin daily for 4–6 weeks; adjust dose to maintain INR 2.0–3.0.

INR, international normalized ratio; LMWH, low-molecular-weight heparin; UFH, unfractionated heparin.

Management of Pregnant Women at Increased Risk for Venous Thromboembolism

Risk factors for thrombosis include a personal history of VTE, known inherited or acquired thrombophilia, obesity, older maternal age, high parity, and prolonged immobilization. The optimal anticoagulation regimens for pregnant women in all clinical settings of VTE have not been fully established, although LMWH, which does not cross the placenta, is gaining widespread use. Compared with UFH, LMWH appears to have a lower risk for inducing osteoporosis and HIT (22). Warfarin is generally avoided in pregnant women, because it carries a risk of teratogenicity when given to a pregnant woman between 6 and 12 weeks of gestation. After parturition, warfarin and heparin are used; both can be given to mothers who are nursing, because they do not appear in breast milk.

Tables 23.7 to 23.12 offer a guide to management options in defined clinical settings. These tables are adapted from Bates et al (22), which has a complete description of thrombotic conditions, including the antiphospholipid syndrome, and appropriate treatments during pregnancy as well as during the postpartum period, when the risk for thrombosis is increased above that during pregnancy.

As parturition approaches, women who are receiving LMWH should plan to discontinue treatment 24 hours before delivery; the drug can be resumed 24 hours after delivery. UFH, which has a half-life of 90 minutes, may well be the preferred anticoagulant for women who require anticoagulation and who have an uncertain time of delivery.

RECOGNITION AND MANAGEMENT OF PERIPHERAL VENOUS AND ARTERIAL DISEASE

The diagnosis and management of two common conditions, postphlebitic syndrome and peripheral arterial disease, are often overlooked by patients and physicians until the conditions are sufficiently severe to require the attention of the vascular surgeon. Early recognition and treatment of both conditions can greatly improve the quality of life for patients and delay disease progression.

TABLE 23.8. *Single Episode of Idiopathic Venous Thromboembolism in Patients Not Receiving Long-Term Anticoagulation*

Treatment During Pregnancy	Treatment During Postpartum Period
Surveillance OR Choice of either: UFH: 5000 U SC every 12 hours (or dose adjusted). If dose adjusted, anti-Xa level of 0.1–0.3 U/ml. or LMWH (enoxaparin): 40 mg SQ daily or BID	Begin anticoagulation with UFH or LMWH and then overlap with warfarin. Warfarin to be given daily for 4–6 weeks; adjust dose to maintain INR 2.0–3.0.

NR, international normalized ratio; LMWH, low-molecular-weight heparin; SQ, subcutaneous; UFH, unfractionated heparin.

TABLE 23.9. *Single Episode of Venous Thromboembolism and Thrombophilia (Confirmed Laboratory Finding) in Patients Not Receiving Long-Term Anticoagulation*

Treatment During Pregnancy	Treatment During Postpartum Period
Surveillance OR Choice of either: UFH: 5000 U SQ every 12 hours (or dose adjusted). If dose adjusted, anti-Xa level of 0.1–0.3 U/ml. or LMWH (enoxaparin): 40 mg SQ daily or BID	Begin anticoagulation with UFH or LMWH and then overlap with warfarin. Warfarin daily for 4–6 weeks; adjust dose to maintain INR 2.0–3.0.

NR, international normalized ratio; LMWH, low-molecular-weight heparin; SQ, subcutaneous; UFH, unfractionated heparin.

TABLE 23.10. *Women with Thrombophilia and with No Prior Venous Thromboembolism*

Treatment During Pregnancy	Treatment During Postpartum Period
Surveillance OR Choice of either: UFH: 5000 U SQ every 12 hours (no need to dose adjust in this situation), no laboratory monitoring needed. or LMWH (enoxaparin): 40 mg SQ daily	Begin anticoagulation with UFH or LMWH and then overlap with warfarin. Warfarin daily for 4–6 weeks; adjust dose to maintain INR 2.0–3.0.

Women who have antithrombin deficiency or who are compound heterozygotes or homozygous for prothrombin gene mutation or factor V Leiden must have prophylaxis with UFH or with LMWH.
INR, international normalized ratio; LMWH, low-molecular-weight heparin; SQ, subcutaneous; UFH, unfractionated heparin.

TABLE 23.11. *Multiple Episodes of Venous Thromboembolism and/or Women Receiving Long-Term Anticoagulation Therapy*

Treatment During Pregnancy	Treatment During Postpartum Period
Choice of either: UFH: Dose adjust SQ every 12 hours to target a midinterval aPTT into therapeutic range. or LMWH: (enoxaparin): 40 mg SQ BID or 1mg/kg BID	Warfarin—resume long-term therapy with appropriate monitoring of INR.

aPTT, activated partial thromboplastin time; INR, international normalized ratio; LMWH, low-molecular-weight heparin; SQ, subcutaneous; UFH, unfractionated heparin.

TABLE 23.12. *Treatment of Venous Thromboembolism During Pregnancy*

Treatment During Pregnancy	Treatment During Postpartum Period
Choice of either: LMWH (enoxaparin): 1 mg/kg every 12 hours, anti-Xa level of 0.6–1.0 U/ml, measured 4 hours after injection or IV UFH: Bolus followed by a continuous infusion. Monitor aPTT levels. Stop 24 hours prior to labor; if high risk may stop 4–6 hours prior to delivery.	Treatment depends on the time of thrombosis during pregnancy. LMWH can be used or warfarin can be initiated while the patient is receiving LMWH or UFH. Treatment in the postpartum period should be continued for at least 6–8 weeks (total duration of therapy should be 6 months).

aPTT, activated partial thromboplastin time; LMWH, low-molecular-weight heparin; UFH, unfractionated heparin.

POSTPHLEBITIC SYNDROME (POSTTHROMBOTIC SYNDROME OR VENOUS INSUFFICIENCY)

Hematologists and internists are well trained to diagnose and manage acute VTE; however, additional attention needs to be given to postphlebitic syndrome, which occurs in as many as 20% to 50% of patients within 1 to 2 years after an episode of DVT (23). Postphlebitic syndrome develops because of venous hypertension, which results from obstruction and damage to the venous valves, usually caused by DVT. The syndrome manifests as chronic pain in the affected leg, as well as edema and hyperpigmentation of the skin, and painless ulcers on the medial malleolar area in severe cases. The diagnosis is primarily clinical; duplex scanning can be used if the symptoms increase in severity and if surgery is contemplated. More extensive testing is often requested by the vascular surgeon.

According to one report, the application of graduated compression stockings prevents or slows the progression of the postphlebitic syndrome (24). However, in the presence of arterial insufficiency, stockings may not be advisable, and therefore patients who are elderly or have known atherosclerosis may need to be assessed to develop an appropriate treatment plan (discussed in Peripheral Arterial Disease). Application of graduated compression stockings should be initiated within 2 to 3 weeks after the first DVT and continued for at least 2 years and for as long as 5 years. Because stockings lose elasticity, they should be replaced every 6 months.

The degree of venous insufficiency can be classified according to the Clinical, Etiologic, Anatomic, Pathophysiologic system (CEAP), with the "C" category being the one primarily used. This category is further subdivided into C0, no visible disease; C1, telangiectasis; C2, varicose veins; C3, edema; C4, skin changes without ulcers; C5, skin changes with healed ulcers; and C6, skin changes with active ulcers.

RECOMMENDATIONS FOR MANAGEMENT OF POSTPHLEBITIC SYNDROME

Minimal Symptoms

Graduated stockings with moderate compression (15 to 20 mm Hg) or leg elevation at the end of the day is recommended. An effective way for the patient to reverse or relieve the symptoms of venous hypertension is to elevate both legs above the level of the heart for 30 minutes 3 or 4 times daily. During the night leg elevation can be achieved by elevating the foot of the bed (using blocks placed under the bed if necessary).

Mild to Moderate Symptoms (Edema, Aching, or Heaviness of Legs)

Graduated stockings with firm compression (20 to 30 mm Hg) are recommended; extra firm is also available (30 to 40 mm Hg) with or without nighttime pneumatic device.

Patients who have had ulcer formation should wear stockings daily throughout the entire day. Nonelastic stockings that are composed of multiple layers attached by Velcro (CircAid) can also be used and may be easier to apply.

Consultation with Vascular Surgeons

Surgical procedures are available for patients who have active ulcers that do not respond to therapy or who have varicose veins in addition to postphlebitic syndrome.

Peripheral Arterial Disease

Peripheral arterial disease (PAD) is present in approximately 12% of the adult population over the age of 50 years and in 20% of individuals over the age of 70 years (25). The presence of PAD indicates systemic atherosclerosis and is associated with carotid and coronary disease. Risk factors for PAD are as for atherosclerosis: smoking, hyperlipidemia, hypertension, diabetes, and advanced age. Clinically, the diagnosis of PAD should be suspected in patients who complain of intermittent claudication, which can increase in severity to chronic pain at rest. Pain from claudication usually involves one or both calves, develops with walking, and resolves within minutes of resting. The more severe manifestation of PAD, chronic limb ischemia, causes pain during the night at bed rest. The differential diagnosis of PAD includes diabetic neuropathy, reflex sympathetic dystrophy, osteoarthritis, and spinal stenosis.

Evaluation of the patient includes, in addition to a careful history and physical examination, measurement of the systolic pressures with a Doppler ultrasound instrument in both lower legs compared with the upper extremities to calculate the ankle brachial index (ABI; Table 23.13).

Treatment

Treatment of PAD addresses the underlying risk factors such as hyperlipidemia, diabetes mellitus, smoking, and hypertension. Patients who smoke should receive counseling and sustained support for smoking cessation. Patients may require statins (with or without niacin) for management of hyperlipidemia (with the goal of reducing low-density lipoprotein [LDL] cholesterol to less than 70 mg/dL) and antihypertensive agents for control of blood pressure. No specific antihypertensive is specifically superior in PAD; however, the angiotensin converting enzyme (ACE) inhibitor ramipril may have

TABLE 23.13. *Measurement and Interpretation of the Ankle/Brachial Index*

Measurement can be made with a blood pressure cuff and hand-held Doppler.
   The systolic blood pressure is measured in both arms (brachial); the higher of the two arm pressures is used in the denominator of the ankle/brachial Index (ABI).
   The systolic blood pressure is then recorded for the right and left ankles, using the dorsalis pedis pulses (DP) and the posterior tibial pulses (PT).

$$\text{Right ABI} = \frac{\text{higher } \textbf{right} \text{ ankle pressure (DP or PT)}}{\text{higher arm pressure}}$$

$$\text{Left ABI} = \frac{\text{higher } \textbf{left} \text{ ankle pressure (DP or PT)}}{\text{higher arm pressure}}$$

Interpretation of results:
ABI 0.00–0.41: Severe peripheral vascular disease (PAD) (this range of values is measured in patients with critical limb ischemia)
ABI 0.41–0.90: Mild to moderate PAD
ABI 0.91–1.30: Normal (patients with complaints of leg pain on exertion could undergo repeat measurement of ABI after treadmill testing)
ABI >1.30: Noncompressible vessel suggests calcification and other tests may be required

vascular benefits in addition to lowering blood pressure. Thus, as a class, the ACE inhibitors should be considered when the antihypertensive regimen is chosen.

Patients with diabetes mellitus are at especially high risk for PAD. Although maintaining glycemic control is essential for reduction of the rate of progression of the complications of diabetes, intensive control of the blood glucose level does not confer benefit with respect to improvement in PAD symptoms. Aspirin at a dose of 81 to 325 mg per day may be effective in reducing the risk of other vascular events.

Clopidogrel, an inhibitor of adenosine diphosphate (ADP)-induced platelet aggregation, used at a dose of 75 mg daily may be even more effective than aspirin in preventing ischemic events in patients with PAD as described in the Clopidogrel versus Aspirin in Patients at Risk of Ischemic Events (CAPRIE) trial (25). Prescribing physicians should know that thrombotic thrombocytopenic purpura occurs, albeit rarely, in patients receiving clopidogrel. Current guidelines developed by the American Heart Association and the American College of Cardiology provide detailed treatment approaches to the patient with PAD (26).

Treatment for Relief of Claudication

Graded exercise therapy under the care of a nurse or trained technician reduces symptoms of claudication. Exercises are usually performed in 1-hour sessions on a treadmill. Cilostazol (Pletal, Otsuka America Pharmaceutical, Rockville, MD), a drug that increases the intracellular concentration of cyclic adenosine monophosphate (cAMP) by inhibiting phosphodiesterase 3, was approved by the FDA in 1999 for treatment of patients with symptoms of claudication. Although cilostazol has multiple functions, such as inhibiting platelet aggregation and inducing vasodilatation, its mode of action in relieving symptoms in patients with PAD is not well understood. When taken at the usual dose of 100 mg orally twice daily, the most common side effect is headache. The drug should not be used in patients with congestive heart failure.

Endoscopic techniques, such as laser-assisted angioplasty and balloon angioplasty, are increasingly used in patients who require surgical intervention. Localized thrombolytic therapy, as well as rheolytic thrombectomy, in which a suction catheter removes the occlusive thrombus, can be used in patients with an acute arterial thrombosis. Knowledge of the techniques available for the recognition and management of PAD and of options available to patients with chronic or acute arterial occlusion allows the hematologist to serve as a more effective member of the consultation team for patients with multiple vascular comorbidities.

REFERENCES

1. O'Shea SI, Ortel TL. Issues in the utilization of low-molecular-weight heparins. Semin Hematol 2002;39:172–178.
2. Geerts WH, Pineo GF, Heit JA. Prevention of venous thromboembolism. Chest 2004;126: 338S–400S.
3. Levine MN, Lee AYY, Kakkar AK. From Trousseau to targeted therapy: new insights and innovations in thrombosis and cancer. J Thromb Haemost 2003;1:1456–1463.
4. Mismetti P, Laporte S, Darmon JY, et al. Meta-analysis of low-molecular-weight heparin in the prevention of venous thromboembolism in general surgery. Br J Surg 2001;88:913–930.
5. Bergqvist D, Agnelli G, Cohen AT, et al. Duration of prophylaxis against venous thromboembolism with enoxaparin after surgery for cancer. N Engl J Med 2002;346:975–980.
6. Rasmussen MS. Does prolonged thromboprophylaxis improve outcome in patients undergoing surgery? Cancer Treat Rev 2003;29(Suppl 2):15–17.
7. ENOXACAN Study Group. Efficacy and safety of enoxaparin versus unfractionated heparin for prevention of deep vein thrombosis in elective cancer surgery: a double-blind randomized multicentre trial with venographic assessment. Br J Surg 1997;84:1099–1103.
8. Goldhaber SZ. Deep vein thrombosis and pulmonary embolism. In Kitchens C, Alving B, Kessler C, eds. Consultative Hemostasis and Thrombosis, 2nd Ed. Philadelphia: W.B. Saunders; 2007: 245–256.

9. Rickles FR, Levine M. Thrombosis and cancer: In Kitchens C, Alving B, Kessler C, eds. Consultative Hemostasis and Thrombosis, 2nd Ed. Philadelphia: W.B. Saunders; 2007:389–403.
10. Agnelli G, Piovella F, Buoncristiani P, et al. Enoxaparin plus compression stockings compared with compression stockings alone in the prevention of venous thromboembolism after elective neurosurgery. N Engl J Med 1998;339:80–85.
11. Goldhaber SZ, Dunn K, Gerhard-Herman M, et al. Low rate of venous thromboembolism after craniotomy for brain tumor using multimodality prophylaxis. Chest 2002;122:1933–1937.
12. Nurmohamed MT, van Riel AM, Henkens CM, et al. Low-molecular-weight heparin and compression stockings in the prevention of venous thromboembolism in neurosurgery. Thromb Haemost 1996;75:233–238.
13. Samama MM, Cohen AT, Darmon JY, et al. A comparison of enoxaparin with placebo for the prevention of venous thromboembolism in acutely ill medical patients. Prophylaxis in Medical Patients with Enoxaparin Study Group. N Engl J Med 1999;341:793–800.
14. Wen PY, Marks PW. Medical management of patients with brain tumors. Curr Opin Oncol 2002;14:299–307.
15. Dickinson LD, Miller LD, Patel CP, et al. Enoxaparin increases the incidence of postoperative intracranial hemorrhage when initiated preoperatively for deep venous thrombosis prophylaxis in patients with brain tumors. Neurosurgery 1998;43:1074–1081.
16. Walsh-McMonagle D, Green D. Low-molecular-weight heparin in the management of Trousseau's syndrome. Cancer 1997;80:649–655.
17. Hirsch J, Raschke R. Heparin and low-molecular-weight heparin. Chest 2004;126:188S–203S.
18. Lee AYY, Levine MN, Baker RI, et al. Low-molecular-weight heparin versus a coumarin for the prevention of recurrent venous thromboembolism in patients with cancer. N Engl J Med 2003; 349:149–153.
19. Papadopoulos S, Flynn JD, Lewis DA. Fondaparinux as a treatment option for heparin-induced thrombocytopenia. Pharmacotherapy 2007;27:921–926.
20. Horne MK III, Chang R. Thrombosis related to venous access devices. In Kitchens C, Alving B, Kessler C, eds. Consultative Hemostasis and Thrombosis, 2nd Ed. Philadelphia: W.B. Saunders; 2007:553–559.
21. Rosenthal D, Wellons ED, Lai KM, et al. Retrievable inferior vena cava filters: initial clinical results. Ann Vasc Surgery 2006;20;157–165.
22. Bates S, Greer IA, Pabinger I, et al. Venous thromboembolism, thrombophilia, antithrombotic therapy, and pregnancy. Chest 2008;133:8446–8865.
23. Kahn SR, Ginsberg J. Relationship between deep venous thrombosis and the postthrombotic syndrome. Arch Intern Med 2004;164:17–26.
24. Prandoni P, Lensing AWA, Prins MH, et al. Below-knee elastic compression stockings to prevent the postthrombotic syndrome. Ann Intern Med 2004;141:249–256.
25. Hiatt WR. Medical treatment of peripheral arterial disease and claudication. N Engl J Med 2001; 344:1608–1621.
26. Hirsch AT, Haskal ZJ, Hertzer NR, et al. ACC/AHA 2005 guidelines for the management of patients with peripheral arterial disease (lower extremity, renal, mesenteric, and abdominal aortic). Executive summary. J Am Coll Cardiol 2006;47:1239–1312.

24

Blood Transfusion

Firoozeh Alvandi and Harvey G. Klein

BLOOD CELL ANTIGENS

Red blood cell (RBC) antigens have varying biochemical, phenotypic, and immunologic character-istics. Based on these characteristics, they have been assembled into blood group systems. The best known and most clinically important are ABO, Rh, Kell, Kidd, and Duffy.

The *antiglobulin* or *Coombs' test* (see below) provides a method by which alloantibodies against antigens may be detected and compatible blood units identified. When a clinically important alloanti-body is present in a recipient's serum, *antigen-negative blood* must be selected. If the alloantibody is against a very high frequency antigen (present in greater than 90% of individuals) or when multiple al-loantibodies are present, procurement of compatible blood may be difficult or impossible. In some cases, the presence of red cell autoantibodies makes all units (including those of the patient) appear in-compatible and masks the presence of alloantibodies.

Naturally occurring antibodies such as anti-A and/or anti-B are present in the absence of prior sen-sitizing stimulus, whereas development of most other alloantibodies requires prior sensitization.

- Blood group A individuals have naturally occurring anti-B.
- Blood group B individuals have naturally occurring anti-A.
- Blood group O individuals have naturally occurring anti-A and anti-B.
- Blood group AB individuals have neither anti-A nor anti-B.

LABORATORY DETERMINATION OF MAJOR BLOOD GROUPS

An individual's blood group is determined by performing a *forward* and *reverse grouping* (*"ABO typing"*).

In forward grouping, reagents of known antibody specificity (anti-A or anti-B) are added to the pa-tient's red blood cells of unknown phenotype (A, B, AB, or O), and the mixtures are examined for vis-ible agglutination; the absence of agglutination on combining the patient's cells with reagent anti-A and anti-B indicates that the patient's cells have neither the A nor the B antigen, and thus the patient's blood group is O on forward grouping.

In reverse grouping, the patient's serum of unknown antibody (anti-A and/or anti-B) content is added to reagent cells of known phenotype (A, B, or O), and the mixtures are examined for visible ag-glutination; the presence of agglutination on combining the patient's serum with reagent cells of A and B phenotype indicates that the patient's serum contains both anti-A and anti-B antibodies, and thus the patient's blood group is O on reverse grouping.

The forward and reverse groups must be consistent: if the patient forwards as blood group O, he or she must also reverse as blood group O. A specific blood group may not be assigned with certainty until any ABO discrepancy is resolved.

Some common causes of apparent ABO discrepancies are (i) presence of A or B subgroups, (ii) missing/weakly reacting antibodies or weak expression/absence of expected antigens (as may occur in profoundly immune suppressed and debilitated individuals, newborns, or in some patients post-hematologic stem cell transplant), (iii) presence of unexpected or nonspecific antibodies such as cold reactive autoantibodies, (iv) interfering substances such as Wharton's jelly from the umbilical cord of a newborn, or (v) hyperproteinemic states causing rouleaux formation.

ANTIGLOBULIN TEST

The antiglobulin test uses antibodies to human globulins to detect the presence of antibody (or complement) on the RBC surface or in a patient's serum.

The direct antiglobulin test (DAT), or the direct Coombs' test, detects antibody or complement that is coating RBC and may be positive in a variety of settings, including hemolytic transfusion reactions (for which it is the single most important assay), hemolytic disease of the newborn, autoimmune hemolytic anemia (including secondary to medical drugs), after administration of immune globulins (passively acquired), and post marrow or organ transplant (donor's lymphocytes producing antibody to red cells of the recipient).

A positive DAT does not necessarily indicate in vivo hemolysis or shortened RBC survival. False-positive results may occur with hypergammaglobulinemia because rouleaux formation may be mistaken for agglutination.

The indirect antiglobulin test (IAT), or indirect Coombs' test, is the method used in the antibody screen portion of a "type and screen" and in the serologic cross-match (patient serum and donor/reagent red cells). The IAT detects antibody present in the serum but not bound to the RBC. When the IAT is positive, antibody specificity must be identified and the corresponding antigen always avoided in transfusions. A negative antibody screen (IAT) does not necessarily indicate absence of alloantibodies: the titer of antibody may be below the level of detection or the antibody may be directed against a low incidence antigen (present in less than 10% of individuals), not present on reagent testing cells but expressed on patient cells. A negative IAT does not guarantee that blood is compatible, nor does a weak IAT indicate that hemolysis is likely to be mild. Regardless, a positive IAT demands further investigation.

In autoimmune hemolytic anemia, in which the antibody may be present in the serum and on the RBC of the patient, both the DAT and IAT may be positive.

BLOOD COMPATIBILITY

In general, blood components that contain more than 2 mL of RBC must be compatible with the patient's plasma. Particular attention is paid to Rh type because less than 1 mL of RBC, a volume found in most platelet concentrates, is sufficient to sensitize an Rh-negative patient (1). Plasma-containing components, including platelet preparations, should be ABO compatible with the patient's RBC when possible to prevent passive antibodies in the plasma from causing hemolysis of recipient red cells (Table 24.1).

The most basic practical application of blood group serology involves the selection of compatible blood. The absence or presence of blood cell antigens can have important biological and clinical implications.

TABLE 24.1. *Compatibility of Recipient Blood with Donor Blood Components*

Patient ABO Group	Whole Blood	Red Blood Cells	Platelets	Plasma	Cryoprecipitate
O	O	O	Any (O preferred)	O, A, B, AB	N/A
A	A	A or O	Any (A preferred)	A or AB	N/A
B	B	B or O	Any (B preferred)	B or AB	N/A
AB	AB	AB, A, B, or O	Any (AB preferred)	AB	N/A

Compatible blood takes time to prepare. In an emergency, group O RBC may be released uncross-matched with the consent of the requesting physician; testing will be completed after release. Group-specific red cells (group A for group A patient, and so on) and an abbreviated cross-match can be prepared in 15 minutes. Fully tested red cells can be prepared in 45 to 60 minutes; cryopreserved RBC and fresh-frozen plasma (FFP) may take longer.

Alloimmunized patients pose a particular problem; patient blood specimens should be submitted well in advance of elective procedures for a "type and screen," which will identify most compatibility difficulties. After 3 days, a new sample will be needed to detect newly appearing antibodies, especially when the patient has been pregnant or transfused within the previous 3 months.

ABO INCOMPATIBILITY IN TRANSPLANT SETTINGS

Hematopoietic stem cell (HSCT) transplantation relies on compatibility at the major histocompatibility locus, so that selection of the recipient-donor pair is determined by similarity of human leukocyte antigens (HLA) at the expense of ABO compatibility. Because HLA and ABO genes are inherited independently, some (20% to 40%) of these transplants will be ABO incompatible (1).

Whereas ABO incompatibility does not appear to impact graft failure, mismatches can cause immediate hemolysis, delayed RBC engraftment, or delayed hemolysis based on the nature of ABO incompatibility between the recipient and donor (2–5).

Minor Incompatibility

Donor's serum contains antibodies against RBC antigens of the recipient (e.g., recipient blood group A, B, or AB and donor blood group O, and so forth). Prior to infusion of the stem cell preparation, plasma containing anti-A and anti-B can be removed to prevent immediate postinfusion hemolysis of the recipient's RBC. Of minor ABO-incompatible transplant recipients, 10% to 15% may experience abrupt onset of hemolysis 7 to 10 days posttransplant when immune-competent B lymphocytes in the graft mount a response against the recipient RBC antigens. Hemolysis may be severe or even fatal unless recognized promptly.

Major Incompatibility

Recipient's serum contains antibodies against the RBC antigens of the donor (e.g., recipient group O and donor group A, B, or AB; recipient group A or B and donor group AB). Hemolysis of RBC in the stem cell preparation upon infusion may occur if the graft is not processed to remove RBC prior to infusion. Posttransplant, the recipient may produce antibodies against donor red cell antigens for months, especially with nonmyeloablative regimens. RBC engraftment and erythropoiesis may be delayed, resulting in red cell aplasia (5,6).

Minor and major (bidirectional) incompatibility between the donor and recipient occurs when each has antibodies against the ABO blood group antigens of the other (such as recipient's blood group is A and that of the donor is B, or vice versa).

Table 24.2 describes appropriate transfusion management during transplantation. All transfusions must be irradiated.

Rh Incompatibility

Rh incompatibility occurs in 10% to 15% of stem cell transplants. Transfusion practice is analogous to that of major and minor ABO incompatibility, but the consequences are less severe.

For Rh-negative recipients of Rh-positive hematopoietic stem cell preparations, RBC from the donor should be removed to decrease risk of alloimmunization similar to ABO major incompatibility.

For Rh-positive recipients from Rh-negative donors previously alloimmunized to the Rh antigen, monitor the patient for signs of delayed hemolysis (as in minor incompatibility).

TABLE 24.2. *Transfusion in Minor and Major ABO Incompatible Transplants*

Minor Mismatch

		PHASE I		PHASE II		PHASE III
RECIPIENT	DONOR	All components	RBC	Platelets	FFP	All components
A	O	Recipient group	O	A; *AB; B; O*	A; *AB*	Donor group
B	O	Recipient group	O	B; *AB; A; O*	B; *AB*	Donor group
AB	O	Recipient group	O	AB; *A; B; O*	AB	Donor group
AB	A	Recipient group	A	AB; *A; B; O*	AB	Donor group
AB	B	Recipient group	B	AB; *B; A; O*	AB	Donor group

Major Mismatch

		PHASE I		PHASE II		PHASE III
RECIPIENT	DONOR	All components	RBC	Platelets	FFP	All components
O	A	Recipient group	O	A; *AB; B; O*	A; *AB*	Donor group
O	B	Recipient group	O	B; *AB; A; O*	B; *AB*	Donor group
O	AB	Recipient group	O	AB; *A; B; O*	AB	Donor group
A	AB	Recipient group	A	AB; *A; B; O*	AB	Donor group
B	AB	Recipient group	B	AB; *B; A; O*	AB	Donor group

Minor and Major Mismatch

		PHASE I		PHASE II		PHASE III
RECIPIENT	DONOR	All components	RBC	Platelets	FFP	All components
A	B	Recipient group	O	AB; *A; B; O*	AB	Donor group
B	A	Recipient group	O	AB; *B; A; O*	AB	Donor group

Phase I = From time patient is prepared for hematopoietic progenitor cell transplant.
Phase II = From initiation of myeloablative therapy from the time DAT is negative and isohemagglutinins against donor are no longer detectable (for RBC) or when the recipient's erythrocytes are no longer detectable.
Phase III = After the forward and reverse type of the patient are consistent with donor ABO group.
Italicized blood groups indicate next best choice in order of preference.
All cellular components should be irradiated.
Modified from Brecher ME, ed. *Technical Manual*, 15th Ed. Bethesda, MD: AABB Press; 2005:600, with permission; and from Friedberg RC, Andrzejewski C. Transfusion therapy in hematopoietic stem cell transplantation. In Mintz PD, ed. *Transfusion Therapy: Clinical Principles and Practice*, 2nd Ed. Bethesda, MD: AABB Press; 2005.

BLOOD COMPONENTS AND DERIVATIVES

Blood Components and Transfusion Therapy

Blood components can be separated from whole blood by centrifugation or by apheresis. Approximately 29 million blood components (RBCs, platelets, plasma, cryoprecipitate) are transfused annually in the United States.

As with any medical treatment, blood transfusion requires informed consent. Patients must be advised of the indications and common adverse events as well as any potential alternatives to allogeneic transfusion. Most adverse transfusion reactions occur in the first 15 minutes. Administration of blood products should start slowly under close observation. The time of transfusion should not exceed 4 hours as the risk of bacterial growth increases with time at room temperature; if transfusion is anticipated to take longer, the transfusion service can divide the unit into smaller aliquots. See Table 24.3 for blood component administration.

Whole blood and other cellular blood components may be infused with isotonic solutions: USP 0.9% NaCl (normal saline) and certain Food and Drug Administration (FDA) approved electrolyte solutions. Cellular blood products must never be infused with hypertonic or hypotonic solutions, solutions containing glucose or calcium such as D5W (5% dextrose in water) or lactated Ringer's; hemolysis, clotting, or agglutination of RBC may result if cellular blood components are infused with hypertonic or hypotonic solutions. Medications should never be added to blood components.

TABLE 24.3. *Blood Component Administration per NIH Practice**

	Whole Blood	Packed RBC	Granulocytes	Platelets	Plasma
ADULTS					
First 15 minutes **Subsequently**	2 mL/min 100–230 mL/hr	2 mL/min 100–230 mL/hr	2 mL/min 75–100 mL/hr	2–5 mL/min 200–300 mL/hr	2–5 mL/min 200–300 mL/hr
PEDIATRIC					
First 5 minutes	N/A	N/A	N/A	5% of total volume† ordered for transfusion	5% of total volume† ordered for transfusion
First 15 minutes	5% of total volume† ordered for transfusion	5% of total volume† ordered for transfusion	5% of total volume ordered for transfusion	N/A	N/A
Subsequently	Variable (as tolerated)	2–5 mL/kg/hr	Over 2–3 hours (for a 200 mL product)	As tolerated	1–2 mL/min

*Flow rates are guidelines to be adjusted to patient tolerance.
†Volume ordered for pediatric transfusion should be based on the child's weight (10–15 mL blood product/kg); excludes granulocyte transfusion.

Blood components should be infused through standard 170–260 μm infusion filters to remove any clots that form during storage. An approved infusion pump may be used for strict control of transfusion rate; nonapproved pumps may damage or hemolyze cells.

Warming devices with internal monitors have been designed for blood to avoid transfusion of large volumes of cold fluid. Blood components should never be warmed in uncertified devices (like microwave ovens or water baths) as lethal hemolysis may occur.

Bedside leukoreduction filters may be used when leukoreduction is indicated for whole blood, packed RBCs, and platelets that have not been leukocyte reduced prior to storage. Blood should filter by gravity. Hypotensive reactions have been associated with bedside leukoreduction, especially in patients receiving angiotensin converting enzyme (ACE) inhibitors. *Granulocyte concentrates must never be infused through leukoreduction filters—these filters are designed to remove white blood cells.* See Table 24.4 for indications for additional modifications to blood components.

Storage conditions for different blood components vary and are designed to maximize preservation and effectiveness. Red cells are refrigerated (at 1–6°C) for up to 42 days. Platelets are stored at room temperature and become outdated in 5 days. Plasma components are stored frozen for a year (at −18°C) or more (at −65°C), but must be thawed before use and are often not immediately available. If transfusion of a component is not started, the blood should be returned to storage (or blood bank) within 30 minutes of issue to minimize wastage. Also, blood components should not be stored in unmonitored refrigerators in nursing units or surgical suites as the risk for administration of blood components to the wrong patient increases when blood is stored in satellite refrigerators.

As with any medical treatment, blood transfusion requires informed consent. Patients must be advised of the indications and common adverse events as well as any potential alternatives to allogeneic transfusion. Patients with religious concerns about blood transfusion must be informed of any human-derived contents in any products that may be administered, allowing them to make an informed decision.

Whole Blood

A unit of whole blood typically has a volume of 450 to 500 mL and a hematocrit of 35% to 45%. Whole blood is rarely available and infrequently used. Indications include acute hypovolemia with red cell loss, massive transfusion, and exchange transfusion. Whole blood is not indicated for chronic anemia (in which blood volume is often increased).

Whole blood is not a source of functional platelets or granulocytes, which deteriorate in less than 24 hours at refrigerator temperatures.

Red Blood Cells

Red blood cells (RBC) are separated from whole blood by centrifugation. A unit of RBC contains approximately 200 mL and a hematocrit of 60% to 80%. In general, 1 unit of packed RBC will increase the hemoglobin (Hb) by 1 g/dL in an average-sized adult. In the average pediatric patient, transfusion of 8 to 10 mL/kg of RBC is expected to increase hemoglobin by 3 g/dL. Hb determination is frequently used to determine the transfusion trigger. However, the decision to transfuse should be based on assessment of symptoms, coexisting or underlying medical conditions, and the cause of the anemia. The single adequately powered prospective study (intensive care unit [ICU] patients) and numerous observational studies indicated that patients with cardiovascular disease are particularly sensitive to anemia and do better at a higher Hb level (7,8).

RBC are indicated for treatment of symptomatic anemia. In general, patients are transfused if the Hb falls below 6 g/dL, and transfusion is rarely considered when it exceeds 10 g/dL; the interval between these values is the area of controversy. Practice guidelines support an Hb level of less than 7 g/dL as generally acceptable for the initiation of RBC transfusion in symptomatic patients (8,9). Patients at particular risk of bleeding (thrombocytopenia, recent hemorrhage) should be maintained at a higher Hb.

RBC should not be transfused for volume expansion or nutritional purposes. Transfusion is rarely indicated in otherwise treatable anemia, including anemia associated with B_{12}, iron, or folate deficiency; if symptoms are severe, these patients may benefit from a single-unit transfusion as the underlying cause is corrected.

Platelets

Platelets may be separated from whole blood shortly after collection (random donor or whole blood-derived platelet concentrates) or collected by apheresis (single donor or apheresis platelets). A therapeutic dose of platelets for an adult is 1 unit of platelets (5.5×10^{10} platelets) per 10 kg of body weight, which should increase the platelet count in an average-sized adult by approximately 5000/μL. Each apheresis (single-donor) platelet product is expected to contain approximately 3×10^{11} platelets, roughly equivalent to 4 to 6 units of random donor platelets. Indications for use are the same for both preparations, except for immunized refractory patients who may require single-donor HLA-matched and compatible platelets. Single-donor platelets offer the additional advantage of decreased donor exposure and a lower risk of bacterial sepsis.

Indications for platelets include bleeding associated with thrombocytopenia, rapid decrease in platelet counts, qualitative platelet defects, or as prophylaxis for major bleeding in severely thrombocytopenic patients.

Platelets are not indicated for bleeding unassociated with thrombocytopenia (except for the unusual patient with a clinically significant platelet function defect), other defects in hemostasis (such as factor deficiencies), or platelet dysfunction caused by many common medications (aspirin, penicillins, nonsteroidal anti-inflammatory drugs [NSAIDs]).

TABLE 24.4. *Indications for Additional Modifications of Cellular Blood Components*

Leukoreduction	Irradiation (Red Blood Cells, Platelets, Granulocytes)	Washing (Plasma Removal)	Volume Reduction	Freezing-Deglycerolization (Red Blood Cells)
Description Filtration of component after collection, at bedside, or removal of WBC during automated collection for a 3 log (99.9%) WBC reduction Final WBC content $\leq 5 \times 10^6$	**Description** Gamma irradiation (cesium or cobalt) of cellular component with 2500 cGy to inactivate viable lymphocytes within component	**Description** Component washed with sterile normal saline to remove >98% of plasma proteins, electrolytes, and antibodies WBC content 5×10^8	**Description** Removal of plasma from cellular components (mainly platelets; RBC concentrates have very little plasma)	**Description** Addition of glycerol and freezing generally within 6 days of collection (depending on the additive solution used at the time of collection and glycerolization-freezing method used)
Purpose Reduction of febrile nonhemolytic transfusion reactions (FNHTR) Reduction of CMV transmission (CMV-safe) Reduction of HLA alloimmunization	**Purpose** Prevention of transfusion-associated graft-versus-host disease	**Purpose** Prevention of allergic reactions Decrease risk of hyperkalemia	**Purpose** Reduction of circulatory overload Removal of antibodies	**Purpose** Long-term storage of autologous or allogeneic rare blood phenotypes
Indications Patients who have experienced an episode of FNHTR Alternative to CMV-seronegative components (from donor tested negative for CMV) for at-risk patients such as neonates and transplant patients	**Indications** Recipients of bone marrow/hematopoietic stem cell transplants Recipients of transfusion from blood relatives Patients on immunosuppressive regimens, particularly with purine analogues Patients with congenital immunodeficiencies and certain malignancies Patients with B-cell malignancies Hodgkin's lymphoma	**Indications** Patients who experience recurrent severe allergic reactions (not responsive to premedication with antihistamines) IgA deficient patients when IgA-deficient component is not available Recipients at risk from hyperkalemia such as newborns and fetuses receiving intrauterine transfusions	**Indications** Patients with expanded plasma volume such as those with normovolemic chronic anemia, thalassemia major, sickle cell disease, congestive heart failure Pediatric, elderly, and other patients susceptible to volume overload	**Indications** Patients with rare blood phenotypes or multiple alloantibodies
			Comments Platelets must be used within 4 hours of volume reduction because of decrease in amount of plasma/volume remaining for optimal platelet metabolism	**Comments** May *not* be feasible for red blood cells with certain abnormalities such as HbS, hereditary spherocytosis, and PNH Depending on the method of glycerolization-freezing used, open or closed system, postdeglycerolization shelf life may be 24 hours or 2 weeks, respectively

Comments
Equivalent to CMV
seronegative
components

*Not effective and not
indicated for prevention of
transfusion-associated
graft-versus-host disease*

Intrauterine transfusion

Premature infants,
especially those
undergoing
extracorporeal
membrane oxygenation

Granulocyte transfusions

Comments
RBC shelf life is decreased
to 28 days (if greater
than the original
expiration date), but
platelet or granulocyte
shelf life is not affected

*Not indicated for
prevention of FNHTR and
unnecessary for patients
with aplastic anemia
(despite ATG therapy) or
patients with HIV in the
absence of other
indications for irradiation
(above)*

May be effective when
ABO identical blood is
not available for patients
with paroxysmal
nocturnal hemoglobinuria
(PNH)

Comments
Washing results in a
15%–20% loss of red
cells or platelets

Red blood cells must be
used within 24 hours and
platelets must be used
within 4 hours of
washing because of
increased risk of
contamination
associated with opening
of a closed system

*Not equivalent to
"leukoreduced"*

*Not equivalent to washing
for prevention of allergic
reactions*

*Not equivalent
to "leukoreduced" (may
remove >95% of WBC)*

ATG, antithymocyte globulin; CMV, cytomegalovirus; HIV, human immunodeficiency virus; HLA, human leukocyte antigen; RBC, red blood cells; WBC, white blood cells.

TABLE 24.5. *Guidelines for Platelet Transfusion per National Institutes of Health Practice**

Patient Population	Threshold
Stable aplastic anemia patients	<10,000/μL or bleeding
General oncology patients	<10,000/μL
Stable nononcology patients	<10,000/μL
Posthematopoietic stem cell transplant	<10,000/μL
Aplastic anemia patients receiving ATG	<20,000/μL
Patients undergoing invasive procedures	<50,000/μL
Neurosurgery patients	<100,000/μL

*Prophylaxis of stable patients assumes no additional hemostatic defect or anatomic lesion (recent surgery, documented ulcer).
ATG, antithymocyte globulin.

Platelets are usually contraindicated in thrombotic thrombocytopenic purpura (TTP), because thrombosis is a greater risk than hemorrhage. However, patients with TTP who develop life-threatening hemorrhage may benefit from a cautious trial of platelets.

The threshold for prophylactic platelet transfusion varies based on the patient's underlying condition and likelihood of hemorrhage. A threshold of 10,000/μL is effective in preventing morbidity and mortality from bleeding in stable oncology patients undergoing chemotherapy. A platelet count greater than 50,000/μL is desirable prior to invasive procedures and in the immediate postprocedure period. Platelet counts closer to 100,000/μL may be prudent for patients at high risk of intracranial hemorrhage, such as those with cerebral leukostasis, or when undergoing neurosurgical or ocular procedures. Stable chronically thrombocytopenic patients, such as those with aplastic anemia or myelodysplasia, may tolerate platelet counts as low as 5000/μL in the absence of complicating factors including fever, infection, and additional defects in hemostasis (1).

More aggressive support is indicated for patients who are unstable—febrile, infected, receiving multiple medications—especially if the platelet counts are decreasing (Table 24.5) (1,10).

Platelet transfusions should be monitored by a 1- to 24-hour posttransfusion platelet or complete blood count (CBC) to assess response and guide subsequent transfusion therapy. A corrected count increment (CCI) may be used to determine the increase in platelet count in an individual postplatelet transfusion:

$$CCI = \frac{(Posttransfusion\ platelet\ count^* - pretransfusion\ platelet\ count) \times body\ surface\ area^{**}}{Number\ of\ platelets\ transfused^{***}}$$

*Posttransfusion platelet count, expressed per microliter, is best obtained 15 minutes to 1 hour posttransfusion

**Body surface area = the square root of [(height in cm × weight in kg)/3600], expressed in meters squared

***Expressed as multiples of 1×10^{11}

An absolute posttransfusion increment of 10,000/μL or greater (approximately 2,000/μL per unit of random donor platelets) in an average-sized adult corresponds to a CCI of 5000.

Platelet Refractoriness

Patients who respond poorly to repeated platelet infusions are considered refractory. Posttransfusion platelet counts (1 hour and 24 hour) are critical. Failure to achieve a CCI of 5000 or greater is cause to suspect platelet refractoriness. Refractoriness may be immune or nonimmune mediated.

Nonimmune-mediated causes of platelet refractoriness include fever, infection, splenomegaly, disseminated intravascular coagulation (DIC), massive bleeding, and medications that enhance platelet destruction; more likely to affect the 24-hour, rather than the 1-hour, posttransfusion count.

Immune-mediated causes of platelet refractoriness include repeated transfusions, especially with nonleukocyte-reduced platelets and multiparity (alloimmunization to HLA and human platelet antigens); detected by the 1-hour posttransfusion count.

Platelets and granulocytes also have antigens to which an antigen-negative individual may become alloimmunized.

In practice, the distinction between immune- and nonimmune-mediated platelet refractoriness is less clear. When immune-mediated platelet refractoriness is suspected and CCI is less than 5000 after each of two platelet transfusions, the following steps should be taken. ABO-compatible fresh (less than 72 hours in storage) platelets should be used for two subsequent transfusions. If CCI does not exceed 5000, HLA antibody screen should be performed to detect alloantibodies, or commercial platelet compatibility tests should be performed. If HLA antibodies are detected, HLA-compatible platelets should be tried. When alloantibodies with broad specificity are found (for HLA A and B loci) platelets from HLA-matched donors are indicated. Cross-match compatible platelets may be beneficial when HLA antibody status of the recipient cannot be determined, HLA-matched platelets cannot be obtained, or when the patient is refractory to HLA-matched platelets (up to 40% to 50% of cases). Corticosteroids, washed platelets, or intravenous immunoglobulin (IVIg) have not proved useful in the treatment of refractoriness.

Granulocytes

Granulocytes are collected by apheresis for specific patients, from donors who are mobilized prior to collection with corticosteroids and/or cytokines (granulocyte colony-stimulating factor [G-CSF]) to enhance collection.

Granulocytes can be stored at room temperature for only up to 24 hours postcollection. Granulocyte collections have a volume of 250 mL and contain plasma, approximately 30 mL RBC, and variable amounts of mononuclear leukocytes and platelets. Granulocyte concentrates should be ABO, Rh, and RBC cross-match compatible. The minimal therapeutic dose is greater than 1×10^{10} granulocytes/unit; however, granulocyte increments are unlikely to be measured unless three to four times this number are infused (1).

Granulocytes are indicated for neutropenia in patients with expected marrow recovery who have an absolute neutrophil count (ANC) of less than 0.5×10^9/L and documented infection not responding to appropriate antibiotics after 24 to 48 hours, or defective granulocyte function despite normal counts (as in chronic granulomatous disease). Infants with bacterial sepsis whose granulocyte counts are less than 3×10^9/L with postmitotic neutrophils comprising less than 10% of their nucleated marrow cells, may benefit from granulocyte transfusions (1).

A 1- to 6-hour posttransfusion CBC with differential for determination of ANC may help assess efficacy. The posttransfusion increment in ANC varies based on the granulocyte content of the transfused unit. Because granulocytes traffic to the lungs before equilibrating in peripheral blood, a 6-hour posttransfusion increment may be higher than a 1-hour posttransfusion ANC. If the patient's ANC fails to reach expected levels or if a reaction occurs, investigation, including an HLA antibody screen and tests for antibodies to human neutrophil antigens (HNA), is indicated.

Granulocyte transfusion is not indicated in the absence of the above criteria and is contraindicated in patients with prior severe pulmonary reactions to HLA or HNA or serologic HLA or HNA incompatibility (alloimmunization). Alloimmunized patients may develop chills, fever, rigors, shortness of breath, wheezing, pulmonary infiltrates, cyanosis, and hypotension (6,11); rigors and fever may respond to intravenous meperidine (25 mg). Pulmonary toxicity may be exacerbated when granulocytes and amphotericin B are administered in close temporal proximity (12). At the National Institutes of Health (NIH), amphotericin B administration and granulocyte transfusions are separated by at least 4 hours.

Granulocyte concentrates may contain leukocyte-associated pathogens such as cytomegalovirus (CMV), a particular concern for immunosuppressed stem cell transplant recipients, solid organ transplant recipients, neonates undergoing extracorporeal membrane oxygenation, and low-birth-weight and premature infants.

Granulocyte transfusion therapy should be evaluated after an initial course of four infusions and then periodically. While granulocyte transfusions decrease the length of bacterial infection, proof that granulocyte transfusions decrease mortality in any situation has been elusive.

Fresh Frozen Plasma

Plasma separated from whole blood or collected by apheresis and frozen within 8 hours is labeled *fresh frozen* plasma (FFP). FFP contains most plasma proteins at the time of thaw at about the same concentration as at the time of collection. The volume of a unit of plasma is approximately 200 mL.

By convention, 1 mL of FFP is expected to provide 1 unit of activity of all factors (except labile factors V and VIII). In practice, individual units may vary in content. To increase factor levels by 20%, the dose used in replacement of coagulation factors is approximately 10 to 20 mL/kg in adults (equivalent to approximately 4 to 6 units of FFP).

FFP is indicated in the correction of multiple clotting factor deficiencies in patients who are bleeding or scheduled for an invasive procedure, replacement of factors consumed in DIC, coagulation factor deficiencies caused by liver disease, coagulation factors diluted by replacement fluids during massive transfusion, replacement fluid in the treatment (plasma exchange) of thrombotic thrombocytopenic purpura (TTP), rapid reversal of warfarin (Coumadin) effect, and replacement of congenital factor deficiencies when the specific factor concentrate is not available (as for replacement of factors II, V, X, XI).

An international normalized ratio (INR) greater than 1.6 or activated partial thromboplastin time (aPTT) greater than 1.5 times the upper range of normal (factor level activity less than 30%) is a guide to consider treatment (9,13).

FFP is not indicated for volume expansion or protein replacement in nutritional deficiencies; crystalloids and colloids and synthetic volume expanders can be used for that purpose without exposing the recipient to transfusion-associated acute lung injury (TRALI) or infectious disease risks.

Cryoprecipitate

Cryoprecipitate (cryo) is the cold-insoluble portion of plasma containing high-molecular-weight glycoproteins. Ordinarily stored frozen, cryoprecipitate can be kept at room temperature for up to 6 hours; on pooling, it must be transfused within 4 hours. Compatibility testing is unnecessary. A unit of cryoprecipitate is usually less than 15 mL of plasma and contains more than 80 international units (IU) of factor VIII (antihemophilic factor), more than 150 mg of fibrinogen, and approximately 30% of the factor XIII of the original plasma; cryoprecipitate also contains von Willebrand complex activity. One unit of cryoprecipitate can increase fibrinogen in an average adult by 5 to 10 mg/dL. A therapeutic dose for an adult is 80 to 150 mL of cryoprecipitate (8 to 10 units pooled).

Cryoprecipitate is indicated for the treatment of fibrinogen deficiency, dysfibrinogenemia, factor XIII deficiency, DIC, and urgent treatment of hemophilia A and von Willebrand disease in the absence of factor VIII concentrate or recombinant factor VIII. Cryoprecipitate has also been used to correct the platelet defect of uremic bleeding, although with variable success.

The dosage of cryoprecipitate depends on the underlying deficiency and on the plasma volume of the patient. To determine the number of bags of cryoprecipitate to replace fibrinogen:

$$\frac{(\text{Desired fibrinogen level mg/dL} - \text{initial fibrinogen level mg/dL}) \times \text{patient's plasma volume dL}^{*}}{250 \text{ mg (fibrinogen per cryo bag)}}$$

*The plasma volume for an average adult = (1 − percent hematocrit/100) × patient weight in kg × 70 mL/kg. For infants and children under 40 kg, the plasma volume = (1 − percent hematocrit/100) × patient weight in kg × 80 to 85 mL/kg.

Cryoprecipitate is not called for in the absence of specific hemostatic abnormality for which it is indicated (see previous text) or for which specific factor concentrates/recombinant factor preparations (e.g., factor VIII) are available.

Hematopoietic Stem and Progenitor Cells

Hematopoietic stem and progenitor cells and umbilical cord blood are commonly collected and stored by blood banks. *Progenitor or stem cells* that were originally derived from bone marrow harvests are now often collected from the peripheral blood, referred to as peripheral blood stem cells

(PBSC), via apheresis for reconstitution of hematopoiesis and immune function in patients with a variety of malignancies and immune disorders.

The number of circulating progenitor cells is increased by mobilizing the donor with hematopoietic growth factors, most often G-CSF, or in autologous transplants, a combination of chemotherapy and growth factors. The degree of mobilization and the probability of a successful collection are best predicted by measuring circulating cells that express the membrane glycoprotein CD34, a marker for stem cells. Where this assay is not available, total white blood cell (WBC) and mononuclear cell count have been used (14,15).

Standard collections of allogeneic PBSC involve 3 to 4 hours per apheresis procedure, during which approximately 10 L of blood are processed. Two to four collections are usual, but large volumes of 25 to 30 L are more efficient and are used increasingly to allow complete collections with a single procedure (16).

While PBSC apheresis collections are generally well tolerated, side effects associated with the several-day administration of growth factor are common: bone pain, headache, fatigue, insomnia, and gastrointestinal disturbances usually respond to administration of acetaminophen or NSAIDs, and cease after the growth factor injections. Vascular complications and citrate toxicity are not unlike those experienced in other long apheresis procedures (see below). With cell mobilization, splenomegaly occurs frequently and splenic rupture has been reported as a rare complication; PBSC donors should be advised to refrain from contact sports for a few weeks after the last mobilization (17).

PBSC grafts are infused as fresh collections or stored frozen with the cryoprotectant dimethyl sulfoxide (DMSO) in liquid nitrogen. Thawed cells infused with DMSO may cause nausea, vomiting, fever, dyspnea, and anaphylaxis. Reactions are dose dependent and may be lessened by prophylactic antihistamines. PBSCs carry the risk of transfusion-transmitted infectious agents and are tested in the same manner as are other blood components. However, given their highly specialized use and their life-saving potential, exceptions are made to donor selection criteria normally used for allogeneic blood collections, with concurrence of the treating physician and the recipient.

Adequate cell dose for engraftment depends on whether the procedure is an autograft, a related, or an unrelated allograft. Cell dose, cell source, and patient characteristics are all important variables. The dose of stem cells for unrelated donors (National Marrow Donor Program) is 2 to 4 $\times$ 10^8 nucleated cells per kilogram of recipient weight (18), with 2 to 4 $\times$ 10^6 CD34+ cells per kilogram of recipient weight deemed as an adequate dose for transplantation and doses of greater than 5 $\times$ 10^6 CD34+ cells per kilogram of recipient weight associated with more rapid engraftment (18). Lower doses may be adequate in related donor settings, but engraftment of both leukocytes and platelets correlates with CD34 cell content.

Cord blood frozen in liquid nitrogen is obtained from the placenta during the third stage of delivery or postdelivery, with the consent of the mother, and stored in liquid nitrogen. The component volume is usually 50 to 100 mL and may be further reduced by removing red cells and plasma. HLA type is determined and used as a search criterion for cord blood. The small volumes and yields of CD34+ progenitor cells currently make cord blood most suitable for children and smaller adults, although simultaneous infusion of two and even three cord blood units have resulted in successful engraftment for larger adults (19). PBSCs stored in liquid nitrogen likely remain stable for many years, but maximum safe storage periods have not been determined. Recipients of minor mismatched cord blood seem less likely to make red cell alloantibodies than do recipients of mismatched marrow or PBSC.

Blood Derivatives

Derivatives or *blood products* are produced commercially by fractionation of plasma and include colloids such as albumin and plasma protein fraction, immune globulins, coagulation factor concentrates, and a variety of orphan proteins such as α-1-antitrypsin and antithrombin (Table 24.6).

Rh Immune Globulin

Rh immune globulin (RhIg) is available in intramuscular (IM) form and intravenous (IV) form.

TABLE 24.6. Selected Blood Derivatives

Derivative	Indications	Cautions	Derivation	Content
Albumin 5% solution	**Hypovolemia** Volume expansion **Acute liver failure** Osmotic pressure Binding excess bilirubin **Cardiopulmonary bypass surgery** Hemodilution	Patients at risk of hypervolemia	Pooled human plasma concentrated by fractionation and treated to nearly eliminate risk of virus transmission Osmotically and oncotically equivalent to plasma	At least 95% albumin and the remainder globulins and other proteins 145 mEq/L sodium
Albumin 25% solution	**Maintenance of plasma colloid osmotic pressure** Can be given 24 hours after extensive burns treated initially with crystalloids **Binding excess free bilirubin** Can decrease risk of kernicterus when given prior to exchange transfusion for hemolytic disease of the newborn	Patients at risk of hypervolemia Hyperoncotic	Pooled human plasma concentrated by fractionation and treated to nearly eliminate risk of virus transmission Hyperoncotic	At least 95% albumin and the remainder globulins and other proteins 145 mEq/L sodium
PPF* (Available only as 5% solution)	**Similar to 5% albumin**	Hypotension Administration at greater than 10 mL/min, especially in patients taking angiotensin converting enzyme (ACE) inhibitors **Contraindication** Intra-arterial administration in cardiopulmonary bypass setting	Similar to 5% albumin	At least 83% albumin and the remainder globulins and other proteins 145 mEq/L sodium

| IVIg[†] | **Prophylaxis**
Passive immunity and passive antibody
Replacement
Primary immunodeficiencies
Immunomodulation
Some autoimmune disorders (e.g., refractory ITP)
Treatment of certain infectious disorders
Pediatric HIV infection, CMV interstitial pneumonitis posthematopoietic transplantation
Thrombocytopenia related to HIV
Neurological disorders
Guillain-Barré syndrome and chronic inflammatory demyelinating polyneuropathy
Relative indications
Posttransfusion purpura
Neonatal alloimmune thrombocytopenia
Refractory warm type autoimmune hemolytic anemia | Attenuated vaccines should not be administered in close temporal association with attenuated vaccines (3 months)
Rapid administration
IgA deficiency
IgA-deficient patients must receive immune globulins from IgA deficient donors only
Route of administration
Intramuscular immune globulins must never be administered intravenously
Intravenous immune globulins should not be administered intramuscularly | Pooled human plasma concentrated by fractionation and treated to nearly eliminate risk of virus transmission | 90% IgG, trace IgM, trace IgA
Half life in preparation: 18–32 days |

Other plasma derivatives include antithrombin complex, protein C concentrate, C1-esterase inhibitor, α-1-proteinase inhibitor, and factor XIII (currently not licensed in the United States), which are indicated for the corresponding specific deficiencies.

From Klein HG, Anstee DJ. *Mollison's Blood Transfusion in Clinical Medicine*, 11th Ed. Oxford: Blackwell Publishing Ltd; 2005.
*Plasma protein fraction.
[†]Intravenous immune globulin.
CMV, cytomegalovirus; HIV, human immunodeficiency virus; ITP, immune thrombocytopenic purpura.

RhIg is indicated in the prevention of alloimmunization of Rh-negative recipients exposed to Rh-positive RBC and in the prevention of development of anti-D by pregnant Rh-negative women with Rh-positive fetuses and subsequent hemolytic disease of the newborn. There is a greater than 90% success in preventing Rh alloimmunization in pregnancy; failure is usually because of missed or insufficient injections. RhIg is used in the treatment of immune thrombocytopenic purpura (ITP) in Rh-positive patients only (intravenous RhIg).

Intramuscular RhIg is used in Rh-negative subjects after exposure to small-volume Rh-positive RBC (with platelet transfusions or the accidental transfusion of an Rh-positive unit of RBC). RhIg IV is used for large volume exposures.

Use of RhIg in males and postmenopausal females depends on the magnitude of exposure, the possibility the individual may require transfusion in the future, and the likelihood that the individual will form antibody (anti-D). For large exposures requiring many doses of RhIg, treatment may not be feasible, especially if the patient is unlikely to become pregnant, form antibody (debilitated because of hematologic malignancy such as leukemia, or solid tumors), or to be retransfused.

RhIg dose should be calculated based on the RBC volume transfused in the event of erroneous transfusion and transfusion of platelets or granulocytes that contain Rh-positive red blood cells, and based on the amount of Rh-positive fetal red blood cells in the maternal circulation in the event of fetal-maternal hemorrhage during pregnancy. A full dose of RhIg contains 300 μg of anti-D to cover an exposure of 15 mL of Rh-positive RBC and is usually administered to postpartum women within 72 hours of delivery and to pregnant women after amniocentesis or chorionic villus sampling performed at more than 34 weeks of gestation. A minidose contains 50 μg of anti-D to cover an exposure of 2.5 mL of Rh-positive RBC and is administered after delivery or abortion of a fetus at less than 12 weeks of gestation or after amniocentesis or chorionic villus sampling at less than 34 weeks of gestation.

The half-life of RhIg is 21 days. Additional RhIg should be administered in situations where there is expected ongoing risk of fetomaternal hemorrhage or in nonobstetric cases with additional transfusion of products containing Rh-positive RBC 21days or more after the last dose of RhIg.

If RhIg has not been given within 72 hours of a sensitizing event, it should still be administered as soon as the need is recognized for up to 28 days. The mechanism of action of RhIg is unknown (20).

RhIg is not indicated for use in Rh-positive individuals (except in the treatment of Rh-positive ITP patients), Rh-negative individuals who have developed anti-D from prior exposure, pregnancy in Rh-negative females with known Rh-negative fetuses or newborns, or in Rh-negative patients with ITP.

Derivative and Recombinant Coagulation Factors

Recombinant and plasma-derived coagulation factors provide a concentrated source of the desired factor in a fraction of volume of FFP. Recombinant factors contain no other human-derived products and no risk of viral disease transmission (Table 24.7).

TRANSFUSION REACTIONS AND ADVERSE SEQUELAE

Any adverse response to blood component transfusion is considered a transfusion reaction. Most reactions occur at the beginning or during transfusion. Others, including development of alloantibodies, iron overload, and some parasitic and viral infections, do not become apparent for months or years.

Because most transfusion reactions occur within 15 minutes, early, close monitoring of vital signs and status may prevent more severe reactions. If a reaction is suspected, the infusion should be halted, the transfusion service notified, appropriate samples collected, and the patient continued to be monitored.

Transfusion reactions are generally classified as hemolytic versus nonhemolytic and acute versus delayed. Hemolytic reactions may be immune-mediated or nonimmune-mediated (Table 24.8).

Acute Hemolytic Transfusion Reaction (Immune-Mediated)

Acute hemolytic transfusion reactions may be severe and fatal. Most result from ABO blood group incompatibility between patient plasma and donor RBC and may involve mistransfusion of a unit (or several units) of blood intended for another patient.

TABLE 24.7. *Selected Coagulation Factor Preparations*

Coagulation Factor	Content	Indications	Risks and Cautions
Recombinant factor VIIa* (rVIIa)	Activated coagulation factor VII	**Licensed use:** Refractory hemophilia A or B High factor VIII or IX inhibitor levels in hemophilia A or B bleeding episodes in patients with factor VII deficiency **Used successfully:** Severe bleeding refractory to other therapy Glanzmann's thrombasthenia	Increased risk of thrombosis, particularly in patients with DIC and atherosclerotic cardiovascular disease Allergic reactions Hypertension
Factor VIII concentrate	Factor VIII Humate P (CSL Behring, King of Prussia, PA) has vWF	Hemophilia A Factor VIII deficiency (other than hemophilia A) von Willebrand disease	Development of factor VIII inhibitor (10% of severely hemophilic patients) Viral transmission potential (small) Hemolysis (passive anti-AB antibodies)
Recombinant factor VIII	Factor VIII ReFacto (Wyeth, Madison, NJ) (B domain deleted preparation) does not contain human albumin	Hemophilia A	Albumin-containing preparations have small risk of viral transmission Allergic reactions
Factor IX complex (Prothrombin complex)	Specified amount of concentrated factor IX, and variable amounts of activated factors II, VII, and X, and protein C	Hemophilia B Factor X deficiency (rare) Factor VII deficiency (rare)	Increased risk of thrombosis in liver disease Viral transmission (small) Hemolysis (passive anti-AB antibodies)
Coagulation factor IX	Purified factor IX and nontherapeutic amounts of factors II, VII, and X	Hemophilia B	Less risk of thrombosis than with factor IX concentrate Viral transmission potential (small) Hemolysis (passive anti-AB antibodies)
Recombinant factor IX	Factor IX	Hemophilia B	Less risk of thrombosis than with factor IX concentrate Allergic reactions

*Hemostatic agent
DIC, disseminated intravascular coagulation; vWF, von Willebrand factor.

TABLE 24.8. *Transfusion Reactions*

	Acute/Severe	Delayed/Potentially Severe	Other
Immunologic	Acute hemolytic transfusion reaction Sickle cell hemolytic transfusion syndrome Anaphylaxis Transfusion-related acute lung injury	Delayed hemolytic transfusion reaction (red blood cell antigen alloimmunization) Human leukocyte antigen alloimmunization Transfusion-associated graft versus host	Mild allergic/ urticarial reaction Posttransfusion purpura Febrile non-hemolytic transfusion reaction
Nonimmunologic	Bacterial sepsis Circulatory overload Air embolism	Viral transmission Parasitic transmission Prion transmission Hemosiderosis	Angiotensin con-verting enzyme inhibitor-related hypotension

Presentation: Fever, chills, flank/back pain, dyspnea, chest pain, anxiety, and when severe, hypotension, renal failure, shock, and death

Mechanism: ABO incompatibility resulting from destruction of transfused RBC by preformed, naturally occurring isohemagglutinins (anti-A and/or anti-B antibodies) of the immunoglobulin M (IgM) class in the recipient's plasma. Intravascular hemolysis caused by complement fixation by IgM and hemoglobin is cleared by the kidneys: causing the patient's plasma to become pink and the urine may have a red-brown tinge. Severe hemolysis may result in anemia. Cytokine release contributes to renal failure, hypotension, shock, and DIC.

Evaluation: Submit to the blood bank:

- The infusion set, the implicated unit, and any units transfused within 4 hours of the reaction
- Blood specimens from the patient for repeat ABO group and Rh type determination, cross-match, and DAT (usually positive); assessment of other parameters such as hematocrit (decreased), lactate dehydrogenase (increased), haptoglobin (decreased), and bilirubin levels (increased usually by 6 hours) (1) as indices of hemolysis
- First posttransfusion voided urine to examine for hemoglobinuria
- Transfusion reaction report detailing the events, signs/symptoms, and documenting the patient's pre-transfusion and posttransfusion vital signs

Management: Transfusion must be stopped and disconnected at the hub of the needle and intravenous access maintained with physiologic saline. Blood pressure and renal blood flow should be maintained with fluids and pressors; diuresis should be induced to maintain urine output at greater than 100 mL/hr (6,21). Further transfusion should be withheld until the cause of the reaction is determined. Coagulation status should be monitored.

Prevention: Meticulous clerical check of the blood unit and patient identification. In case of error in patient identification, immediate steps must be taken to insure that a second patient does not receive the wrong unit.

Passive Antibody Infusion

Severe acute hemolysis can occur if large volumes of ABO-incompatible plasma (usually group O FFP or apheresis platelets into group A patient) are infused. Recognition and management of acute anemia is ordinarily sufficient.

Sickle Cell Hemolytic Transfusion Syndrome

Patients with sickle cell anemia are at increased risk from hemolytic transfusion reactions. More profound anemia may develop because of autologous red cell destruction in addition to the destruction of incompatible transfused RBC, and to suppression of erythropoiesis after transfusion (hyperhemolytic syndrome) (1,21,22). Transfusion-associated hemolysis may mimic a severe posttransfusion pain crisis and may be exacerbated by factors such as decreasing hemoglobin, complement activation, and increased oxygen consumption with fever. Additional transfusion may result in exacerbation of the syndrome. In the United States, inherent differences in RBC antigen phenotypes between patients with sickle cell anemia (almost exclusively of African descent) and the majority of blood donors (primarily non-African) place patients with sickle cell anemia at increased risk of alloantibody formation and immune hemolysis. In addition, patients with sickle cell disease are often chronically and heavily transfused. Phenotyping of the red cells of patients with sickle cell anemia in the early stages of transfusion therapy helps to manage alloimmunization and suspected transfusion reactions.

Delayed Hemolytic Transfusion Reaction

Delayed hemolytic transfusion reactions (DHTR) occurs within days to weeks posttransfusion in patients who have been immunized previously (primary immunization) by transfusion or pregnancy. Because its manifestation may be mild and symptoms delayed in onset, DHTR may not be immediately recognized and is therefore likely underreported (21). Death is rare. The importance of recognizing these reactions is to document antibody formation and so prevent severe hemolysis from future transfusions.

Presentation: Fever with or without chills, decreasing hematocrit, hyperbilirubinemia, and jaundice. Subtle decrease in hemoglobin may be the only clinical manifestation. DAT is usually positive. Hemoglobinuria is rare because hemolysis is extravascular.

Mechanism: Repeat stimulation and accelerated (anamnestic) appearance of the antibody in a previously alloimmunized patient upon re-exposure to the offending antigen.

Management: Close monitoring of the patient's Hb level for evidence of continuing hemolysis and supportive therapy.

Prevention: Future transfusions must be antigen-negative for the corresponding implicated antibody even if antibody is no longer detectable. Notification of the patient is necessary to prevent future reactions (as by antibody card or bracelet).

Other Causes of Hemolysis

Other causes of hemolysis temporally associated with transfusion that may mimic hemolytic transfusion reactions include drug-induced hemolysis, mechanical and thermal hemolysis, and hemolysis related to bacterial contamination of the RBC unit. Drug-induced hemolysis may present with anemia, positive DAT, elevated LDH and bilirubin. Hemolysis may be either intravascular or extravascular, so that haptoglobin may be decreased and hemoglobinemia and hemoglobinuria present. Hemolysis may result from administration of blood with hypotonic solutions (D5W, hypotonic saline, distilled water) or medications. Mechanical hemolysis may result from prosthetic heart valves and other intravascular devices and transfusion through small-bore catheters. Thermal hemolysis results from exposure of red cells to cold (ice, temperatures below 1–6°C, use of unmonitored refrigerators) or to temperatures above 42°C (malfunction of blood warmers or unmonitored unconventional blood warming methods); the DAT should be negative in these cases; some of these reactions have been fatal.

Anaphylactic Transfusion Reactions

Anaphylactic transfusion reactions may occur after very small amounts of blood containing plasma are transfused. Although rare, anaphylactic reactions may be rapidly fatal. Sensitized IgA-deficient patients are particularly susceptible to anaphylaxis on receiving plasma containing IgA.

Presentation: Sudden onset of flushing, chills, vomiting, diarrhea, initial hypertension followed by hypotension, generalized edema, coughing, stridor, laryngeal edema, and progression to respiratory distress and shock. Fever is not a feature of anaphylaxis.

Mechanism: IgE-mediated response to transfused proteins.

Management: Discontinue transfusion and use standard measures for anaphylaxis: epinephrine, corticosteroids, circulatory support. Anti-IgA or antibody to a subspecies must be demonstrated to confirm the diagnosis.

Prevention: Usually not predictable or preventable. Subsequent transfusions to IgA deficient patients should come from IgA-deficient donors. If IgA-deficient blood components are not available, patients may benefit from receiving blood products that are depleted of plasma, such as washed RBC and platelets or frozen-deglycerolized RBC.

Transfusion-Related Acute Lung Injury

Transfusion-related acute lung injury (TRALI) is noncardiogenic pulmonary edema associated with transfusion of plasma-containing blood components, which includes practically all blood components. Previously believed to be underreported (21), it has an estimated frequency of 1:5000 transfusions and a mortality rate of 6% to 10% (1).

Presentation: Acute respiratory insufficiency, tachycardia, dyspnea, hypotension, oxygen desaturation (O_2 saturation <90% on room air), chills, rigors, fever with 1°C to 2°C temperature increase, and a bilateral pulmonary infiltration (white-out) by chest radiograph in the absence of heart failure or elevated central venous pressure, and unrelated to other causes of acute lung injury (21,23). Reaction occurs during or within 6 hours (most commonly after 2 hours) of transfusion. Hypoxemia may require intubation (70% to 75% of cases) (21). Symptoms subside rapidly; chest radiograph becomes normal/returns to baseline 96 hours; clinical recovery in 48 to 96 hours.

Mechanism: Reaction of antineutrophil antibodies and/or anti-HLA class I and II antibodies to the corresponding antigens between donors and recipients, occurring in the pulmonary vasculature and resulting ultimately in endothelial damage. Transfused *donor* antibodies are responsible in the majority of cases; multiparous females are more likely to be HLA/HNA alloimmunized, as are donors who have themselves been transfused. Antibodies from the *recipient* against cells in the donor plasma are implicated in approximately 5% of cases. In 10% of cases, no donor or recipient antibodies are identified.

A second possible pathophysiologic mechanism of TRALI is the "two-hit" theory, which suggests an interaction between primed pulmonary leukocytes in patients with underlying illness (in proinflammatory states) and biologically active response modifiers (lipids, cytokines) introduced by transfusion.

Management: Discontinue transfusion and provide supportive care.

Prevention: A patient who has experienced TRALI is not necessarily at increased risk for development of TRALI with future transfusions, unless receiving blood from the same donor. Implicated donors are ordinarily deferred indefinitely. Many blood centers now draw plasma preferentially from male donors to reduce the risk from multiparous female donors (24).

Circulatory Overload

The symptoms of circulatory overload or hypervolemia with blood transfusion are similar to TRALI. Unlike TRALI, circulatory overload is associated with central venous pressure elevation and cardiac failure. Pulmonary edema in circulatory overload is cardiogenic in origin and may result in the development of or exacerbation of preexisting congestive heart failure. In the absence of other complicating factors, circulatory overload is rarely fatal. Children, the elderly, those with compromised cardiac, renal, or pulmonary function, and patients in states of plasma volume expansion (normovolemic chronic anemia, thalassemia major, and sickle cell disease) are at particular risk (6,21).

Presentation: Cough, dyspnea, cyanosis, orthopnea, chest discomfort, rales, headache, distension of jugular veins, restlessness, and tachycardia

Management: Discontinue transfusion and administer supportive care (oxygen, diuresis, phlebotomy), if necessary.

Prevention: Patients at risk should receive smaller aliquots of blood infused at slower rates (1 mL/kg per hour to 4 mL/kg per hour) in as concentrated a form as possible.

Transfusion-Associated Graft-versus-Host Disease

Transfusion-associated graft-versus-host disease (TAGVHD) is a rare but severe adverse outcome of transfusion. Immunocompromised poststem cell or organ transplant patients, those with congenital immune deficiencies, patients with certain malignancies (particularly lymphomas and some tumors such as rhabdomyosarcoma, glioblastoma, neuroblastoma), and blood relatives (especially first-degree) of donors are at particularly high risk of TAGVHD. Absent these circumstances or associations, patients with acquired immune deficiency (such as human immunodeficiency virus [HIV]) and aplastic anemia patients do not need irradiated blood products (1,6,21). See also Table 24.4.

Presentation: Rash, diarrhea, hepatitis, mucositis, and pancytopenia; mortality approaches 90% with rare reports of survival (1,21).

Mechanism: Lymphocytes from an immune-competent donor engraft, recognize the patient's antigens as foreign and initiate an immune response.

Management: Supportive; no specific measures have proved effective.

Prevention: Gamma irradiation (at 2500 cGy) or X-irradiation of blood components. *Leukoreduction does not prevent TAGVHD.*

Bacterial Contamination and Sepsis

The initial symptoms of bacterial contamination occur during or several hours posttransfusion and include chills and fever. Temperature increase is less marked in patients premedicated with antipyretics or receiving corticosteroids.

Mild septic reactions may be initially obscured by underlying conditions that predispose the patient to fever or manifest similar signs and symptoms (6,21).

Presentation: Rigors and shaking chills, fever, nausea, vomiting, abdominal cramp, bloody diarrhea, hemolysis, hemoglobinuria, severe hypotension, and rapid progression to circulatory compromise, renal failure, shock, and DIC. Not all contaminated blood products result in clinically detectable sepsis, and fewer yet are fatal.

Common sources of bacterial contamination are subclinical/unrecognized bacteremia in the donor or skin contaminants at the phlebotomy site. Commonly implicated in RBC contamination are bacteria that survive the cold storage conditions, such as *Yersinia* and *Pseudomonas*. Platelets stored at room temperature are the component most susceptible to bacterial growth. Contamination occurs in approximately 1:5000 collections, sepsis in 1:50,000 transfusions, and death in 1:500,000 transfusions (25). More than half of bacterial contaminations of platelets are caused by skin flora, Staphylococci, Streptococci, *Propionibacterium*; many species are not implicated in serious transfusion reactions (6,21,25). Currently, the residual risk of septic transfusion reaction from platelets is estimated to be more than twice as high for whole blood-derived platelets, not tested by culture method, than for culture-negative apheresis platelets; 1:33,000 versus 1:75,000 (26). The highest mortality is usually associated with blood components contaminated with endotoxin-producing gram-negative bacteria.

Evaluation and management: Transfusion must be stopped. All transfusion units and blood component bags transfused within 4 hours should be returned to the blood bank for culture. Blood samples from both the blood component unit(s) and the patient should be sent for culture.

Prevention: Strict hygienic practice from collection to processing, storage, and administration of the component, and transfusion of blood components within the allotted 4 hours.

Mild Allergic/Urticarial Transfusion Reactions

Allergic transfusion reactions are relatively common, do not generally progress to anaphylaxis, are rarely lethal, and do not necessarily recur with subsequent transfusions.

Presentation: Localized erythema, pruritus, flushing, and urticaria, usually near the IV site. Severe urticaria and pruritus may be the initial signs of anaphylaxis.

Mechanism: Release of histamine and other anaphylotoxins.

Evaluation and management: Mild allergic reactions generally resolve when transfusion is temporarily stopped, and symptoms improve with administration of oral or parenteral antihistamines. In *mild allergic reactions* (hives only), transfusion with the same unit may be resumed, at a slower rate and with close monitoring of the patient. Transfusion reaction evaluation is generally not necessary.

Prevention: Mild allergic reactions are considered atopic reactions and generally unpredictable. There is no method to prescreen for all possible offending antigens. Premedication with antihistamines ameliorates mild allergic reactions in patients with previous reactions.

Posttransfusion Purpura

Posttransfusion purpura (PTP) is a profound thrombocytopenia that may occur after transfusion with any blood component.

Presentation: Abrupt decline in the platelet count within days to 2 to 3 weeks posttransfusion, which is usually self-limited and resolves within 2 to 3 weeks without treatment.

Mechanism: Antibodies against platelet-specific antigens (most commonly antihuman platelet antigen 1a [HPA-1a]) to which the patient may have become sensitized as a result of pregnancy or prior transfusion.

Management: Usually self-limited, but IVIg is effective. Transfusion with platelets negative for the implicated antigen is generally considered not beneficial during the PTP episode, but antigen-negative components will prevent recurrence. Family members provide a good source of donors if antigen-negative blood is otherwise not available. Severe PTP that does not resolve spontaneously, and if refractory to high-dose IVIG, may respond to plasmapheresis (1,21).

Hypotension Associated with Transfusion

Mechanism: Transient isolated hypotension that resolves after discontinuation of transfusion may be caused by activation of bradykinin and associated with use of bedside leukoreduction filters and apheresis procedures (especially with albumin replacement) (21). Patients receiving ACE inhibitors are at particular risk since ACE inhibitors block normal metabolism of bradykinin.

Evaluation and Management: Anaphylaxis, acute hemolytic transfusion reaction, TRALI, and bacterial contamination (sepsis) must be excluded.

Prevention: Avoid bedside leukoreduction (especially for patients taking ACE inhibitors).

Febrile Nonhemolytic Transfusion Reaction

Febrile nonhemolytic transfusion reactions (FNHTR) are defined by a greater than 1°C increase in temperature. FNHTR is a diagnosis of exclusion, made after consideration of acute hemolytic transfusion reaction, TRALI, and sepsis and determination that the symptoms are not related to the patient's underlying medical condition or medications. The incidence of FNHTR varies among patient populations and depends on the age and type of blood component and a variety of donor and recipient factors. Platelets are more likely to be implicated than are RBC or FFP, and older blood components more than fresh, leukocyte-reduced components (because cytokines accumulate during storage). The incidence is higher in multiply transfused patients (21).

Presentation: Chills, fever, rigors, which may be preceded by headache, nausea, and chilliness; the patient may also experience tachycardia, tachypnea, and general discomfort. Patients who sustain significant fever with transfusion are likely to have repeated reactions.

Mechanism: Interaction of antibodies in the recipient against donor leukocytes or platelets (antigens) and subsequent monocyte activation; cytokines accumulated in blood component bag during storage and pyrogens passively transferred from the donor to the recipient in the blood component.

Evaluation and management: As with a hemolytic reaction. Antipyretics may be administered.

Prevention: Leukoreduction (especially prestorage leukoreduction), removal of plasma in extreme situations, and premedication with antipyretics.

Hemosiderosis

Hemosiderosis or iron overload occurs in patients who receive repeated RBC transfusions (usually more than 50). One unit of RBC typically contains 200 to 250 mg of iron.

Presentation: Typical "bronzing" of skin, hepatomegaly, hepatic fibrosis and malfunction, diabetes and other endocrine gland dysfunction, and cardiac failure.

Mechanism: Accumulation of iron in the skin and internal organs. One unit of RBC typically contains 200 to 250 mg of iron.

Evaluation and management: Iron studies and iron chelation or phlebotomy when appropriate.

Prevention: Consider chelation for more than 50 unit red cell burden; red cell exchanges using apheresis help delay iron accumulation in patients with sickle cell disease (6).

TABLE 24.9. *Estimated Risk of Transfusion Transmission of Viral Diseases in the United States with Current Testing*

Virus	Risk Per Transfusion
HIV 1 and 2	1:2,000,000–3,000,000
Hepatitis C	1:2,000,000–3,000,000
Hepatitis B	1:200,000–500,000
HTLV I and II	1:2,000,000 (cellular components)
West Nile virus	Seasonal and regional variability

From Stramer SL. Current risks of transfusion-transmitted agents: a review. Arch Pathol Lab Med 2007;131:702–707; and Dodd, RY, Notari EP IV, Stramer SL. Current prevalence and incidence of infectious disease markers and estimated window-period risk in the American Red Cross blood donor population. Transfusion 2002;42:975–979.
Ranges in table reflect estimates from various sources.
HIV, human immunodeficiency virus; HTLV, human T-lymphotropic virus.

Transfusion-Transmitted Infections

Current testing of donor blood prior to release of blood components includes:

• *Antibodies* to HIV types 1 and 2 (anti-HIV-1/2); hepatitis C virus (HCV) (anti-HCV); hepatitis B core antigen (anti-HBc); human lymphotropic virus types I and II (anti-human T-cell leukemia virus [HTLV] I/II)
• *Surface antigen:* Hepatitis B surface antigen (HBsAg)
• *Nucleic acid testing (NAT)* for HIV; HCV; West Nile virus (WNV)

With current mandated testing, the estimated risk of transmission of viral infections per transfusion is reported in Table 24.9 (27). Blood is also tested by *RPR* for the detection of *Treponema pallidum* bacterium, the causative agent of syphilis, and by enzyme-linked immunoassay for the detection of *Trypanosoma cruzi* parasite, the causative agent for Chagas' disease.

Other infectious agents and diseases transmissible by transfusion (28,29) for which the blood supply is not currently routinely tested include hepatitis A virus, parvovirus B19, and dengue virus; parasitic diseases (not as common in the United States) including malaria, babesiosis, and leishmaniasis; the protozoal disease toxoplasmosis, which affects mainly immunocompromised patients; and prions (protein particles) responsible for the transmission of variant Creutzfeldt-Jacob disease (vCJD) (30).

Alternatives to Allogeneic Blood Transfusion

Alternatives to the use of blood component therapy are available and may be particularly useful for bleeding patients who refuse allogeneic blood component or blood product transfusions (usually for religious beliefs) or bleeding patients unresponsive to appropriate transfusion therapy. Examples of alternatives to allogeneic blood transfusion (6,31) are listed in Table 24.10. Indications for use of some pharmaceutical hemostatic agents (1,32) are summarized in Table 24.11.

Massive Transfusion

Massive transfusion is the administration of blood components over a 24-hour period in amounts that equal or exceed the total blood volume of the patient. After transfusion of one or more blood volumes, an abbreviated RBC cross-match (see general concepts) is performed to provide RBC more rapidly. Group O, Rh-negative or Rh-positive blood, depending on the age and gender of the patient, or ABO/Rh-specific blood are effective and relatively safe ways to obtain blood urgently.

TABLE 24.10. *Examples of Alternatives to Allogeneic Blood Transfusion*

Preoperative	Intraoperative	Postoperative
Autologous Blood Collection	**Blood Salvaged from a Sterile Surgical Field**	**Blood Recovered from Drainage**
Donor's Hb should meet or exceed 11 g/dL	Use in oncologic procedures is controversial	Used primarily with cardiac and orthopedic surgery*
Donor must be at no increased risk of bacterial infection	Gross contamination of surgical field with malignant cells constitutes a relative contraindication	Blood recovered is generally dilute (hematocrit of approximately 20%) and may be partially hemolyzed
Donations up to every 5 days with last collection no later than 72 hours prior to procedure	Blood salvaged/processed by devices that collect, centrifuge, wash, and concentrate red blood cells	Transfusion should start within 6 hours of initiation of collection*,†
Autologous blood subject to same shelf-life limitations as allogeneic blood components	May be stored at room temperature for 4 hours from the end of collection and at 1–6°C for up to 24 hours if refrigeration began within 4 hours from completion of processing†	
Unit(s) may be frozen until used	**Acute Normovolemic Hemodilution**	
Prevents Transmission of viral infections; Red blood cell antigen alloimmunization; Some transfusion reactions	Whole blood is collected from patient and replaced with crystalloid or colloid and reinfused after cessation of major blood loss, or sooner if indicated	
Risk of bacterial contamination and of clerical error leading to transfusion of ABO incompatible units not decreased significantly*	May be stored at room temperature up to 8 hours or refrigerated at 1–6°C up to 24 hours after collection†	
	Other Blood Components	
	Examples include platelet-rich and platelet-poor plasma and cryoprecipitate intended for transfusion or for topical use	
	Must be stored at room temperature and administered before the patient leaves the operating room†	

*From Brecher ME, ed. Technical Manual, 15th Ed. Bethesda, MD: AABB Press; 2005.
†From Santrach P, ed. Standards for Perioperative Autologous Blood Collection and Administration, 2nd Ed. Bethesda, MD: AABB Press; 2005:18–19, Reference Standard 5.1.7A.

Adequate intravascular blood volume and blood pressure may be maintained initially with colloids (albumin, plasma protein fraction) or crystalloids (lactated Ringer' solution or normal saline). Transfusion of packed RBC may become necessary after a loss of more than 25% to 30% of the blood volume, depending on the rate of blood loss, tissue perfusion and oxygenation status of the patient (33). Transfusion of blood components based on fixed ratios or algorithms should be avoided.

TABLE 24.11. *Selected Pharmacologic Hemostatic Agents*

Agent	Indications	Nonindications and Adverse Effects	Administration and Preparations
rFVIIa*	Licensed use: Refractory hemophilia A or B High factor VIII or IX inhibitor levels in hemophilia A or B Off-label use: Severe bleeding refractory to other therapy Glanzmann's thrombasthenia Bleeding with need for rapid reversal of warfarin anticoagulants	Potential for thromboembolic events in patients predisposed to thrombosis No suitable assay for monitoring drug efficacy; laboratory values do not correlate with hemostatic effectiveness	**Usual dose:** 90 μg/kg repeated every 2 hrs (Doses of 30–120 μg/kg have been used) Half-life: 2–3 hrs
Vitamin K	Vitamin K deficiency resulting in coagulopathy (factors II, VII, IX, X) Reversal of warfarin anticoagulation when prolonged effectiveness is desired and simple discontinuation of warfarin is not feasible	Not effective for urgent reversal of warfarin or correction of vitamin K-dependent factors Intravenous administration associated with anaphylaxis (rare), which may be fatal	Intravenous (IV) faster effect than subcutaneous (SC) or oral (PO) Solution and tablet forms: 0.5–20 mg
Protamine	Neutralization of anticoagulation from unfractionated heparin (displaces antithrombin III and complexes heparin) After cardiac bypass surgery in patients who have received unfractionated heparin	Possible heparin rebound because of shorter half-life of protamine compared with heparin Requires close monitoring of coagulation parameters Hypotension Increased pulmonary artery pressure Allergic reactions Dosing should not exceed 100 mg in 2 hours	Immediate onset of action 1 mg of protamine neutralizes 80–100 USP heparin Half-life: 2 hrs Activated clotting time used to monitor effectiveness and determine dosing
Conjugated Estrogens	Coagulopathy related to uremia, GI bleeding associated with angiodysplasia (Osler-Weber-Rendu syndrome), end-stage renal disease, von Willebrand disease	Not useful when immediate hemostasis is required May be associated with gynecomastia, weight gain, and dyspepsia	Onset of effect within 6 hrs and duration of up to 2 weeks Maximum effectiveness between 5–7 days **Usual dose:** IV: 0.6 mg/kg Patch: 50–100 μg/24 hrs PO: 50 mg
DDAVP*	Bleeding associated with: Hemophilia A; von Willebrand disease; Bernard-Soulier disease; aspirin ingestion; platelet hemostasis; defects where other treatment options are not effective	Not useful in type 2B von Willebrand disease because of thrombocytopenia and increased affinity of vWF for platelets May be associated with hyponatremia when administered with hypotonic fluids	Peak response IV within 1 hr and duration of up to 12 hrs **Usual dose:** IV: 0.3 μL/kg in 50 mL normal saline (in 10 mL normal saline for

(continued)

TABLE 24.11. *Selected Pharmacologic Hemostatic Agents (continued)*

Agent	Indications	Nonindications and Adverse Effects	Administration and Preparations
		Electrolytes and volume should be closely monitored Hypertension, facial flushing, nausea, increased risk of myocardial infarction in cardiac surgery patients Tachyphylaxis with repeated administration	children weighing <10 kg) over 30 min SC: 0.3 µg/kg Intranasal: 300 µg (adults)

AMCA[†]/ EACA[‡]	Excessive fibrinolysis:
	  Congenital α2-antiplasmin deficiency
	  GI and uterine bleeding where antifibrinolytic action is needed
	Some acquired causes of fibrinolysis (e.g., cardiac bypass surgery)
	May be useful as irrigation in intractable bleeding from the bladder
	Amegakaryocytic and peripheral immune mediated thrombocytopenia
	AMCA: Used in patients with hemophilia A and B during dental procedures along with fibrin sealant and DDAVP
		Contraindicated in thrombotic disorders with fibrinolysis (DIC) or active intravascular clotting
		Reduce dose in renal insufficiency
		EACA: May be associated with rhabdomyolysis (myonecrosis) with prolonged usage
		AMCA has less GI discomfort than EACA
			AMCA is 10-fold more potent than EACA
			Usual dose:
			EACA: 2–4 g/ 3–4 hrs
			Total of 10–24 g/ 24 hrs
			AMCA: 1 g/6–8 hrs
			Total of 3–4 g/ 24 hrs
			Half-life for both: 2–10 hrs

Aprotinin	Antifibrinolytic and anticoagulant properties Intravenous preparations approved for use as a hemostatic in cardiac bypass surgery Off-label use: Liver transplant/other procedures associated with large volumes of blood loss	Anaphylaxis 10,000 kallikrein inhibitory units IV test dose should be given prior to surgery Renal insufficiency, myocardial infarction, and stroke may be increased Possibility of vCJD transmission (because of derivation from bovine lung)	**Usual dose:** Initial loading dose of 2 million kallikrein inhibitory units (KIU) followed by continuous infusion of 250,000–500,000 KIU/hr Cardiac bypass surgery: Additional 2 million KIU may be added to bypass pump prime Half-life: 7 hrs

From Klein HG, Anstee DJ. Mollison's Blood Transfusion in Clinical Medicine, 11th Ed. Oxford: Blackwell Publishing Ltd; 2005; and Bolan CD, Klein HG. Blood component and pharmacologic therapy of hemostatic disorders. In Kitchens C, Kessler C, Alving BM, eds. Consultative Hemostasis and Thrombosis. 22nd Ed. Philadelphia: Elsevier; 2007:461–490.
*1-deamino-8-D-arginine vasopressin (desmopressin); †tranexamic acid; ‡ε-aminocaproic acid.
DIC, disseminated intravascular coagulation; GI, gastrointestinal; vCJD, variant Creutzfeldt-Jakob disease; vWF, von Willebrand factor.

Adverse Sequelae of Massive Transfusion

Adverse sequelae of massive transfusion include dilution and/or consumption of hemostatic constituents of blood. Platelet count, prothrombin time (PT), PTT, and fibrinogen levels should be determined frequently. Generally a platelet count of greater than 50,000/μL (80,000 to 100,000/μL for neurologic surgery, ophthalmologic surgery, or cardiopulmonary bypass), PT or PTT of less than 1.5 times normal range, and a fibrinogen concentration of greater than 80 to 100 mg/dL are considered adequate for maintenance of hemostasis (9,33). Combinations of low values seen during massive transfusion may require replacement therapy. Hypothermia, acidosis, hypocalcemia, and other biochemical disturbances may occur and electrolytes, particularly potassium and calcium, should be monitored (1,33). Hypocalcemia secondary to citrate accumulation may occur when large volumes of blood are administered at rapid rates (more than 100 mL/min), especially in the presence of liver and renal dysfunction (1,33).

Disseminated Intravascular Coagulation

DIC probably complicates massive transfusion less often than suspected, but DIC is associated with shock, independent of blood loss or transfusion. Laboratory coagulation test results are consistent with a consumptive coagulopathy. Transfusion management of DIC is supportive while the underlying cause is addressed. Cryoprecipitate should be administered when fibrinogen levels are below 80 mg/dL. Other components, such as platelets may be necessary, especially if bleeding is severe. Usually massive transfusion, even in trauma settings, requires only replacement of platelets (34). If multiple factors are consumed, plasma factor levels of above 30% can be achieved with an FFP dose of 10 to 20 mL/kg (1,33).

IMMUNOHEMATOLOGIC DISORDERS

Hemolytic Disease of the Newborn

Hemolytic disease of the newborn (HDN) is the destruction of fetal erythrocytes by maternal IgG antibodies that cross the placenta and react with a paternally derived antigen present on the fetal RBC. Although traditionally associated with Rh antibodies (anti-Rh$_0$D), other antibodies including anti-A, anti-B, and anti-K:1 have been implicated and may cause significant HDN.

In *mild cases,* the newborn is asymptomatic, and laboratory findings of a positive DAT and mild bilirubinemia are the only abnormalities.

Severe cases may result in intrauterine death (hydrops fetalis, erythroblastosis fetalis). There is a high risk of *kernicterus* caused by high unconjugated bilirubin.

Treatment: Intrauterine RBC transfusion (in severe cases) using compatible (with the mother's antibody), irradiated, CMV-negative, sickle-negative RBC suspended in 5% albumin or FFP. Usually a two-blood-volume exchange removes approximately 25% of excess bilirubin, provides albumin to which excess bilirubin can bind, and removes antibody and approximately 70% of RBC coated with antibody. Additional exchange transfusions may be necessary if level of bilirubin continues to rise.

Neonatal Alloimmune Thrombocytopenia and
Maternal Immune Thrombocytopenic Purpura

Neonatal Alloimmune Thrombocytopenia

Neonatal alloimmune thrombocytopenia (NAIT), the platelet equivalent of HDN, is the destruction of platelets that carry paternally derived antigens by maternal antibodies that cross the placenta. As with HDN, NAIT may vary in severity from very mild and asymptomatic thrombocytopenia to life-threatening bleeding, and it may occur in utero or in the neonatal period. The vast majority of NAIT is associated with antibody (IgG) against the common platelet antigen HPA-1a (PL^{A1}), especially in the presence of HLA DRw52a phenotype (1).

NAIT is usually self-limiting and resolves within 2 to 3 weeks. If NAIT is suspected, often as a result of a previous affected pregnancy, cordocentesis to determine platelet counts may be performed in conjunction with administration of compatible platelets (maternal platelets or platelets known to be negative for the implicated antigen).

With in utero NAIT, IVIg is given with or without weekly corticosteroid administration to the mother (1 g/kg) until delivery. If there is a high risk of intracranial hemorrhage, platelet transfusion is performed immediately prior to delivery. When compatible platelets are unavailable, high-dose IVIG has been administered to the neonate with variable effectiveness. An increase in platelet counts within 24 to 48 hours may be seen in patients who respond (6).

Maternal Immune Thrombocytopenic Purpura

In *maternal* ITP, antibodies related to maternal ITP such as IgG (as in NAIT) are implicated and have broad specificity. The degree of thrombocytopenia is milder than that associated with NAIT. There is a lower risk of fetal or neonatal intracranial hemorrhage. Maternal platelets and random donor platelets may be equally effective or ineffective. IVIg may also be beneficial. Maternal ITP usually resolves in days to weeks (upon clearance of maternal antibodies from the neonate's circulation).

Autoimmune Hemolytic Anemias

Autoimmune hemolytic anemias (AIHA) are characterized by the presence of antibodies against the individual's own RBC antigens (autoantibodies), resulting in accelerated destruction of these RBC. AIHA may be associated with autoimmune disorders, infections, medications, or malignancies, or it may be primary. The laboratory hallmark is the positive DAT, indicating the presence of autoantibody directed against red cells. Antibody may also be present in the serum so that positive DAT and IAT may coexist, making identification of underlying alloantibodies and compatibility testing difficult.

Warm Autoimmune Hemolytic Anemia

Warm AIHA is about four times as common as hemolysis from cold-reacting antibodies. The implicated antibody is usually IgG and reacts with all cells, although occasionally a warm autoantibody will appear to have specificity against Rh antigens and several others. Patients with compensated warm AIHA require no specific treatment but should be investigated for an underlying condition such as systemic lupus erythematosus or a lymphoproliferative disorder. In children, viral illness may be accompanied by transient AIHA. Medications, particularly purine nucleoside analogues, are commonly associated with warm AIHA. Warm-reacting autoantibodies may be present only as a laboratory finding, or they may cause severe, even life-threatening hemolysis; these antibodies react optimally at 37°C in vitro. Patients are often totally asymptomatic, but some present with fatigue, jaundice, or mild anemia. Moderate splenomegaly occurs in about one third to one half of the cases and hepatomegaly in one third of the patients. Hemolysis is usually not severe and is mainly extravascular (35).

Laboratory findings include a positive DAT, spherocytes on the blood smear, elevated unconjugated bilirubin and LDH as indices of cell turnover, and high reticulocyte count. Rarely, reticulocytopenia may be seen, either because of inadequate bone marrow response or because the autoantibody reacts with red cell precursors as well as with mature cells.

Red cell alloantibodies developed as a result of previous transfusions or pregnancies, found in approximately one third of patients with AIHA, are capable of causing severe hemolytic transfusion reactions. Broadly reactive autoantibody may mask underlying alloantibodies and make procurement of compatible blood difficult.

Occasionally hemolysis may result in severe anemia accompanied by changes in mental status and coma. This medical emergency requires immediate transfusion even when compatible blood cannot be obtained. The term "least incompatible" has not been adequately defined, does not correlate to clinical events, and would be best abolished (35).

Treatment with oral glucocorticoids (prednisone at 60 mg per day) is helpful in more than half of the cases, and splenectomy is effective in approximately half of those who are refractory to steroids.

Immunosuppressive regimens and IVIg may benefit selected patients (35). Refractory AIHA, especially when associated with lymphoproliferative disease, may respond to the monoclonal antibody rituximab (see below).

Cold Agglutinin Syndrome

Cold-reacting antibodies are common and usually of no significance, but some cold agglutinins, especially those with very high titer at 4°C but broad thermal amplitude (reactivity up to 30°C) may result in cold agglutinin syndrome (cold hemagglutinin disease). IgM is the immune globulin classically implicated. Cold agglutinin syndrome may be primary (cause undetermined) or secondary to a viral infection or lymphoproliferative disorder. Acute cold agglutinin syndrome may be associated with Mycoplasma pneumonia and infectious mononucleosis, is seen mostly in children and young adults, and tends to be transient and self-limited. Chronic cold agglutinin syndrome may be associated with lymphoma, chronic lymphocytic leukemia, and Waldenström's macroglobulinemia. Patients may present with acrocyanosis and hematuria precipitated by cold, and/or severe pain in the nose, ears and distal extremities upon cold exposure. Severe anemia is rare in the chronic form.

Transfusion is rarely necessary, but when performed, the typing specimen must be kept at body temperature from the time of phlebotomy through the testing procedure. Up to 50% of transfused cells may be destroyed by autoantibodies of the patient even when blood warmers are used.

Treatment with corticosteroids and splenectomy is not effective, and most patients do well simply by avoiding exposure to the cold. Rituximab, a monoclonal antibody targeted against the B lymphocyte CD20 antigen, appeared useful when administered as four weekly infusions in a small number of patients (35).

Paroxysmal Cold Hemoglobinuria

Paroxysmal cold hemoglobinuria (PCH) is a rare autoimmune hemolytic anemia that results from a biphasic IgG antibody (Donath-Landsteiner antibody). Originally associated with untreated syphilis, it is now found most often with viral infections in children. The Donath-Landsteiner antibody binds to the RBC at cold temperatures and causes intravascular hemolysis as complement is fixed at warmer temperatures, accounting for the paroxysms of hemoglobinuria. Anemia associated with PCH is usually transient and self-limited over 2 to 3 weeks. If transfusion support becomes necessary, cross-match–compatible blood may be found if the antibody is not reactive at temperatures above 4°C. Unavailability of compatible RBC should not preclude transfusion in life-threatening anemia associated with hemolysis, despite shortened survival of the transfused RBC (1,6,35).

Therapeutic Apheresis in the Management of Immunohematologic Disorders

Apheresis is the process by which selected components or substances in blood are removed from the circulation and the remainder of the blood returned to the patient. Apheresis is used to collect routine blood components (platelets, plasma, stem cells) and for the therapeutic removal of undesirable components and substances from the circulation, and is achieved through automated machines. See Table 24.12 for commonly accepted indications for therapeutic apheresis for hematologic disorders, endorsed by the American Association of Blood Banks and /or the American Society for Apheresis (ASFA) (36,37).

The kinetics of most intravascular substances indicate that exchange of 1 to 1.5 plasma volumes results in the highest efficiency removal with progressively decreased efficiency with each additional consecutive exchange. The volume of blood processed in order to attain the desired apheresis effect depends on the nature of the specific component, including its intravascular distribution and concentration in the particular patient. The patient's total blood volume determines the safe extracorporeal blood volume (which should not exceed 15% of blood volume). Small patients may require that the machine be primed with saline or blood.

Apheresis is generally safe, especially for normal component donors. Complications mainly relate to vascular access, hemodynamic changes (especially for patients with cardiovascular disease), and a variable loss of blood components. Risks associated with apheresis are usually associated with a patient's underlying disease.

TABLE 24.12. *Recommendation for Therapeutic Apheresis in Hematologic Disorders*

Category I Accepted as standard first-line or primary therapy
Cryoglobulinemia (plasma exchange)
Cutaneous T-cell lymphoma (photopheresis)
Erythrocytosis or polycythemia vera (phlebotomy/cytapheresis)
Hyperviscosity in monoclonal gammopathies (plasma exchange)
Leukocytosis (cytapheresis)
Sickle cell disease – life/organ threatening complications (red cell exchange)
Thrombocytosis – symptomatic (cytapheresis)
Thrombotic thrombocytopenic purpura (plasma exchange)

Category II Generally accepted as adjunctive or supportive therapy
ABO-incompatible hematopoietic progenitor cell/marrow transplantation (plasma exchange recipient)
Coagulation factor inhibitors (plasma exchange)
Cryoglobulinemia with polyneuropathy (plasma exchange)
Graft-versus-host disease – skin (photopheresis)
Idiopathic (autoimmune) thrombocytopenic purpura (immunoadsorption)
Malaria or babesiosis – severe (red cell exchange)
Myeloma, paraproteins, or hyperviscosity (plasma exchange)
Myeloma with acute renal failure (plasma exchange)
Polyneuropathy with IgM, with or without Waldenström's (plasma exchange)
Posttransfusion purpura (plasma exchange)
Red cell alloimmunization in pregnancy* (plasma exchange)
Sickle cell disease – primary/secondary prophylaxis/iron overload prevention (red cell exchange)

Category III No clear indication based on conflicting or insufficient evidence of efficacy or favorable risk-to-benefit ratio; sometimes used as a last resort
Aplastic anemia or pure red blood cell aplasia (plasma exchange)
Autoimmune hemolytic anemia (plasma exchange)
Catastrophic antiphospholipid syndrome
Graft-versus-host disease – nonskin (photopheresis)
Hemolytic disease of the newborn (plasma exchange)
Hemolytic uremic syndrome – atypical (plasma exchange)
Platelet alloimmunization and refractoriness (plasma exchange or immunoadsorption)
Multiple myeloma with polyneuropathy (plasma exchange)
Thrombocytosis – prophylactic (cytapheresis)

*If fetus <20 weeks gestation and previous severely affected pregnancy
Modified from Smith JW, Weinstein R, Hillyer KL, et al. Therapeutic apheresis: a summary of current indication categories endorsed by the AABB and the American Society for Apheresis. Transfusion 2003;43:820–822 and from Szczepiorkowski ZM, Bandarenko N, Kim HC, et al. Guidelines on the use of therapeutic apheresis in clinical practice—evidence-based approach from the apheresis applications committee of the American Society for Apheresis. J Clin Apher 2007;22:106–175.

Plasma exchange may result in a 30% or more decrease in platelet counts (38). Platelet transfusion may be required for patients with low platelet counts and hemostatic problems. Cellular blood component counts return to normal after a few days and proteins and electrolytes reequilibrate within hours, although fibrinogen may remain below baseline levels after 72 hours (39). Plasma exchange may also reduce blood levels of certain medications, especially those bound to plasma proteins or those with a long plasma half-life (40). Hypotension may occur as a result of volume shifts and bradykinin activation from blood contact with plastic (6,40); withhold ACE inhibitors, which potentiate this effect, should be withheld from patients for 24 to 48 hours prior to an apheresis procedure.

Citrate is used to prevent coagulation of blood in the circuit and may result in *citrate toxicity:* binding of calcium and decreased levels of ionized calcium. Citrate toxicity symptoms include mild perioral tingling and discomfort, chest tightness, and tetany in severe cases; if symptoms do not subside with adjustment of citrate and whole blood flow rates, administration of oral calcium (as chewable tablets) or intravenous calcium gluconate (more common) or calcium chloride (for large volume apheresis procedures) helps prevent hypocalcemia and the accompanying syndromes (41).

Therapeutic Apheresis (Cytapheresis and Plasmapheresis)

Thrombocytapheresis

Increased platelet counts, particularly in myeloproliferative disorders in which platelets are qualitatively abnormal as well, may be associated with bleeding or thrombosis.

Patients with elevated platelets who are symptomatic (as in essential thrombocytosis or polycythemia rubra vera) or hemorrhage (chronic myelogenous leukemia [CML]) may have immediate benefit from therapeutic cytapheresis. Generally plateletpheresis is a first-line therapy for thrombocytosis (platelet counts greater than 500,000/μL) in symptomatic patients. Each procedure will lower the count 30% to 50%. Cytoreductive chemotherapy should be initiated simultaneously, because plateletpheresis is not effective long term (37,40).

Leukocytapheresis (Leukapheresis)

Malignant leukocytosis or hyperleukocytosis (immature white blood cell counts of greater than 100,000/μL), in association with some leukemias, can result in leukostasis in the central nervous system, kidneys, and lungs. Symptoms may occur with rapidly rising blast cells at counts less than 100,000/μL, especially in acute myeloid leukemia (AML) and CML.

Changes in mentation, dizziness, blurred vision, hypoxia, or respiratory symptoms constitute a medical emergency. Therapeutic leukapheresis can reduce the leukocyte count by 30% to 50% in hours. Symptoms may abate promptly. Reduction of the white cell count permits cytoreductive chemotherapy by abrogating fever, increased uric acid, renal failure, and electrolyte imbalances of the acute cytolysis syndrome. Chemotherapy with hydroxyurea or a similar agent should be initiated concurrently because repeated leukocytapheresis may not control hyperleukocytosis.

Photopheresis (Extracorporeal Photochemotherapy)

Photopheresis is the separation of the patient's leukocytes by apheresis for extracorporeal treatment with the chemotherapeutic agent 8-methoxy-psoralen (8-MOP) and photoactivation by ultraviolet A (UVA) light for subsequent reinfusion to the patient. It is effective in the treatment of cutaneous T-cell lymphoma, allograft rejection, posthematopoietic stem cell transplant GVHD, scleroderma, and other autoimmune diseases. The mechanism of action is not fully understood; it may possibly be related to apoptosis of pathogenic T lymphocytes and antigen-presenting cells or anti-idiotype cytotoxic T-cell response (1,40). The use of 8-MOP is contraindicated in patients with light-sensitive disorders such as xeroderma pigmentosa, albinism, and certain porphyrias (40).

Erythrocytapheresis/Red Cell Exchange

Red cell exchange involves the removal of abnormal red cells. The patient's RBC are replaced with stored RBC. Erythrocytapheresis may be used to reduce red cell mass acutely in symptomatic (visual disturbances, confusion, lethargy, hemorrhage, threatened stroke, thrombosis of abdominal vasculature) patients with excessive polycythemia (37,40). Saline or colloid volume replacement is administered to maintain isovolemia.

Red Cell Exchange and Sickle Cell Anemia

Red cell exchange may be used acutely to treat complications of sickle cell disease (37) including acute chest syndrome, stroke, retinal infarction, priapism, and hepatic crisis, or as protracted or chronic treatment for the prevention of recurrent complications such as stroke and severe painful crises, and for reduction of iron overload secondary to transfusion (40).

In the perioperative setting, simple transfusion or a single red cell exchange prevents morbidity associated with sickle cell disease. The goal is to achieve hemoglobin A of more than 50%. Transfusion and exchange have been used to treat sickle complications during pregnancy, but routine use is unnecessary. Exchange transfusion can raise hemoglobin A to levels difficult to achieve with simple transfusion and may benefit patients in the third trimester for preeclampsia, sepsis, and preoperative management (40).

Red Cell Exchange and Parasitemia

Red cell exchange has been used as antiparasitic treatment in malaria to decrease the circulating parasite load when it exceeds 5% (42).

Plasmapheresis

Plasmapheresis may be used to collect plasma for transfusion or manufacturing of plasma derivatives, or to remove undesirable substances from the circulation. Colloids or saline (plasma with TTP) are administered to maintain isovolemia. See Tables 24.12 and 24.13 for common indications for therapeutic plasmapheresis (36,37).

Thrombotic Microangiopathies

TTP and hemolytic uremic syndrome (HUS) belong to a spectrum of thrombotic microangiopathies: TTP may be associated with prominent neurologic symptoms; HUS presents with a more prominent renal component. Characteristic findings of TTP include fever, renal impairment, neurologic symptoms such as change in mental status, seizures or coma, thrombocytopenia (platelet counts less than $30,000/\mu L$), and hemolytic anemia with schistocytes.

TTP results from the accumulation of ultralarge von Willebrand factor multimers caused by congenital absence or immune mediated (IgG) interference with the vWF-cleaving metalloprotease

TABLE 24.13. *Category I and II Recommendations for Therapeutic Plasma Exchange*

Category I	Category II
ABO-incompatible renal allograft (plasma exchange recipient)	ABO-incompatible hematopoietic progenitor cell/marrow transplantation (plasma exchange recipient)*
Acute inflammatory demyelinating polyradiculoneuropathy	Acute central nervous system inflammatory demyelinating disease
Antiglomerular basement membrane antibody disease	Coagulation factor inhibitors
Chronic inflammatory demyelinating polyradiculoneuropathy	Cryoglobulinemia with polyneuropathy
Cryoglobulinemia	Idiopathic (autoimmune) thrombocytopenic purpura
Demyelinating polyneuropathy with IgG and IgA	Familial hypercholesterolemia
Familial hypercholesterolemia (selective adsorption)	Lambert-Eaton myasthenia syndrome
Hyperviscosity with monoclonal gammopathy	Mushroom poisoning
Myasthenia gravis	Myeloma, paraproteins, or hyperviscosity
Sydenham's chorea	Myeloma with acute renal failure
Thrombotic thrombocytopenic purpura	Pediatric autoimmune neuropsychiatric disorders (PANDAS)
	Phytanic acid storage disease
	Polyneuropathy with IgM (with or without Waldenstrom's)
	Posttransfusion purpura
	Rapidly progressive glomerulonephritis
	Rassmussen's encephalitis
	Renal transplantation – antibody-mediated rejection/HLA desensitization
	Rheumatoid arthritis – refractory (immunoadsorption)

Modified from Smith JW, Weinstein R, Hillyer KL, et al. Therapeutic apheresis: a summary of current indication categories endorsed by the AABB and the American Society for Apheresis. Transfusion 2003;43:820–822 and from Szczepiorkowski ZM, Bandarenko N, Kim HC, et al. Guidelines on the use of therapeutic apheresis in clinical practice—evidence-based approach from the apheresis applications committee of the American Society for Apheresis. J Clin Apher 2007;22:106–175.
*Removal of RBC from the hematopoietic progenitor cell/marrow.
HLA, human leukocyte antigen; RBC, red blood cells.

ADAMTS13 (1,40). When TTP and HUS-like syndromes are associated with immunosuppressive agents (typically vinca alkaloids, mitomycin, bleomycin, BL22, cisplatin, tacrolimus, and cyclosporin A), they do not respond well to therapeutic plasma exchange (TPE).

TPE is first-line therapy for the treatment of TTP and a last resort for HUS. TPE should be performed promptly after diagnosis of TTP. The effectiveness of TPE in TTP depends on the removal of ultralarge vWF multimers and reduction of the IgG antibodies against vWF-cleaving protease. Plasma (FFP) is the fluid replacement of choice in TPE for TTP and also replaces the vWF-cleaving protease. TPE is often done daily, then tapered until platelet counts stabilize at more than 100,000/µL for 2 consecutive days. Response can be monitored by clinical assessment and laboratory measurements (platelet count, LDH, extent of schistocytosis).

Platelet transfusion is generally discouraged because patients suffer from thrombosis rather than bleeding. However, platelet transfusion may be necessary for life-threatening hemorrhage (6).

Immune (Autoimmune) Thrombocytopenic Purpura

ITP involves destruction of platelets by IgG autoantibodies. In its acute form, typically seen in children after a viral infection, ITP is usually self-limited. In adults, ITP is more chronic, and TPE has been used to treat severe cases refractory to corticosteroids and high-dose IVIg.

Anti-Rh immune globulin is effective in Rh-positive patients. Therapeutic plasmapheresis in combination with steroids may result in fewer relapses and decreased need for splenectomy (40).

Coagulation Factor Inhibitors

Plasmapheresis can lower inhibitor titers in patients who experience uncontrollable hemorrhage or prevent bleeding from invasive procedures. TPE may be used to treat coagulation factor inhibitors (factor VIII, IX inhibitors).

Dysproteinemias

Complications of paraproteinemias of multiple myeloma, Waldenström's macroglobulinemia, and cryoglobulinemia respond to TPE. Hyperviscosity syndrome with mental status changes, mucosal and gastrointestinal bleeding, retinopathy, and hypervolemia constitutes a medical emergency. Hyperviscosity responds to even small volume exchanges, but procedures need to be repeated until the paraprotein is controlled with chemotherapy (40).

REFERENCES

1. Klein HG, Anstee DJ. Mollison's Blood Transfusion in Clinical Medicine, 11th Ed. Oxford: Blackwell Publishing Ltd; 2005.
2. Mielcarek M, Leisenring W, Torok-Storb B, et al. Graft-versus-host disease and donor-directed hemagglutinin titers after ABO-mismatched related and unrelated marrow allografts: evidence for graft-versus-plasma cell effect. Blood 2000;96:1150–1156.
3. Worel N, Greinix HT, Keil F, et al. Severe immune hemolysis after minor ABO-mismatched allogeneic peripheral blood progenitor cell transplantation occurs more frequently after nonmyeloablative than myeloablative conditioning. Transfusion 2002;42:1293–1301.
4. Griffith LM, McCoy JP, Bolan CD, et al. Persistence of recipient plasma cells and antidonor isohaemagglutinins in patients with delayed donor erythropoiesis after major ABO incompatible nonmyeloablative haematopoietic cell transplantation. Br J Haematol 2005;128:668–675.
5. Bolan CD, Leitman SF, Griffith LM, et al. Delayed donor red cell chimerism and pure red cell aplasia following major ABO-incompatible nonmyeloablative hematopoietic stem cell transplantation. Blood 2001;98:1687–1694.
6. Brecher ME, ed. Technical Manual, 15th Ed. Bethesda, MD: AABB Press; 2005.
7. Hébert PC, Wells G, Blajchman MA, et al. A multicenter randomized, controlled clinical trial of transfusion requirements in critical care. N Engl J Med 1999;340:409–417.

8. Majdpour C, Spahn DR, Weiskopf RB. Anemia and perioperative red blood cell transfusion: a matter of tolerance. Crit Care Med 2006;34:S102–S108.

9. Practice guidelines for blood component therapy: Report by American Society of Anesthesiologists Task Force on Blood Component Therapy. Anesthesiology 1996;84:732–747.

10. Schiffer CA, Anderson KC, Bennett CL, et al. Platelet transfusion for patients with cancer: clinical practice guidelines of the American Society of Oncology. J Clin Oncol 2001;19:1519–1538.

11. Stroncek DF, Leonard K, Eiber G, et al. Alloimmunization after granulocyte transfusions. Transfusion 1996;36:1009–1015.

12. Wright DG, Robichaud KJ, Pizzo PA, et al. Lethal pulmonary reactions associated with the combined use of amphotericin B and leukocyte transfusions. N Engl J Med 1981;304:1185–1189.

13. Administration Development Task Force of the College of American Pathologists. Practice parameter for the use of fresh frozen plasma, cryoprecipitate, and platelets. JAMA 1994;271:777–781.

14. Haas R, Mohle R, Fruehauf S, et al. Patient characteristics associated with successful mobilizing and autografting of peripheral blood progenitor cells in malignant lymphoma. Blood 1994;83:3787–3794.

15. Fruehauf S, Haas R, Conradt C, et al. Peripheral blood progenitor cell (PBPC) counts during steady-state hematopoiesis allow to estimate the yield of mobilized PBPC after filgrastim (R-metHuG-CSF)-supported cytotoxic chemotherapy. Blood 1995;85:2619–2626.

16. Bolan CD, Carter CS, Wesley RA, et al. Prospective evaluation of cell kinetics, yields, and donor experiences during a single large-volume apheresis versus two smaller volume consecutive day collections of allogeneic peripheral blood stem cells. Br J Haematol 2003;120:801–807.

17. Stroncek D, Shawker T, Follmann D,et al. G-CSF-induced spleen size changes in peripheral blood progenitor cell donors. Transfusion 2003;43:609–613.

18. Snyder EL, Haley NR, eds. Cellular Therapy: A Physician's Handbook, 1st Ed. Bethesda, MD: AABB Press; 2004:11–23.

19. Brunstein CG, Wagner JE. Cord blood transplantation for adults. Vox Sang 2006;91:195–205.

20. ACOG Practice Bulletin. Prevention of Rh D alloimmunization. Number 4, May 1999 (replaces educational bulletin Number 147, October 1990). Clinical management guidelines for obstetrician-gynecologists. American College of Obstetrics and Gynecology. Int J Gynecol Obstet 1999; 66:63–70.

21. Popovsky MA, ed. Transfusion Reactions, 3rd Ed. Bethesda, MD: AABB Press;2007.

22. Petz LD, Calhoun L, Shulman IA, et al. The sickle cell hemolytic transfusion reaction syndrome. Transfusion 1997;37:382–392.

23. Toy P, Popovsky MA, Abraham E, et al. Transfusion-related acute lung injury: definition and review. Crit Care Med 2005;33:721–726.

24. Eder AF, Herron R, Strupp A, et al. Transfusion-related acute lung injury surveillance (2003–2005) and the potential impact of the selective use of plasma from male donors in the American Red Cross. Transfusion 2007;47:599–607.

25. Eder AF, Kennedy JM, Dy BA, et al. Bacterial screening of apheresis platelets and the residual risk of septic transfusion reactions: the American Red Cross experience (2004–2006). Transfusion 2007;47:1134–1142.

26. Stramer SL. Current risks of transfusion-transmitted agents: a review. Arch Pathol Lab Med 2007;131:702–707.

27. Dodd, RY, Notari EP IV, Stramer SL. Current prevalence and incidence of infectious disease markers and estimated window-period risk in the American Red Cross blood donor population. Transfusion 2002;42:975–979.

28. Dodd RY. Transmission of parasites by blood transfusion. Vox Sang 1998;74(Suppl 2):161–163.

29. Alter HJ, Stramer SL, Dodd RY. Emerging infectious diseases that threaten the blood supply. Semin Hematol 2007;44:32–41.

30. Health Protection Agency Press Statement: Fourth case of transfusion-associated vCJD infection in the United Kingdom. Euro Surveill 2007;12:E070118.4.

31. Santrach P, ed. Standards for Perioperative Autologous Blood Collection and Administration, 2nd Ed. Bethesda, MD: AABB Press; 2005:18–19, Reference Standard 5.1.7A.

32. Bolan CD, Klein HG. Transfusion medicine and pharmacologic aspects of hemostasis. In Kitchens C, Kessler C, Alving BM, eds. Consultative Hemostasis and Thrombosis. New York: Harcourt Health Sciences; 2007:461–484.

33. Spence RK, Mintz PD. Transfusion in surgery, trauma, and critical care. In Mintz PD, ed. Transfusion Therapy Clinical Principles and Practice. Bethesda, MD: AABB Press, 2005:203–232.
34. Counts RB, Haisch C, Simon TL, et al. Hemostasis in massively transfused trauma patients. Ann Surg 1979;190:91–99.
35. Petz LD, Garratty G, eds. Immune Hemolytic Anemias, 2nd Ed. Philadelphia: Churchill Livingstone; 2004.
36. Smith JW, Weinstein R, Hillyer KL, et al. Therapeutic apheresis: a summary of current indication categories endorsed by the AABB and the American Society for Apheresis. Transfusion 2003;43:820–822.
37. Szczepiorkowski ZM, Bandarenko N, Kim HC, et al. Guidelines on the use of therapeutic apheresis in clinical practice—evidence-based approach from the apheresis applications committee of the American Society for Apheresis. J Clin Apher 2007;22:106–175.
38. Rogers RL, Johnson H, Ludwig R, et al. Efficacy and safety of plateletpheresis by donors with low-normal platelet counts. J Clin Apheresis 1995;10:194–197.
39. Flaum MA, Cuneo RA, Appelbaum FR, et al. The hemostatic imbalance of plasma-exchange transfusion. Blood 1979;54:694–702.
40. McLeod BC, ed. Apheresis: Principles and Practice, 2nd Ed. Bethesda, MD: AABB Press; 2003.
41. Bolan CD, Cecco SA, Wesley RA, et al. Controlled study of citrate effects response to IV calcium administration during Allogeneic peripheral blood progenitor cell donation. Transfusion 2002;42:935–946.
42. White NJ. The treatment of malaria. N Engl J Med 1996;335:800–806.

SUGGESTED READINGS

Eder AF, Chambers LA. Noninfectious complications of blood transfusion. Arch Pathol Lab Med 2007;131:708–718.
Gottschall J. Blood Transfusion Therapy: A Physician's Handbook, 8th Ed. Bethesda, MD: AABB Press; 2005.
McLeod BC. Therapeutic Apheresis: A Physician's Handbook, 1st Ed. Bethesda, MD: AABB Press, 2005.
Osby MA, Saxena S, Nelson J, et al. Safe handling and administration of blood components: review of practical concepts. Arch Pathol Lab Med 2007;131:690–694.
Roseff SD. Pediatric Transfusion: A Physician's Handbook, 1st Ed. Bethesda, MD: AABB Press; 2003.
Snyder EL, Haley NR, eds. *Cellular Therapy: A Physician's Handbook.* 1st Ed. Bethesda, MD: AABB Press; 2004.
Stramer SL. Current risks of transfusion-transmitted agents: a review. Arch Pathol Lab Med 2007;131: 702–707.
Szczepiorkowski ZM, Bandarenko N, Kim HC, et al. Guidelines on the use of therapeutic apheresis in clinical practice—evidence-based approach from the apheresis applications committee of the American Society for Apheresis. J Clin Apher 2007;22:106–175.

25

Hemochromatosis

Susan F. Leitman and Charles D. Bolan

EPIDEMIOLOGY

Classic hereditary hemochromatosis, also known as HFE-hemochromatosis, is an autosomal-recessive disorder caused by inappropriate dietary absorption of iron and abnormal iron cycling. It is characterized by progressive accumulation of iron in tissues, particularly the liver, pancreas, heart, endocrine organs, and skin, which may lead to end-stage organ damage, usually during or after middle age (1–3). It is one of the most common single-gene disorders in Caucasians of northern European descent, with an incidence of 1 in 200 and a carrier rate of 1 in 10 persons. However, the clinical penetrance of the disorder is highly variable, and only a minority of affected persons develops severe or life-threatening organ dysfunction (4,5).

Genetic Basis for Classic Hemochromatosis: HFE Mutations

- Mutations in *HFE*, an MHC class-I like gene on chromosome 6, are found in nearly 90% of persons with the clinical phenotype and 100% of affected persons with a strong family history of the disorder (6,7).
- Substitution of tyrosine for cysteine at amino acid 282 of the *HFE* gene product (C282Y) is considered the founder mutation. Linkage disequilibrium studies demonstrate that the mutation originated recently, within the past 2000 years. A single copy of the C282Y allele occurs with highest frequency in northwestern European populations, reaching 14% in areas of Great Britain (Table 25.1). Allele frequency decreases in a north-to-south and west-to-east direction across Europe, and the ancestral haplotype may have been of Viking or Celtic origin; it is extremely rare in African and Asian populations. Homozygosity for C282Y is seen in 64% to 96% of persons with clinical hemochromatosis.
- A second HFE mutation, replacement of histidine by aspartate at residue 63 of the HFE protein (H63D), is frequently found on the non-C282Y-containing chromosome of individuals with clinical hemochromatosis who are heterozygous for C282Y (6). H63D is an older mutation with a wider population distribution, having an allele frequency of 5% to 14% throughout Europe and Asia. It appears to be a genetic polymorphism without much clinical impact in the absence of another genetic or environmental factor. Compound heterozygosity for C282Y/H63D is seen in 4% to 7% of persons with a hemochromatosis phenotype.
- More than 20 additional polymorphisms in HFE have been described. Of these, only the S65C mutation appears to have clinical impact and may cause mild iron overload when compound heterozygous with C282Y or H63D.

PATHOPHYSIOLOGY

Because iron excretion in the gut is fixed at 1 mg per day, normal iron balance must be maintained by meticulous control of iron absorption in the intestine and iron release from macrophages. These are modulated in response to body iron stores and the erythropoietic demand for iron.

TABLE 25.1. *Frequency of HFE Genotypes in the U.S. Caucasian Population*

Genotype	Frequency (Percent)
C282Y/C282Y	1 in 200 (0.5%)
C282Y/wt	1 in 7–12 (8%–14%)
H63D/H63D	1 in 40 (2.5%)
H63D/wt	1 in 4 (25%)
S65C/wt	1 in 25 (4%)

wt, wild type.

Hepcidin: Key Regulator of Iron Homeostasis

Hepcidin, a liver-derived peptide hormone, is a key negative regulator of iron release into the plasma by intestinal enterocytes, macrophages, hepatocytes, and placental cells (8). It binds to and causes internalization and degradation of the cell surface iron exporter, ferroportin (9). Hepcidin excess decreases intestinal iron absorption and macrophage iron release and may cause iron-deficiency anemia. Hepcidin deficiency promotes intestinal iron absorption and leads to tissue iron overload. Hepcidin gene expression is enhanced by iron overload and inflammation and is suppressed by anemia and hypoxia. Although hepcidin is ordinarily induced by dietary iron loading, its expression is inappropriately reduced in all forms of inherited hemochromatosis (10,11).

Iron Overload Disorders and Hepcidin Deficiency

Hepcidin deficiency plays a central role in the pathogenesis of the inherited hemochromatosis disorders, including those caused by mutations in the HFE gene, the hemojuvelin gene *(HJV)*, the transferrin receptor 2 gene *(TfR2)*, and hepcidin itself *(HAMP)* (Table 25.2). Hemojuvelin acts as a coreceptor in the bone morphogenetic protein (BMP) pathway, interacting with BMP ligands and BMP type I and II receptors to generate an active signaling complex (10). This complex activates a Smad receptor signaling cascade and translocation of a Smad complex to the nucleus, where it increases *HFE* transcription. *HJV* and *HAMP* mutations are critical components in the same common pathway; their negative effect on hepcidin expression is associated with severe iron loading in childhood, or juvenile hemochromatosis.

HFE Localization and Function

HFE is highly expressed in Kupffer cells of the liver and in tissue macrophages. Binding to $\beta2$ microglobulin ($\beta2$m) allows expression of HFE/$\beta2$m on the cell surface (12), where it forms a stable complex with transferrin receptor 1 (TfR1). The C282Y mutation prevents formation of a disulfide bond in HFE, disabling $\beta2$m binding and preventing cell surface expression. Disruption of the HFE/$\beta2$m/TfR1 complex and mutations in *TfR2* are associated with adult-onset iron overload. HFE and TfR2 may regulate hepcidin expression by enhanced iron transport into the cell (endocytosis of

TABLE 25.2. *Classification of Iron Overload Disorders*

Primary (Genetic) Hemochromatosis	Secondary Hemochromatosis
Type 1: Classical/hereditary hemochromatosis (HFE gene)	1. Transfusional siderosis
Type 2: Juvenile hemochromatosis (severe phenotype)	2. Congenital anemia with
2a. Hemojuvelin mutations (HJV gene, 1q-linked)	ineffective erythropoiesis
2b. Hepcidin mutations (HAMP gene)	(thalassemia, red cell enzyme
Type 3. Transferrin receptor-2 deficiency (TfR2 gene)	deficiencies)
Type 4. Ferroportin deficiency (IREG-1 gene)	3. Acquired sideroblastic and
Type 5. African iron overload	dyserythroblastic anemias

TABLE 25.3. *Body Iron Distribution*

	Men (g)	Women (g)
Hemoglobin (red cells)	3.0	2.4
Storage iron (liver)	1.0	0.4
Myoglobin and respiratory enzymes (muscle)	0.3	0.2
Total nonhemochromatosis adult	4.4	3.1
Total hemochromatosis adult	5–20	4–10

diferric transferrin), by upstream regulation of hepcidin, or as weak coreceptors for BMP-SMAD signaling. According to this model, it might be possible to treat hemochromatosis by hepcidin replacement.

The most common form of secondary hemochromatosis is transfusional iron overload: 1 mL of red cells contains about 1 mg of iron. Inappropriate absorption of iron in the gut may also occur in association with ineffective erythropoiesis. In this case, the erythropoietic stimulus to decrease hepcidin levels overrides the effect of iron overload on increasing hepcidin expression.

Iron Homeostasis

The distribution of body iron is shown in Table 25.3, with a comparison of iron stores in the normal state and in subjects with hemochromatosis.

- ***Excess Iron and Tissue Injury.*** When the capacity for iron storage is exceeded, excess tissue iron causes cellular damage by catalyzing the formation of oxyradicals (13). Oxidative damage to lipids, proteins, carbohydrates, and DNA may lead to widespread impairment in cell function and integrity. In particular, lipid peroxidation may result in impaired membrane-dependent mitochondrial and lysosomal function. Oxidative injury to DNA, particularly in hepatocytes, may predispose to mutagenesis and cancer.
- ***Nontransferrin Bound Iron.*** Nontransferrin bound iron (NTBI) represents "free iron in serum." NTBI enters cells freely, independent of receptor-mediated uptake. NTBI levels are low or undetectable at transferrin saturation (TS) below 40% and increase linearly with TS levels above 40% to 50%. NTBI and its intracellular labile iron counterpart may be the direct mediators of oxidant stress (13).

CLINICAL FEATURES AND DIAGNOSIS OF HFE-HEMOCHROMATOSIS

Prior to the availability of biochemical and genetic screening tests, HFE-hemochromatosis was identified by damage to the liver, pancreas, heart, and joints, and was diagnosed by demonstrating increased iron stores on liver biopsy. The "classic triad" of cirrhosis, diabetes, and skin pigmentation appeared in many publications and textbooks (1). Patients typically presented with:

- Severe liver disease because of hepatic fibrosis or cirrhosis
- Cardiac failure and refractory arrhythmias
- Polyendocrine failure: insulin-dependent diabetes and hypogonadotrophic hypogonadism
- Debilitating symmetric polyarthritis
- Grayish skin pigmentation

It is now recognized that this severe clinical phenotype is relatively rare and only develops in 1% to 4% of untreated C282Y homozygotes over their lifetime (4). Between 40% and 60% of C282Y

TABLE 25.4. *Clinical Features of HH: Historical versus Current*

Historical Description	Current Common Presentation
Liver disease	Fatigue
Skin "bronzing"	Arthropathy
Diabetes	Impotence (men)

homozygote males and 60% and 80% of homozygote females will remain asymptomatic or have minimal clinical manifestations throughout their lives; of the 40% to 50% who do develop symptoms that affect quality of life, arthritis, fatigue, and sexual dysfunction are the most common complaints (Table 25.4) (14,15).

New Diagnostic Definition

In the current era of molecular testing, recognizing that clinical penetrance can be highly variable, the diagnosis of hemochromatosis is established by the detection of two mutated HFE alleles. This definition does not require active symptoms or signs of illness or the presence of iron overload. Four stages of the disorder are recognized (16):

1. Genetic predisposition with no other abnormality (age 0 to 20, 0 to 5 g tissue iron storage)
2. Iron overload without symptoms (age >20, >5 g iron storage)
3. Iron overload with early symptoms (age >30, >8 g iron storage)
4. Iron overload with organ damage (age >40, 10 to 20 g iron storage)

Common Clinical Presentation

The most common clinical presentation of hereditary hemochromatosis (HH) is with nonspecific symptoms, and therefore practitioners should have a low threshold for ordering serum transferrin saturation and ferritin studies in patients with unexplained chronic fatigue, arthralgias or arthritis, sexual dysfunction, hepatomegaly, or elevated liver function studies (alanine aminotransferase [ALT]). Because such symptoms are easily overlooked, the single most common event currently leading to a diagnosis of hemochromatosis is the incidental detection of an abnormal laboratory test result, either an elevated transferrin saturation, serum ferritin, or ALT. In patients with hemochromatosis diagnosed with fatigue on presentation, screening laboratory tests to evaluate possible concomitant thyroid disease should be obtained.

Typical findings related to the most common clinical signs and symptoms of hemochromatosis are shown in Table 25.5. It is difficult to assign a frequency to these symptoms, because there is a continuum of increasing frequency with increasing age and with male versus female sex (16). Arthritis is the clinical feature with the greatest impact on quality of life (17). In contrast to significant cardiac abnormalities described in patients with hemochromatosis who presented with very high iron prior to the advent of more frequent screening and the availability of a genetic test, heart disease now is generally absent or clinically insignificant in newly diagnosed, asymptomatic patients (18).

The considerable variability in clinical penetrance of C282Y homozygosity, both in rate of accumulation of iron stores and appearance of organ dysfunction, may be due to environmental, lifestyle, and genetic factors (Table 25.6).

LABORATORY TESTING

Once the clinical suspicion of hemochromatosis is raised, the diagnosis should be confirmed by laboratory testing.

TABLE 25.5. *Clinical and Laboratory Features of HH (C282Y Homozygotes)*

Sign/Symptom	Frequency	Features
Fatigue	30%–50%	May be related to liver disease, endocrine dysfunction
Arthritis	30%–60%	Major quality of life feature; more likely in subjects with higher iron burden at presentation. Symmetric, degenerative noninflammatory osteoarthritis; radiographic features include sclerosis, joint space narrowing, subchondral cysts, osteophytes, osteopenia. Chondrocalcinosis (pseudogout) and gout more common than in non-HH population. Disproportionate involvement of hands and feet, with MCP and MTP joints commonly affected. Hip replacement more common than in age-adjusted non-HH population.
Sexual dysfunction	30%–50%	Excess iron deposited in anterior pituitary and testes. Reduced shaving, loss of libido, erectile dysfunction, gynecomastia in men. Low free testosterone levels, inappropriately low LH and FSH. Testosterone replacement therapy may restore libido and potency.
Skin changes	10%–20%	Grayish or gray-brown hue; bronzing is rare
Hepatomegaly	10%–20%	Portal circulation leads directly from GI tract to liver; liver is first site of iron deposition; hepatic iron loading precedes other organs; 70% of all HH-related deaths are because of liver disease.
Hypothyroidism	10%–15%	Primary hypothyroidism; thyroid gland fibrotic; elevated TSH
Elevated TS	>80%	TS >50% in 94% of men and 82% of women over age 40
Elevated ferritin	>60%	Ferritin >normal in 90% of men and 60% of women over age 40
Elevated ALT	0%–25%	Influenced by other factors: alcohol, drugs, obesity

GI, gastrointestinal; HH, hereditary hemochromatosis; LH, luteinizing hormone; MCP, metacarpophalangeal; MTP, metatarsophalangeal; TS, transferrin saturation; TSH, thyroid-stimulating hormone.

1. **Confirmatory laboratory tests**
   - ***Serum iron, transferrin, and transferrin saturation***: transferrin is the major iron transport protein in plasma. Several assay methods for transferring saturation (TS) exist: most accurate is direct colorimetric analysis of serum iron (SI) combined with nephelometric assay of transferrin, wherein TS = molar concentration of iron divided by twice the molar concentration of transferrin. Less expensive but also less robust methods include chemical analyses of

TABLE 25.6. *Factors Influencing Clinical Penetrance*

Factors That Accelerate Iron Overload	Factors That Lessen Iron Overload and Organ Damage
Environmental/Lifestyle	
• Alcohol use	• Blood donation
• Oral iron supplementation	• Multiparity/menorrhagia (women)
• Dietary habits (meat-rich diet)	• Dietary habits (vegetarian diet, tea)
• Exogenous estrogen, vitamin C	
Genetic/Acquired Disorders	
• Hepatitis B or C infection (HBV, HCV)	
• Nonalcoholic steatohepatitis (NASH)	
• Porphyria cutanea tarda (PCT)	
• Alpha-1 antitrypsin deficiency (AAT)	
• Mutations in hepcidin, ferroportin, transferrin receptor, other genes	

total serum iron binding capacity (TIBC) and unbound iron capacity (UIBC). Saturation of serum iron binding capacity is measured by dividing the serum iron by either TIBC (SI/TIBC) or by the sum of iron and UIBC [(SI)/(SI + UIBC)]. Normal range for TS is 15% to 45%.

- **Serum ferritin:** major intracellular iron storage protein and is measured immunologically. It estimates the degree of iron overload and the size of mobilizable iron stores (1ug/L ferritin = 7–8 mg stored iron; e.g., 1000 ug/L ferritin = 7000–8000 mg stored iron). It is used to determine pace of initial phlebotomy therapy. Normal levels are <350 ug/L in men and <120 ug/L in women.
- **HFE genotype:** definitive diagnostic test. It assesses predisposition to serious illness and is useful for family counseling.

2. **Ancillary laboratory tests**

- *Alanine aminotransferase (ALT)*: to assess degree of liver injury
- *CBC*: obtain baseline hemoglobin and red cell mean corpuscular volume (MCV), which can be monitored during therapy (decrease in MCV is an indicator of iron-limited erythropoiesis).
- *Blood glucose and electrolytes*
- *Total and free testosterone*: as indicated by symptoms
- *Thyroid function tests*: as indicated by symptoms
- *Alpha fetoprotein*: as baseline for subsequent monitoring for liver cancer
- *Serologic tests for exposure to hepatitis B and C (HBsAg and anti-HCV)*: active viral hepatitis worsens liver injury; useful to guide vaccine administration

Role of Liver Biopsy

Liver biopsy is generally not required for diagnosis. Although it previously served as the criterion standard for both diagnosis and prognosis, the diagnosis is now more safely and reliably made with use of the HFE genotype (16).

Indications for biopsy include confirmation of a high clinical suspicion of cirrhosis; for example, when the ferritin >3000 ug/L, hepatomegaly and/or signs of portal hypertension are present (large spleen, low platelets), or the ALT does not normalize with phlebotomy.

Biopsy is also indicated if: (i) concomitant hepatitis B (HBV) or hepatitis C (HCV) infection are present, (ii) in the diagnostic workup of elevated ferritin and ALT, with normal HFE genotype, and (iii) to evaluate mass lesions seen on radiographic imaging studies.

Histologic Findings

Histologic findings include marked increase in hepatocellular iron, with relative sparing of Kupffer cells. Iron is distributed in a decreasing gradient from the periportal to the centrilobular areas. With progressive damage, portal fibrous expansion, bridging fibrosis with piecemeal necrosis, and macro- or micronodular cirrhosis may be seen. Hepatic iron index (hepatic iron concentration/56 × age) >1.9 (in absence of transfusional siderosis) strongly suggests iron overload is because of hemochromatosis rather than other causes.

Radiographic and Other Tests

Skeletal films are performed to evaluate symptomatic joints. *Liver ultrasound* is useful in workup of non-HH causes of elevated ferritin and may show steatosis. It is important in surveillance for liver cancer. *Computed tomography (CT) and/or magnetic resonance imaging (MRI) of liver* are not indicated diagnostically but are useful for suspected liver cancer. *Superconducting quantum interference device (SQUID) assessment* provides the most sensitive noninvasive quantitative assessment of iron stores but has limited availability.

POPULATION SCREENING

The clinical course of HH meets the definition of a disorder for which population screening should be performed (2,3):

1. High prevalence in selected populations
2. Burden of disease (clinical penetrance) high enough to warrant medical and public attention
3. Prolonged presymptomatic phase, during which detection and treatment lead to reductions in morbidity and mortality (early detection prevents complications and improves outcomes)
4. Availability of reliable, accurate, easily available, and inexpensive screening tests
5. Treatment is effective, safe, inexpensive, and easily accessible

Thus, the costs of widespread testing and preventive treatment are considered favorable (more effective and less expensive) than delaying until development of late symptoms, particularly as the early, presenting symptoms are nonspecific, are often not recognized as being caused by hemochromatosis, and are associated with a 5- to 10-year delay until accurate diagnosis.

Laboratory Screening

- *Transferrin saturation*: The single best screening test is the serum TS: it is inexpensive, widely available, and highly sensitive and specific for the presence of the C282Y HFE allele (19). The decision threshold at which confirmatory testing should be initiated ranges from TS values of 45% to 62%, depending on whether sensitivity or specificity is preferred (Table 25.7). Because TS is affected by dietary and diurnal variation, an elevated valued should be confirmed by a second TS after an overnight fast, in the absence of oral iron supplements. Phenotype screening with TS is not advised until age 20 to 30, as iron burdens are generally low below this age (16). An algorithm for workup of persons detected through screening programs is shown in Figure 25.1.
- *Ferritin screening*: Ferritin is an acute phase reactant; levels rise with inflammation, infection, and non-HH liver disease. Lack of sensitivity and specificity make it a less reliable screening test.
- *Genotype screening*: A 1998 consensus conference decided against widespread population screening using genetic tests. The high cost of genetic tests and variable clinical penetrance of HH, coupled with concerns over stigmatization, discrimination, and insurability, led to rejection of this approach at the time (20). Passage of the Genetic Information Nondiscrimination Act (GINA) by the U.S. Congress in July 2008, however, has led to a reconsideration of the role of genetic screening in targeted populations, such as Caucasian males above age 20.

Screening of Family Members of C282Y Homozygotes

- *Screening of children:* The most cost-effective test is HFE genotype; biochemical screening is also acceptable. Testing should be delayed until age 20 to 30. If fewer than two children are involved, the best approach may be genotyping of the other parent (21).

TABLE 25.7. *Diagnostic Yield of Transferrin Saturation Screening*

Gender	TS Decision Threshold (%)	Sensitivity (Detection rate)	Specificity (False positive)
Male	≥50	94%	7%
	≥60	86%	1.5%
Female	≥50	82%	5%
	≥60	67%	0.6%

Further evaluation is recommended if TS 0.55% to 62% in men and 0.45% to 50% in women.
TS, transferring saturation.

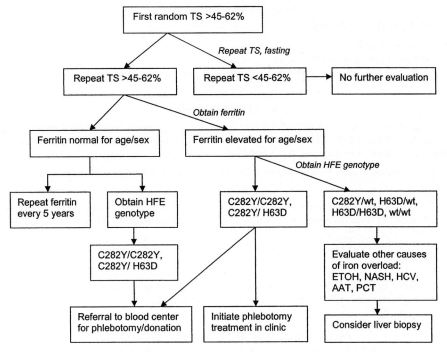

FIG. 25.1. Decision tree for hemochromatosis population screening.

- *Screening of siblings:* All siblings should be counseled to undergo either genetic or phenotypic screening. The most cost-effective test is HFE genotype, but phenotypic screening with combination of TS and ferritin is also acceptable (21).

TREATMENT

Phlebotomy Therapy

Phlebotomy therapy includes the periodic removal of 1 unit (500 mL) of whole blood. It has been the safe and inexpensive standard of care for past 50 years (22). One unit of whole blood removes 200 to 250 mg of iron. Double red cell collection by apheresis removes 360 mL of packed red cells (400 to 420 mg of iron) and may be particularly useful in blood center setting.

There has been controversy regarding treatment indications for patients with modest iron burdens. However, patients generally desire treatment and are eager and willing to be blood donors. The therapy is safe, accessible, and prevents late organ damage. Referral to the blood center shifts the argument in favor of treatment as there is a double benefit, to the patient and to the community, and the care is maximally efficient and provided free of charge.

Guidelines for Plebotomy Therapy

Phase 1: Iron Depletion

Pace

Initiate phlebotomy at 1- to 4-week intervals, depending on ferritin, hemoglobin, ALT, gender, and weight. As iron depletion approaches, decrease pace to monthly.

Target of "De-ironing" Therapy

Several assays may be used:

- Ferritin <30 ug/L
- Transferrin saturation <30%
- Decrease in red cell mean corpuscular volume (MCV) to 3% below prephlebotomy level (23)

Monitoring Parameters

Prephlebotomy fingerstick hemoglobin or hematocrit (+/− venous complete blood count [CBC]) should be performed at each visit to avoid anemia. Ferritin should be performed every 4 to 8 weeks initially, then ferritin +/− TS every 1 to 2 treatments once ferritin is <100 ug/L.

Safety Guide

Threshold hemoglobin for therapeutic bleed is ≥12.5 g/dL (hematocrit ≥38%). In general, do not bleed below this level; defer therapy for 1 to 4 weeks until hemoglobin recovers. Iron deficiency is not necessary during treatment; anemia should be avoided.

General Guide

For initial ferritin of 500 to 1500, patients generally require 10 to 30 bleeds to achieve iron depletion. If initial ferritin >2000 ug/dL, may require >40 to 50 bleeds.

Phase II: Preventing Reaccumulation (Maintenance)

Pace

In maintenance therapy, 500 mL should be removed every 8 to 26 weeks (mean, 10 to 12 weeks), depending on gender, weight, age, and dietary habits. This is usually a lifelong requirement, although some subjects reaccumulate iron very slowly.

Goals of Maintenance Therapy

Goals of maintenance therapy include ferritin 30 to 50 ug/L, transferrin saturation <50%, and hemoglobin >12.5 g/dL.

Monitoring Parameters

Prephlebotomy fingerstick hemoglobin or hematocrit (+/− venous CBC) should be performed at each visit, and ferritin and/or TS every one to two treatments.

Evaluation of Anemia During Phlebotomy Therapy

Persistent hemoglobin <12.5 g/dL despite elevated ferritin levels may be due to occult bleeding or may have an endocrine cause, which should be evaluated with thyroid function studies and testosterone levels (men). If concomitant disorder of erythroid production is present (thalassemia, renal insufficiency) and urgent need for phlebotomy exists, weekly erythropoietin may be helpful. Anemia may also be due to development of liver cancer.

Arthritis, Endocrine Replacement, Vaccinations, and Cancer Surveillance

- *Arthritis:* responds moderately well to nonsteroidal anti-inflammatory agents. Joint aspiration should be performed to exclude gout or pseudogout in acutely inflamed joints. Orthopedic evaluation should

be conducted for joint replacement for severe chronic hip, knee, or ankle pain. Cumulative incidence of major joint replacement in C282Y +/+ HH subjects is 30% by age 70.
- ***Testosterone replacement***: consider in men with symptomatic sexual dysfunction and low testosterone levels.
- ***Hepatitis A and B vaccination***: should be given as prophylaxis against future hepatic injury in unexposed patients
- ***Liver Ultrasound***: surveillance for hepatocellular cancer. Repeat every 6 months if cirrhosis documented by biopsy.

Dietary and Lifestyle Counseling

- Avoid oral iron supplements
- Limit alcohol intake to protect the liver
- Consume red meat in moderation, but major change in dietary habits is not required. Iron stores are most efficiently controlled by adjusting frequency of bleeds rather than reducing intake of iron-rich foods.
- Avoid raw shellfish until iron depletion achieved (avoid *vibrio vulnificus*)

If ALT is elevated, discontinue alcohol intake until iron depletion is completed and ALT is normal and consider discontinuation of medications with potential hepatic toxicity.

PROGNOSIS AND RESPONSE TO THERAPY

If cirrhosis is not present, long-term survival is unchanged from non-HH population (24). If cirrhosis is present, risk of hepatic cancer is increased and persists for life: 18.5% of subjects with cirrhosis will develop liver cancer, which may not be detected until 5 to 10 years after iron depletion. Overall incidence of hepatic cancer is 100-fold greater in HH than in non-HH subjects and accounts for 10% to 30% of HH-related deaths. Progression of cirrhosis due to HH is slower than in other types of cirrhosis (alcoholic, viral); however, HH subjects undergoing liver transplant for end-stage liver disease or liver cancer have a higher than average peritransplant mortality.

The response to phlebotomy varies by tissue site (Table 25.8).

HEMOCHROMATOSIS SUBJECTS AS BLOOD DONORS

- **Regulatory issues:** The Food and Drug Administration (FDA) allows blood centers to obtain a "variance" from federal code to permit blood from HH subjects to be made available for transfusion into others, even if collected more frequently than 56-day interval.
- **FDA requirements:** FDA requirements state phlebotomy must be performed under a physician's direction, without charge regardless of whether subjects qualify as donors, and with periodic laboratory monitoring.

TABLE 25.8. *Response to Phlebotomy Therapy in Hemochromatosis*

Complication	Prevents	Reverses or Improves
Arthropathy	Unknown	Partly, if initiated early in course
Fatigue	Yes	Yes, to a variable degree
Skin graying	Yes	Yes
Liver fibrosis	Yes	Partly, if initiated early in course
Cirrhosis	Yes	No; but portal hypertension may improve
Cardiomyopathy	Yes	Partly, if initiated early in course
Diabetes	Yes	No
Hypogonadism	Yes	No
Hypothyroidism	Yes	No

- **Logistics and safety**
  - 75% of all HH subjects meet allogeneic donor eligibility criteria
  - 55% of HH subjects were blood donors prior to knowledge of their diagnosis
  - Potential HH-donor contribution estimated at 1 to 2 million red cell units per year in the United States
  - Recent rapid increase in number of U.S. blood centers with FDA-approved variances to allow HH subjects to be blood donors (142 centers, October 2008)
  - HH subjects documented to be safe, reliable donors (23)
- **Advantages of phlebotomy care in the blood center:** free, consistent, accessible, and convenient treatment; increased patient satisfaction (avoid frustration of knowing blood will be discarded), and it helps alleviate national blood shortages.

FUTURE CHALLENGES

The process of molecular discovery is rapidly leading to a more comprehensive understanding of the role of HFE protein in iron homeostasis. At the same time, the availability of a genetic test has focused increased public and medical attention on hemochromatosis. Robust population screening studies are currently in progress to more accurately determine clinical penetrance, both for early as well as late complications. It is hoped that increased emphasis on educational campaigns to foster prompt recognition of early symptoms by primary care providers will complement or perhaps even alleviate the need for targeted screening programs. Better appreciation of the advantages of referral to the blood center may improve the quality and accessibility of care and also confer a benefit to the general public health.

REFERENCES

1. Bothwell TH, MacPhail AP. Hereditary hemochromatosis: etiologic, pathologic, and clinical aspects. Semin Hematol 1998;35:55–71.
2. Bomford A. Genetics of hemochromatosis. Lancet 2002;360:1673–1681.
3. Tavill AS. Diagnosis and management of hemochromatosis: AASLD practice guidelines. Hepatology 2001;33:1321–1328.
4. Beutler E. Penetrance in hereditary hemochromatosis. The HFE Cys282Tyr mutation as a necessary but not sufficient cause of clinical hereditary hemochromatosis. Blood 2003;101:3347–3350.
5. Ajioka R, Kushner JP. Clinical consequences of iron overload in hemochromatosis patients. Blood 2003;101:3351–3354.
6. Feder JN, Gnirke A, Thomas W, et al. A novel MHC class I-like gene is mutated in patients with hereditary haemochromatosis. Nat Genet 1996;13:399–408.
7. Jazwinska EC, Cullen LM, Busfiled F, et al. Haemochromatosis and HLA-H. Nature Genetics 1996;14:249–251.
8. Ganz T. Hepcidin, a key regulator of iron metabolism and mediator of anemia of inflammation. Blood 2003;102:783–788.
9. Nemeth E, Tuttle M, Powelson J, et al. Hepcidin regulates cellular iron efflux by binding to ferroportin and inducing its internalization. Science 2004;306:2090–2093.
10. Babitt JL, Huang FW, Wrighting DM, et al. Bone morphogenetic signaling by hemojuvelin regulates hepcidin expression. Nat Gen 2006;38:531–539.
11. Bridle KR, Frazer DM, Wilkins SJ, et al. Disrupted hepcidin regulation in HFE-associated haemochromatosis and the liver as a regulator of body iron homeostasis. Lancet 2003;361:669–673.
12. Feder JN, Penny DM, Irrinki A, et al. The hemochromatosis gene product complexes with the transferrin receptor and lowers its affinity for ligand binding. Proc Natl Acad Sci USA 1998;95:1472–1477.
13. Brissot P, Loreal O. Role of nontransferrin bound iron in the pathogenesis of iron overload and toxicity. In Hershko C, ed. Iron Chelation Therapy. New York: Kluwer Academic/Plenum Publishers; 2002:45–53.

14. Olynyk JK, Cullen DJ, Aquilia S, et al. A population-based study of the clinical expression of the hemochromatosis gene. N Engl J Med 1999;341:718–724.
15. Bulaj ZJ, Ajioka RS, Phillips JD, et al. Disease-related conditions in relatives of patients with hemochromatosis. N Engl J Med 2000;343:1529–1535.
16. Adams P, Brissot P, Powell LW. EASL International Consensus Conference on Haemochromatosis-Part II. Expert document. J Hepatol 2000;33:487–496.
17. Adams P, Speechley M. The effect of arthritis on the quality of life in hereditary hemochromatosis. J Rheumatol 1996;23:707–710.
18. Shizukuda Y, Bolan C, Tripodi D, et al. Left ventricular systolic function during stress echocardiography in subjects with asymptomatic hereditary hemochromatosis. Am J Cardiol 2006:98:694–698.
19. Bradley LA, Haddow JE, Palomaki GE: Population screening for hemochromatosis: expectations based on a study of relatives of symptomatic probands. J Med Screen 1996; 3:171–177.
20. Burke W, Thomson E, Khoury MJ, et al. Hereditary hemochromatosis. Gene discovery and its implications for population-based screening. J Am Med Assoc 1998;280:172–178.
21. El-Serag HB, Inadomi JM, Kowdley KV. Screening for hereditary hemochromatosis in siblings and children of affected patients. Ann Int Med 2000;132:261–269.
22. Barton JC, McDonnell SM, Adams PC, et al. Management of hemochromatosis. Ann Intern Med 1998;129:932–939.
23. Leitman SF, Browning JN, Yau YY, et al. Hemochromatosis subjects as allogeneic blood donors: a prospective study. Transfusion 2003;43:1538–1544.
24. Niederau C, Fischer R, Purschel A, et al. Long-term survival in patients with hereditary hemochromatosis. Gastroenterology 1996;110:1107–1119.

26

Consultative Hematology

Pierre Noel

HEMATOLOGIC COMPLICATIONS OF PREGNANCY

Anemia in Pregnancy

During normal pregnancies, plasma volume increases by 40% to 60%, and red cell mass increases by 20% to 40%. The hematocrit typically drops to 30% to 32%; lower limit of normal for hemoglobin drops to 11 g/dl in the first trimester and 10 g/dl in the second and third trimesters. The most common forms of anemia of pregnancy in North America are iron and folate deficiency anemias. The Centers for Disease Control (CDC) estimated that 12% of all women ages 12 to 49 years were iron deficient in 1999 through 2000.

One thousand milligrams of additional iron are required during pregnancy. The normal 500 mg iron storage pool is insufficient, and iron deficiency anemia develops unless iron supplementation occurs throughout pregnancy. The recommended daily allowance for iron during pregnancy is 27 mg of elemental iron. CDC recommends routine low-dose iron supplementation (30 mg of elemental iron daily) for all pregnant women, beginning at the first prenatal visit. Calculations of dosage for iron preparations should be based on the amount of iron in each preparation: Ferrous sulfate contains 20% elemental iron, ferrous gluconate 12%, and ferrous fumarate 33%. Low values of serum iron and ferritin are reliable indicators of iron deficiency in pregnancy. The consequences of maternal iron deficiency on the neonate are controversial. Mild to moderate maternal iron deficiency anemia is not associated with significant anemia in the fetus (1).

Folate needs are increased during pregnancy. Folate deficiency is associated with anemia, neural tube defects, and cleft palate. Neural tube closure occurs during the fourth week of pregnancy; folate supplementation needs to be given prior to conception to prevent neural tube defects. Most prenatal vitamins contain both folate and iron.

Sickle Cell Disease in Pregnancy

Women with sickle cell anemia are part of the high-risk pregnancy group. With modern obstetric and perinatal care, maternal mortality is less than 1% and perinatal mortality is less than 15%.

Prophylactic red cell transfusions are associated with fewer maternal painful episodes, but they have no impact on maternal morbidity, birth weight, gestational age, fetal distress, or perinatal mortality.

Maintenance transfusions should be given to women who are symptomatic of vasoocclusive or anemia-related problems or when signs of fetal distress are present.

Thrombocytopenia in Pregnancy

Platelet count decreases by approximately 10% during pregnancy; most of this decrease occurs in the third trimester.

The most common cause of thrombocytopenia is incidental thrombocytopenia of pregnancy (75%), followed by thrombocytopenia complicating hypertensive disorders of pregnancy (20%), and finally immunologic disorders of pregnancy (5%).

Thrombocytopenia of less than 100,000/μl in the first trimester of pregnancy is most consistent of immune thrombocytopenic purpura. Thrombocytopenia of over 70,000/μl occurring late during the second trimester or during the third trimester in the absence of hypertension or proteinuria most likely represents incidental thrombocytopenia of pregnancy. Platelet-associated immunoglobulin G (IgG) is elevated in both incidental thrombocytopenia of pregnancy and immune thrombocytopenic purpura.

It is important in any patient with thrombocytopenia to consider human immunodeficiency virus (HIV), systemic lupus erythematosus, and thrombocytopenia associated with antiphospholipid antibodies in the differential diagnosis (2).

Incidental Thrombocytopenia of Pregnancy

The platelet count in incidental thrombocytopenia usually remains above 100,000/μl. Incidental thrombocytopenia usually develops in the third trimester and is not associated with neonatal thrombocytopenia. The likelihood of a more serious cause of thrombocytopenia increases once the platelet count drops below 70,000/μl. The pathogenesis of incidental thrombocytopenia is not clearly defined but may involve a combination of hemodilution and decreased platelet half-life.

Incidental thrombocytopenia remains a diagnosis of exclusion. The diagnosis is made by observing no other physical or laboratory abnormality in patients with no antecedent history of immune thrombocytopenia. Women with incidental thrombocytopenia should receive standard obstetrical care.

Immune Thrombocytopenic Purpura

Immune thrombocytopenic purpura (ITP) is the most common cause of severe thrombocytopenia in the first trimester of pregnancy. An antecedent history of ITP or autoimmune disorder makes the diagnosis more likely. The nadir platelet count in ITP usually occurs in the third trimester.

Patients with platelet counts greater than 20,000/μl and with no evidence of bruising or mucosal bleeding generally do not require treatment in the first two trimesters of pregnancy. A platelet count of >50,000/μl is felt to be safe for normal vaginal delivery or cesarean section. Although there is no consensus, a platelet count of >80,000/μl is felt to be sufficient for epidural anesthesia. The bleeding time is not an accurate predictor of risk of bleeding in these situations. Optimal first-line therapy for ITP in pregnant patients is controversial. Corticosteroids are the least expensive option, but they have been associated with pregnancy-induced hypertension, gestational diabetes, osteoporosis, excessive weight gain, and premature rupture of fetal membranes. The placenta metabolizes 90% of the administered dose of prednisone; serious fetal side effects are unlikely. Prednisone is initiated at a dose of 1 mg/kg/day (based on the prepregnancy weight) and subsequently tapered to the minimum hemostatically effective dose. Intravenous IVIg should be considered if the maintenance dose of prednisone is in excess of 10 mg/day. IVIg given at a dose of 1 g/kg (based on prepregnancy weight) is associated with a response in over 60% of patients; the response lasts on average 1 month.

In patients refractory to corticosteroids and IVIg, splenectomy should be considered. Splenectomy is best performed in the second trimester of pregnancy. Splenectomy in the first trimester may induce labor, and splenectomy in the third trimester may be technically difficult. Splenectomy has been successfully performed laparoscopically during pregnancy. High-dose methylprednisolone and intravenous anti-D have been used in small series of refractory patients. Experience with immunosuppressive and cytotoxic agents during pregnancy is limited. Danazol and vinca alkaloids are best avoided. Interventions that raise maternal platelet count are not effective in raising that of the fetus.

The use of nonsteroidal anti-inflammatory drugs should be avoided postpartum in patients with platelet counts <100,000 /μl. Thromboprophylaxis should be considered in all women with a platelet count >50,000/μl if they have undergone surgical delivery, are immobilized for a prolonged amount of time, or have acquired or congenital thrombophilia.

Neonatal mortality is less than 1% in ITP; 5% of neonates will have a platelet count of <20,000/μl. Most hemorrhagic events in neonates occur 24 to 48 hours after delivery at the nadir of the platelet count. There is no evidence that cesarean section is safer for the neonate than vaginal delivery. The mode of delivery should be decided on the basis of obstetric indications. Maternal platelet count, maternal platelet antibody levels, or a history of maternal splenectomy for ITP are not accurate predictors of neonatal platelet counts. The most accurate predictor of fetal thrombocytopenia is a history of thrombocytopenia at delivery in a prior sibling. Fetal scalp blood sampling and cordocentesis have been abandoned.

A cord platelet count should be determined following delivery in every neonate. Thrombocytopenic neonates should be followed closely following delivery; the platelet count nadir may not occur before 2 to 5 days. Neonates presenting with clinical bleeding or a platelet count <20,000μl should be managed with IVIg 1 g/kg. Life threatening bleeding can be managed with a combination of IVIg and platelet transfusions.

Preeclampsia and the Hemolysis, Elevated Liver Enzyme Levels, and a Low Platelet Count Syndrome (HELLP)

Preeclampsia is defined as hypertension and proteinuria (>300 mg protein/24 hours) occurring after 20 weeks of gestation. Preeclampsia occurs in 5% of all pregnancies; it accounts for 18% of maternal deaths in the United States and is more frequent in nulliparous women or multiparous women with new partners. Thrombocytopenia develops in 50% of patients with preeclampsia. Endothelial damage and activation of the coagulation system with thrombin generation may explain the thrombocytopenia. D-dimers and thrombin-antithrombin complexes are increased in patients with thrombocytopenia. Aspirin prophylaxis does not reduce the incidence of either preeclampsia or HELLP.

The criteria for HELLP syndrome (**h**emolysis, **e**levated **l**iver **e**nzymes, and **l**ow **p**latelets) include:

- microangiopathic hemolytic anemia
- increased transaminases
- thrombocytopenia (<100,000/μl)

HELLP occurs in up to 10% of women with severe preeclampsia. The syndrome usually occurs in white, multiparous women above the age of 25 years. Maternal mortality is 1%, and fetal mortality is 10% to 20%. Fetal mortality is attributed to placental ischemia, abruption of the placenta, immaturity. and intrauterine asphyxia. Neonatal thrombocytopenia can occur in both preeclampsia and HELLP. The mechanism of neonatal thrombocytopenia remains unclear. There is a 3% risk of recurrence of HELLP in subsequent pregnancies.

The definitive treatment for eclampsia and HELLP is delivery of the fetus. Management focuses on stabilization of the patient and maturation of the fetal lung. The presence of multiorgan dysfunction, fetal distress, or a gestational age greater than 34 weeks warrants immediate delivery. Coagulopathy resulting from preeclampsia-associated disseminated intravascular coagulation (DIC) occurs in 20% of patients. The clinical manifestations of preeclampsia and HELLP resolve within a few days of delivery. Rarely HELLP syndrome can present postpartum. If the manifestations worsen or persist after 1 or 2 days, plasma exchange is indicated.

Acute fatty liver of pregnancy (AFLP) is associated with hypertension and proteinuria in 50% of patients. Microangiopathic hemolytic anemia and thrombocytopenia are not prominent in this syndrome. Patients usually have a prolonged prothrombin time, a low fibrinogen, and low antithrombin levels.

Thrombocytopenic Purpura and Hemolytic Uremic Syndrome

Thrombocytopenic purpura/hemolytic uremic syndrome (TTP/HUS) occurs in only 0.004% of pregnancies. The classic pentad of symptoms of TPP include microangiopathic hemolytic anemia, thrombocytopenia, neurologic abnormalities, fever, and renal dysfunction.

The classic pentad is present in only 40% of patients. Pregnancy is a precipitating factor for TTP. The mean time of onset of TTP is 23.5 weeks of pregnancy. Plasma therapy is recommended for the management of the pregnant patient with TTP. Delivery is recommended only for patients who do not respond to plasma exchange. Pregnancy termination is not considered therapeutic in TTP or HUS.

Ultralarge von Willebrand factor (VWF) multimers are found in TTP; this is thought to be secondary to the deficiency of a specific VWF-cleaving protease, identified as ADAMTS13. The deficiency can be congenital or acquired. All cases of idiopathic TTP to date have been associated with severe

TABLE 26.1. *Pregnancy-Associated Microangiopathies*

Diagnosis	Preeclampsia	HELLP	PP-HUS	TTP
Time of onset	>20 weeks	>34 weeks	Postpartum (90%)	< 24 weeks
MAHA	No	Yes	Yes	Yes
Thrombocytopenia	Yes	Yes	Yes	Yes
Coagulopathy	No	20%	No	No
Renal failure	Rare	Rare	Yes	Possible
Liver disease	No	Yes	No	No
Hypertension	Yes	Possible	Possible	Possible
Effect of delivery on disease	Yes	Yes	None	None

HELLP syndrome, hemolysis, elevated liver enzymes, and low platelets; MAHA, microangiopathic hemolytic anemia; PP-HUS, postpartum hemolytic uremic syndrome; TTP, thrombotic thrombocytopenic purpura.

protease deficiency; secondary TTP can occur in the context of a normal protease. Idiopathic TTP is associated with an IgG inhibitory auto-antibody directed against ADAMTS13 in 60% of cases.

Reduced VWF-cleaving protease is not specific for TTP; reduced levels are seen in the third trimester of pregnancy as well as uremia, acute inflammation, malignancy, and diffuse intravascular coagulation.

The mean time of onset of HUS is 26 days following delivery. Patients with HUS present with microangiopathic hemolytic anemia and acute renal failure. The VWF levels are usually elevated, while multimer analysis may or may not show ultralarge multimers. Deficiency of VWF-cleaving protease is usually not associated with this syndrome.

Several women with a familial history of pregnancy-associated HUS have developed their first episode of HUS during pregnancy, and HUS has occurred in such patients with the use of oral contraceptives. Postpartum HUS is associated with a poor prognosis. Plasma therapy is less effective in reversing renal failure in pregnancy-associated HUS. Nevertheless, a trial of plasma exchange is indicated. Dialysis and other supportive care measures may also need to be initiated (Table 26.1) (3).

Diffuse Intravascular Coagulation

Placental abruption is the most common cause of DIC (Table 26.2). Placental abruption has an increased incidence in cocaine addicts. Amniotic fluid embolism is associated with cardiopulmonary collapse and a mortality of 85%. The incidence of DIC complicating placental abruption and dead fetus syndrome has decreased with advances in ultrasonography and prenatal care.

Fetal death syndrome is recognized by ultrasonography; delivery of the dead fetus removes the source of tissue thromboplastin release. Blood component support and the use of antithrombin-3 have been useful in the management of the coagulopathy.

TABLE 26.2. *Causes of Obstetrical Disseminated Intravascular Coagulation*

Placental abruption
Fetal death syndrome
Amniotic fluid embolism
HELLP syndrome
Clostridial sepsis
Sepsis
Major obstetrical hemorrhage

HELLP syndrome, hemolysis, elevated liver enzymes, and low platelets.

Placental abruption is managed with blood component support followed by delivery. Antithrombin-3 and activated protein C have been used with success in this disorder. Transient DIC occurs in patients undergoing hypertonic saline abortions; the DIC usually resolves once the fetus is delivered. Clostridial sepsis following abortions is associated with DIC and poor clinical outcome.

Venous Thromboembolic Disease in Pregnancy

The incidence of venous thromboembolic disease (VTE) is increased two- to fourfold during pregnancy and is higher in patients undergoing cesarean delivery. Proven deep venous thrombosis occurs with similar frequency in each of the three trimesters. Venous thrombi occur predominantly in the left leg, partly because of the compression of the left iliac vein by the right iliac artery as they cross.

Hemodynamic changes causing venous stasis and hypercoagulabity most likely play a role in the increased risk of VTE during pregnancy. Hypercoagulability is thought to be secondary to an increase in fibrinogen, factor VIII, and VWF as well as a decrease in protein S, the development of acquired protein C resistance, and reduced fibrinolytic activity.

Inherited thrombophilias and antiphospholipid antibodies increase the risk of VTE during pregnancy (4,5).

Diagnosis of Venous Thromboembolic Disease in Pregnancy

The diagnosis of VTE during pregnancy is complicated by the potential fetal oncogenicity and teratogenicity associated with the use of ionizing radiation for diagnostic purposes. Compression ultrasonography (CU) of the entire proximal venous system to the trifurcation should be performed as the initial test for suspected deep vein thrombosis in pregnancy. A normal CU does not exclude a calf deep vein thrombosis (DVT). The CU needs to be repeated at day 2 and day 7 to rule out an extending calf-vein thrombosis. A limited venogram with fetal shielding can be used in equivocal cases. When iliac DVT is suspected, pulsed Doppler should be used. If the results of pulsed Doppler are negative or equivocal, magnetic resonance venography (MRV) or venography should be considered.

In patients with suspected pulmonary emboli (PE) during pregnancy, a V/Q lung scan should be performed. If the results of the V/Q scan are equivocal, bilateral compression ultrasounds should be performed. In cases where the diagnosis cannot be established by V/Q scan and CU, pulmonary angiography should be considered. There is controversy regarding the use of spiral computed tomography (CT) in pregnancy.

D-dimer levels increase with gestational age and during preterm labor as well as with abruptio placentae and gestational hypertension. These characteristics reduce the test's usefulness during pregnancy.

Treatment of Venous Thromboembolic Disease in Pregnancy

Unfractionated heparin (UFH), low-molecular-weight heparin (LMWH), and danaparoid do not cross the placenta; therefore, the risk of fetal bleeding or teratogenicity is not present. Heparin-induced thrombocytopenia, bleeding, and heparin-induced osteoporosis are more common with UFH than with LMWH.

Direct thrombin inhibitors such as hirudin and pentasaccharide have not been evaluated during pregnancy. Hirudin crosses the placenta; there is published data suggesting that pentasaccharide does not cross the placenta. Coumarin derivatives cross the placenta and have been associated with fetal bleeding and teratogenicity. Central nervous system abnormalities have been associated with the use of coumarin derivatives in every trimester of pregnancy. Nasal hypoplasia and/or stippled epiphyses have been associated with the use of coumarin derivatives between the 6th and 12th week of pregnancy.

The activated partial thromboplastin time (APTT) response to UFH is blunted in pregnancy because of increased factor VIII levels and increased heparin-binding proteins. This blunted response may lead to heparin overdosing. Measuring anti-FXa levels may obviate this problem. LMWH have less nonspecific binding to heparin-binding proteins; hence, they have a more predictable dose-response than UFH.

UFH and LMWH are not secreted in breast milk. Clinical evidence suggests that warfarin sodium is not excreted in breast milk and that it is safe to breastfeed while taking warfarin sodium.

The initial dose of LMWH is based on the patient weight. Because of variation of weight and glomerular filtration rate during pregnancy, it is recommended to monitor anticoagulation by performing monthly anti-FXa levels. LMWH should be discontinued 24 hours prior to elective induction of labor and neuroaxial anesthesia. Intravenous UFH can be initiated in patients at high risk for thrombosis and discontinued 4 to 6 hours prior to the time of expected delivery. LMWH can usually be restarted within 12 hours of delivery.

UFH is usually initiated by an intravenous bolus followed by a continuous infusion. The continuous infusion is usually continued for 5 days prior to transitioning to adjusted-dose subcutaneous UFH. The APTT should be maintained within therapeutic range. Anti-FXa levels can be obtained to prevent overanticoagulation. Adjusted-dose subcutaneous UFH can be used for the remainder of pregnancy with weekly midinterval monitoring of the APTT. The subcutaneous heparin should be discontinued 24 hours prior to elective induction of labor. Intravenous UFH can be used in patients at high risk for thrombosis and discontinued 4 to 6 hours prior to the time of expected delivery. UFH can usually be restarted within 12 hours of delivery.

UFH or LMWH should be continued for at least 4 days after initiation and Coumadin until the International Normalized Ratio (INR) has been therapeutic $\geq$ to 2.0 for 2 consecutive days.

Prophylactic Anticoagulation in Patients with a Previous History of Venous Thromboembolic Disease

More than half of thromboembolic events in pregnancy are related to thrombophilias (Table 26.3). Intrauterine fetal growth retardation, stillbirth, abruption, and severe preeclampsia have also been linked to thrombophilias. There are conflicting reports on the association between thrombophilias and recurrent early abortions (<10 weeks).

Patients with idiopathic VTE who are pregnant or plan to become pregnant should undergo screening for thrombophilias. Patients with history of fetal loss, abruption, severe preeclampsia, and intrauterine fetal growth retardation should also be screened for thrombophilias.

Patients with thrombophilia and an idiopathic VTE (not associated with a temporary risk factor such as surgery, trauma, and/or prolonged immobilization) should be prophylactically anticoagulated during pregnancy as well as postpartum. The management of the pregnant patient with thrombophilia without a previous VTE is controversial; the evidence for prophylaxis is more compelling in patients with antithrombin III deficiency and in patients with antiphospholipid antibodies.

Thrombophilias and Recurrent Miscarriage

Recurrent miscarriage is defined as three consecutive spontaneous abortions of an intrauterine pregnancy of less than 20 weeks gestation. Anticardiolipin antibodies have been linked with recurrent

---

TABLE 26.3. *Most Common Thrombophilias*

Inherited
- Factor V Leiden
- Prothrombin G20210A mutation
- 4G/4G mutation of the plasminogen activator inhibitor gene (PAI-I)
- Thermolabile variant of methylenetetrahydrofolate reductase, the most common cause of homocystinemia
- Antithrombin III deficiency
- Protein C deficiency
- Protein S deficiency

Acquired
- Antiphospholipid antibody

TABLE 26.4. *Causes of Anemia in Malaria*

Intravascular rupture of parasitized red cells
Hypersplenism
Autoimmune hemolysis (50% of patients have a positive direct
  Coombs)
Reticulocytopenia (Anemia of chronic disease)
Dyserythropoiesis (Cytokine mediated)
Secondary bacterial, fungal, or viral infections
Nutritional anemias

miscarriage. There is insufficient data to include inherited thrombophilias in the evaluation of women with recurrent miscarriage (6).

Prednisone, low-dose aspirin, UFH, LMWH, and intravenous immunoglobulin have been used in the management of this problem. Prednisone was found to be equally effective to low-dose subcutaneous UFH in preventing pregnancy loss but was associated with an increased incidence of side effects. UFH and aspirin have been shown to be superior to aspirin alone in preventing pregnancy loss. LMWH can be used instead of UFH. The optimal dosage of UFH and LMWH remain to be defined.

Hematologic Manifestations of Tropical Disease

Malaria

Anemia is a serious complication of malaria, especially *P. falciparum* infection. The prevalence and degree of anemia depends on the nutritional and immune status of the patient. The degree of anemia cannot be explained entirely by intravascular rupture of parasitized red cells. Several mechanisms are involved in the anemia of malaria (Table 26.4). *P. vivax* and *P. ovale* invade only reticulocytes, *P. malaria* invades only mature red cells, and *P. falciparum* invades red cells of all ages. The proportion of cells parasitized in *P. vivax* malaria rarely exceeds 1%, whereas as many as 50% of red cells may be parasitized in *P. falciparum* infections (7–9).

P. vivax uses the Duffy antigen as a receptor for junction formation during invasion. *P. falciparum* does not use the Duffy antigen as a receptor for invasion. Sialic acid residues of glycophorin A and B serve as invasion receptors for *P. falciparum*. Certain inherited defects confer resistance to parasitization by malarial organisms (Table 26.5).

There are two major clinical patterns in malaria: (i) acute malaria in the nonimmune, and (ii) recurrent malaria. Acute malaria is associated with a rapid drop in hemoglobin. Recurrent malaria is associated with splenomegaly, less severe anemia, and only scanty asexual forms and some gametocytes in the peripheral blood smear (Table 26.6). In tropical areas, anemia tends to be more prevalent and most

TABLE 26.5. *Protective Genetic Alterations*

Southeast Asian ovalocytosis (Autosomal dominant, 27 base pair deletion in the band 3 gene).
Heterozygotes for beta-thalassemias (Protection against *P. falciparum*)
HbE, HbS
Hereditary persistence of fetal hemoglobin
Glucose-6-phosphate dehydrogenase deficiency
Duffy-null phenotype (The Duffy antigen receptor for chemokines serves as a receptor for red cell invasion by *P. vivax*. Individuals who are Duffy-null are resistant to vivax malaria.)
Glycophorin A deficient phenotypes [En(a-), M^k] (Glycophorins are important ligands for the attachment and invasion of *P. falciparum* merozoites).
Glycophorin B deficient phenotypes [S-s-U-]
CD35 (Knops antigen) variants (CD35 is involved in the resetting of *P. falciparum*–infected red cells with uninfected cells)

TABLE 26.6. *Hematologic Manifestations of Malaria*

	Acute malaria (Nonimmune)	Recurrent malaria
Drop in hemoglobin	Drop in Ht within 24–48 hours of onset of symptoms	Chronic
Severity of anemia	Hemoglobin can drop down to 2 g/dl	2 g/dl lower than noninfected controls
Neutrophils	Neutrophilia in the first 2 days, followed by neutropenia for 1 to 2 weeks, followed by neutrophilia	May be decreased because of hypersplenism
Monocytes	Monocytosis	Variable
Lymphocytes	Lymphocytosis	Variable
Platelets	Thrombocytopenia	May be decreased because of hypersplenism
Hypersplenism	No	Yes

severe in children from 1 to 5 years of age and during pregnancy. Pregnant women who are nonimmune to *P. falciparum* develop severe malaria during pregnancy with high rates of abortion, premature delivery, and perinatal and maternal mortality. In women who are immune, extravascular hemolysis and secondary folic acid deficiency play a major role in the pathogenesis of anemia. The extravascular hemolysis in immune women peaks during the second trimester and is associated with progressive splenomegaly.

Hyperreactive malarial splenomegaly (HMS) is characterized by splenomegaly, hypersplenism, a polyclonal B-lymphocyte proliferation, high IgM levels, and raised titers of antibodies against the predominant species of malaria. Sickle cell trait is protective against HMS. Patients with HMS have a persistence of malaria-induced IgM lymphocytotoxic antibodies, which reduce the numbers of T-suppressor lymphocytes and permit the proliferation of B-lymphocytes. HMS has been associated with the development of splenic lymphoma with villous lymphocytes. Fifteen percent of patients with HMS will develop significant lymphocytosis, which may be mistaken for chronic lymphocytic leukemia.

Visceral Leishmaniasis, (Kala-Azar)

Visceral leishmaniasis (VL) is caused by one of three species of *L. donovani* complex. *L. donovani* is transmitted by phlebotomine sandflies. VL can also be transmitted through sexual contact, blood transfusions, and congenital transmission.

Leishmania donovani infects macrophages throughout the reticuloendothelial system. Patients develop irregular fever, weight loss, hepatosplenomegaly, pancytopenia, and hypergammaglobulinemia. The pancytopenia is secondary to hypersplenism and is worsened by folic acid deficiency. Monocytosis and lymphocytosis are typically present. Chronic VL infection can be associated with marrow hypoplasia, gelatinous transformation, dyserythropoiesis, and myelofibrosis.

African Trypanosomiasis (Sleeping Sickness)

African Trypanosomiasis (AT) is endemic in sub-Saharan Africa. Trypanosoma brucei gambiense and Trypanosoma brucei rhodanese are the etiologic agents. The tsetse fly is the vector. The infection is associated by the proliferation of macrophages and lymphocytes. Patients typically develop splenomegaly, pancytopenia secondary to hypersplenism, polyclonal hypergammaglobulinemia, monocytosis, and lymphocytosis.

Helminth Infections

Eosinophilia is present during the invasive migrating phase of hookworms, Strongyloides, and Ascaris. Hookworm is second only to malaria as an infectious cause of anemia. The daily loss of blood

TABLE 26.7. *Iron Deficiency Associated with Helminth Infections*

Helminth	Site of Blood Loss
Trichuriasis (whipworm)	Intestinal bleeding
Urinary Schistosomiasis	Bladder
Intestinal Schistosomiasis	Colon

in the gut is 0.03 to 0.05 ml for each Necator americanus worm and 0.15 to 0.23 ml for each A. duodenale worm. The development of iron deficiency is related to the dietary intake of iron, the size of the iron stores, and the hookworm load. Iron depletion is more common in women, during pregnancy, and in children. Less frequent causes of iron deficiency are outlined in Table 26.7.

Clonal Eosinophilic Disorders

Blood eosinophilia is defined as an eosinophil count superior to 450/µl. Eosinophils are much more abundant in tissues than in the peripheral blood. Sustained eosinophilia is associated with end-organ damage in some patients. The majority of patients with sustained eosinophilia do not sustain end-organ damage (Table 26.8) (10).

IL-5, IL-3, and granulocyte monocyte colony stimulating factor (GM-CSF) both stimulate eosinophil production and inhibit eosinophil apoptosis. Eotaxin-1, eotaxin-2, and RANTES (regulated on activation T cell expressed and secreted) are chemotactic cytokines, causing eosinophils to migrate into tissues. Eosinophils are the source of multiple cytokines (IL-2, IL-3, IL-4, IL-5, IL-7, IL-13, IL-16, TNF-alpha, TGF-beta, and RANTES). Eosinophils are also the source of cationic proteins such as eosinophil cationic protein, eosinophil peroxidase, major basic protein, eosinophil-derived neurotoxin, and Charcot-Leyden crystal lysophospholipase.

When the blood eosinophil count is greater than 1500/µl for a period of 6 months, and end-organ damage can be demonstrated, in the absence of a clonal abnormality or a reactive cause, the term idiopathic hypereosinophilic syndrome can be applied.

TABLE 26.8. *End-Organ Damage Associated with Hypereosinophilia*

End-Organ	Eosinophil Granule Proteins	Clinicopathologic Manifestations
Heart	Peroxidases, eosinophil major basic protein, eosinophil cationic protein	Constrictive pericarditis, fibroplastic endocarditis, endomyocardial fibrosis, myocarditis, intramural thrombus formation, mitral and tricuspid regurgitation, coronary arterial thrombi
Nervous system	Eosinophil-derived neurotoxin	Mononeuritis multiplex, paraparesis, central nervous system dysfunction, cerebellar involvement, recurrent subacute encephalopathy, cerebral infarction, seizures, eosinophilic meningitis
Lungs		Infiltrates, fibrosis, pleural effusions, pulmonary nodules
Skin		Angioedema, urticaria, papulonodular lesions, mucosal ulcerations (buccal and genital)
Eyes		Retinal vasculitis, microthrombi
Gastrointestinal/hepatic		Ascites, diarrhea, gastritis, colitis, pancreatitis, hepatitis, hepatic nodules
Muscle/joints		Destructive arthritis, effusions, arthralgia, myositis

TABLE 26.9. *Diseases Commonly Associated with Eosinophilia*

1. Infectious (Helminth, protozoa, fungi, HIV, HTLV-1)
2. Allergic diseases (Asthma, atopic dermatitis, allergic rhinitis, urticarias, allergic drug reactions)
3. Respiratory tract disorders (Hypersensitivity pneumonitis, Loeffler's syndrome, allergic bronchopulmonary aspergillosis, tropical pulmonary eosinophilia)
4. Endocrinologic disorders (Addison's disease)
5. Gastrointestinal disorders (Inflammatory bowel disease, eosinophilic gastroenteritis)
6. Cutaneous and subcutaneous disorders (Atopic dermatitis, eosinophilic cellulitis, scabies, episodic angioedema with eosinophilia, chronic idiopathic urticaria, recurrent granulomatous dermatitis, eosinophilic fasciitis)
7. Immunodeficiency syndromes
8. Connective tissue disease (Churg-Strauss and cutaneous necrotizing eosinophilic vasculitis)
9. Neoplastic (Lymphomas, T-ALL, T- cell lymphoproliferative disorders, solid tumors)
10. Myeloid leukemias and myeloproliferative disorders (Acute eosinophilic leukemia, myelomonocytic leukemia with eosinophilia, chronic myelomonocytic leukemia with eosinophilia, chronic myeloid leukemia)
11. Idiopathic hypereosinophilic syndrome
12. Cytokines (IL-2, GM-CSF)
13. L-tryptophan and toxic oil syndrome

GM-CSF, granulocyte macrophage colony-stimulating factor; HIV, human immunodeficiency virus; HTLV-1, human T-cell leukemia virus; IL-2, interleukin 2; T-ALL, T-cell acute lymphoblastic leukemia.

Helminthic infections are the most common cause of eosinophilia worldwide; atopic disorders are the most common cause in industrialized countries. Clonal eosinophilic disorders account for only a small proportion of all eosinophilia cases (Table 26.9).

Sustained hypereosinophilia, whether reactive or clonal, can lead to end-organ damage. The factors playing a role in determining who will develop end-organ damage are unclear. The workup of a patient with eosinophilia is influenced by the patient's geographic origin and his/her travel history. Serial stool examinations for ova and parasites may need to be supplemented by endemically relevant serologies and occasionally tissue biopsies. A clonal eosinophilic disorder needs to be investigated in patients without evidence of infectious or reactive causes of eosinophilia. Clonal eosinophilic disorders can be subdivided into (i) clonal T-cell disorders, (ii) clonal myeloid disorders, and (iii) cases in which clonality is suspected but cannot be proven (idiopathic hypereosinophilic syndrome [IHES]). The number of patients classified as having IHES is decreasing as our diagnostic tools are improving (Table 26.10).

The clonality of eosinophils can be demonstrated by the expression of a single alloenzyme of glucose-6-phosphate dehydrogenase in purified eosinophils from female heterozygotes. Polymerase chain reaction amplification of the human androgen receptor gene locus (HUMARA) can also be used to document clonality of eosinophils in female patients. Analysis of Wilms' tumor gene expression has been used to differentiate clonal form reactive eosinophilic disorders in both males and females.

T-Cell Clonal Disorders

IL-5 overproduction by TH2 lymphocytes has been demonstrated in both clonal and reactive hypereosinophilic disorders. Aberrant clones of T-lymphocytes are found in 25% of patients with clonal hypereosinophilic disorders. The aberrant phenotypes are heterogeneous ([CD3+,CD4+,CD8-], [CD3+,CD4-,CD8+], [CD3+,CD4-,CD8-], [CD3-,CD4+]). In most cases, an activated T-cell phenotype is present with expression of CD25 and HLA-DR. In 50% of cases a clonal rearrangement of the T-cell receptor gene (beta) or (gamma) can be found. T-cell lymphomas develop in a portion of these patients.

Patients with aberrant CD4+,CD3- T cells producing high levels of IL-5, IL-4, IL-13 typically present with skin manifestations, lack of severe end-organ involvement, and have elevated IgE levels and polyclonal hypergammaglobulinemia.

TABLE 26.10. *Clonal Hypereosinophilic Disorders*

Clonal T-cell disorders
- T-ALL
- T-cell lymphomas
- Aberrant T-cell clones ([CD3+, CD4+, CD8−], [CD3+, CD4−, CD8+], [CD3+, CD4−, CD8-], [CD3−, CD4+])

Clonal myeloid disorders
- Acute leukemias (M2 AML with eosinophilia, M4 Eo AML with inv(16) (p13;q22), t(16;16) (p13;q22)
- Chronic myelomonocytic leukemias with eosinophilia
- Myeloproliferative disorders with eosinophilia (polycythemia vera, chronic myelogenous leukemia, essential thrombocytosis, agnogenic myeloid metaplasia)
- Systemic mast cell disease with eosinophilia
- FIP1L1-PDGFRα hypereosinophilic disorders

Clonal hypereosinophilic disorders
The evaluation of patients with suspected clonal hypereosinophilic disorders should include:
- CBC-differential and peripheral blood smear
- Chemistry group
- Serum IgE
- B12
- Serum tryptase (Increased in mast cell disease with eosinophilia and the myeloproliferative variant of FIP1L1-PDGFRα hypereosinophilic disorders.)
- Peripheral blood flow cytometry (Used to identify an aberrant population of T-lymphocytes.)
- T-cell receptor gene (beta) or (gamma) rearrangement studies
- HIV serology
- CT scans of the chest, abdomen, and pelvis
- Bone marrow aspirate and biopsy (with reticulin and tryptase staining of the biopsy)
- Bone marrow cytogenetics
- PCR for FIP1L1-PDGFRA fusion gene and/or CHIC2 fluorescent in situ hybridization

---

AML, acute myeloid leukemia; CBC, complete blood count; CT, computed tomography; HIV, human immunodeficiency virus; IgE, immunoglobulin E; PCR, polymerase chain reaction; T-ALL, T-cell acute lymphoblastic leukemia.

The optimal treatment of patients with aberrant T-cell clones remains unclear. Corticosteroids have been associated with some responses. Interferon-alpha has in vitro antiapoptotic effects on the clonal CD4+,CD3- population and may increase the risk of lymphomatous transformation. The role of cyclosporine and chlorodeoxyadenosine in the management of these disorders is being evaluated.

Acute Leukemias

Acute eosinophilic leukemia is rare. Cyanide-resistant peroxidase can be used to identify eosinophilic blasts. In M2 acute myeloid leukemia (AML) with eosinophilia, the eosinophils have abnormal appearance. Myelomonocytic leukemia (M4-Eo) with eosinophilia is associated with inv (16) (p13;q22) and t(16;16) (p13;q22). The core binding factor-beta is a transcription factor is located at 16q22 and the smooth muscle myosin heavy chain is located at 16p13. The eosinophils in M4Eo frequently have a dysplastic appearance.

Chronic Myelomonocytic Leukemia-Eo

The two predominant subtypes of chronic myelomonocytic leukemia (CMML) with eosinophilia involve, respectively, platelet-derived growth factor receptor beta (PDGFR-β) and fibroblast growth factor receptor 1 (FGFR1). In both subtypes fusion oncoproteins are constitutively activated and are able to activate downstream stimulatory and antiapoptotic pathways.

Chronic Myelomonocytic Leukemia-Eo Subtypes

PDGFR-β Subtype

- Age 50 to 60
- Male predominance (>90%)
- Monocytosis, eosinophilia, splenomegaly
- Imatinib responsive
- t(5;12) (q33;p13) ETV6-PDGFR-β, t(5;7) (q33;q11.2) HIP1-PDGFR-β, t(5;10) (q33;q21) H4/D10S170-PDGFR-β, t(5;17) (q33;p13) Rabaptin 5- PDGFR-β

FGFR1 Subtype

- Median age: 32
- Male: female ratio (1.5:1)
- Associated with lymphoblastic lymphoma transformation (B and T)
- Not responsive to Imatinib
- t(8;13) (p11;p12) ZNF198-FGFR1, t(8;9) (p12;q32-34) FAN-FGFR1, t(6;8) (q27;p12) FOP-FGFR1

FIP1L1-PDGFRα Hypereosinophilic Disorders

FIP1L1-PDGFR-α is a constitutively activated tyrosine kinase that was first described in a patient with hypereosinophilic syndrome with an interstitial deletion on chromosome 4q12. The FIP1L1-PDGFRα in hypereosinophilic disorders is inhibited by imatinib and is more sensitive to inhibition (100 mg per day) than BCR-ABL in chronic myeloid leukemia (CML) (300 to 400 mg per day). The large majority of patients with the FIP1L1-PDGFR-α obtain a clinical remission with imatinib within 3 weeks of initiating therapy. Long-term follow-up of these patients is not yet available. The optimal dosage and duration of treatment remains to be defined. Resistance to imatinib is associated with a T6741 mutation in PDGFR-α; this mutation occurs in the adenosine triphosphate (ATP)-binding region of PDGFR-α at the same position as the T3151 mutation in BCR-ABL (11,12).

The myeloproliferative variant of hypereosinophilic syndrome associated with the FIPL1-PDGFR-α fusion tyrosine kinase is characterized by elevated serum tryptase levels, increased atypical mast cells in the bone marrow, and tissue fibrosis. Clinical improvement, resolution of eosinophilia, reversal of bone marrow fibrosis, hypercellularity, and disappearance of spindle-shaped marrow mast cells are seen in all patients treated with imatinib (300 to 400 mg per day) within 4 to 8 weeks of initiation of therapy. Molecular remission occurs in the majority of patients. Cardiac dysfunction is not altered by therapy, indicating that early initiation of therapy prior to cardiac dysfunction may be preferable.

Treatment of Clonal Hypereosinophilic Disorders

The treatment of hypereosinophilia is aimed at reducing the eosinophil count and preventing end-organ damage. It is important to fully evaluate the patient prior to initiating therapy. Imatinib is the treatment of choice in hypereosinophilic disorders associated with the FIP1L1-PDGFR-α fusion protein as well as CMML-Eo associated with PDGFR-β fusion proteins. Interferon-alpha is used in steroid-resistant patients with idiopathic hypereosinophilic syndrome; it may increase the incidence of lymphomatous transformation in some patients with clonal T-cell disorders.

In patients with idiopathic hypereosinophilia, in which a constitutively activated tyrosine kinase cannot be found; corticosteroids represent the first-line therapy. Both corticosteroids and cyclosporine will inhibit IL-2 gene transcription factors NF-AT and AP-1 and inhibit IL-5 production by peripheral lymphocytes. Cyclosporine and chlorodeoxyadenosine (2-CDA) can be used to minimize the side effects of long-term steroid therapy. Hydroxyurea and interferon-alpha have been used in steroid-resistant patients. The role of imatinib as front-line therapy in patients without FIP1L1-PDGFR-α fusion proteins remains unclear. Allogeneic transplantation has been used in treatment-resistant patients with progressive disease.

TABLE 26.11. *Neutropenia Classification*

Intrinsic disorders
 • Congenital
 • Acquired
Extrinsic disorders
 • Immune neutropenias
 • Neutropenia associated with autoimmune disorders
 • Neutropenia associated with large granular lymphocytes
 • Hypersplenism
 • Neutropenia associated with infectious diseases
 • Drug-related neutropenias
 • Nutritional deficiencies (B12, folate, copper)

Evaluation of Neutropenia

Neutropenia is defined as a decrease in neutrophils below $1500/\mu l$. Severe neutropenia is defined as a decrease in neutrophils below $500/\mu l$. In patients of African origin, the neutrophil count may normally be as low as $1000/\mu l$.

Neutropenias can be divided into intrinsic disorders of the hematopoietic system and secondary forms. The secondary forms are caused by extrinsic factors such as immune causes, hypersplenism, infections, and drugs (Table 26.11) (13,14).

Intrinsic Disorders

Congenital Neutropenias

Congenital neutropenias include Kostmann syndrome, cyclic neutropenia, congenital immunodeficiency syndromes, as well as several other rare syndromes that will not be discussed in this chapter.

Kostmann syndrome is an autosomal-dominant disorder presenting in the newborn. Characteristic findings include neutrophils below $200/\mu l$, monocytosis, anemia, thrombocytosis, splenomegaly, and evidence of maturation arrest in the marrow at the promyelocyte level. The accelerated apoptosis of neutrophilic precursors is secondary to a mutation of neutrophil elastase. Ninety percent of children with Kostmann syndrome respond to G-CSF. Evolution to myelodysplasia and acute leukemia occurs in some patients. It is unclear if G-CSF increases this risk.

Cyclic neutropenias can be a congenital (autosomal-dominant congenital disorder) or acquired disorder in association with clonal large granular lymphocyte syndrome. Congenital cyclic neutropenia is associated with mutations of the neutrophil elastase gene at the enzyme active site, which leads to accelerated apoptosis of neutrophils. Characteristically, patients present with cycles of neutropenia every 21 days. The neutropenia can be severe and last 3 to 6 days. Fever, mucosal ulcers, and lymphadenopathy can occur during the nadir of the cycles. G-CSF is very useful in the management of cyclic neutropenia.

Congenital immunodeficiency syndromes frequently associated with neutropenia include X-linked agammaglobulinemia, X-linked hyperimmunoglobulin M syndrome, and reticular dysgenesis (15).

Acquired Intrinsic Disorders

Acquired intrinsic disorders include leukemias, myelodysplastic syndromes, lymphoproliferative disorders, aplastic anemia, neutropenia of prematurity, and chronic idiopathic neutropenia.

Chronic idiopathic neutropenia occurs in both children and adults. The neutropenia in some patients can be severe. Patients have negative antineutrophil antibodies, normal marrow cytogenetics, and either normocellular marrows or marrows showing decreased in postmitotic cells. The prognosis is excellent; patients do not progress to myelodysplasia or leukemia. A proportion of these patients may have autoimmune neutropenia with undetectable antineutrophil antibodies. G-CSF is effective in increasing the neutrophil count.

Extrinsic Disorders

Immune Neutropenias

Alloimmune neonatal neutropenia occurs when maternal antibodies cross the placenta and react with the infant's neutrophils. In isoimmune neutropenia, the mother produces an antibody to the paternal CD16 isotype that is different from hers.

Autoimmune neutropenia is diagnosed in patients with isolated neutropenia who have detectable antineutrophil antibodies.

Neutropenias Associated with Autoimmune Disorders

In systemic lupus erythematosus, the neutrophils have increased amounts of IgG and immune complexes on their surface, leading to their rapid turnover. Marrow cellularity and granulocytic maturation are usually normal.

Patients with Felty's syndrome have deforming rheumatoid arthritis, splenomegaly, and elevated rheumatoid factor titers. The neutropenia in Felty's is thought to be antibody mediated. In a proportion of patients with Felty's the neutropenia is secondary to the presence of clonal large granular lymphocytes.

Neutropenia Associated with Large Granular Lymphocyte Syndrome

Large granular lymphocyte (LGL) syndrome is caused in the majority of cases by an expansion of either T-lymphocytes or natural killer (NK) cells. The NK-cell subtype is more aggressive and accounts for 15% of cases; 40% of LGL cases are associated with other diseases such as rheumatoid arthritis.

The T cells in clonal large granular lymphocyte syndrome express the CD3-TCR complex and rearrange TCR genes. These cells are thought to represent in vivo activated cytotoxic T cells. Clonal LGLs express high levels of Fas ligand. Normal neutrophil survival is regulated by the Fas-Fas ligand apoptotic system. The neutropenia in clonal LGL syndrome is mediated by dysregulated expression of Fas ligand.

Neutropenia Associated with Infectious Diseases

The most common cause of acquired neutropenia is infection. Gram-negative septicemia, staphylococcus aureus, typhoid fever, paratyphoid fever, tularemia, and brucellosis can cause neutropenia. Infectious hepatitis, influenza, measles, Colorado tick fever, mononucleosis, cytomegalovirus, Kawasaki disease, HIV, and Parvovirus B19 can also cause neutropenia. Parvovirus B19 is frequently associated with transient neutropenia and can cause protracted leucopenia in immunosuppressed patients. Neutropenia is seen in over 70% of patients with acquired immunodeficiency syndrome and can be associated with hypersplenism and the presence of antineutrophil antibodies.

Drug-Induced Neutropenias

The second most common cause of neutropenia is medication exposure. Approximately 70% of agranulocytosis cases in the United States are attributed to medications. Procainamide, antithyroid drugs, and sulphasalazine are most commonly implicated. An exhaustive list of drugs causing neutropenia is outside the scope of this book.

Three pathogenetic mechanisms for isolated neutropenia include dose-dependent inhibition of granulopoiesis, immune-mediated destruction of neutrophils and their precursors, and direct toxic effect on marrow granulocytic precursors (Table 26.12).

The onset of neutropenia is rapid (1 to 2 days) in immune-mediated destruction of neutrophils and variable with agents causing either direct toxic effect or dose-dependent inhibition. Immune-mediated destruction of neutrophils and their precursors occurs by two mechanisms. In the hapten-mediated mechanism, the agent acts as a hapten to induce antibody formation and needs to be present for

TABLE 26.12. *Mechanisms of Drug-Induced Isolated Neutropenia*

Dose-dependent inhibition of granulopoiesis
• β-lactam antibiotics, carbamazepine, valproic acid
Immune-mediated destruction of neutrophils and neutrophil precursors
• Agent acts an hapten to induce antibody formation, complement fixation, and neutrophil destruction: Penicillin, gold, cephalosporins, antithyroid drugs
• Immune complex related: Quinidine
Direct toxic effect on marrow granulocytic precursors
• Sulfasalazine, captopril, phenothiazine, clozapine.
• Chemotherapy drugs seldom cause isolated neutropenia

neutropenia to occur. In the immune complex mechanism, once the immune complex is formed it does not require continued drug presence for neutrophil destruction.

REFERENCES

1. Burrows RF. Haematological problems in pregnancy. Curr Opin Obstet Gynecol 2003;15:85–90.
2. McCrae K. Thrombocytopenia in pregnancy: differential diagnosis, pathogenesis, and management. Blood Rev 2003;17:7–14.
3. Allford SL, Hunt BJ, Rose P, et al. Guidelines on the diagnosis and management of the thrombotic microangiopathic haemolytic anaemias. Br J Haematol 2003;120:556–573.
4. Ginsberg JS, Bates SM. Management of venous thromboembolism during pregnancy. J Thromb Haemost 2003;1:1435–1442.
5. Bates SM, Ginsberg JS. How we manage venous thromboembolism during pregnancy. Blood 2002;100:3470–3478.
6. Lockwood CJ. Inherited thrombophilias in pregnant patients: detection and treatment paradigm. Obstet Gynecol 2002;99:333–340.
7. Fleming AF. Hematologic diseases. In Strickland GT, ed. Hunter's Tropical Medicine and Emerging Infectious Diseases, 8th Ed. Philadelphia: Saunders; 2000:34.
8. Wickramasinghe SN, Abdalla SH. Blood and bone marrow changes in malaria. Baillieres Clin Haematol 2000;13:277–299.
9. Chitnis CE. Molecular insights into receptors used by malaria parasites for erythrocyte invasion. Curr Opin Hematol 2001;8:85–91.
10. Brito-Babapulle F. The eosinophilias, including the idiopathic hypereosinophilic syndrome. Br J Haematol 2003;121:203–223.
11. Cools J, DeAngelo DJ, Gotlib J, et al. A tyrosine kinase created by fusion of the PDGFRA and FIP1L1 genes as a therapeutic target of imatinib in idiopathic hypereosinophilic syndrome. N Engl J Med 2003;348:1201–1214.
12. Klion AD, Noel P, Akin C, et al. Elevated serum tryptase levels identify a subset of patients with a myeloproliferative variant of idiopathic hypereosinophilic syndrome with tissue fibrosis, poor prognosis, and imatinib responsiveness. Blood 2003;101:4660–4666.
13. Boxer L, Dale DC. Neutropenia: causes and consequences. Semin Hematol 2002;39:75–81.
14. Palmblad J, Papadaki HA, Eliopoulos G. Acute and chronic neutropenias. What is new? J Intl Med 2001;250:476–491.
15. Ancliff PJ. Congenital neutropenia. Blood Rev 2003;17:209–216.

27

Interpretation of Standard Hematologic Tests

Roger Kurlander and Geraldine P. Schechter

AUTOMATED COMPLETE BLOOD COUNT

The complete blood count complete blood count (CBC) is a critical tool in clinical evaluation of hematopoiesis, hemostasis, and host immunity. The informed hematologist should have at least a general understanding of how high-volume automated counters make their measurements and familiarity with the errors caused by the more common preanalytic and analytic problems.

PREANALYTIC ARTIFACTS

The automated instruments designed to perform the CBC are extremely accurate and reproducible in assaying properly collected normal specimens. However, reliability can be compromised by problems during sample collection or storage.

ARTIFACTS ASSOCIATED WITH BLOOD COLLECTION

The CBC requires anticoagulated whole blood, and even minimal blood coagulation during collection can markedly affect the results. Clots consume platelets and trap other cell types, depressing the reported values. Most counters contain a clot detector, but some clots elude detection by this device. Samples collected from indwelling catheters are particularly prone to clotting and to inadvertent dilution with intravenous fluids. Incomplete filling of ethylene diamine tetraacetic acid (EDTA) or citrate tubes with blood can also cause artifacts by exposing cells to toxic quantities of anticoagulant and excessively hypertonic conditions.

STORAGE ARTIFACTS

Measurements of white blood cell, red blood cell, and platelet counts and hemoglobin concentration are relatively stable for at least 3 days in EDTA-treated samples stored at room temperature (1). However, EDTA increases the mean platelet volume (2) and alters fine detail of white cell morphology on a blood film within 2 to 3 hours. Mean corpuscular volume (MCV) and red cell distribution width (RDW) are affected within 4 to 8 hours and the accuracy of automated WBC differentials after about 24 hours (2,3). While these time intervals do not pose a problem for samples analyzed on site, accuracy of some parameters can be compromised by delays in processing mailed specimens.

ANTICOAGULANT-ASSOCIATED ARTIFACTS

EDTA, the anticoagulant normally used for CBC samples, causes platelet clumping or platelet-leukocyte "satellite" formation in about 0.1% of normal samples. Either of these artifacts will falsely depress the automated platelet count and may elevate the white count. In some published studies, 15% of patients referred for low platelets were found to have this pseudothrombocytopenia (4).

Whenever unexpected thrombocytopenia is encountered, the tube should be inspected for evidence of clotting, and a blood film should be examined for evidence of platelet agglutination or adherence to leukocytes. If clumping is absent, a manual estimate of the platelet count should also be made from the peripheral blood film and compared with the automated counts (see below). In most institutions this sequence is triggered automatically by the clinical pathology laboratory when new thrombocytopenia is recognized. Despite these efforts, clotting or agglutination artifacts may be difficult to detect. Clinically suspicious results should be repeated, preferably in duplicate in tubes containing EDTA and sodium citrate, an anticoagulant that usually does not cause rapid platelet agglutination. Platelet counts obtained from citrate tubes must be multiplied by 1.1 to correct for sample dilution by the liquid anticoagulant. Correction of thrombocytopenia by collection in citrate establishes the diagnosis of EDTA-associated pseudothrombocytopenia. However, some patients' platelets will also clump in citrate tubes. In rare cases, an accurate count can only be obtained if blood is added directly into the platelet diluting fluid and counted immediately.

INTERPRETATION OF THE AUTOMATED CBC

The basic methods used to generate an automated CBC were developed almost 50 years ago, but new technologic tools are being continuously incorporated into each new generation of counters to improve their reliability. The following discussion reviews generally how the elements in the CBC are measured and how the results may be influenced by interfering factors. It must be stressed, however, that each specific instrument uses its own proprietary methods of analysis. Consequently, performance characteristics vary substantially (5,6). Hematologists need to be familiar with the specific strengths and limitations of the instruments used by the clinical laboratories at their institution as well as the local laboratory policies for evaluating abnormal samples.

Red Cell Parameters

Automated counters measure hemoglobin concentration, red blood cell concentration (RBC count), and MCV directly from patient samples. Automated counters usually derive other parameters by mathematical manipulation of these primary values.

Hemoglobin concentration is measured spectrophometrically after the red cells are osmotically or chemically lysed, and the released hemoglobin is modified (using cyanide or less toxic agents) to assure quantitative measurement. While this method is usually extremely reliable, any condition that alters plasma turbidity or color can artifactually increase hemoglobin values (Table 27.1). Such interference also causes telltale elevations in the mean corpuscular hemoglobin concentration (MCHC). The laboratory often can compensate for interference using spun plasma to adjust the baseline, but it is prudent to use the RBC count or hematocrit in lieu of hemoglobin to monitor red cell status in this setting.

The RBC count is obtained either by measuring pulses of electrical impedance produced by the passage of cells between precisely positioned electrodes within an aperture and/or by measuring the absorption or scatter of light by cells passing through an optical cell. Each brand of automated counters has its own protocol for distinguishing red cells from leukocytes and platelets based on size, resistance to osmotic lysis, and other factors. Because automated counters sample large numbers of cells, RBC counts are usually much more accurate and sensitive than are manual counts, but instruments are vulnerable to the following problems. Red cell agglutination within the test tube caused by cold or warm reactive antibodies or rouleaux formation can artifactually reduce the red cell count because clumped cells cannot be properly identified and counted. In some counters, white blood cells (WBC) are included along with erythrocytes in the RBC count. Extreme leukocytosis therefore, particularly a WBC of more than 500,000 per microliter, can falsely increase the RBC count and the calculated hematocrit derived from the RBC count. Because red cells are detected in part based on size, RBC counts in patients with extremely small or fragmented red cells may be artifactually low.

TABLE 27.1. *Sources of Potential Artifact in Red Cell Parameters of the Complete Blood Count Red Blood Cell Count*

• Extreme leukocytosis with WBC >100,000/μl (particularly small lymphocytes) increases values.
• Autoagglutination, rouleaux formation, and cold agglutinins decrease values.

Hemoglobin
Each of the following may falsely increase the level:
- High triglycerides (more than 700 mg/dl)
- Plasma hemoglobin because of in vivo hemolysis
- Extreme leukocytosis (usually WBC >50,000/μl)
- Hyperbilirubinemia (greater than 30 mg/dl)

MCV
- Leukocytosis (WBC >50,000/μl)
- Autoagglutinins, rouleaux formation, or cold agglutinins
- Clinical conditions (such as diabetes and hypernatremia) that alter plasma osmolality may change MCV by swelling or dehydrating red cells during automated counting*.

Hematocrit
- Factors interfering with the MCV and RBC count will affect the hematocrit.

MCH
- Factors interfering with the RBC count and hemoglobin will affect the MCH.

MCHC
- Factors interfering with the hemoglobin and hematocrit will affect the MCHC.

*Hyperosmolarity associated with substances that do not cross the cell membrane (e.g., urea, ethanol) does not alter the MCV.
MCH, mean corpuscular hemoglobin; MCHC, mean corpuscular hemoglobin concentration; MCV, mean corpuscular volume; RBC, red blood count; WBC, white blood count.

In the past, when the CBC was performed manually, the spun hematocrit was the most direct technique for monitoring the erythroid component in blood. The automated counter, however, computes the hematocrit indirectly by multiplying the MCV (see below) by the RBC count. While less direct than measurement of blood hemoglobin concentration, the hematocrit is usually reliable, but it is vulnerable to several recognized artifacts (Table 27.1). The clinical laboratory usually can identify and correct for such interference before reporting, but results deviating from the "rule of 3" (hemoglobin in g/dl × 3 = hematocrit in % ± 3%) deserve special scrutiny looking for undetected interference with the MCV or the RBC.

Red cell indices were developed to help recognize deviations in the size and hemoglobin content of erythrocytes. The MCV is measured either electronically by analyzing the shape of the impedance spike produced during cell counting or optically by monitoring light scattering by individual cells. While usually an accurate measure of mean red cell size, the MCV is relatively insensitive to the presence of small numbers of abnormal cells found during the early stages of a microcytic or macrocytic anemia. The mean corpuscular hemoglobin (MCH), calculated by dividing the hemoglobin concentration by the RBC count, usually provides similar information. Because the MCV, the red blood cell count, and the hemoglobin concentration are all vulnerable to artifact (Table 27.1), in some situations one or even both indices may be invalid.

The automated MCHC, the hemoglobin concentration divided by the hematocrit, has more limited clinical utility. In part because of balanced technical artifacts, in most machines it is slow to deviate from the normal range, even in patients with iron deficiency anemia, until erythropoiesis is severely affected. High values of the MCHC are usually artifactual (Table 27.1), but levels greater than 36 fmol are characteristic of spherocytosis and should prompt examination of the blood film.

RDW (Red cell distribution width) is a measure of the variability in size within the red cell population. The precise mathematical equation used for calculation varies with the specific instrument, but in all cases elevated values indicate anisocytosis. For casual observers, the RDW is more reliable than inspection of the blood film for detecting this characteristic (7). Although nonspecific, an elevated RDW is valuable for alerting the clinician and laboratory to abnormalities in red cell morphology. When markedly increased, inspection of the blood film is essential because findings with very different implications (for example anisocytosis and red cell fragmentation) can cause equivalent elevations.

Because the RDW is sensitive to the presence of small subpopulations of large or small cells, it is more useful than the MCV for the early detection of nutritional deficiencies of iron, cobalamin, or folate. On the other hand, the RDW often remains normal in thalassemia. The combination of a high or normal RBC count, a low MCV, and a normal RDW is a common pattern in patients with thalassemia trait (8). Attempts to use the RDW in conjunction with the MCV to classify anemias have not been widely accepted because they tend to be unreliable in complex settings.

White Blood Cell Parameters

White Blood Cell Counts

The white blood cell (WBC) count is measured using the same impedance and optical methods used to count red cells and platelets. Because there are approximately 1000-fold more red cells and 40-fold more platelets than white cells, it is essential for the automated counter to distinguish between cell types. To facilitate the process, red cells are usually destroyed by osmotic lysis before white cell counting. Residual red cells or platelets are excluded from the count by selective gating based on size and granularity. Automated counting is faster, more reproducible, and usually more accurate than the older manual methods, particularly in counting leukopenic samples. In the absence of interference (see below), counters can quantitate WBC counts as low as 100 cells per μL. However, hematologists should be aware of several potential sources of interference that may influence automated WBC counts measured by older or smaller automated counters (Table 27.2).

Automated leukocyte differentials

Subclassifying leukocytes is more difficult than simply counting them. To distinguish the different types of peripheral blood leukocytes, each manufacturer has developed its own proprietary combination of impedance-based, optical, and/or histochemical methods. Depending on the sophistication of the counter, a three-part, five-part (neutrophil, lymphocyte, monocyte, eosinophil, and basophil), or

TABLE 27.2. *Artifacts Affecting White Blood Count and Platelet Counting*

Factors that may increase the WBC count
- Nucleated red blood cells
- Lysis-resistant red cells
- Platelet clumps
- Cryoglobulins

Factors that may increase the platelet count
- WBC fragmentation
- Extreme red cell microcytosis
- Rbc fragments
- Cryoglobulinemia

Factors that decrease the platelet count
- Platelet clumps
- Platelet satellitism

WBC, white blood count.

more than five-part differential count may be generated. These are quite accurate in characterizing white cells from normal controls or patients with qualitatively normal white cell morphology.

In patients with hematologic disease or qualitative leukocyte abnormalities, automated differentials may still be accurate, but reliability can no longer be assumed. One of the most important tasks for the instrument is to identify and flag abnormalities in leukocyte size, granularity, and other features for morphologic review. Because neither automated counters nor laboratory technologists are infallible, the hematologist should personally review the white cell differential of new patients with complex clinical findings and not rely on the reported laboratory values.

The automated calculation of the absolute granulocyte counts plays an extremely important role in grading chemotherapy-induced toxicity. Fortunately, chemotherapy usually does not cause changes that interfere with neutrophil recognition by the sophisticated automated instruments used in central laboratories. With only occasional exceptions, which can be identified based on machine flags, the absolute granulocyte counts obtained are sufficiently accurate for making clinical decisions.

Platelet Monitoring

Similar to the RBC and WBC counts, the platelet count is measured by impedance- and/or optical-based techniques. Platelets are distinguished from red cells by size and in some cases by resistance to osmotic lysis. As noted earlier, clumping is a frequent cause of error in the platelet counting and sometimes falsely elevates the white blood cell count. Conversely, small white or red cell fragments, or protein precipitates may artifactually increase the platelet count (Table 27.2).

Automated counters are more accurate than older manual counting methods in monitoring thrombocytopenia and often can accurately count less than 10,000 platelets per microliter. On occasion, it may be difficult even with advanced optical techniques to distinguish true platelets from debris derived from precipitated proteins or cell fragments. One manufacturer has developed a fluorescently labeled anti-CD61 (platelet-specific) monoclonal antibody reagent for use with their instrument to improve the accuracy of the platelet count in samples with extensive interference.

Mean Platelet Volume

The mean platelet volume (MPV) is routinely measured by automated analyzers. The MPV has modest value as a measure of increased platelet turnover and/or activation because young platelets are larger. However, the MPV may increase rapidly during the first 2 hours after collection because of shape changes and swelling in EDTA, and there are not well-developed reference standards for comparing values from different institutions (2). Consequently, the routine MPV included in the automated CBC is of limited usefulness.

The Peripheral Blood Film

Verification of Automated Results in the Clinical Pathology Laboratory

When an automated counter flags one or more CBC parameters it implies some aspect of the measurement(s) is atypical but not necessarily invalid. For some flags, inspection of the blood film is sufficient to verify that the value of the parameter in question was measured correctly. For example, when thrombocytopenia is newly noted, a laboratory technologist will scan the blood film for evidence of platelet clumping before releasing the results. When the WBC or platelet count is flagged, the automated value will be compared with a manual estimate obtained by counting the average number of platelets present in 5 to 10 oil immersion high-power (1000×) fields (hpf) and/or the number of leukocytes in a similar number of low power (100×) fields (lpf). The selected fields are chosen from representative regions that contain an even monolayer of cells, avoiding the edge of the film. The platelet count and leukocyte count are estimated by using the formulas (1,2):

Platelet count (platelets/mm^3) = average platelets per hpf × 15,000
Leukocyte count (cells/mm^3) = average leukocytes per lpf × 250

Although manual counts have limited precision, they will be reported in place of the automated result when a source of machine interference can be identified or the automated result deviates from manual estimates beyond the laboratory's acceptable limits. This process of manual verification remains an important and time-consuming laboratory responsibility. In a recent review of practice in a broad range of institutions, slide inspection or manual differentials were performed for 10% to 50% of CBC samples with a median rate of 26.7% (9). Given the fallibility of automated counts and differentials, a clear discrepancy between platelet or leukocyte frequencies on a blood film and the automated value should alert the clinician to the possibility of undetected machine error.

Evaluation of Red Cell Abnormalities

Blood film inspection by a skilled observer may permit the detection of abnormal cells in the early stages of macrocytic anemia and iron deficiency before red cell indices and the RDW become abnormal. In practice, however, serum iron, cobalamin, and folate levels are far more valuable than inspection of the blood film in the diagnosis of uncomplicated mild deficiency states.

The film plays a more important role in the evaluation of other types of anemia. While detection of anisocytosis, poikilocytosis, or polychromasia often does not lead to a specific diagnosis, their severity usually reflects the seriousness of the disorder. More important is the recognition of characteristic abnormalities such as sickled cells, dacryocytes, spherocytes, schistocytes, echinocytes, acanthocytes, or intracellular parasites. These can critically influence the direction of an anemia evaluation, and in some cases the finding itself is diagnostic.

Evaluation of White Cell Disorders

Automated cell counters are proficient in detecting the presence of large immature myeloid and lymphoid cells, but the blood film remains one of the most important tools in diagnosing hematologic malignancies. Morphologic findings alone may be sufficient to make a diagnosis in some patients with myeloproliferative, myelodysplastic, or lymphoproliferative disorders. In other cases, the peripheral blood findings must be supplemented with ancillary data obtained from flow cytometric, cytogenetic, and histochemical studies.

Automated counters are unlikely to identify small malignant lymphoid cells that would be readily recognizable by a skilled observer based on the presence of nuclear clefts or irregularities in nuclear contour. In the absence of lymphocytosis, samples containing such cells may not be flagged at all. Automated counters are also not useful in detecting qualitative findings such as granulocyte hypogranularity, a "left" shift to immaturity in granulocytic maturation, Pelger-Huet cells, toxic granulation, or Döhle bodies. Inspection of the film remains essential when there is a high clinical suspicion of a leukocyte abnormality or hematologic malignancy, even if the automated differential is reported as normal.

Quantitation of Bands

A shift to the left in the myeloid series—an increased proportion of immature forms—is a common finding during the early response to stress. The band count historically has been used to quantitate this phenomenon. The band count is performed manually by grading 1000 neutrophils on a Romanowsky-stained peripheral blood film. The result is expressed in percent or as an absolute number. From a technical viewpoint the band count is an imprecise, poorly reproducible assay because of high interobserver differences in band identification and inadequate sample of cells counted (10). Despite its limitations, the band count is still used in some settings as an aid in identifying early stages of acute bacterial infection or severe systemic illness, particularly in infants and the elderly (11).

Evaluation of Platelet Disorders

Routine inspection of platelet morphology is indicated in evaluating patients with thrombocytopenia or suspected platelet function disorders. The role of the film in detecting platelet clumping has been described above, but abnormalities in platelet morphology can also be helpful. The presence of large platelets suggests accelerated platelet turnover. Giant platelets (larger than a red cell) may indicate an inherited syndrome (Bernard-Soulier disease, Alport's syndrome, May-Hegglin anomaly) or an acquired myelodysplastic or myeloproliferative syndrome. Hypogranular platelets suggest the congenital "gray platelet" syndrome or a myelodysplastic syndrome.

THE RETICULOCYTE COUNT

Erythrocytes newly released from the bone marrow contain intracellular RNA, which usually disappears within 1 day. These cells are designated reticulocytes based on the presence of RNA-containing reticulum recognizable microscopically after supravital staining with appropriate dyes. The reticulocyte count plays a very important role in the evaluation of anemia because it is a noninvasive indicator of new red cell production by the bone marrow.

Reticulocyte Counting Methods

Reticulocytes can be counted microscopically by scoring 1000 new methylene blue-stained red cells, but automated optical and fluorescent methods that detect the uptake of an RNA-binding dyes by red cells have largely replaced the older manual method. Both approaches generate similar values (approximately 1% of red cells from normal individuals are reticulocytes), but the automated technique, with its more standardized criteria and larger samples, is more precise.

Both methods are vulnerable to interference from intracellular organisms, basophilic stippling, and other artifacts (see Table 27.3). These artifacts are often flagged by the automated counter or noted during the course of manual counting. Nonetheless, whenever a reticulocyte count seems inappropriately high in the clinical context, microscopic inspection of a standard blood film and/or of a reticulocyte preparation is warranted to identify potentially relevant causes for interference.

Interpretation of the Reticulocyte Count

The significance of the reticulocyte percentage is highly dependent on the red cell count of the patient. To provide a more quantitative picture of new red blood cell production, reticulocyte levels are now commonly expressed as an absolute count by using the expression: Absolute reticulocyte count = % reticulocytes × RBC count /100.

The relationship between the absolute reticulocyte count and bone marrow production is not linear in patients who have severe anemia or who are receiving an erythropoiesis-stimulating agent. A highly stimulated marrow not only makes more new cells but also releases them more quickly. The resulting stress reticulocytes (12), which are larger, more polychromatophilic, and more RNA-rich than normal steady state forms, may stain with supravital dyes for up to 3 days. Because these cells survive longer, the absolute reticulocyte count will overestimate the true rate of reticulocyte production. Attempts to take into consideration the impact of prolonged reticulocyte survival by calculating a corrected reticulocyte production index have not been validated rigorously or used widely in clinical practice. While the relationship between reticulocytosis and marrow production can not be defined precisely, the implication is that a modestly elevated absolute reticulocyte count may still represent an inadequate marrow red cell response in a patient with severe anemia and high numbers of stress erythrocytes.

TABLE 27.3. *Findings That Can Artifactually Increase the Reticulocyte Count*

- Howell-Jolly bodies
- Basophilic stippling
- Red cell parasites including malaria, babesiosis
- Giant platelets

Immature Reticulocyte Fraction

Automated reticulocyte counters not only count the number of reticulocytes but also the amount of RNA per reticulocyte. This information allows the machine to distinguish normal reticulocytes from the more RNA-rich stress forms. At least two distinct subpopulations containing intermediate and high amount of RNA have been identified and comprise the immature reticulocyte fraction (IRF).

This parameter is not used extensively in the routine diagnosis or management of anemia, but it is a sensitive tool for detecting the early phases of red cell response to erythropoiesis-stimulating agents (13) and early bone marrow recovery after chemotherapy or stem cell transplantation. In the latter setting, elevations in the IRF usually precede and predict early myeloid recovery 1 to 2 days later (14). In some settings, this information can be useful in clinical management—for example, in anticipating future blood product needs. Although each of the commonly used automated hematology counters can measure the IRF, the performance characteristics and normal limits vary considerably between instruments. Physicians must become familiar with the normal limits of the instrument used to generate the IRF before using it in clinical management.

Reticulocyte Hemoglobin Content

Because normal red cell survival is 120 days, most circulating red cells are more than 1 month old. Consequently, the standard red cell indices are an insensitive tool for monitoring changes in erythropoiesis. By selectively measuring the hemoglobin content of reticulocytes, the youngest subset of red cells, modern automated hematology counters can more selectively address current marrow function. For example, reticulocyte hemoglobin content, designated CHr, diminishes rapidly as accessible iron stores are exhausted, making early iron deficiency readily detectable in blood donors undergoing repeated phlebotomy, iron-depleted dialysis patients receiving erythropoietin for the treatment of anemia, or iron-stressed women during the late stages of pregnancy (15). Although the available information suggests measurements of reticulocyte hemoglobin content can be useful in several common clinical settings, unfortunately, most of the clinical data documenting the value of this parameter were obtained using a single automated hematology counter, the Bayer Advia (Leverkusen, Germany). Analogous information (the Retic-He) with different normal limits is generated by the Sysmex XE-2100 (Sysmex Corporation, Kobe, Japan), but other commonly used counters as yet do not provide a measurement of this parameter.

INTRAVENOUS BONE MARROW ASPIRATE/BIOPSY

Indications for the Aspirate and Biopsy

The hematologist, unlike many subspecialists in internal medicine, can safely perform a biopsy on the organ of interest in an outpatient setting. The procedure, however, involves some expense and discomfort for the patient and should be reserved for situations where the findings may influence clinical care. Common indications for the procedure are considered below.

Evaluation of Neutropenia, Thrombocytopenia, or Pancytopenia

In the evaluation of patients with unexplained persistent or severe thrombocytopenia and granulocytopenia, bone marrow aspirate and biopsy may establish or rule out diagnoses such as aplastic anemia, myelodysplastic syndrome, marrow replacement by nonhematopoietic cells, or hemophagocytosis. Bone marrow studies are sometimes also obtained in the evaluation of prolonged pancytopenia after intensive chemotherapy for cancer to determine simultaneously for early evidence of marrow recovery or marrow replacement by malignancy as the cause for delayed recovery.

There is no clear consensus as to the role of bone marrow evaluation in patients with isolated thrombocytopenia or granulocytopenia suggestive of an autoimmune or drug-induced process. Because the findings are nonspecific, the study is sometimes omitted in patients with classic clinical features of autoimmune disease. On the other hand, it is of definite value when the picture is atypical and potentially compatible with another diagnosis.

Evaluation of Anemia in the Absence of Thrombocytopenia or Neutropenia

The bone marrow study has a limited role in the evaluation of isolated anemia. Most patients with iron, cobalamin or folate deficiency, hemoglobinopathy, anemia of inflammation, renal insufficiency, gastrointestinal blood loss, thyroid disease, or hemolytic anemia can be diagnosed using the clinical examination and blood tests without a marrow examination. In patients with unexplained anemia, particularly if requiring transfusions, a bone marrow study is appropriate. The yield of new diagnoses in patients with persistent anemia and multifactorial chronic disease is low, but the study does occasionally reveal an unexpected treatable diagnosis.

The assessment of iron stores in patients with chronic inflammation represents a common and difficult problem. Serum assays to define iron status are often confusing (see below), and as a last resort Prussian blue stainable marrow iron stores are often used as a criterion standard. This approach may not resolve the uncertainty. In a recent study the authors reviewed the findings from 108 patients who were diagnosed as iron depleted based on the absence of stainable iron on a bone marrow study. A reevaluation of the marrow films and sections revealed 19 cases with technically inadequate iron stains, usually because of hypocellularity. In a more detailed review of 37 of the remaining 89 patients who had full clinical data and adequate serum iron studies available, 18 (48%) had other clinical and laboratory data arguing strongly against the diagnosis of iron deficiency (16).

When stainable marrow iron is demonstrated, tissue iron stores can be assumed to be adequate. As discussed below this finding does not assure that the patient can appropriately mobilize these stores for use in erythropoiesis. For example, when hepcidin levels are elevated by chronic inflammation iron will be trapped in the macrophages and unavailable for hemoglobin synthesis. The absence of stainable iron suggests depleted iron stores. It must be stressed, however, that the sensitivity of method depends heavily on the quantity of sample obtained; to obtain maximal yield, at least seven separate spicules should be evaluated for stainable iron (17).

Detection of Marrow Infiltration with Neoplasm, Infectious Organisms,
Fibrosis, or Other Processes

Marrow aspiration and biopsy are extremely valuable in staging and serially monitoring patients with malignancies such as multiple myeloma, lymphoma, and aleukemic leukemia, which diffusely invade the bone marrow compartment. Marrow studies may also be valuable in screening for metastatic spread of nonhematologic malignancies, such as small cell carcinoma of the lung, which diffusely metastasize to bone marrow early in the course of disease. However, given the focal nature of the lesions in most nonhematologic cancers, radiologic or nuclear medicine techniques are more sensitive and reliable tools for detecting metastases.

Bone marrow studies can also identify infectious agents, especially mycobacteria and fungi. Occasionally metabolic disorders such as Gaucher's disease and infiltrative disorders such as amyloidosis may also be discovered, but biochemical tests or less invasive biopsies are preferable.

Methodology

Choice of Sites

In adults, the posterior iliac crest is the site of choice for marrow aspiration and biopsy. The anterior iliac crest is a reasonable alternative when obesity, local irradiation, or local skin conditions preclude a posterior approach. Aspiration from the sternum also can be performed safely by experienced operators, but it is less well accepted by patients and more vulnerable to local complications because major vessels and thoracic structures lie nearby. Sternal aspiration may be justified when an iliac approach is not possible.

Bone Marrow Aspiration

The aspiration is performed, after appropriate local anesthesia, by advancing a specially designed 14- to 16-gauge needle fitted with an obturator through the cortex into the medullary space. After the obturator is removed, marrow is aspirated using a syringe and negative pressure. Individual marrow particles are spread on a glass slide and stained with Romanowsky stains. The final product, similar to a peripheral blood film, is particularly useful in identifying abnormalities in cellular morphology. The cell suspensions obtained are also valuable for cytogenetic, molecular, and flow cytometric analyses.

At the time of aspiration, unused marrow particles (or the aspirate clot itself) can also be fixed in a standard preservative to prepare an aspirate (or clot) section, which is stained with hematoxylin and eosin, or other stains in the same way as a bone marrow biopsy (see below). The major limitation of the marrow aspirate is its vulnerability to sampling error. Marrow may be inaspirable because of hypercellularity, hypocellularity, or the presence of reticulum or collagen fibrosis. Aspirates are less reliable than marrow biopsies in detecting marrow involvement with malignancy and are not useful at all to detect myelofibrosis or granulomas.

Bone Marrow Biopsy

This procedure is performed using a larger needle (such as the Jamshidi needle), which can cut a cylinder of bone from the medullary space. In practice, after administering local anesthesia, the needle is advanced through the skin and bone cortex with the obturator in place to prevent unwanted material from entering the needle bore. Once the tip has entered the medullary space, the obturator is removed and the needle advanced until the desired length of specimen (usually 1–2 cm) is captured. The needle is rotated extensively to release the captured sample and withdrawn. The sample is ejected from the needle by using a metal probe and then fixed, decalcified, sectioned, and stained with hematoxylin and eosin, histochemical stains (for reticulin, collagen, iron), or a wide variety of immunohistochemical stains. Because of the required decalcification process, iron stains and some immunohistochemical stains may be falsely negative.

It is almost always possible to obtain a biopsy specimen, even when hematopoietic cells have been totally replaced by fibrous tissue or tumor. Hematoxylin and eosin-stained biopsy sections show less cytoplasmic and nuclear detail than Romanowsky-stained aspirate films but provide other essential information about marrow architecture and cellularity.

Risks and Contraindications of Marrow Aspiration and Biopsy

Hemorrhage is the most frequent serious complication of the procedure and fortunately is rare. In a British survey of complications from 54,890 biopsies, there were 14 instances of serious hemorrhage with 1 death, and 6 instances requiring transfusion (18). This may underestimate the risk, because cases with complications may go unreported.

Thrombocytopenia is common in patients requiring bone marrow aspirate/biopsy, and the procedure is routinely done in patients with platelet counts below 50,000/μL without incident. Platelet function defects (such as those associated with aspirin administration, myeloproliferative disorders, or disseminated intravascular coagulation) may increase the risk of local bleeding in severely thrombocytopenic patients. Prolonged local pressure to the puncture site may be sufficient to attain hemostasis, but platelet transfusion or desmopressin acetate may be necessary if bleeding after the procedure is persistent.

Risks are much greater in patients with major bleeding disorders such as hemophilia or active fibrinolysis associated with severe liver disease. In these instances, factor replacement and meticulous local care after the procedure are essential. Anticoagulation poses an intermediate level of risk. Where practical, anticoagulation should be reversed before bone marrow procedures are performed. Heparin or enoxaparin anticoagulation can be reversed by withholding drug for 6 and 12 hours, respectively. If the procedure cannot be delayed, warfarin-treated patients with an international normalized ratio (INR) in excess of 2 should receive fresh frozen plasma at the time of the procedure or, failing this, should be very carefully monitored postprocedure to assure adequate hemostasis.

Local infection is usually preventable by use of sterile technique and proper local care after the procedure. There are rare reports of broken needles sometimes requiring surgical removal (18). Traumatic fracture of the sternum with damage to underlying structures is a rare but serious complication, which is of particular concern when there is underlying structural damage secondary to malignancy. Sternal aspirates should be avoided in patients with multiple myeloma.

Interpretation of the Aspirate and Biopsy

In reporting results the interpreter should always indicate the site of acquisition and methodically review at least the following elements.

Marrow Cellularity

Estimates of cellularity are best obtained by inspection of a marrow biopsy. Because it can vary focally, larger specimens are particularly valuable in this regard. Marrow cellularity decreases with age; an approximate rule of thumb is that the normal percent cellularity can be estimated by subtracting patient age from 100. Inappropriately low cellularity suggests marrow damage, and high cellularity is consistent with a proliferative disorder, reaction to stress, or the use of growth factors.

Rough estimates of cellularity can sometimes be obtained from an aspirate but may be misleading, particularly when the marrow is inaspirable (a "dry tap"). The failure to obtain an aspiration specimen may reflect a markedly hypercellular ("packed") marrow or myelofibrosis, but dry taps are sometimes encountered in the absence of obvious hematologic disorder, presumably because of unappreciated technical problems.

Megakaryocyte Number and Appearance

Normocellular biopsy or aspirate specimens should contain multiple megakaryocytes per low power ($100\times$) field. An increase in megakaryocytes is consistent with increased turnover secondary to peripheral destruction, a response to inflammation, iron deficiency, cancer, or myeloproliferative/myelodysplastic disorders. Reduced megakaryocyte numbers may reflect a primary marrow disease such as aplastic anemia, amegakaryocytic thrombocytopenia, or suppression secondary to chemotherapy.

Normal megakaryocytes are large cells containing multilobated (three or more) attached nuclei. The presence of substantial numbers of smaller cells or megakaryocytes with less than three lobes suggests either a shift to the left in megakaryocyte maturity because of increased platelet turnover or dysplasia. The presence of megakaryocytes with a single nucleus or with multiple small separated nuclei associated with mature cytoplasm is particularly suggestive of myelodysplasia.

Myeloid to Erythroid Ratio

This distribution can be estimated by inspection of an aspirate or biopsy specimen and quantitated more precisely by counting 300 to 500 cells from a marrow aspirate sample. There are often substantial local variations in myeloid to erythroid (M:E) ratio; hence, it is important to sample multiple areas within the sample. In normal adults, the M:E ratio varies from 1:1 to approximately 3:1. A ratio below 1:1 implies too much erythroid or too little myeloid activity; levels above 4:1 suggest the opposite. The implications of the M:E ratio must always be judged in the context of the overall cellularity, the qualitative appearance of the affected cells, and the clinical setting.

Marked erythroid hyperplasia, a low M:E ratio in a cellular marrow, suggests an erythroid response to anemia (particularly to hemolysis), megaloblastic anemia, myelodysplasia, or erythropoietin administration.

Marked erythroid hypoplasia with rare giant erythroblasts suggests parvovirus-induced pure red cell aplasia. It may also be due to autoimmunity or an adverse effect to a medication. Myeloid hyperplasia may reflect a host response to physiologic stress, infection, exogenous growth factors, or a myeloproliferative disorder.

Myeloid hypoplasia with a "maturation arrest" (an absence of myeloid precursors beyond the promyelocyte or myelocyte stage) may reflect drug-induced or autoimmune agranulocytosis.

Myeloid and Erythroid Morphology

The disruption of the normal maturation sequence (with a complete maturation arrest or a marked shift to the left), the presence of excess numbers of blasts, or dysplastic changes affecting at least two of the three major hematopoietic cell lines suggest a serious hematologic disorder such as leukemia, myelodysplasia, or megaloblastosis. Other changes such as a mild shift to the left or mild megaloblastic changes are more nonspecific.

Lymphocytes and Plasma Cells

There is substantial normal variation in the number of lymphocytes encountered in a marrow specimen, and these elements may be distributed diffusely or in well-defined lymphoid aggregates. Paratrabecular lymphoid collections (collections immediately adjacent to bony trabeculae) are of greatest concern, because they are common in follicular lymphoma. When immunohistochemical stains are performed, benign lymphoid collections typically contain more T cells than B cells. Monotonous B cell-rich lymphoid collections are more likely because of clonal B-cell lymphoproliferative disorders.

Plasma cells usually constitute less than 2% of marrow cells; however, increases are commonly noted in a variety of inflammatory diseases, benign monoclonal gammopathy, and multiple myeloma. It may be difficult to distinguish reactive from neoplastic plasma cells in a routine aspirate film. Extensive multinuclearity and the presence of plasma cell collections of greater than 5 to 10 cells are all features suspicious for malignancy. The percentage of plasma cells in patients with reactive plasmacytosis caused by inflammation or liver disease may reach 20% to 30%, and hypocellular marrows are often rich in plasma cells. To diagnose myeloma with confidence from the routine aspirate, it is helpful to see marked atypia of plasma cell morphology including conspicuous variation in cell size and immature nuclei with nucleoli. These features are easier to appreciate in the marrow aspirate than in the marrow biopsy. Immunohistochemical staining for intracellular kappa and lambda chains within plasma cells in the marrow biopsy and/or immunofixation studies of serum and urine are needed to establish the presence of a monoclonal disorder. Once clonality is established, distinguishing between benign monoclonal gammopathy and multiple myeloma may require additional clinical and laboratory data (see Chapter 17). The presence of concentrated collections of plasmacytoid lymphocytes suggests Waldenstrom's macroglobulinemia or lymphoplasmacytic lymphoma.

Other Cells

Malignant cells of epithelial or mesenchymal origin adhere more tightly together and aspirate poorly, forming tightly clumped groups of unusually large cells with a very high nuclear-cytoplasmic ratio. Such clumps may be rare; therefore, when screening an aspirate for malignant cells, the whole slide should be scanned at low power including the leading edge of the film. Tumor cells can also be readily identified in marrow biopsies, and specialized immunohistochemical stains can sometimes help identify the site of origin.

Iron Stores

When marrow iron is markedly increased, yellow granules of hemosiderin may be seen in Romanowsky and hematoxylin and eosin preparations. Prussian blue stain, which specifically detects iron, is necessary to appreciate lesser iron stores and the iron granules in erythroid cells. Macrophage iron is most easily recognized within marrow particles, while the few small iron granules in normal maturing erythroid precursors are best seen where the cells are separated from the particles. Ringed sideroblasts, the hallmark of sideroblastic anemias, are erythroid precursors bearing coarse iron granules immediately surrounding at least half the circumference of the nucleus because of accumulation of iron within mitochondria. They are always abnormal, implying anomalous porphyrin synthesis. Sideroblastic anemias may be caused by a congenital abnormality, nutritional deficiency of pyridoxine, exposure to a toxin (especially lead or alcohol) or medication, or myelodysplasia.

Additional Studies

As described in other chapters, flow cytometry, cytogenetics, fluorescent in situ hybridization (FISH), and other molecular diagnostic studies have an increasingly important role in diagnosis and monitoring of hematologic disorders. To cite only a few of the many emerging uses of these techniques when applied to bone marrow derived specimens: cytogenetics and FISH often play a central role in defining the molecular defect in myeloid malignancies, and immunohistochemical stains and molecular studies assessing T- and B-cell receptor rearrangements are often critical in documenting clonality in lymphoid malignancies.

SERUM TESTS TO EVALUATE NUTRITIONAL AND HYPOPROLIFERATIVE ANEMIAS

Serum Iron and Total Binding Capacity Assays

Serum iron is measured by automated chemical assays following dissociation from transferrin (19,20). Total iron binding capacity (TIBC), which is mainly because of binding to transferrin, is usually measured by the addition of excess iron to the sample. Unbound iron is removed by absorption, and the iron bound to protein is again dissociated and measured by the serum iron assay. In some laboratories, unsaturated iron binding capacity or transferrin levels may be measured directly. Measurement of serum iron can be falsely elevated in specimens containing hemoglobin (hemolysed specimens) and also for many hours after blood transfusion. The percent saturation of transferrin by iron is calculated by dividing the serum iron by the total iron binding capacity and then multiplying by 100. Iron deficiency is associated with low serum iron and elevated serum total iron binding capacity and therefore low iron saturation of transferrin. Although total iron binding capacity falls in patients with anemia of inflammation/chronic disease, the levels of serum iron and the percent iron saturation in patients with severe chronic inflammation/chronic disease and with iron deficiency anemia frequently overlap. The high TIBC levels (more than 300 μg/dL) in patients with uncomplicated iron deficiency are helpful in distinguishing the two entities; however, when they coexist the TIBC is frequently low (see ferritin and transferrin receptor assays below). Elevated serum iron levels occur in multiple conditions including hemolysis, megaloblastic and sideroblastic anemias, pure red cell aplasia, iron overload states because of genetic hemochromatosis, transfusion hemosiderosis, chronic liver disease, and chronic alcoholism. A rise in the serum iron into the normal range 1 to 2 hours after ingestion of 325 mg ferrous sulfate in the form of a tablet or elixir indicates appropriate bioavailability and normal small bowel absorption (21).

Soluble Transferrin Receptor

A truncated form of tissue transferrin receptor, soluble transferrin receptor is measured by a "sandwich-type" enzyme-linked immunoassay. Serum transferrin receptor levels are elevated in states of increased erythropoiesis such as hemolytic anemias, megaloblastic anemia, thalassemia, and also in iron deficiency anemia. Transferrin receptor levels are decreased when erythropoiesis is reduced as in aplastic anemia and renal insufficiency. The assay is reported to distinguish iron deficiency from the anemia of chronic inflammation/disease (22,23); however, overlap in receptor levels between the two conditions is often noted. The ratio of the serum transferrin receptor level to the ferritin level or to log ferritin level may be more useful in distinguishing between the two entities (22). Elevated transferrin receptor levels observed in some patients with anemia of inflammation likely reflect limited availability of functional iron pools for erythropoiesis rather than depleted iron stores (24,25). An automated immunoturbidimetric assay has been reported to be superior to two commonly used enzyme-linked immunoassays methods in predicting iron deficiency (26). As discussed previously, changes in reticulocyte hemoglobin content, which is a direct measure of new red cell hemoglobinization, may be the most dynamic and sensitive measure of functional iron availability during active hematopoiesis.

Serum Ferritin

The ferritin assay is most useful clinically at the extremes: low values (<20 ng/mL) reflect storage iron depletion, and very high levels may indicate iron overload states resulting from genetic hemochromatosis, liver disease, or transfusion hemosiderosis. Because ferritin is an acute phase reactant, even very high levels above 5000 ng/mL may be seen with severe inflammatory states (such as disseminated fungal disease) as well as in iron overload. Patients with both iron deficiency in the setting of inflammation or liver disease often have serum ferritin levels in the normal range, usually not exceeding 100 ng/mL (23). In the presence of concurrent inflammation or liver disease, ferritin levels may not accurately gauge the response to iron chelation therapy in patients with transfusion hemosiderosis.

Serum Vitamin B12 (Cobalamin)

Serum vitamin B12 is generally assayed by an enzyme-linked competitive binding assay most frequently based on binding to intrinsic factor (19,20). Serum levels below 100 pg/mL are almost invariably associated with cellular cobalamin deficiency as reflected by elevated serum methylmalonic acid levels (see below) (27). Fifty percent of patients with cobalamin levels between 100 and 200 pg/mL and up to 10% of patients between 200 and 300 pg/mL have elevated methylmalonic acid levels indicating cellular deficiency. Above 300 pg/mL, only 0.1% have tissue cobalamin deficiency. Low cobalamin levels in patients without evidence of tissue deficiency presumably indicate early depletion of cobalamin stores or reduced levels of transcobalamin I binding protein (the major cobalamin binding protein in the plasma). Clinical conditions where myeloid cells, the major producer of transcobalamin I, are severely depleted such as aplastic anemia may result in low serum cobalamin levels. Patients with myeloma and human immunodeficiency virus (HIV) infection frequently have unexplained low levels of cobalamin, which also may reflect reduced myeloid mass. Elevated levels are seen after treatment with parenteral vitamin B_{12}, in patients with hepatic necrosis, or because of increases in B_{12} binding proteins associated with myeloproliferative disorders, particularly chronic myeloid leukemia.

Serum Methylmalonic Acid

Methylmalonyl dehydrogenase is a cobalamin-dependent enzyme required for transformation of methylmalonate into succinate in mammalian cells. Methylmalonic acid is assayed by gas-liquid chromatography or mass spectrometry (20). Serum and urine methylmalonic acid increase in more than 95% of patients with cellular cobalamin deficiency. Some patients with low serum cobalamin and normal serum methylmalonic acid levels presumably have depleted stores without frank cobalamin deficiency. In renal insufficiency, reduced methylmalonic acid excretion can lead to elevated serum levels in the absence of cellular cobalamin deficiency. A diagnosis of cellular cobalamin deficiency can be confirmed by demonstrating a decrease in serum methylmalonic acid levels after initiation of cobalamin treatment.

Serum Homocysteine

Deficiency of folic acid or cobalamin prevents the methylation of homocysteine to form methionine and leads to increased serum homocysteine levels, which can be measured by ion exchange chromatography (20). Cellular cobalamin deficiency usually causes elevated levels of both methylmalonic acid and serum homocysteine, but in 5% of cobalamin-deficient patients only serum homocysteine will be elevated. In usual practice, it is not cost effective to use homocysteine to confirm cellular deficiency of cobalamin or folate. Indeed, homocysteine levels are more often obtained for the clinical evaluation of arterial or venous hypercoagulability (see Chapter 22). Other causes of elevated levels of homocysteine include renal insufficiency and inherited abnormalities in the enzymes required for the folic acid cycle and sulphur amino acid metabolism.

Serum Intrinsic Factor Antibody Assay

A positive result in this assay is highly specific for a diagnosis of malabsorption of cobalamin because of autoimmune depletion of intrinsic factor (pernicious anemia), but the sensitivity of the serum assay is less than 50%.

Serum and Red Cell Folate Assays

These levels are determined by a competitive receptor-binding assay (20). Serum folate levels reflect recent dietary intake, while red cell folate levels reflect body folate stores at the time when the red cell was formed. Because cobalamin is required for cellular uptake of folate, reduced red cell folate levels are found with either folate or cobalamin deficiency; therefore, a serum cobalamin level is always required to interpret a low red cell folate level. Red cell folate is measured from a hemolysate prepared from whole blood, and elevated levels of serum folate may therefore affect the red cell folate value. Elevated serum folate is found in cobalamin deficiency states and following treatment with folic acid. The assessment of folic acid deficiency with serum and red cell folate assays is not cost effective, because it is easily treated. While folate deficiency was previously common in nutritionally deficient individuals, folate addition to products made with flour has made deficiency infrequent in the United States. Cobalamin levels, however, are essential in the evaluation of patients with presumed folate deficiency, because folic acid replacement may improve the anemia but not the potentially irreversible neurologic complications of cobalamin deficiency.

Serum Erythropoietin

In patients with refractory anemia because of marrow failure, markedly elevated erythropoietin levels (over 1000 U/mL) usually predict failure of recombinant erythropoietin therapy. This immunoassay can therefore be useful in identifying a subset of patients unlikely to benefit from therapy with erythropoiesis-stimulating agents. On the other hand, it is not worthwhile to assay erythropoietin levels in anemic patients with renal insufficiency, malignancy, or inflammation because erythropoietin levels in these conditions are invariably low (under 100 U/mL). Erythropoietin assays that are sensitive to low levels are useful for distinguishing polycythemia vera from other causes of erythrocytosis. Patients with polycythemia vera have levels below the normal range indicating autonomous erythroid proliferation. Erythropoietin levels in patients with secondary polycythemia may be elevated but often are within the normal range. Erythropoietin levels may elevate following phlebotomy treatment of patients with secondary erythrocytosis.

TESTS FOR THE EVALUATION OF ABNORMAL HEMOGLOBINS AND HEMOLYTIC ANEMIAS

Hemoglobin Electrophoresis

Methods used to differentiate and quantitate abnormal hemoglobins and the minor hemoglobins include alkaline electrophoresis on cellulose acetate membranes, acid citrate agar gel electrophoresis, isoelectric focusing (IEF), and high-performance liquid chromatography (HPLC) (28). Clinical laboratories traditionally have used cellulose acetate or agarose gel electrophoresis at pH 8.6 to screen patient samples and to identify the common hemoglobins A, S, and C. When aberrant hemoglobins are observed, levels are quantified by using densitometry (Fig. 27.1). The minor hemoglobins F and A_2 are

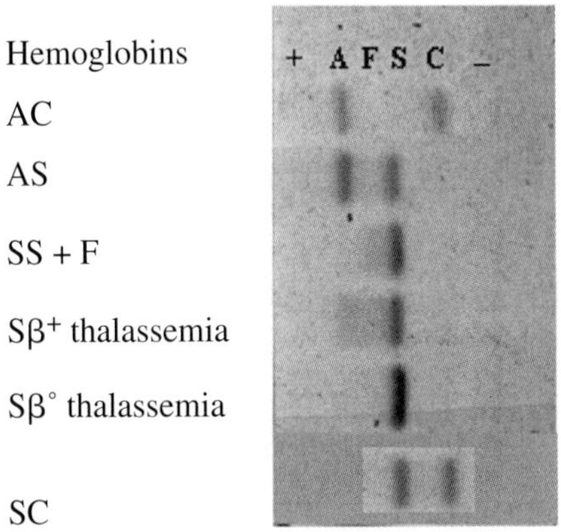

Hemoglobins

AC

AS

SS + F

Sβ⁺ thalassemia

Sβ° thalassemia

SC

FIG. 27.1. Hemoglobin electrophoresis, cellulose acetate, pH 8.6.

also separated by this method; however, their levels in adults cannot be measured accurately by densitometry. Because a number of common G and D hemoglobins comigrate with Hb S, a solubility test is routinely used to confirm the presence of S (see below). Acid citrate agar electrophoresis (which also separates hemoglobins A, S, C, and F) is routinely used for secondary confirmation because (unlike electrophoresis at pH 8.6) it can distinguish Hb D (containing mutated beta globin chains) and Hb G (containing mutated alpha globin chains) from Hb S. Citrate agar electrophoresis can also distinguish Hb C from Hb E and Hb O Arab, variants that comigrate with C on alkaline electrophoresis.

Alkaline electrophoresis is not useful for neonatal screening because it does not cleanly separate Hb F from Hb A. IEF and HPLC are used in neonatal screening programs because they have greater power than cellulose acetate or acid agar electrophoresis in screening for atypical variant hemoglobins. These methods, however, are more expensive and require greater expertise for interpretation.

Sickle Solubility Test

The insolubility of deoxygenated Hb S in a concentrated phosphate buffer can be exploited to confirm that a hemoglobin with the appropriate electrophoretic mobility is actually Hb S. Because the solubility test cannot distinguish between sickle trait and sickle cell disease, it is not a useful to diagnose sickle cell disease in clinical settings.

Sickle Cell Prep

Red cells from individuals with sickle cell trait or homozygous S will take on the sickle shape when deoxygenated. This test has been replaced by the sickle cell solubility test to confirm the presence of Hb S. It also does not distinguish sickle cell trait from sickle cell disease.

Hb A_2 Quantitation

HPLC is the method of choice for this measurement (28). Column chromatography is also frequently used; however, it is unreliable in the presence of Hb S. Elevated levels of Hb A_2 above 3.5% will generally confirm a diagnosis of β-thalassemia trait; the clinician should be aware that iron deficiency will reduce the Hb A_2 level. Patients with α-thalassemia trait have normal levels of Hb A_2.

Hb F Quantitation

Many clinical laboratories continue to use the alkali-denaturation test to quantitate the percentage of Hb F. This test exploits the persistent solubility of Hb F under alkaline conditions that precipitate most other hemoglobins. After treatment with alkali, the residual Hb F can be separated by filtration and quantified spectrophotometrically. The assay is accurate with samples containing as much as 10% to 15% hemoglobin F but will often underestimate higher levels for which HPLC-based methods are more accurate.

Hb F Cells

Hb F can also be measured immunologically to determine the amount of Hb F in red cells and distinguish high Hb F containing cells ("F cells") from red cells containing low levels of Hb F (see Chapter 4).

Tests for Unstable Hemoglobins

Unstable hemoglobins such as Hb Zurich and Hb Koln can be recognized by their propensity to precipitate when hemolysates are exposed to heat (50°C) or to 17% isopropanol. Unstable hemoglobins may also be detected by the formation of Heinz bodies (denatured hemoglobin) in intact red blood cells after exposure to oxidizing conditions. These purple inclusions, located near the red cell membrane, are detected microscopically after incubating red cells with supravital stains such as brilliant cresyl blue or new methylene blue (see Chapter 3).

Glucose-6-Phosphate Dehydrogenase

Both qualitative and quantitative tests are used in clinical laboratories to detect G6PD deficiency. These tests depend on the generation of NADPH from NADP. The most common screening test is the fluorescent spot test which depends on the intrinsic fluorescence of NADPH. Reticulocytes from individuals with the most common variant of G6PD deficiency seen in the United States (G6PD A-) have much higher quantities of enzyme than mature red cells. Deficiency can be missed in A-deficient if reticulocytosis has developed in response to hemolysis produced by an oxidant chemical or drug. Heinz bodies (denatured hemoglobin, see above) can also be recognized in this setting. Female heterozygotes may also escape detection by screening tests (29).

Serum Haptoglobin

This hemoglobin-binding protein can be assayed by nephelometric or turbidimetric methods. Haptoglobin is an acute phase reactant, but its main usefulness is that very low levels are an indicator of acute or chronic hemolysis. Free hemoglobin bound to haptoglobin is cleared by the reticuloendothelial system in less than 30 minutes. The in vivo hemolysis of as little as 50 mL of red blood cells will deplete the blood of haptoglobin. In the absence of continuing hemolysis, it will take at least 5 days to regenerate to normal levels. The normal range varies widely because of genetic differences in the alpha chains. Rare patients have very low haptoglobin levels on a genetic basis. Patients with severe liver disease may have a decrease in haptoglobin because of failure of hepatic synthesis.

Urine Hemosiderin

In patients with chronic intravascular hemolysis such as paroxysmal nocturnal hemoglobinuria or cardiac valve hemolysis, renal excretion of hemoglobin leads to uptake of heme with subsequent accumulation of hemosiderin in the renal tubular cells. After staining the urine sediment for hemosiderin with Prussian blue, microscopic evaluation of the sediment will demonstrate blue-stained renal casts, indicating iron deposition in the tubular cells.

HEMOSTASIS AND COAGULATION ASSAYS

Activated Partial Thromboplastin Time

This assay measures the time required to initiate clotting after citrated plasma is incubated with calcium, a partial thromboplastin (a lipid source devoid of tissue factor), and a surface activating agent. Automated instruments detect clot initiation mechanically or based on turbidimetric changes. The activated partial thromboplastin time (aPTT) is particularly sensitive to deficiencies of factors VIII and IX but will also be prolonged because of deficiencies of factors XII, XI, X, V, and II and fibrinogen. Mild reductions in factor VIII (above 30% to 50%) and fibrinogen (over 100 mg) may not be detected by this assay (30). The aPTT is prolonged by anticoagulants (antithrombins such as heparin, hirudin, argatroban, bivalirudin, melagatran), factor-specific antibodies (most commonly against factor VIII), and lupus anticoagulants. Persistence of a prolonged aPTT in 1:1 mixing studies (50% patient plasma mixed with 50% normal plasma) suggests the presence of an antibody. Detection of antibodies against factor VIII may require incubation of the 1:1 mix with normal plasma for 1 hour at 37°C to allow antibody to bind to factor VIII. The presence of lupus anticoagulants can be confirmed by demonstrating correction of a prolonged aPTT by the addition of phospholipid.

Unfractionated heparin therapy is monitored using the aPTT to avoid subtherapeutic or supratherapeutic levels. Although the sensitivity of the many available partial thromboplastins to heparin (as well as the instruments used) vary, a recent study suggests an aPTT test to control ratio of 2.0 to 3.0 is a good target range for therapeutic heparin levels (31). Some laboratories monitor heparin levels by its capacity to inhibit antifactor Xa. The aPTT is not sensitive to low molecular weight heparins (LMWH). When monitoring of LMWH is indicated (e.g., in patients with renal insufficiency, obesity, or pregnancy), an anti-Xa assay for the specific LMWH must be used.

Spurious results of the aPTT are usually because of poorly filled tubes, high hematocrit causing a low plasma to citrate ratio, delays in delivery of sample to the laboratory, or contamination with intravenous fluids or heparin.

Prothrombin Time

The prothrombin time (PT) is sensitive to deficiencies of factors VII, V, X, II, and fibrinogen (30), and therefore it is valuable in assessing liver function and monitoring warfarin therapy. Inherited deficiencies of these factors are uncommon and autoantibodies are rare. Some lupus anticoagulants may affect the PT as well as the aPTT. Rarely, exposure to bovine thrombin will trigger the development of antithrombin and antifactor V antibodies. The international normalized ratio (INR) has been useful in standardizing the control of warfarin therapy. The INR is the ratio of the patient PT to the mean normal PT raised to the power of the International Sensitivity Index (ISI). Commercial thromboplastins are calibrated and given an ISI value, which reflects their sensitivity to warfarinized plasma. It may be misleading to use the INR to describe the prolongation of the PT in a patient not receiving warfarin. The PT is vulnerable to the same preanalytic artifacts described above for the aPTT assay.

Activated Clotting Times

Activated clotting times (ACT) are used on site in cardiac surgery and cardiac catheterization procedures.

Thrombin Time

The thrombin time is prolonged by low fibrinogen levels or the presence of heparin, paraproteins, dysfibrinogens, or fibrin(ogen) split products (30). The reptilase time is prolonged by similar molecules but is insensitive to heparin.

Specific Factor Assays

Specific factor assays are based on the ability of patient plasma to correct clotting times of specific factor-deficient plasma in PTT or PT-based assays (see Chapter 20).

Euglobulin Clot Lysis

Euglobulin, a plasma precipitate containing fibrinogen, plasminogen, and plasminogen inhibitor without most fibrinolysis inhibitors, is prepared from the patient sample and clotted with thrombin. The time required for clot lysis is then determined. Because euglobulin lacks inhibitors, clot lysis normally occurs quite rapidly (within 90 to 300 minutes). Abnormally short lysis times occur in states of hyperfibrinolysis such as severe liver disease but may also simply reflect poor clot formation because of hypofibrinogenemia.

D-Dimer

This immunologic assay detects fibrin split products that are cross-linked because of the action of thrombin and factor XIIIa. Elevated levels indicate extensive local fibrin formation (deep vein thrombosis, pulmonary emboli, pneumonia) or disseminated intravascular coagulation. The value of a positive value in predicting localized thrombosis is poor; a negative study (depending on the sensitivity of the assay) is more helpful in ruling out thrombosis (32). A positive D-dimer level has been also used to predict recurrence of thrombosis after treatment of an initial unprovoked thrombosis (33); however, factors such as age and sex are also important to consider along with the D-dimer level (34).

Fibrinogen

Fibrinogen levels are routinely determined by using a thrombin time-based assay, but chemical or immunologic methods may also be used (30). Fibrinogen can also be estimated from clot density assessment during prothrombin time measurements. Because fibrinogen is an acute phase reactant, levels are frequently raised in patients with inflammation and malignancy. Decreased levels are found with disseminated intravascular coagulation, the hemophagocytic syndrome, advanced liver disease, treatment with asparaginase, or rarely as an inherited condition.

Bleeding Time

This in vivo test of platelet function is useful in evaluation of patients with normal platelet counts and suspected platelet dysfunction. In the modified Ivy technique, a template is used to make two incisions on the volar surface of the forearm parallel to the antecubital fold, while a blood pressure cuff applied to the upper arm is inflated to 40 mmHg. Blood is gently removed from the incisions every 30 seconds. It is not useful in evaluating patients with thrombocytopenia; they will have long bleeding times. The bleeding time is affected by the skill of the technologist and the depth of the incision. Because it is not reproducible and not a reliable predictor of hemorrhagic risk, it is not valuable as a general screening test. Its use should be limited to the evaluation of patients requiring an invasive procedure who are suspected to have inherited platelet function defects such as von Willebrand disease or significant acquired disorders that affect platelet function such as severe renal insufficiency, myeloproliferative disorders, or drug-induced platelet dysfunction (30). Automated in vitro instruments have been developed that may be more reliably used as a screening test for platelet function abnormalities; a widely used one is the platelet function analyzer PFA-100 (Dade Behring, Deerfield, Illinois) (30).

TESTS FOR HYPERCOAGULABILITY

Antithrombin, Protein C, and Protein S

Functional assays of these proteins are more sensitive to deficiency than are antigen-based assays. Patients heterozygous for an inherited defect in one of these factors typically have only modest reductions from the lower limit of normal in factor levels. Nevertheless, they may be at significant risk of venous hypercoagulability (particularly in patients with antithrombin deficiency). Acquired deficiency of antithrombin occurs in disseminated intravascular coagulation, liver disease, heparin therapy, and extensive thrombosis. Acquired deficiency of protein C and S occurs with vitamin K deficiency, warfarin therapy, and extensive thrombosis. Free protein S deficiency occurs in patients with increased C4b-binding protein secondary to inflammation. These assays should not be performed in the setting of acute venous thromboembolism.

Activated Protein C Resistance

Abnormality of this aPTT-based assay is mainly associated with the inherited polymorphism factor V Leiden.

Lupus Anticoagulants

These acquired antibodies to β2-glycoprotein I, a protein with a high affinity for phospholipid, can be associated with both arterial and venous hypercoagulability. On the other hand, positive assays are frequently seen in otherwise healthy individuals and may be transient. The functional assays (dilute Russell viper venom test, platelet neutralization test) may be more sensitive to thrombosis risk than are the serologic tests for anticardiolipin antibodies (see Chapters 20 and 22).

Factor V Leiden and Prothrombin G 20210A

The assays for these mutations are DNA-based and therefore are not affected by the presence of acute venous thromboembolism.

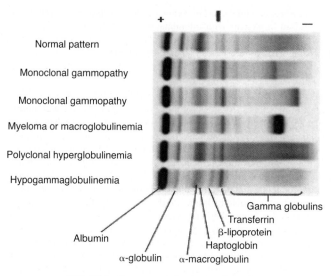

FIG. 27.2. Serum protein electrophoresis.

TESTS FOR EVALUATION OF PATIENTS WITH HEMATOLOGIC MALIGNANCIES

Serum Protein Electrophoresis

Electrophoresis separates proteins mainly on the basis of electric charge. When normal plasma proteins are electrophoresed on cellulose acetate or now more commonly on agarose films and stained with a protein binding dye, six zones appear. Albumin, α_1, α_2, and two β globulins appear as five discrete bands, and γ globulins migrate as a more diffuse, electrophoretically heterogeneous band (Fig. 27.2 and Table 22.4). Monoclonal immunoglobulins (M paraproteins) are recognized because they

TABLE 27.4. *Plasma Protein Migration Patterns on Standard Protein Electrophoresis*

Albumin zone
  Albumin
Alpha₁ zone
  Alpha₁-antitrypsin
  Alpha₁-lipoproteins (high-density lipoproteins [HDL])
Alpha₂ zone
  Alpha₂-macroglobulin
  Haptoglobin
  Ceruloplasmin
Beta zone
  β-Lipoprotein (low-density lipoprotein)
  Transferrin
  C3 (complement)
Gamma zone
  Fibrinogen (in incompletely clotted specimens)
  IgA
  IgM
  IgG

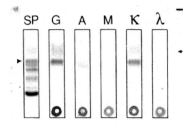

FIG. 27.3. Immunofixation illustrating an IgG kappa monoclonal protein. The *arrowhead* points to the putative monoclonal band in the SP lane stained with a protein binding dye. Staining in the remaining lanes indicates the presence of products reacting with specific antibodies directed against IgG (G), IgA (A), and IgM (M) heavy chains, and Ig kappa (κ) and lambda (λ) light chains. Small *arrow* on the right indicates origin.

form discrete bands ("spikes") in the β or γ globulin regions. The concentration of the proteins in normal or paraprotein bands can be determined by densitometry. When hyperglobulinemia is detected by routine total protein and albumin measurements, protein electrophoresis is essential to distinguish between reactive polyclonal from monoclonal processes (Fig. 27.3). When a putative monoclonal band is noted in an electrophoretic pattern, immunofixation (see below) studies are required to confirm the product is truly a monoclonal immunoglobulin with a single heavy chain and, more important, a single light chain. Alternatively, quantitation of heavy and light chains and capillary zone electrophoresis may be used to confirm a monoclonal process. The presence of a monoclonal immunoglobulin is consistent with the presence of a plasma cell or lymphoid malignancy or light chain-related amyloidosis but is not diagnostic. Most monoclonal proteins of concentrations below 3 g/dL in serum are not associated with clinical or pathologic evidence of malignancy and are referred to as monoclonal gammopathy of unknown significance (MGUS) because of the potential for malignant transformation. Occasional individuals exhibit two monoclonal proteins ("diclonal" gammopathy) either representing the products of two separate clones, or, if both bands contain the same heavy and light chain, two products of a single clone with differing electrophoretic mobilities possibly because of multimer formation. Patients with marked polyclonal gammopathy, for example due to HIV or liver disease, may have multiple small discrete bands termed oligoclonal gammopathy. The majority of the γ-globulin in these individuals is polyclonal.

M paraproteins of greater than 3.0 g/dL usually reflect the presence of a plasma cell dyscrasia. The concentration of M protein in the plasma (or urine) is a marker of tumor burden in myeloma and macroglobulinemia patients, and serial monitoring by electrophoresis is extremely important in assessing response to therapy. For this determination to be reliable, the M paraprotein must be quantitated separately from polyclonal immunoglobulins.

Urine Protein Electrophoresis

Light chain excretion must be examined in patients with hypogammaglobulinemia or other findings suspicious of a plasma cell dyscrasia. Approximately 15% of patients with myeloma excrete monoclonal light chains in the urine (Bence Jones proteinuria) in the absence of any detectable M protein in the serum. For screening, a random urine specimen is concentrated if required and electrophoresed on cellulose acetate or agar films. Discrete bands are then assayed by immunofixation to confirm that they represent intact monoclonal immunoglobulins or free light chains. If a paraprotein is found, serial 24-hour urine collections are useful in monitoring tumor burden and response to therapy.

Immunofixation

Immunofixation has replaced immunoelectrophoresis to confirm monoclonality of discrete bands noted in the β or γ globulin regions of the electrophoresis. Antibodies against the γ, α, μ heavy chains and the κ and λ light chains are layered separately on membranes containing the electrophoresed samples. A monoclonal immunoglobulin will form immunofixation bands with antibodies against one heavy chain class and/or one light chain type (Fig. 27.3). IgM and IgA proteins are more likely to be found close to the β globulin region; IgG proteins may be found in any area of the β and γ globulin zones. Free light chains are seen on serum protein electrophoresis only in myeloma patients with severe renal failure or in instances where the light chains form spontaneous tetramers too large for renal clearance. The uncommon IgD and very rare IgE myelomas should be suspected when a serum paraprotein binds only an anti-light chain antibody.

Serum Free Light Chain Assay

This nephelometric automated immunoassay depends on the use of antibodies to κ and λ light chains that react with epitopes that are exposed in free light chains but hidden in the intact monoclonal immunoglobulins. Because of its superior convenience and comparable sensitivity to urine electrophoresis, it is being used frequently to monitor response to treatment of light chain myeloma and amyloidosis (35,36). The assay also has diagnostic and prognostic utility in amyloidosis, monoclonal gammopathy, and smoldering multiple myeloma (37).

Quantitative Serum Immunoglobulins

Quantitative serum immunoglobulins are measured with an automated nephelometric or turbidimetric immunoassay; this assay is most useful for quantitating normal immunoglobulins rather than M paraproteins. Because the measurement can be affected by changes in immunoglobulin molecular weight, IgA M proteins that form multimers and monoclonal IgM pentamers with a propensity to disassociate into smaller-molecular-weight species can produce erroneous results.

Serum Cryoglobulins

The most critical step in this test is the treatment of the specimen before it reaches the laboratory. The blood should be drawn into a preheated syringe or warm tube, transported to the laboratory at 37 °C, and kept at this temperature until the serum is separated from the clot. The serum is then refrigerated at 4°C and examined after 24 hours. A precipitate that dissolves when the tube is rewarmed to 37°C indicates a serum cryoglobulin. Electrophoresis and immunofixation of the separated and redissolved cryoprecipitate will reveal the immunoglobulins involved in the cryoglobulin formation. Cryoglobulins may be (i) a monoclonal immunoglobulin, usually IgM; (ii) a monoclonal IgM that binds to polyclonal IgG (has rheumatoid factor activity); or (iii) polyclonal IgM bound to polyclonal IgG.

Serum Viscosity

The Ostwald viscosimeter measures viscosity by comparing the time required for serum and water to flow through a capillary tube at 37°C. Normal serum is 1.4 to 1.8 times more viscous than water. Symptoms resulting from hyperviscosity generally occur when the relative viscosity exceeds 6 but may occur with a relative viscosity as low as 3 or 4.

Serum β_2-Microglobulin

Serum β_2-microglobulin is a small protein noncovalently linked with class I human leukocyte antigen (HLA) molecules. Serum levels are measured by nephelometric immunoassay. Elevated levels may be found in inflammatory conditions, renal failure (because of failure of excretion), and in lymphoid and plasma cell malignancies. High serum β_2-microglobulin is an important prognostic feature indicating advanced disease and poor response to therapy in myeloma and certain lymphomas. In myeloma, elevated β_2-microglobulin levels predict early relapse following autologous transplantation. Serum levels are not useful, however, to follow chemotherapy responsiveness in myeloma because of the lack of specificity.

Serum Lactic Dehydrogenase

This protein is measured by an automated enzyme activity-based assay. The normal range varies depending on the type of assay. Elevated serum levels reflect necrosis of cells rich in the enzyme. The most marked elevations (more than five times normal) usually are noted with severe megaloblastic anemia, intravascular hemolytic anemia, or hemophagocytic syndromes. Similar levels can be seen in acute leukemia and lymphomas often as harbingers of tumor lysis syndrome. An elevated serum level is a risk factor in the International Prognostic Index for non-Hodgkin's lymphoma. Distinguishing the five isoenzymes of lactic dehydrogenase is seldom useful in diagnosing hematologic disorders.

Serum Uric Acid

Serum uric acid is measured by an automated enzyme assay. Elevated serum levels, particularly over 10 mg/dL in patients with hematologic malignancies, should raise concern for increased cell turnover (tumor lysis syndrome) and incipient renal compromise because of uric acid precipitation. Hypouricemia may occur in Hodgkin disease and in Fanconi syndrome associated with interstitial renal disease caused by Bence Jones (light chain) proteinuria.

NEUTROPHIL EVALUATION

Marrow Granulocyte Reserve

Marrow granulocyte reserve may be assessed by the hydrocortisone stimulation test (38) or by the response to filgrastim (39). In the hydrocortisone stimulation test, the absolute neutrophil concentration is measured before administering 200 mg hydrocortisone intravenously and again 3, 4, and 5 hours later. A failure of the neutrophil concentration to increase by at least 1600 neutrophils per microliter indicates poor marrow granulocyte reserve. Similarly, the failure of the absolute granulocyte level to rise above 5000 per microliter 24 hours after a subcutaneous injection of 5 µg/kg filgrastim indicates increased risk for chemotherapy-induced febrile neutropenia.

Leukocyte Alkaline Phosphatase

This assay is an inexpensive cytochemical test of peripheral blood neutrophils used to screen patients with leukocytosis suggesting a diagnosis of Philadelphia chromosome-positive chronic myelogenous leukemia. The assay depends on the enzyme's ability to cleave a dye, which then stains the cells. Individual neutrophils are scored by the intensity of staining as 0 to 4+, and the sum of the scores of 100 cells are tallied. Neutrophils from patients with chronic myelogenous leukemia or paroxysmal nocturnal hemoglobinuria have low levels of leukocyte alkaline phosphatase (<10 Kaplow units). Neutrophils from patients with reactive leukocytosis and polycythemia vera have elevated scores (>80 Kaplow units). Patients with other myeloproliferative disorders may have normal, low, or high levels. This assay has been largely replaced by the FISH assay for BCR-ABL in peripheral blood neutrophils or cytogenetic analysis of the bone marrow. The availability of highly effective therapy for chronic myelogenous leukemia warrants the use of the more specific, albeit expensive FISH assay (40) (see Chapter 13).

REFERENCES

1. Gulati GL, Hyland LJ, Kocher W, et al. Changes in automated complete blood cell count and differential leukocyte count results induced by storage of blood at room temperature. Arch Pathol Lab Med 2002;126:336–342.
2. Thompson CB, Diaz DD, Quinn PG, et al. The role of anticoagulation in the measurement of platelet volumes. Am J Clin Pathol 1983;80:327–332.
3. Narayanan, S. Preanalytical issues in hematology. Lab Medizin 2003;27:243–248.
4. Silvestri F, Virgolini L, Savignano C, et al. Incidence and diagnosis of EDTA-dependent pseudothrombocytopenia in a consecutive outpatient population referred for isolated thrombocytopenia. Vox Sang 1995;68:35–39.

5. Ward PC. The CBC at the turn of the millennium: an overview. Clin Chem 2000;46:1215–1220.

6. Bourner G, Dhaliwal J, Sumner J. Performance evaluation of the latest fully automated hematology analyzers in a large, commercial laboratory setting: a four-way, side-by-side study. Lab Hematol 2005;11:285–297.

7. Simel DL, DeLong ER, Feussner JR, et al. Erythrocyte anisocytosis. Visual inspection of blood films vs. automated analysis of red blood cell distribution width. Arch Intern Med 1988;148: 822–824.

8. Bessman JD, Feinstein DI. Quantitative anisocytosis as a discriminant between iron deficiency and thalassemia minor. Blood 1979;53:288–293.

9. Novis DA, Walsh M, Wilkinson D, et al. Laboratory productivity and the rate of manual peripheral blood smear review: a College of American Pathologists Q-Probes study of 95,141 complete blood count determinations performed in 263 institutions. Arch Pathol Lab Med 2006;130: 596–601.

10. Cornbleet PJ. Clinical utility of the band count. Clin Lab Med 2002;22:101–136.

11. Al-Gwaiz LA, Babay HH. The diagnostic value of absolute neutrophil count, band count, and morphologic changes of neutrophils in predicting bacterial infections. Med Princ Pract 2007; 16:344–347.

12. Crouch JY, Kaplow LS. Relationship of reticulocyte age to polychromasia, shift cells, and shift reticulocytes. Arch Pathol Lab Med 1985;109:325–329.

13. Chuang CL, Liu RS, Wei YH, et al. Early prediction of response to intravenous iron supplementation by reticulocyte haemoglobin content and high-fluorescence reticulocyte count in haemodialysis patients. Nephrol Dial Transplant 2003;18:370–377.

14. Torres A, Sánchez J, Lakomsky D, et al. Assessment of hematologic progenitor engraftment by complete reticulocyte maturation parameters after autologous and allogeneic hematopoietic stem cell transplantation. Haematologica 2001;86:24–29.

15. Mast AE, Blinder MA, Dietzen DJ. Reticulocyte hemoglobin content. Am J Hematol 2008;83: 307–310.

16. Barron BA, Hoyer JD, Tefferi A. A bone marrow report of absent stainable iron is not diagnostic of iron deficiency. Ann Hematol 2001;80:166–169.

17. Hughes DA, Stuart-Smith SE, Bain BJ. How should stainable iron in bone marrow films be assessed? J Clin Pathol 2004;57:1038–1040.

18. Bain BJ. Bone marrow biopsy morbidity and mortality. Br J Haematol 2003;121:949–951.

19. Henry JB. Clinical Diagnosis and Management by Laboratory Methods, 20th Ed. Philadelphia: W.B. Saunders; 2001.

20. Burtis CA, Ashwood ER, Bruns DE, eds. Tietz Textbook of Clinical Chemistry and Molecular Diagnostics, 4th Ed. Saint Louis: Elsevier Saunders; 2006.

21. Beutler E, Hoffbrand AV, Cook JD. Iron deficiency and overload. Hematology Am Soc Hematol Educ Program 2003;40–61.

22. Punnonen K, Irjala K, Rajamaki A. Serum transferrin receptor and its ratio to serum ferritin in the diagnosis of iron deficiency. Blood 1997;89:1052–1057.

23. Beutler E, Hoffbrand AV, Cook JD. Iron deficiency and overload. Hematology (Am Soc Hematol Educ Program) 2003:40–61.

24. Siebert S, Williams BD, Henley R, et al. Single value of serum transferrin receptor is not diagnostic for the absence of iron stores in anaemic patients with rheumatoid arthritis. Clin Lab Haematol 2003;25:155–160.

25. Brugnara C. Iron deficiency and erythropoiesis: new diagnostic approaches. Clin Chem 2003; 49:1573–1578.

26. Pfeiffer CM, Cook JD, Mei Z, et al. Evaluation of an automated soluble transferrin receptor (sTfR) assay on the Roche Hitachi analyzer and its comparison to two ELISA assays. Clin Chim Acta 2007;382:112–116.

27. Stabler SP, Allen RH, Savage DG, et al. Clinical spectrum and diagnosis of cobalamin deficiency. Blood 1990;76:871–881.

28. Chui DHK, Steinberg MH. Laboratory diagnosis of hemoglobinopathies and thalassemias. In Hoffman R, ed. Hematology: Basic Principles and Practices. Philadelphia: Elsevier, Churchill Livingstone; 2005:2687–2695.

29. Beutler E. Glucose-6-phosphate dehydrogenase deficiency. A historical perspective. Blood 2008;111:16–24.
30. Rand JH, Senzel L. Laboratory evaluation of hemostatic disorders. In Hoffman R, ed. Hematology: Basic Principles and Practices. Philadelphia: Elsevier, Churchill Livingstone; 2005: 2001–2008.
31. Bates SM, Weitz JI, Johnston M, et al. Use of a fixed activated partial thromboplastin time ratio to establish a therapeutic range for unfractionated heparin. Arch Intern Med 2001;161:385–391.
32. Rathbun SW, Whitsett TL, Raskob GE. Exclusion of first-episode deep-vein thrombosis after-hours using D-Dimer. Blood Coagul Fibrinolysis 2007;16:795–800.
33. Palareti G, Cosmi B, Legnani C, et al. D-Dimer testing to determine the duration of anticoagulation therapy. N Engl J Med 2006;355:1780–1790.
34. Baglin T, Palmer CR, Luddington R, et al. Unprovoked recurrent venous thrombosis: prediction by D-Dimer and clinical risk factors. J Thromb Haemost 2008;6:577–582.
35. Bradwell AR, Carr-Smith HD, Mead GP, et al. Highly sensitive, automated immunoassay for immunoglobulin free light chains in serum and urine. Clin Chem 2001;47:673–680.
36. Bradwell AR, Carr-Smith HD, Mead GP, et al. Serum test for assessment of patients with Bence Jones myeloma. Lancet 2003;361:489–491.
37. Kyle RA, Rajkumar SV. Monoclonal gammopathy of unknown significance and smouldering multiple myeloma: emphasis on risk factors for progression. Br J Haematol 2007;139:730–743.
38. Mason BA, Lessin L, Schechter GP. Marrow granulocyte reserves in black Americans. Hydrocortisone-induced granulocytosis in the "benign" neutropenia of the black. Am J Med 1979;67:201–205.
39. Hansen PB, Johnsen HE, Ralfkiaer E, et al. Blood neutrophil increment after a single injection of rhG-CSF or rhGM-CSF correlates with marrow cellularity and may predict the grade of neutropenia after chemotherapy. Br J Haematol 1993;84:581–585.
40. Tkachuk DC, Westbrook CA, Andreef M, et al. Detection of bcr-abl in chronic myelogenous leukemia by in situ hybridization. Science 1990;250:559–562.

28

Basic Principles and Clinical Applications of Flow Cytometry

Thomas A. Fleisher

Flow cytometry is a technology used routinely in most hematology laboratories. Its entry into the mainstream of clinical laboratory analysis has been aided by the increasing availability of monoclonal antibody reagents that define cell surface proteins as markers of cell lineage, differentiation, maturation, and/or activation. Instrument design advances have yielded benchtop cytometers with fixed optics that linked with new developments in fluorochrome chemistry enable a wide range of clinical applications. In addition, proficiency testing is now available in support of these clinical applications through the College of American Pathologists (CAP) as mandated by the Clinical Laboratory Improvement Amendment of 1988 (CLIA88). The major advantage that flow cytometry provides is its capacity to assess multiple measurements (parameters) on large numbers of individual cells. Flow cytometric studies have extended the understanding of hematopoietic cell development, differentiation, activation, and apoptosis. In addition, they have provided important information regarding hematologic malignancies, insight into reconstitution after stem cell transplantation, and understanding of cell defects that result in immune deficiencies. Overall, flow cytometry has played an important role in the diagnosis and characterization of a number of hematologic disorders.

The basic design of a flow cytometer involves four major elements: optics, fluidics, electronics, and computer (with specific software) (1,2). The optical system utilizes one or more light sources, typically one (or several lasers) that produces monochromatic light and serves as the excitation beam(s). At the opposite side of the optical bench, light generated from the cells that have intersected the excitation beam is collected; filters and dichroic mirrors set in fixed locations are linked to photodetectors to allow quantitation of the emitted light at specific wavelengths. To ensure that all cells analyzed experience consistent exposure to the excitation beam, the fluidic system must maintain the cells in a consistent location as they move sequentially through the beam; to accomplish this result, the cell suspension is injected into a flowing stream of sheath fluid that hydrodynamically focuses the inner stream of cells within the outer sheath fluid stream (1). The intersection of the cells with the excitation light beam(s) produces characteristic and cell-specific light scatter (nonfluorescent) signals; additional fluorescent signals are generated by fluorochromes that typically are linked to specific reagents that bind antigens present on or within the cells of interest. The various light signals (parameters) are collected by the optical bench, while instrument design determines the number of parameters collected per cell. The two reagent-independent (nonfluorescent) parameters are forward angle light scatter, as a marker of cell size, and side angle light scatter, as an index of cellular regularity/granularity. The combination of these two parameters allows for discrimination among the three major types of leukocytes as well as evaluation of red blood cells and platelets in whole blood samples (3).

The fluorescent data collected by a flow cytometer are the result of either cell surface or intracellular binding of specific monoclonal antibodies conjugated directly to fluorochromes or detected with secondary reagents conjugated to fluorochromes, as well as reagents that are inherently fluorescent. Fluorochromes are excited by light of a defined wavelength and emit light of lower energy (longer wavelength). There are currently many different fluorochromes used in clinical flow cytometry, including fluorescein isothyacyanate (FITC), phycoerythrin (PE), peridin chloryphyl protein (PercCP), and allophycocyanin (Table 28.1). More recently, combinations of two fluorochromes linked to each other

TABLE 28.1. *Fluorochromes Used Commonly in Clinical Flow Cytometry*

Fluorochrome	Flow cytometer		Maximum Emission (nm)
	Excitation (nm)	Excitation (nm)	
Fluoroscein isothyocyanate (FITC)	490	488	519
Phycoerythrin (PE)	480–565	488	578
Peridin chlorophyll protein (PerCP)	488	488	678
Allophycocyanin (APC)	650	633	660
PE-Cy5*	480–565	488	667
PE-Cy5.5*	480–565	488	695
PE-Cy7*	480–565	488	785
APC-Cy5.5*	650	633	695
APC-Cy7*	650	633	785

*Dual (tandem) fluorochrome—first of pair excites the second fluorochrome.

have been developed; they depend on the transfer of energy from the first fluorochrome to excite the second fluorochrome (Table 28.1). These tandem fluorochromes extend the range of emission wavelengths available from one excitation beam. The availability of multiple fluorochromes that absorb light of the same wavelength but emit light at different wavelengths means that multiple reagents can be used simultaneously with a single light source to yield a multicolor study. A second light source is present in most current clinical instruments to facilitate additional colors extending the range of multicolor studies. Research flow cytometers and the availability of a host of new fluorochromes have greatly extended multicolor limits with recent descriptions of 10 "color" clinical studies (4). In the research setting, there is the potential of defining 131,072 (2^{17}) subpopulations from 17 "color" studies. Extended multicolor (polychromatic) studies require complex color compensation and data management processes that typically involve sequential evaluation.

The clinical application of flow cytometry in hematology saw its earliest use as a supplement to the morphologic classification of leukemias and lymphomas, affording not only lineage information but also the state of differentiation and/or maturation (5,6). In addition, flow cytometry provided the best prognosticator in human immunodeficiency virus (HIV) infection based on absolute CD4 T-cell numbers (7). More recently, flow cytometry has proven important in characterizing hematopoietic stem cells, defining immune deficiencies and certain red blood cell-related disorders, evaluating platelets, and characterizing other cells (8–12). Flow cytometry also can be used to look inside the cell as well as at the cell surface. Fixation and permeabilization facilitate intracellular entry of reagents to determine the presence of specific proteins and to assess functional characteristics (13). This chapter is directed at basic concepts of flow cytometry, including data presentation and interpretation, followed by a brief review of applications for hematologists.

DATA PRESENTATION AND INTERPRETATION

Current flow cytometers generally yield graphic displays of the cell frequency versus the light intensity for one or more parameters by means of specific computer software. Figure 28.1 shows a single parameter histogram that reflects the quantitative distribution of cells (y-axis) versus signal strength (light intensity) of a single parameter (x-axis). Alternatively, the signal intensity of two parameters can be plotted versus cell frequency, using either a dot plot (Fig. 28.2A) or a contour plot (Fig. 28.2B). When evaluating multiple parameters (i.e., colors) the data are typically evaluated by using sequential two color displays, each reflecting the progressive subdivision of specific cell subpopulations working off of the prior data set. Typically, 10,000 to 20,000 events are collected to provide sufficient numbers of cells for meaningful data relative to the subpopulations of interest. However, when the cell or cells of interest are in low abundance, such as evaluating hematopoietic stem cells (CD34$^+$) in peripheral blood or detecting minimal residual disease in leukemia, larger total numbers of cells must be collected (8,14).

FIG. 28.1. Single parameter histogram, a distribution plot of CD3 fluorescence intensity (x-axis) versus number of events/cells (y-axis) evaluating lymphocytes.

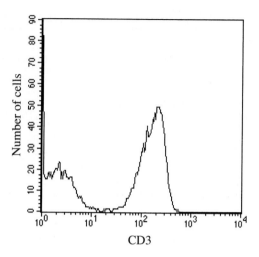

Distinguishing a positive signal is usually based on defining background signals from either unstained cells (no monoclonal antibody added) or cells that have been incubated with fluorochrome-conjugated irrelevant antibody. By convention, the negative-positive discriminator includes either 99% or 98% of all cells based on one of the background conditions described above; cells that emit a signal above this discriminator are scored as positive for binding to the specific reagent(s) added to the cell suspension. Some circumstances may require modification or alternative interpretation, and not all positive cells for a specific marker are necessarily part of the same cell population or subpopulation, reflecting the heterogeneity of cell surface protein expression.

The data generated by the computer are only as good as the instrument settings, reagents, and cell preparation used. To prevent reporting invalid data, certain standards must be met (15). First, optimal instrument performance is integral to a quality control program utilizing standard software and methods. The use of validated reagents is also part of good laboratory practices, while the quality of the cell preparation can be assessed using the nonfluorescent parameters, forward and side angle light scatter,

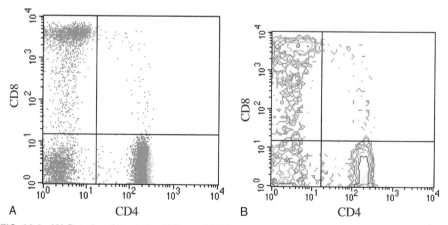

FIG. 28.2. (A) Dot plot of two-color (CD4 and CD8) staining evaluating lymphocytes. Frequency of events is reflected by the number of dots. **(B)** Contour plot of two-color (CD4 and CD8) staining evaluating lymphocytes. Frequency of events is reflected by the contour levels.

to confirm the presence of the population of interest. Each major blood cell type has distinctive features in this scatter plot. Platelets are obviously smaller than all other blood cells and heterogeneous in size, characteristics that can be confirmed in comparison to red blood cells. Erythrocytes have a characteristic appearance based on forward and side angle light scatter (Fig. 28.3A), which is similar to that of lymphocytes. However, because of the large difference in frequency of circulating erythrocytes and leukocytes, there is no practical concern of lymphocytes contaminating erythrocytes (a collection of 10,000 erythrocytes normally would include less than 20 lymphocytes). In contrast, the presence of erythrocytes makes evaluation of lymphocytes virtually impossible, because their scatter properties overlap and erythrocytes are in far greater abundance. Consequently, the study of lymphocytes (leukocytes) in a whole blood sample typically involves a red blood cell lysis step to eliminate erythrocytes (Fig. 28.3B). Following successful red cell lysis, a three-part differential is observed with normal lymphocytes representing the smallest (forward angle light scatter) and most regular/agranular (side angle scatter) cells, granulocytes are slightly larger (forward angle scatter) and show substantial granularity (side angle scatter), and monocytes fall between these two cell types (Fig. 28.3B). The two less prevalent granulocytes differ in their location on a scatter plot, with eosinophils typically falling within the granulocyte population, while basophils overlap with lymphocytes. Hematopoietic stem cells are

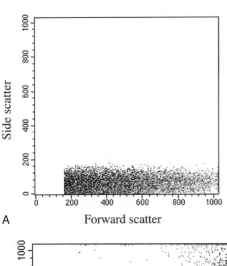

FIG. 28.3. (A) Dot plot of forward scatter (x-axis) versus side scatter (y-axis) on nonlysed whole blood sample. **(B)** Dot plot of forward scatter (x-axis) versus side scatter (y-axis) on lysed whole blood sample demonstrating a three-part leukocyte differential.

FIG. 28.4. CD8 histogram evaluating lymphocytes.

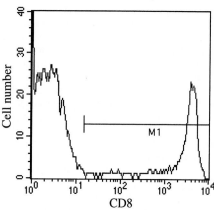

normally found in the lymphocyte area of the scatter plot. These scatter relationships are all based on normal cells and are used to confine the evaluation to the cells of interest, a process referred to as gating. It is important to recognize that the cell relationships noted above do not necessarily apply in cases of hematopoietic malignancy. Standard practice is to confirm the accuracy of the three-part differential using the pan-leukocyte monoclonal antibody, CD45, in combination with the myelomonocytic specific antibody, CD14. Alternatively, CD45 can be included in each staining combination as a specific lymphocyte identifier (characteristically bright staining) when red cell lysis is inadequate or substantial numbers of nonlymphocytes contaminate the lymphocyte gate (16). Malignant cells also may differ in their staining characteristics with a variety of reagents, including CD45 expression.

The interpretation of fluorescent data based on a monoclonal antibody's binding reflects the biology of its particular cognate cell surface protein. When the monoclonal reagent identifies exclusively one cell population, data interpretation is unambiguous, as for the pan-T-cell marker CD3 shown in Figure 28.1. In this example, when the evaluation is confined to lymphocytes (typically using a lymphocyte gate generated by the scatter signals), there clearly are two populations: CD3 negative cells (B and natural killer [NK] lymphocytes) and CD3 positive T cells. In other situations, biologic variability in surface protein expression impacts data interpretation; examples are shown in Figures 28.4 and 28.5. In both histograms, there are at least three cell populations: cells negative for the marker, cells showing intermediate fluorescence, and cells that have bright fluorescence. In Figure 28.4, the CD8 intermediate cells are predominantly NK cells, while the bright staining cells are primarily CD8 positive T cells. In Figure 28.5A, the CD4 intermediate staining cells are monocytes while the bright staining cells are T cells, with the former being present only in very small numbers with proper gating on lymphocytes (Fig. 28.5B). The finding of low-density CD4 expression on monocytes helps to explain HIV infection of this cell lineage.

Many monoclonal antibodies, individually or in combination, can serve to distinguish cells of a specific lineage (Table 28.2), and characteristic binding features can be used to direct a flow study to a specific cell population. Nonfluorescent parameters of forward angle and side angle scatter help distinguish among lymphocytes, monocytes, granulocytes, and platelets (3). Within the granulocyte population, neutrophils and eosinophils are discriminated by the differential expression of the complement receptor CD16: neutrophils stain for CD16, while eosinophils are negative (11). Cells of the erythroid lineage can be identified based on the expression of glycophorin. Within the lymphocyte population, lineage specific antibodies differentiate various populations and subpopulations. Hematopoietic stem cells can be identified by the expression of the cell surface protein, CD34; this valuable marker has enabled evaluation and ex vivo isolation of bone marrow or mobilized stem cells for transplantation (8).

Many of the monoclonal reagents used to evaluate hematopoietic elements detect antigens that are not exclusively expressed on one specific cell type, and interpretation of data must incorporate knowledge of different surface protein expression patterns. A combination of additional antibodies often

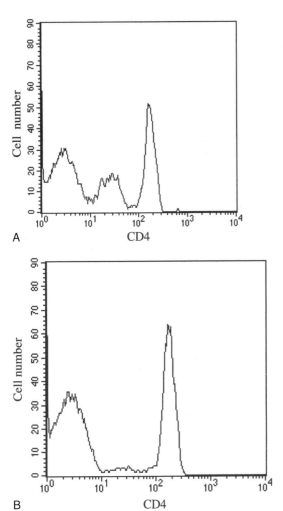

FIG. 28.5. (A) CD4 histogram evaluating mononuclear cells (lymphocytes and monocytes). **(B)** CD4 histogram evaluating only lymphocytes.

clarifies the relative expression of a specific antigen. Cell surface proteins may be altered under different circumstances during the lifecycle of a cell, including preferential expression early and/or late during differentiation and expression in response to cell activation and/or in various states of cell specific function. Protein upregulation implies a range of expression that could include cells that are negative to clearly positive cells, depending on the temporal pattern of expression. The α chain of the interleukin (IL)-2 receptor (CD25) shows such a pattern on T cells (Fig. 28.6), while the interpretation of CD25 expression as an activation marker has been complicated by the identification of T regulatory cells among CD25 expressing CD4+ T cells (17). When the interpretation of positive and negative is visually less clear, consistent interpretation criteria are crucial in order for valid comparison of data between different studies. In some circumstances, isoforms of a specific protein are differentially expressed, and cells may express one or the other isoform or both (Fig. 28.7). Sometimes the use of percentage positive for a specific marker is misleading, as shown in Figure 28.8. The histogram for the unstained cells overlaps significantly with that of stained cells; the histogram overlay demonstrates that there is a shift in the stained cells that would not be adequately reflected by simply scoring cells as positive or negative. Our laboratory typically notes the geometric mean channel

TABLE 28.2. *Commonly Used Leukocyte Antigens Used in Clinical Flow Cytometry Based on Cluster of Differentiation Designation*

CD1a: Cortical thymocytes, dendritic cells, Langerhan cells
CD2: T cells, thymocytes, NK-cell subset
CD3: T cells, thymocytes
CD4: T-cell subset, thymocyte subset, monocytes/macrophages
CD5: T cells, B-cell subset
CD7: Thymocytes, T cells, NK cells, early myeloid cells
CD8: T-cell subset, thymocyte subset, NK-cell subset
CD10: Early B cell, neutrophils, bone marrow stromal cells
CD11b: Monocytes, granulocytes, NK cells
CD11c: Myeloid cells, monocytes
CD13: Myelomonocytic cells
CD14: Monocytes, myelomonocytic cells
CD15: Granulocytes, monocytes, endothelial cells
CD16: NK cells, granulocytes, macrophages
CD19: B cells (from pre-B-cell stage)
CD20: B cells
CD21: Mature B cells, follicular dendritic cells
CD22: Mature B cells
CD23: Activated B cells
CD25: Activated T cells, activated B cells, regulatory T cells
CD27: Memory B cells
CD30: Activated T, B, NK cells, monocytes, Reed-Sternberg cells
CD33: Myeloid cells, myeloid progenitor cells, monocytes
CD34: Hematopoietic precursor cells, capillary endothelium
CD36: Platelets, monocytes/macrophages
CD41: Megakaryocytes, platelets
CD42b: Megakaryocytes, platelets
CD45: Leukocytes
CD45RA: T-cell (naïve) subsets, B cells, monocytes
CD45RO: T-cell (memory) subsets, B-cell subsets, monocytes/macrophages
CD56: NK cells, NK T cells
CD57: NK cells, T-cell subsets, B cells, monocytes
CD61: Megakaryocyte platelets, megakaryocytes, macrophages
CD79a: B cells
CD95 (Fas): Lymphocytes (upregulated after activation), monocytes, neutrophils
CD103: Intestinal epithelial lymphocytes
CD117: Myeloid blast cells, mast cells
Glycophorin: erythrocytes, erythrocyte precursors

CD, cluster of differentiation; NK, natural killer.

(GMC) fluorescence of the unstained and stained cells and then reports the cells to be positive for the specific marker with an increased fluorescence of x-fold over background (based on the quotient of the GMC-stained cells divided by the GMC of unstained cells). These considerations are particularly relevant for many markers used to evaluate malignant cells.

Flow cytometry has been applied to investigate intracellular characteristics and, specifically, the presence of intracellular proteins, both proteins that are ultimately expressed on the cell surface as well as proteins that can only be detected intracellularly (13). In addition, there are a series of reagents that bind to DNA and/or RNA and allow assessment of cell cycle status (18). More recently, intracellular flow cytometry has been applied to measure some functional properties of cells, including the detection of intracellular cytokines following cell stimulation and cell activation-specific processes such as calcium flux, pH changes, and phosphorylation of intracellular signaling proteins (13).

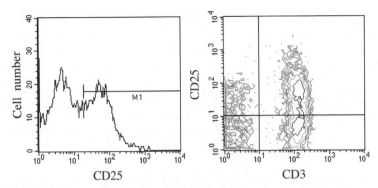

FIG. 28.6. Single parameter histogram of CD25 expression on lymphocytes (*left panel*) and contour plot of CD25 (y-axis) and CD3 (x-axis) expression.

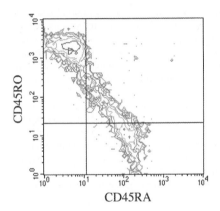

FIG. 28.7. Contour plot of CD45RA and CD45RO expression on CD4$^+$ T cells.

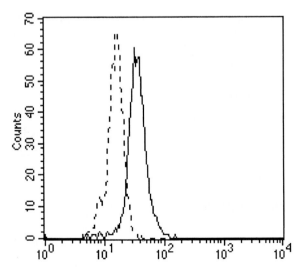

FIG. 28.8. Overlapping control and positively stained histograms.

APPLICATIONS OF FLOW CYTOMETRY IN HEMATOLOGY

Characterization of lymphocytes by flow cytometry in hematologic malignancies is one of the most common applications in the clinical laboratory but is beyond the space constraints of this chapter to explore in detail. The focus of such studies in general is to establish lineage markers and within these to define the specific state of maturation and/or differentiation. In addition, intracellular markers are emerging as useful adjuncts in evaluating certain malignancies; for example, the expression of ZAP70 provides prognostic information in chronic lymphocytic leukemia (19). Applications in nonmalignant diseases are also becoming routine in the clinical laboratory. Flow cytometry remains a critical tool in monitoring disease progression and therapy in HIV infection (7). There are specific lymphocyte findings characteristic of primary immunodeficiencies, including loss of cell populations or subpopulations, the absence of specific cell surface or intracellular proteins, and changes in normal immunologic processes that can be detected by flow cytometry (like the development of memory T cells and/or B cells) (13). Assessment of specific lymphocyte populations and subpopulations is being studied in a variety of disorders characterized by inflammation, with particular attention to expression of activation markers. Reconstitution of the immune system can be monitored by flow cytometry following intensive chemotherapy and stem cell transplantation, now more significant because of the recent focus on immunotherapy and vaccines in experimental treatment protocols for malignancies.

Assessment of leukocytes other than lymphocytes is emerging in the clinical laboratory. Monocytes can be evaluated to define deficiencies associated with defective monocyte surface receptor expression (13). Granulocyte expression of critical adhesion molecules and their capacity to generate reactive oxygen species can be assessed by flow cytometry (13). In addition, granulocyte-specific autoantibodies can be detected. Flow cytometric methods are being used to characterize eosinophils in settings of increased production such as the hypereosinophilia syndrome (16), and basophils have been studied for intracellular cytokine production.

Hematopoietic stem cell identification is dependent on flow cytometry, which is routinely used to characterize and quantitate stem cells in the transplantation setting generally based on CD34 expression together with other cell surface markers (8)—the latter in attempts to identify the pluripotent stem cell. Separation techniques to purify stem cells from either bone marrow or peripheral blood typically utilize CD34 selection methods, and patients are followed by flow cytometric testing posttransplantation to assess donor cell engraftment and donor-host cell chimerism.

The evaluation of erythrocytes by flow cytometry has been applied to cell surface proteins, autoantibodies in hemolytic anemia, and the detection of F cells in fetomaternal hemorrhage and sickle cell anemia (9,20). The detection of glycosylphosphatidylinositol-anchored proteins on erythrocytes and leukocytes by flow cytometry is now the favored method to accurately diagnose paroxysmal nocturnal hemoglobinuria (21).

Flow cytometric evaluation of platelets has been described as a method to study these cells in whole blood, thus eliminating the need for platelet isolation and minimizing cell manipulation (10). This approach allows for the detection of platelet-associated immunoglobulin, assessment for states of platelet activation and aggregation, and detection of reticulated platelets.

SUMMARY

Flow cytometry has been integral in the laboratory assessment of many hematologic disorders. This technology provides a powerful tool to assess simultaneously cell surface and intracellular characteristics. The increasing range of reagents and expanded understanding of cell biology mean that flow cytometry will play an even larger role in the clinical evaluation of various cellular components of the hematologic system.

REFERENCES

1. Givan AL. Flow Cytometry: First Principles, 2nd Ed. New York: Wiley-Liss; 2001.
2. McCoy JP. Basic principles of flow cytometry. Hematol Oncol Clin North Am 2002;16:229–243.

3. Loken MR, Brosnan JM, Bach BA, et al. Establishing optimal lymphocyte gates for immunophenotyping by flow cytyometry. Cytometry 1990;11:453–459.
4. Wood B. 9-color and 10-color flow cytometry in the clinical laboratory. Arch Pathol Lab Med 2006;130:680–690.
5. Szezpanski T, van der Velden VH, van Dongen JJ. Flow cytometric immunophenotyping of malignant lymphocytes. Clin Chem Lab Med 2006;44:111–123.
6. Kussick SJ, Wood BL. Using 4-color-flow cytometry to identify abnormal myeloid populations. Arch Pathol Lab Med 2003;127:1140–1147.
7. Mandy F, Nicholson J, Autran B, et al. T-cell subset counting and the fight against AIDS: reflections over a 20-year struggle. Cytometry 2002;50:39–45.
8. Gratama JW, Krann J, Keeny M, et al. Validation of the single-platform ISHAGE method for CD34(+) hematopoietic stem and progenitor cell enumeration in an international multicenter study. Cytotherapy 2003;5:55–65.
9. Davis BH. Diagnostic utility of red cell flow cytometric analysis. Clin Lab Med 2001;4:829–840.
10. Linden MD, Frelinger AL 3rd, Barnard MR, et al. Application of flow cytometry to platelet disorders. Semin Thromb Hemost 2004;30:501–511.
11. Gopinath R, Nutman TB. Identification of eosinophils in lysed whole blood using side scatter and CD16 negativity. Cytometry 1997;30:313–316.
12. Khan SS, Solomon MA, McCoy JP Jr. Detection of circulating endothelial cells and endothelial progenitor cells by flow cytometry. Cytometry B Clin Cytom 2006;64:1–8.
13. Bleesing JJH, Fleisher TA. Cell function–based flow cytometry. Semin Hematol 2001;38:169–178.
14. Schulman HM, Wells D, Gooley T, et al. The biologic significance of rare peripheral blasts after hematopoietic cell transplantation is predicted by multidimensional flow cytometry. Am J Clin Pathol 1999;112:513–523.
15. Perfetto SP, Ambrozak D, Mguyen R, et al. Quality assurance for polychromatic flow cytometry. Nat Protocol 2006;1:1522–1530
16. Schnizlein-Bick CT, Mandy FF, O-Gorman MRG, et al. Use of CD45 gating in three- and four-color flow cytometric immunophenotyping: guidelines from the National Institute of Allergy and Infectious Diseases, Division of AIDS. Cytometry 2002;50:46–52.
17. Raimondi G, Turner MS, Thomson AW, et al. Naturally occurring regulatory T cells: recent insights in health and disease. Crit Rev Immunol 2007;27:61–95.
18. Darzynkiewiewicz Z, Bedner E, Smolewski P. Flow cytometry in analysis of cell cycle and apoptosis. Semin Hematol 2001;38:179–193.
19. Fleisher TA, Oliveira JB. Functional and molecular characterization of lymphocytes. J Allergy Clin Immunol 2004;114:227–234.
20. Chen JC, Davis BH, Wood B, et al. Multicenter clinical experience with flow cytometric method for fetomaternal hemorrhagic detection. Cytometry 2002;50:285–290.
21. Richards SJ, Hill A, Hillmen P. Recent advances in the diagnosis, monitoring, and management of patients with paroxysmal nocturnal hemoglobinuria. Cytometry B Clin Cytom 2007;72:291–298.

29

Molecular Diagnostics in Hematology

Jaroslaw P. Maciejewski, Lukasz P. Gondek, Carmine Selleri,
and Antonio M. Risitano

The application of molecular biology and genetic techniques has greatly contributed to recent advances in hematology. Many new technologies have found utility in the clinical routine. This chapter illustrates the application of molecular techniques in the diagnosis of hematologic diseases and explains the principles and details of the most commonly used tests. The individual techniques are described in the context of specific applications; many of the methods are applied in a variety of diseases described in specific chapters of this handbook.

Introduction of the polymerase chain reaction (PCR) revolutionized molecular diagnostics in hematology; various modifications of this technique exist. Both DNA and RNA reverse transcribed into cDNA can be used as a template. In the presence of forward and reverse DNA primers that bind to the sequence-specific regions of the target DNA, Taq polymerase extends both strands of the DNA. Repeated cycles of annealing, extension, and denaturation lead to the exponential amplification of the targeted DNA sequence with the specificity provided by the DNA primers (Fig. 29.1).

DETECTION OF GERMLINE GENE MUTATIONS/POLYMORPHISMS

Precise diagnosis of many hematologic diseases or detection of susceptibility to develop complications depends on the identification of mutated genes. Clinically applicable methods mostly involve detection of defined mutations occurring at specific sites within the genes. Currently, most protocols use PCR to amplify the involved gene fragments. For the identification of the presence of individual mutations various methods can be used (Fig. 29.2).

Molecular techniques described in the following are currently used for the routine diagnosis of a number of genetic hematologic diseases including thalassemia and other hemoglobinopathies, hereditary familial hemochromatosis (HFE) gene mutations such as C282Y and H63D, factor V Leiden, prothrombin gene mutations G20210A, and thermolabile C677T 5,10-methylenetatrahydrofolate reductase (1,2). Clearly, similar methods can be applied for the detection of other clinically relevant mutations or polymorphisms.

Restriction Fragment Length Polymorphism Analysis

Prior to the advent of PCR technology, traditional Southern blotting of genomic DNA followed by probe hybridization was used to detect changes in the endonuclease restriction patterns. Currently, restriction fragment length polymorphism (RFLP) analysis is used in conjunction with PCR amplification. Restriction digest can be performed either prior to or after amplification. If a mutation affects the restriction endonuclease digestion patterns, its presence can be easily demonstrated using RFLP analysis. After PCR amplification of a relevant gene fragment that carries a specific mutation, the resulting amplicons are subjected to restriction endonuclease cleavage. Using gel electrophoresis changes in the fragment size can be demonstrated. Through comparison with a wild-type form, heterozygote and homozygote patterns can be easily distinguished. When a fluorochrome labeled primer is used (e.g., 6-carboxyfluorescein; 6-FAM), capillary gel electrophoresis can be applied allowing for high sensitivity and throughput. Detection of HFE mutations by RFLP of PCR products serves as an example for this technique.

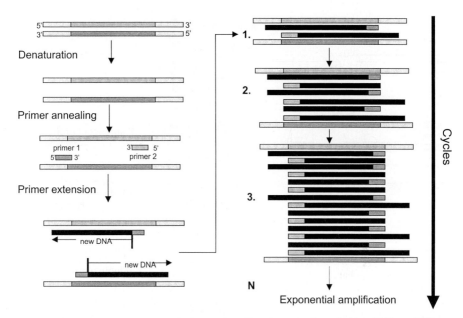

FIG. 29.1. Principle of polymerase chain reaction. Template consists of either DNA or cDNA generated by reverse transcription of mRNA. In the presence of forward and reverse DNA primers that bind to the sequence-specific region of the target DNA, Taq polymerase extends both strands of the DNA such that repeated cycles of annealing, primer extension, and denaturation lead to amplification and accumulation of the targeted newly synthesized DNA sequence with the specificity provided by DNA primers.

Melting Curve Analysis of Polymerase Chain Reaction Products

More recently, a light-cycler PCR method combined with melting curve analysis has been used for the detection of gene mutations allowing for a reduction in the workload and enabling automation. Melting curve analysis exploits the fact that even a single nucleotide mismatch between the labeled probe and the targeted sequence significantly reduces the melting temperature. Consequently, amplicon/probe mismatches will melt off at lower temperatures different than that of matched target DNA.

PCR amplification of specific gene fragments is performed in the presence of a fluorescent DNA probe or probes (anchor and sensor probe) that release light on hybridization to the internal portion of the amplicon containing the potential mutation. After completion of the reaction, the hybridized fragments are denatured; the release of the probe decreases the amount of the emitted fluorescence, a process recorded in the form of a melting curve. The shape of the melting curves identifies the presence of two normal alleles (singular curve), or heterozygotes (two peaks). For mutation homozygotes the curve is shifted, producing a singular characteristic peak. If multiple mutations are present in a gene, specific probes and primers must be applied to detect heterozygotes, homozygotes, and compound heterozygotes.

Allele-Specific Polymerase Chain Reaction

The tetra-primer amplification refractory mutation system (ARMS) PCR is one of the variants of allele-specific PCR; it allows for detection of single nucleotide polymorphisms (SNP) as well as single gene mutations. Two different allele-specific amplicons and a larger (nonallele-specific) control amplicon are generated by a pair of two common (outer) primers and by two allele-specific (inner) primers that have opposite orientation (allele 1-specific primer, antisense and allele 2-specific primer, sense).

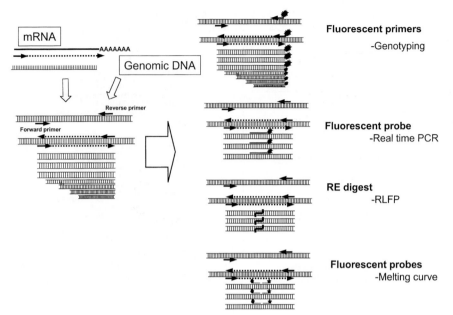

FIG. 29.2. Application of PCR technology for the detection of a gene mutation. Various techniques based on PCR can be used for specific applications in hematology. Fluorescent primers can be used for determining the small differences in the size of the amplified product, a technique called genotyping. Fluorescent probes can also be selected to hybridize between the primer sequences of the template allowing design of real-time PCR. DNA amplicons generated in the process of PCR reactions can be used for restriction endonuclease digestion. If restriction sites for specific enzymes within the amplicon contain a mutation, restriction endonuclease digestion of the PCR product will result in fragments of different sizes, which can be resolved on either capillary or agarose gel electrophoresis. Finally, using specific fluorescent probes that hybridize to the amplified sequences, melting curves can be recorded to distinguish individual alleles. The presence of sequence differences between the probe and template results in different melting curves; these curves are recorded based on the emission of light induced by melting off the fluorescent probes from the template.

Because the common primers are designed so that the mutation is located nearer one of them, the two allele-specific amplicons will have different lengths and thus will be easily separated by gel electrophoresis: wild-type genotype generates two bands on gel electrophoresis, homozygous on two bands, and heterozygous mutation all three bands.

Direct Polymerase Chain Reaction-Based Sequencing

Alternative methods of mutation analysis include direct sequencing of PCR products. Both alleles can be easily identified, and the direct sequencing method has the advantage that it does not target a specific mutation and that all possible sequence differences can be detected.

MOLECULAR DIAGNOSIS OF HEMOGLOBINOPATHIES

Hemoglobinopathies constitute a large group of inherited autosomal-recessive hematologic disorders. While routine laboratory tests and clinical presentation are often sufficient for a proper diagnosis, molecular analysis is mandatory for the confirmation of the defect and precise characterization of the abnormal hemoglobin (3). For example, combinations of specific mutations may greatly affect the phenotype expected in the progeny. Thus, molecular diagnosis may have significant consequences for counseling affected patients, asymptomatic carriers, and prenatal diagnostics.

Traditionally, Southern blotting was used, but recently, PCR-based methods are preferred. Allele-specific oligonucleotide (ASO) hybridization and allele-specific priming are the most commonly applied techniques. The first method relies on hybridization of ASO probes (wild type and mutant) to PCR-amplified genomic DNA. In the dot-blot assay, ASO is labeled, while the reverse dot-blot technique utilizes labeled amplified DNA, allowing for simultaneous screening of multiple mutations. Allele-specific priming is based on the principle that a perfectly matched primer pair amplifies target DNA more efficiently than a mismatched pair. In the amplification refractory mutation system (ARMS), genomic DNA is challenged with both wild-type and mutant primer sets. Multiple mutations may be simultaneously screened in a multiplex PCR assay using fluorescently labeled ARMS primers, producing products of different length that can be detected using an automated DNA analyzer. Large deletions of both the α and β globin gene may be screened using the gap-PCR, with primers complementary to the breakpoint sequences. However, for some deletion mutants, Southern blotting is still standard.

Combining all these approaches in the context of the ethnic- and region-specific distribution of globin mutations, successful molecular identification is possible in more than 90% of cases. Mutations remaining unknown after standard molecular screening may be investigated further by denaturing gradient gel electrophoresis (DGGE) or heteroduplex analysis; nevertheless, complete sequencing of the globin gene represents the best option to identify rare or unknown mutations.

CHROMOSOME DIAGNOSTICS

Metaphase Karyotyping

Traditional cytogenetics, utilizing banding techniques, is performed on chromosomal metaphase spreads. Because mitotic activity is required, metaphase karyotyping is performed after cell culture in the presence of mitogens. For myeloid disorders, either lymphocyte-conditioned media or hematopoietic growth factors are most commonly used, while for lymphoid malignancies, lectins are added. Various banding methods have been utilized for chromosome identification and resolution of individual chromosomal fragments, but G-banding is usual in clinical diagnostics. Characteristic bands result from the biochemical properties of chromatin such as AT and GC content (4–8).

Cellularity and mitotic activity affect the diagnostic yield of the procedure, and the proportion of noninformative spreads varies from disease to disease. In myelofibrosis, marrow is often not aspirable. In aplastic anemia and myelodysplasia, noninformative results are frequent because of the lack of progenitor cells. In such cases, cytogenetic analysis may be also performed on blood specimens.

Approximately 330 chromosomal bands can be distinguished by routine karyotyping, and each band may contain as much as 10^7 base pairs (bp) and a multitude of genes. Classic karyotyping can identify defects of approximately 5 Mb; thus, smaller defects and their locations remain undetected (resolution). The sensitivity level depends on the number of analyzed cells; routinely 20 cells are counted with a detailed analysis of at least 2 cells. Analysis may be more complicated if several clones, each harboring a distinct defect, are present. Depending on the nature of the identified defect, the sensitivity limit is approximately 10% (i.e., identification of 2 abnormal cells) in 20 cells tested.

Both balanced and unbalanced translocations can be identified, but some defects may require a more intricate analysis. Some of the balanced translocations are highly diagnostic; examples are t(9;22) in chronic myelogenous leukemia (CML), t(15;17), inv 16 and t(8;21) in acute myeloid lymphoma (AML), t(15:17) in acute promyelocytic leukemia (APL), t(9;22) and t(12;21) in acute lymphoblastic leukemia (ALL), as well as t(14:18), t(11;14), t(11:18) in lymphomas. Once a specific defect is identified, metaphase karyotyping can be used for monitoring of therapy response (cytogenetic remission); however, the sensitivity of this method is limited (5–8).

Fluorescence In Situ Hybridization

For the targeted detection of specific abnormalities, fluorescence in situ hybridization (FISH) is the most commonly applied method particularly helpful in the characterization of structural chromosomal abnormalities and identification of chromosomes of uncertain origin. However, FISH is not suitable for screening for unknown defects unless a high clinical suspicion exists. FISH does not require cell division, and consequently cell culture and is more sensitive than traditional cytogenetics. FISH provides a more accurate measure for the true frequency of abnormal cells and can be used for the monitoring of minimal residual disease. Identification of the donor versus recipient origin of the blood cell production following hematopoietic stem cell transplantation is another application of this technology (see below). The technique can be applied to blood, marrow, body fluids, tissue touch preparations as well as to paraffin-embedded tissues (5,9).

In FISH, specific fluorescent-labeled single-stranded DNA probes are hybridized to the nuclei of metaphase or interphase cells attached to glass slides. The use of probes labeled with different dyes allows for multicolor FISH on a single slide. Probes can also be designed to identify a specific chromosomal structure, hybridize to multiple chromosomal sequences, and to identify unique DNA sequences. Probes recognizing α-satellite sequences are chromosome specific; in diploid cells both chromosomes are labeled. Chromosome painting probes are derived from whole chromosomes (see also spectral karyotyping [SKY], discussed next). Probes can be derived from unique sequences cloned from specific regions of the genome. Finally, telomeric probes can be used to determine the telomere length based on the intensity of the hybridization.

For balanced translocations, probes spanning individual breakpoints are used. Dual-color/dual-fusion probes or single-fusion/dual-color FISH probes target sequences located at opposite ends of two breakpoints. In addition, two-color break-apart probes recognizing DNA sequences from the 3' and 5' ends of a single gene can be applied. These probes yield combined yellow signal in the normal germline configuration, while two colors are seen when target sequences are separated because of translocation. FISH is more reliable for the detection of duplication of chromosome fragments than deletions. In general, FISH is less sensitive than PCR, with detection limits of 1 of 100 cells. As a result of the false-positive rate, it is not clear whether sensitivity can be increased through routine counting of a higher number of cells.

FISH techniques have been widely applied for the detection of lymphoma-specific translocations, in the diagnosis of CML, myelodysplastic syndrome (MDS), T-cell acute lymphoblastic leukemia (T-ALL), and B-cell acute lymphoblastic leukemia (B-ALL) (Table 29.1) (6,8–10). In addition, FISH is frequently used for intracellular detection of Epstein-Barr virus (EBV) in certain non-Hodgkin's lymphomas, Hodgkin's disease, and aggressive natural killer (NK) cell lymphomas (see later).

TABLE 29.1. *Translocations and Deletions Commonly Detected by Fluorescence in Situ Hybridization*

Disease	Chromosomal Abnormality
CLL/SLL	del13q14, del11q22
LPL	t(9:14)
MZL	t(11:14), t(1:14), t(14:18)
FL	t(14:18)
MCL	t(11:14)
DLBCL	del3q27, t(14:18)
BL	t(8:14), t(2:8), t(8:22)
ALL	t(12:21), t(11q23), t(9:22)
AML	t(11q23), t(8:21), inv(16),
CML	t(9:22)
APL	c(15, 17)

ALL, acute lymphocytic leukemia; AML, acute myeloid leukemia; BL, Burkitt lymphoma; CCL, chronic leukemia/lymphoma; CML, chronic myelogenous leukemia; DLBCL, diffuse large B-cell lymphoma; FL, follicular lymphoma; LPL, lymphoplasmacytoid lymphoma; MCL, mantle cell lymphoma; MZL, marginal zone lymphoma; SLL, small lymphocytic lymphoma.

Spectral Karyotyping

SKY allows for the visualization of all 24 chromosomes and analysis of their structure based on hybridization with multicolor painting probes (11). These probes are derived from individual chromosomes using degenerate primer-based PCR and differentially labeled with fluorochromes. After hybridization to metaphase spreads, a digital camera is used to record the complete emission spectra. As a result, each chromosome-specific probe is distinctively labeled and easily identified. SKY has a much higher precision than traditional cytogenetics and allows for identification of new, previously unidentified reciprocal translocations and defects that cannot be resolved by traditional banding. In one study, SKY allowed detection of new translocations in 35% of cases and resulted in confirmation of the previously known defects and refinement of 35% of diagnoses.

Array-Based Comparative Genomic Hybridization and Single Nucleotide Polymorphisms

Array-Based Comparative Genomic Hybridization

Array-based comparative genomic hybridization (A-CGH) allows for cytogenetic analysis of chromosomal defects that can be applied in many clonal diseases. In this technique, genomic DNA from malignant cells and normal reference DNA are fragmented, differentially labeled with fluorescent dyes, and cohybridized to immobilized DNA probes. Chromosomal imbalances across the genome in tumor DNA can be detected, quantitated, and positionally defined through analysis of the fluorescence intensity of the two different colors. Initially, this analysis was performed on metaphase chromosome preparations (M-CGH). However, the resolution of CGH as applied to metaphase spreads is limited by the standard cytogenetic resolution of approximately 5 Mb, and considerable cytogenetic expertise is required to accomplish such an analysis. Therefore, M-CGH has never become a widely utilized technique and has remained limited to specialist research applications.

Bacterial artificial chromosome (BAC) was originally used to produce CGH arrays. The advent of oligo-array technology made CGH applicable to the study of genomic alterations in human disease. Sixty-mer oligonucleotide probes corresponding to individual SNPs cover the whole genome and include both coding and noncoding regions; thus, an ordered array of DNA segments at high genomic resolution can be generated, circumventing the limitations associated with the use of metaphase preparations as the hybridization template. The fluorescence ratio of the two colors can be compared between different spots representing different genomic regions, providing a genome-wide molecular profile of the sample with respect to regions of the genome that are deleted or amplified (Fig. 29.3A). Resolution is dependent on a combination of the number, size, and map positions of the DNA elements within the array.

Single Nucleotide Polymorphism Array-Based Karyotyping and Genotyping

Recently introduced SNP arrays to study the genetic predisposition of diseases also can be applied for analysis of copy number variation and loss of heterozygosity (LOH). This technique utilizes arrays containing oligonucleotide probes corresponding to SNPs present throughout the human genome (36). Test DNA is fragmented, ligated to universal linkers, amplified with primers corresponding to the linkers, and labeled (Fig. 29.3B). Unlike in CGH, there is no requirement for normal reference DNA. Following hybridization, fluorescence intensity is measured for each spot on the array. After bioinformatic analysis, genotyping calls are possible for each SNP to determine homo- or heterozygozity for each SNP. In addition to genotyping, the copy number for each locus (tagged by a specific SNP probe) can be deduced based on the flouorescence intensity that corresponds to hyper- or hypoploid gene copy number. A whole variety of array designs (bead hybridization or array liquid phase hybridization) platforms are currently available with a density of >1 million markers covering 22 autosomes and the X-chromosome. The average intermarker distance is approximately 10Kb, resulting in a superior resolution. Initially designed for genotyping and whole genome association studies, SNP-A also can be used for karyotyping. As a karyotyping tool, SNP-A allows for a very high resolution (depending on the density of the SNP probes), does not require cell division (no culture and proliferation of cells is needed) but because of the nature of the technology allows for detection of only balanced translocations. When compared with metaphase

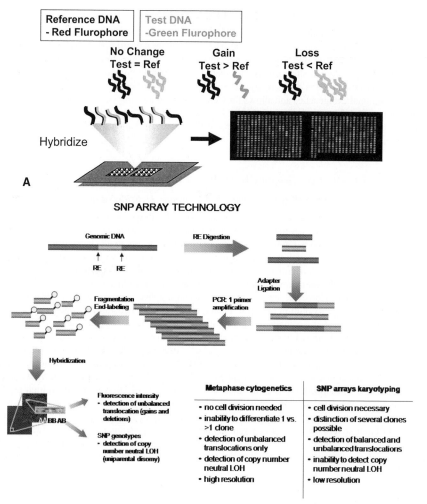

FIG. 29.3. (A) Array-based comparative genomic hybridization (A-CGH). A-CGH consists of hybridization of tester and reference DNA samples that have been differentially labeled with fluorochromes to arrays of sequences corresponding to specific portions of chromosomes. Unbalanced translocations such as deletion or duplication of individual genes (or portions of chromosomes) can be detected based on the disparity between fluorescent spectra emitted by the tester versus reference DNA. Consequently, depending on the number of probes, a very intricate analysis of chromosomes can be performed with regard to the presence or absence of specific DNA segments. **(B)** SNP array-based karyotyping. The principle of the method relies on amplification and labeling of fragmented genomic PCR products with subsequent hybridization to arrays containing oligonucleotide probes homologous to allelic variants of SNPs. Based on the density of the arrays and choice/location of SNPs to be detected various resolution levels can be achieved. Bioinformatic analysis of hybridization results allows for detection of copy number changes (fluorescence intensity) for individual loci as well as loss of heterozygosity that can be a result of deletion or segmental uniparental disomy because of mitotic recombination.

cytogenetics, SNP-A-based karyotyping allows for detection of clonal unbalanced chromosomal defects in higher percentage of patients with hematologic malignancies including MDS, multiple myeloma (MM), AML, and CLL. The additional advantage over metaphase karyotyping and aCGH is the ability to detect copy number neutral LOH (uniparental disomy), present in many solid tumors and myeloid malignancies. The sensitivity of SNP-A karyotyping is relatively low (as it depends on the proportion of clonal cells in the sample), comparable to metaphase karyotyping. In addition to whole genome arrays with various probe densities, customized SNP arrays are available or can be designed for specific applications: targeting nonsynonymous SNPs, particular set of SNPs, or specific regions of the genome (as for the human leukocyte antigen [HLA]-locus).

Because of the high resolution of SNP-A and the convenient microarray format, these methods will likely be introduced into the clinical routine, especially for diseases in which unbalanced translocations are expected (12).

DETECTION AND QUANTITATION OF SOMATIC MUTATIONS AND TRANSLOCATIONS

Polymerase Chain Reaction–Based Analysis of Translocations

PCR has found a wide application to the diagnosis of malignant disorders associated with specific translocations of genetic material (5,7,8). The main advantage of PCR is high specificity and sensitivity, but there is need for immaculate technique to avoid contamination. DNA primers are designed to flank the specific translocated region, producing a PCR product with a characteristic size, while in the absence of the specific translocation the amplification product is not generated. Appropriate controls can be incorporated into the reaction. Because of the higher template copy number per cell, reverse transcriptase real-time PCR may be a more sensitive modification of this technique. In real-time PCR, mRNA of the abnormal transcript is reverse transcribed, and cDNA serves as template for the amplification reaction (Fig. 29.4). Sensitivity and specificity can be further improved by an additional round of amplification with a pair of internal primers, termed nested PCR. The sensitivity of this method approaches 1 malignant cell per 10^6 normal cells, allowing for the assessment of minimal residual disease (MRD) in various conditions (5).

Recently, introduction of the real-time light cycler PCR assay (Fig. 29.4) has led to quantification of the numbers of cells up to one malignant cell per 10^5 normal cells. The reference standard includes a single-copy gene. The principle of real-time PCR consists of target sequence amplification in the presence of fluorochrome-labeled probes. Such probes are designed to target the sequences between the forward and reverse primers. The probe is labeled at the 5′ end with a reporter fluorochrome (6-FAM) and a quencher fluorochrome (6-carboxytetramethyl-rhodamine [TAMRA]) at the 3′ end and is designed to have a higher melting temperature than the extension primers. As long as both fluorochromes are connected through the DNA sequence, no light is emitted. However, the 5′ to 3′ exonuclease activity of Taq polymerase degrades the probe and releases the fluorochromes. Consequently, progression of the reaction can be monitored by the detection of the fluorescent signal generated during the exponential phase of the reaction, and the cycle number at which the reporter dye intensity rises above the background noise. This threshold number is inversely related to the copy number of the target template. Measurement of the frequency of abnormal cells is based on standard curves and is generated with dilution of control cells or DNA/cDNA containing the targeted mutation. The results can be expressed as copy numbers of fusion transcripts per microgram of RNA or as the frequency of abnormal cells. Ubiquitously expressed housekeeping transcripts/genes are commonly incorporated, and the PCR cycle threshold number of the fusion gene is normalized to the value of the housekeeping gene (5).

In clinical practice, PCR technology, including quantitative PCR, has proven predictive of therapy response and relapse. For certain hematologic malignancies with translocations coding for specific targets, cytogenetic and molecular remissions have been defined as specific end points of therapy. Risks of relapse associated with molecular versus cytogenetic remission have been determined. The most common applications of PCR in the detection of disease-defining translocations are for CML (bcr/abl), APL (PML/RARA), mantle cell and follicular lymphomas (cycD1/IgH and IgH/bcl2, respectively), and B-cell lymphoblastic leukemia (bcr/abl, rearranged IgH) (Table 29.2).

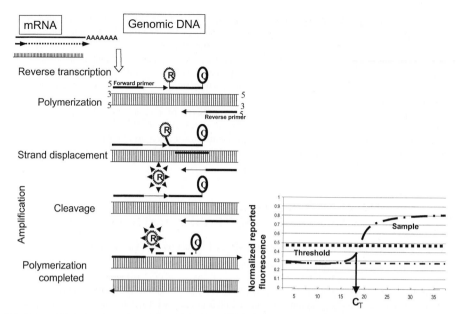

FIG. 29.4. Real-time quantitative PCR. Either cDNA generated from mRNA or DNA can be used as a template. The principle of real-time PCR consists of target sequence amplification in the presence of flurochrome-labeled probes. Such probes are designed to target the sequences between the forward and reverse primer that hybridize to the PCR product accumulated during amplification. The probes are usually labeled with a reporter fluorochrome at the 5′ and a quencher fluorochrome with the 3′ end. Probes are designed to have a higher melting temperature than the extension primer. As long as both fluorochromes are connected through the DNA sequence, no light is emitted. However, the 5′ to 3′ exonuclease activity of Taq polymerase degrades the probe and releases the fluorochromes. Consequently, progression of the reaction can be monitored by the detection of the fluorescent signal generated during the exponential phase of the reaction and the cycle number at which the reporter dye intensity rises above the background noise. This value, also referred to as the threshold number, is inversely related to the copy number of the target template.

Clearly, separate screening for all described abnormalities is too expensive and time consuming to be applied as a global diagnostic battery. Multiple attempts have been made to adapt PCR technology for precise molecular diagnosis associated with individual leukemias and lymphomas. In multiplex PCR, multiple primer pairs are combined to enable detection of several translocations in a single PCR reaction. For example, primer mixtures have been designed to allow for the detection of 28 different translocations, including 80 breakpoints and splice variants, using a limited number of PCR reactions. The introduction of such technologies in clinical practice is hampered by the need for positive controls and limited sensitivity. However, the potential value of more comprehensive screening techniques has been demonstrated in cases that showed PCR positivity for PML/RARA transcripts despite M3 morphology or the cytogenetic presence of t(15:17), and cryptic translocations such as t(12:21) or t(4;11) in ALL, and in AML.

Detection of Somatic Gene Mutations

Acquired mutations of individual genes can lead to the acquisition of a malignant phenotype, and their presence or absence may have clinical significance (5). The principle of PCR-based detection of such mutations is similar to that used for germline mutations (see above). Methods include direct DNA PCR, if the mutation results in a length difference between the amplified fragments (e.g., internal

TABLE 29.2. *Common Translocations Diagnosed by Polymerase Chain Reaction*

Translocation	Fusion Product	Disease
t(9:22)	bcr/abl P190	CML
	bcr/abl P210	ALL
	bcr/abl P230	CNL
t(15:17)	PML/RAR-A	AML-M3
t(8:21)	AML/ETO	AML-M2
inv16	CBF-B/MYH11	AML-M4eo
t(5:12)	TEL/PDGF-R	CMML
t(1:19)	E2A/PBX1	ALL
t(4:11)	MLL/AF4	ALL
t(12:21)	TEL/AML1	ALL
t(14:18)	IgH/bcl2	FL
t(11:14)	bcl1/IgH	MCL
t(11:18)	API2/MLT	MZL
t(2:5)	NPM/ALK	ALCL
t(8:22)	c-myc/Igλ	BL
t(8:14)	c-myc/IgH	BL
t(2:8)	c-myc/Igκ	BL

ALCL, anaplastic large cell lymphoma; ALL, acute lymphocytic leukemia; AML, acute myeloid lymphoma; BL, Burkitt lymphoma; CML, chronic myelogenous leukemia; CMML, chronic myelomonocytic leukemia; CNL, chronic neutrophilic leukemia; FL, follicular lymphoma; MCL, mantle cell lymphoma; MZL, marginal zone lymphoma.

tandem duplication of the FTL-3 gene [13]), wild-type and mutated amplicons will be clearly identified by electrophoresis. When a labeled primer is used for amplification, even small size differences can be resolved by capillary gel electrophoresis. Single nucleotide changes can also be identified when the mutation produces a new or abolishes an existing restriction site. Consequently, after amplification, PCR products are digested with appropriate restriction endonucleases and are subjected to electrophoresis to identify the presence of the mutation (see above RFLP). Again, genotyping with a fluorochrome-labeled primer can be applied.

Allele-specific PCR with primers designed to amplify either the mutated or wild-type allele is a currently the most commonly used method. One of the variant ARMS PCR (see above) allows for distinction between homozygous or heterozygous mutations in one reaction.

In contrast to the detection of germline mutation, using PCR technologies, the proportion of mutated cells in the sample may affect the results of the test: even if 100% of cells carry the mutation, only 50% of the alleles will be affected. The current detection limits of PCR-based techniques can reach 10% of cells carrying the mutation. These methods can be used for known invariant mutations. In contrast, if a gene can be affected by several mutations at various positions, sequencing may be required. Examples of clinically relevant somatic DNA alterations routinely detected by various PCR-based methods include internal tandem duplication of the FLT-3 gene, D835 FLT-3 mutation, p53, Ras, and Jak2 V617F mutations. Of note is that the choice of cellular material used for the detection of single gene mutations may influence the results with regard to the status of homozygous mutations, such as Jak2V617F. In most methods beginning with unfractionated cells, the distinction between heterozygous and homozygous may not be possible because of contamination with wild-type cells.

CLONALITY STUDIES

Where acquired defects (point mutations, translocations) have been identified, they can serve as a suitable marker. However, in many clinical situations such a marker is not available. Consequently, a number of clonality assays have been developed that allow for the diagnosis of oligoclonal or skewed hematopoietic function.

X Chromosome Inactivation Pattern Analysis

X chromosome inactivation pattern (XCIP) analysis is particularly useful in the analysis of disorders without a disease-specific clonality marker (14). XCIP clonality analysis can be informative in a large proportion of female patients. Clearly, clonal/oligoclonal XCIP does not secure the diagnosis of malignancy but may be complementary with other clinical signs and laboratory results.

XCIP is based on the inactivation of one X chromosome in female mammalian cells (14). The inactivation pattern is random, laid down early in embryogenesis, and stably inherited by all daughter cells. The inactivation mechanism includes methylation of certain portions of the DNA. Based on the single-cell theory of malignant disorders, XCIP representation should change in the affected tissue, most significantly in blood. Consequently, the distinction between the two chromosomes made by using a polymorphic marker gene located on X chromosome and differentiation between the active and inactive X chromosomes underlie XCIP clonality analysis. While a disease-specific marker is not required, the pathologic change can be extrapolated from the expected pattern. The most commonly used polymorphic markers include human androgen receptors (HUMARA), phosphoglycerate kinase (PGK), or the fragile X (FRM1) genes. The heterozygosity rate for HUMARA is approximately 90%. Modern XCIP analysis techniques utilize PCR technology.

In the HUMARA assay, DNA is digested with a methylation-sensitive restriction endonuclease, amplified, and the electrophoretic pattern of the amplicons compared with the undigested amplicons. *Hpa*II digests the unmethylated allele and leaves methylated allele available for amplification. Comparison of the intensity of the bands allows extrapolation as to the skewing of the normally equally distributed amplicons of the methylated and unmethylated gene fragment.

In other common assays, single-base or short tandem repeat (STR) polymorphisms in the coding sequences of X chromosomal genes distinguish between the usage of the inactive or active chromosome by RNA based techniques. Reverse transcriptase (RT)-PCR is followed by RFLP of the amplicons.

Interpretation of the results of the XCIP analysis must account for age-rated skewing of inactivation and also for a nonrandom pattern among normal cells that may be encountered in up to 25% of women.

ANALYSIS OF T-CELL RECEPTOR AND IMMUNOGLOBULIN REARRANGEMENT

During T- and B-cell ontogeny, rearrangement of VDJ genes of heavy (H) and light (L) Ig chains and α (A) and β (B) or δ [D] and γ [G] chains of T-cell receptor (TCR), respectively, provides the molecular basis for the heterogeneity of B- and T-cell recognition repertoire (15–17).

For immunoglobulin (Ig) H-chain, there are at least 40 functional variable (VH) gene fragments, 27 diversity (DH) fragments, 6 functional junctional (JH) fragments, and several constant (CH) gene segments. The Igκ gene complex consists of 35 Vκ gene segments, 5 Jκ, and a single Cκ gene. Igλ gene is generated through recombination 30 Vλ segments and 4 Cλ segments all preceded by a Jλ region.

The TCR is a homodimer consisting either of TCR α and β or TCR δ and γ chains. Similar to Ig genes, α and δ chains are encoded by recombined VDJ fragments (65 VB segments, 7 JB fragments, and 2 CB segments, each preceded by a DB region for β chain and 8 VD, 3 DD, and 4 JD gene segments, as well as a single CD region). TCR α and γ chain are generated through recombination of V and J regions. TCR α-chain gene complex consists of more than 50 VA, 61JA, and 1 CA gene segments. The TCR γ gene complex consists of 6 VG and 2 CG segments, each preceded by 2 or 3 JG1 or JG2 gene segments.

During recombination, Ig and TCR gene complexes rearrange and a specific combination VDJ segment is generated. This process is imprecise, and nucleotides may be added or lost from the germline VD and DJ junctions, a mechanism that further adds to the diversity of the TCR and Ig. Addition of nucleotides is mediated by the TdT enzyme. This junctional diversity is responsible for the variability of the complementarity determining region 3 (CDR3) of the IgH and TCRB chain. Because of the triple reading frame, two of three joinings will be out of frame, and translation of a functional protein cannot occur. Indeed, a majority of B cells have rearranged both IgG, and T cells have a biallelic rearrangement of their TCR β and α chains. Postgerminal center B cells also have an additional mechanism of diversity in somatic hypermutation of the Ig V genes. Technically, detection of complete VH-JH rearrangement (as by

PCR amplification) may fail to identify clonality, and assessment of incomplete DH-JH rearrangement may be required.

During B-cell development, the IgH chain rearranges first, followed by the recombination of Igκ and, if nonproductive, Igλ. As a result, all B cells harbor the IgH rearrangement and likely also Igκ rearrangement. The κde is a genetic element included in the Igκ locus and is involved in its inactivation. Consequently, virtually all B cells harbor Igκ rearrangement, which is productive in Igκ+ cells, or nonfunctional in Igλ+ B cells, in which it likely involves Kde rearrangement.

During T-cell development, TCR δ genes rearrange first, followed by TCR γ. TCR β genes rearrange before TCR α. Because δ genes are located within the α locus, TCR α rearrangement results in the deletion of the entire δ locus. This process results in circular excision products, also called TCR excision circle (TREC). TREC are can serve as markers of recent thymic output and may be helpful in certain clinical conditions, such as immune reconstitution after transplantation. Virtually all mature A/B T cells have rearranged TCR γ genes (generally biallelic) but not δ genes, while G/D lymphocytes harbor functional rearrangement of both γ and δ genes, and often incomplete β rearrangement as well.

Ig and TCR rearrangements are not lineage restricted: B and T cells may contain complete or incomplete cross-lineage rearrangements that can be used for assessment of clonality.

Clonal expansion results in overrepresentation of the specifically rearranged Ig or TCR configuration, a property of lymphocytes exploited for the diagnosis of T- and B-cell malignancies. Southern blotting and PCR-based techniques can be used to detect overrepresented, specifically rearranged Ig and TCR genes.

Immunoglobulin and T-Cell Receptor Gene Southern Blotting

Southern blotting detects deleted and translocated gene segments based on changes in the distances between the cleavage sites of restriction enzymes (18). The method takes advantage of combinatorial diversity. DNA from experimental samples is digested with restriction enzymes, separated by electrophoresis, and blotted. Specific bands appear after hybridization with labeled probes corresponding to Ig or TCR gene segments. Optimally designed probes will recognize sequences downstream of the rearranging segments. In a clonal process, specifically rearranged Ig or TCR genes are at high concentration, and the detected bands will differ from the normal germline configuration. In contrast, polyclonal proliferations containing many different rearrangements produce a background pattern visible as a smear of multiple bands.

The sensitivity of Southern blotting is above 10% to 15% of clonal cells present in a polyclonal background. However, the technique is time consuming, requires longer amounts of DNA than PCR, and often is not be feasible, as in tissue biopsies. When DNA probes and restriction enzymes are appropriately selected, Southern blotting may reveal clonal rearrangements that remain undetected by PCR, as some of the V chains may not be included in the consensus Vβ primer mixture used for PCR (see later).

Immunoglobulin and T-Cell Receptor Junctional Region Polymerase Chain Reaction

PCR analysis of Ig and TCR gene segments is based on selective amplification of junctional regions. Amplification is only possible when the Ig or TCR gene are juxtaposed through rearrangement, because the distance between these gene segments in the normal germline configuration is too large for PCR amplification. In contrast to the Southern blot, PCR relies on both the combinatorial and the junctional diversity of the appropriate rearrangements. PCR can be easily applied to blood and tissue specimens including lymph nodes and skin (particularly helpful in the diagnosis of cutaneous T-cell lymphoma). For both IgH and TCR amplification, sets of consensus primers covering the full spectrum of the V regions combined with sets of JB primers are used in multiplex PCR. For B-cell populations, analysis of the IgH rearrangement is most informative, because the IgH locus rearranges first; a complete VH-JH rearrangement is usually investigated. However, as somatic hypermutation within the IgV gene hampers annealing and amplification, analysis of incomplete DH-JH rearrangement may also be helpful in identifying nonproductive partial rearrangement in some immature B cells. Additionally, comprehensive Ig clonality assessment may include analysis of IgL chain, especially the Igκ locus. As discussed above, given the hierarchical rearrangement of IgL, all mature B cells have either a productive or a nonproductive Igκ rearrangement (generally involving the κde element) if cells are Igλ+. Further analysis of the IgL genes may be added to increase the sensitivity of clonality assessment.

For T-cell clonality, analysis of the γ TCR locus has been the paradigm; the main advantage is that the rearrangement of the γ chain occurs early and is present in both α/β and δ/γ cells and in some B cells. Furthermore, the number of primers required for all the possible combinations is small, and junctional diversity is limited compared with other TCR loci. Rearrangement of β genes is a very powerful tool for detection of α/β clonality; even considering the extreme combinatorial diversity, amplification of almost the entire repertoire may be obtained using a relatively limited number of reactions containing appropriate sets of primers. Both complete VB-JB and incomplete DB-JB rearrangements may be studied, increasing the sensitivity of the method; the extreme junctional diversity of the B locus gives high sensitivity to β TCR clonality, even if sophisticated analysis of the PCR product may be required (see below). Analysis of the D locus is relatively easy and may add information on immature T cells and G/D populations but is usually not informative for A/B cells. In contrast, α genes are not very helpful given the extreme complexity of gene segments and concomitant rearrangement of β locus.

Two modifications of PCR are currently used for the detection of clonality: heteroduplex electrophoresis (19) and genescan analysis. In both methods, PCR amplicons are analyzed for fine discrimination and identification of identical products, utilizing different biologic properties of DNA.

Genotyping of rearranged TCR or Ig genes relies on the amplification of the gene fragments with primers that are labeled with a fluorochrome and detection of the labeled products using capillary gel electrophoresis (20). Most capillary electrophoresis-based automated gene sequencers can be adopted for this technique, which allows for resolution of PCR products that usually vary in size by multiples of 3 bp. Under normal circumstances, the amplification products are polyclonal, showing a large number of distinct peaks on capillary electrophoresis tracing. Best results are seen with IgH and TCR B loci, which both have a high frequency of in-frame V-J rearrangements, while for other loci the spacing between peaks is not preserved because of out-of-frame (nonproductive) or incomplete rearrangements. If a monoclonal population is present, a distinct singular peak is present that corresponds to the immunodominant clone. An equivalent technique can be used for the identification of Ig rearrangement. The sensitivity of genotyping is around 5% of malignant (clonal) cells in a cell mixture. As with heteroduplex analysis, frequently a biallelic rearrangement can be detected.

As discussed previously, Ig and TCR clonality can be assessed regardless of the lineage restriction of a putatively clonal population; however, a classic genescan pattern with triplet spacing of peaks is limited to functional in-frame rearrangements. In this case, representation of productive rearrangements may be also obtained by RT-PCR starting from RNA.

Rearranged dominant junctional CDR3 sequences can be sequenced and used for the design of clonotypic PCR primers that uniquely amplify only the malignant clone. Using nested PCR and variable and J primers, further rounds of amplification with a clonotype specific primer (such as an internal J primer) can be added. Such an approach may increase the sensitivity and specificity of detection, especially if utilized in the context of loci with extreme junctional diversity such as TCR β.

The application of TCR and Ig rearrangement analysis include determinations of B- and T-cell clonality in blood, marrow, lymph nodes, and skin lesions for the diagnosis of T-ALL, B-ALL, MM, lymphomas, large granular lymphocyte (LGL) leukemia, and chronic leukemia/lymphoma (CLL). In CLL, Ig rearrangement analysis is a major prognostic marker (see also Chapter 14). Detailed sequencing of clonal IgH may reveal homology to the germline IgV gene. Somatic hypermutations of the IgV gene usually occur after antigen priming and, consequently, the IgV mutation status allows for distinction between pre- and postgerminal center CLL, entities with different clinical behavior.

MOLECULAR DIAGNOSIS OF INFECTIONS IN HEMATOLOGY

Molecular methods are increasingly supplementing serologic and histochemical methods in microbiology (21). Precise detection, localization, and quantitation of the nucleic acids of pathogenic viruses allow for better distinction of individual disease entities and are often used for therapeutic decisions. For instance, detection of EBV activation is essential for early diagnosis and therapy of posttransplant

TABLE 29.3. *Viral Pathogens in Hematologic Maligancies*

Disease	Pathogen
Diffuse large B-cell lymphoma	EBV frequent in immunodeficiency, SV40 proposed
Plasmablastic B-cell lymphoma	EBV
Primary effusion lymphoma	HHV-8, invariant occasional EBV
Diffuse T-cell lymphoma	EBV frequent
Burkitt lymphomas	EBV
Lymphomatoid granulomatosis	EBV occasional
Aggressive NK-cell leukemia	EBV invariant
Extranodal NK/T cell lymphoma	EBV occasional
Angioimmunoblastic T-cell lymphoma	EBV occasional
Lymphoplasmacytic lymphoma	HCV
Hodgkin's lymphoma	EBV certain forms
Posttransplant lymphoproliferative disorder	EBV 90%
Primary CNS lymphoma	EBV 100%
Follicular dendritic sarcoma	EBV occasional
Adult T-cell leukemia	HTLV-1

CNS, central nervous system; EBV, Epstein-Barr virus; HCV, hepatitis C virus; HHV-8, human herpesvirus 8; HTLV-1, human T-cell leukemia virus 1; NK, natural killer; SV40, simian virus 40.

lymphoproliferative disorder. For DNA viruses such as herpesviruses, detection of mRNA transcripts by means of RT-PCR allows diagnosis of active infections, while DNA PCR is positive even when only latent virus in present. Molecular techniques are most often used for the diagnosis to EBV, cytomegalovirus (CMV), human herpes virus-6 (HHV-6), as well as retroviruses such as human T-cell leukemia virus (HTLV-1; Table 29.3) (22,23).

Epstein-Barr Virus

Both PCR and FISH can detect EBV in lymphoid neoplasms (Table 29.3). FISH probes complementary to EBV localize the virus to the malignant cells. Because of its sensitivity and lack of quantitation, DNA PCR may provide positive results without clinical relevance because of the frequency of latent EBV infection in the community. In contrast, quantitative light-cycler PCR assays provide highly precise copy numbers, but they are less sensitive methods. Both TaqMan probes (single-stranded DNA probes that release light on degradation by Taq polymerase; see previous discussion) and beacon probes (DNA probes that release light on conformational change after hybridization to the internal segment of the amplicons) are used. TaqMan PCR is performed as described above for the detection of translocations. Sensitivity levels can be as low as 1 viral copy per 1 to 2×10^5 cells (24). Virus is always cell-associated, and DNA for analysis is extracted from blood leukocytes.

FISH performed with probes detecting EBV-encoded RNA (EBER) is the most commonly applied test for the detection of virus in malignant cells. The sensitivity of this method is related to the high copy number of these transcripts and the ability to detect EBV genome in its latent state (EBER transcription is not dependent on induction of a productive rival lifecycle).

Cytomegalovius

Molecular methods have a wide application in the diagnosis of CMV disease and compete with traditional culture and histochemistry-based techniques. DNA PCR can be used for the detection of the CMV genome, but because of its high sensitivity, results may not be informative in seropositive individuals. CMV is strictly cell-associated, and blood leukocytes are used as a source for DNA. Quantitative PCR utilizing the light cycler technology is the usual method for detection of CMV viremia and titer quantitation. Both beacon and TaqMan probes have been developed (as described for EBV). Based on standard curves with calibrated positive controls, the number of viral genome copies can be precisely calculated (25). CMV can be detected at levels as low as one and as high as 5×10^5 copies per milliliter, correlating well with the antigenemia measured per 2×10^5 leukocytes.

B19 Parvovirus

Serologic methods are informative only in a minority of circumstances. Similar to CMV, B19 PCR may provide a high positivity rate that does not reflect clinically relevant viremia. Because of the extremely high copy number of virions during active infection, B19 can be detected and quantitated in serum using DNA hybridization methods without amplification. Dot-blot hybridization is most suitable to provide quantitation by serial dilution of positive sera with defined B19 genome copy numbers. Viral titer can be determined by comparison to the dilution standards (21).

Other Viruses

In theory, all viruses of known nucleic acid sequence can be detected using PCR. In some clinical circumstances, viral detection may have diagnostic consequences (Table 29.3). For example, herpes virus-6 may be identified in primary effusion lymphomas; presence of adenovirus (type 11) and polyomavirus (BK, JC) DNA may be helpful for diagnosis of hemorrhagic cystitis after bone marrow transplantation.

MOLECULAR DETECTION OF DONOR/RECIPIENT CHIMERISM AFTER STEM CELL TRANSPLANTATION

Determination of the contribution of host versus recipient blood cell production after allogeneic stem cell transplantation has become a standard laboratory test with clinically relevant implications. Several techniques have been devised, including short-tandem repeat (STR) analysis, RFPL, or FISH for X or Y chromosomes. Selection of various cell types for analysis allows for the separate determination of chimerism in individual hematopoietic lineages.

Polymerase Chain Reaction–Based Short-Tandem Repeat Analysis

Highly polymorphic microsatellite STR exist for a large number of human loci. STR sequences show great variability in the number of repeats, their length is inherited, and their pattern may be individually specific (26–29). Examples of such loci include FGA, VWA, TH01, F13A1, and D21S11. A large number of primer pairs allows for amplification of STR from several loci that show biallelic deletion/insertion polymorphisms. Their size patterns enable forensic identity determination and paternity testing.

For bone marrow transplantation, STR for several loci can be amplified in a donor and recipient. Informative loci can be selected for the highest resolution of size differences between the donor and recipient pair. After transplantation, blood is sampled and DNA extracted. Following amplification of informative STR, gel electrophoresis is used to determine the presence of donor and/or recipient bands. When fluorochrome-labeled primers are used, PCR amplicons can be genotyped using capillary gel electrophoresis to precisely resolve the amplified products by size. The areas under the informative peaks are measured, and the percentage of donor chimerism is calculated by the division of donor's peak area by the sum of the areas of the recipient and donor. This calculation can be performed for several informative loci and averaged. The sensitivity of this type of STR analysis permits the detection of 5% of donor/recipient cells for all loci and around 1% for all patients and selected loci. Combining this method with techniques of cell separation allows determination of chimerism within lymphoid or myeloid cells compartments, adding useful information in the setting of nonmyeloablative transplantation.

Short-Tandem Repeat Analysis by Real-Time (Quantitative) Polymerase Chain Reaction

Real-time PCR STR analysis is a more sensitive and highly quantitative method (30–32). Two primer pairs, each specific for the donor and recipient STR alleles, are selected. STR suitable for this analysis have biallelic polymorphism, with both alleles varying by at least two consecutive bases and showing a high level of heterozygosity. The sensitivity of this method can be as low as 0.1%, but there is need for a large selection of labeled primers and probes for identification of the most informative loci.

Restriction Fragment Length Polymorphism Analysis

Many loci within the human genome show significant allelic polymorphism, resulting in changes in endonuclease restriction sites. After enzyme digestion, DNA is electrophoresed. The resulting Southern blot is hybridized with tagged DNA probes derived from the polymorphic loci, resulting in the appearance of donor- and recipient-specific bands if there are allelic differences at the locus.

Fluorescence In Situ hybridization Analysis of Sex Chromosomes

Centromeric X and Y chromosome probes can be used for the detection and quantitation of donor and recipient cells. The assay is informative only in sex-mismatched transplants.

MOLECULAR HUMAN LEUKOCYTE ANTIGEN TYPING

Traditional serologic testing is increasingly replaced by molecular testing that allows for a higher precision and resolution of HLA alleles and polymorphisms (33,34). Molecular analysis of HLA loci resulted in the identification of a large number of new alleles, with new polymorphisms still being added. PCR-based methods and primers have been developed for intermediate-resolution (IR) and high-resolution (HR) level typing. Serologic testing continues to be performed in many institutions for class I and II alleles, but elsewhere serologic testing has been abandoned for class II alleles (35). Serologic testing retains some role, especially for the confirmation of null alleles after molecular testing.

Polymerase Chain Reaction–Based Human Leukocyte Antigen Testing

Two methods have dominated modern HLA testing technology: PCR amplification with sequence-specific primers (SSP) and hybridization with a sequence-specific oligonucleotide probe (SSOP). Allele- or group-level typing is commonly performed using SSP. Group- and locus-specific primers can be used in the first stage of testing followed by allele specific primers. Standardized primer sets have been developed for both IR and HR testing (35).

SSOP testing can be used for the identification of individual alleles or for the detection of single nucleotide polymorphisms (SNPs). In general, SSOP analysis includes differential hybridization of amplicons to specific probes that are designed to match nucleotide sequences at all polymorphic sites of exons 2 and 3. Standardized probe sets have been developed. Several modifications of SSOP hybridization are possible, including membrane- and bead-based fluorometric techniques. For flow cytometric approaches, such as using luminex technology, PCR amplification is performed in the presence of a fluorescently labeled primer pair. The probes are immobilized to polystyrene beads tagged with fluorochromes that can be characterized by a flow cytometric technology using their orange-red emission profile combined with the counterfluorescence of the tagged amplicons. The presence of specific alleles can be identified based on a specific double-fluorescence profile of beads that carry a probe complementary to the amplicon. This assay can be multiplexed to allow a wide screening for many alleles.

SNPs within individual HLA alleles can also be detected using sets of primers designed to investigate polymorphism. This method, also referred to as single nucleotide extension (SNE), can also be multiplexed, similar to SOP.

Finally, for greatest resolution and detection of previously unknown or new polymorphisms, individual region of HLA genes can be PCR amplified and directly sequenced.

REFERENCES

1. Lillicrap D. Molecular diagnosis of inherited bleeding disorders and thrombophilia. Semin Hematol 1999;36:340–351.
2. Arcasoy MO, Gallagher PG. Molecular diagnosis of hemoglobinopathies and other red blood cell disorders. Semin Hematol 1999;36:328–339.
3. Old JM. Screening and genetic diagnosis of haemoglobin disorders. Blood Rev 2003;17:43–53.

4. Spowart G. Mitotic metaphase chromosome preparation from peripheral blood for high resolution. In Gosden JR, ed. Methods in Molecular Biology Chromosome Analysis Protocols. Vol. 29. Totowa, NJ: Humana Press; 1994:1–10.
5. Hokland P, Pallisgaard N. Integration of molecular methods for detection of balanced translocations in the diagnosis and follow-up of patients with leukemia. Semin Hematol 2000;37:358–367.
6. Rowley JD. Cytogenetic analysis in leukemia and lymphoma: an introduction. Semin Hematol 2000;37:315–319.
7. Bernard OA, Berger R. Location and function of critical genes in leukemogenesis inferred from cytogenetic abnormalities in hematologic malignancies. Semin Hematol 2000;37:412–419.
8. Ferrando AA, Look AT. Clinical implications of recurring chromosomal and associated molecular abnormalities in acute lymphoblastic leukemia. Semin Hematol 2000;37:381–395.
9. Gozzetti A, Le Beau MM. Fluorescence in situ hybridization: uses and limitations. Semin Hematol 2000;37:320–333.
10. Kirsch IR, Reid T. Integration of cytogenetic data with genome maps and available probes: present status and future promise. Semin Hematol 2000;37:420–428.
11. Schrock E, Padilla-Nash H. Spectral karyotyping and multicolor fluorescence in situ hybridization reveal new tumor-specific chromosomal aberrations. Semin Hematol 2000;37:334–347.
12. Lichter P, Joos S, Bentz M, et al. Comparative genomic hybridization: uses and limitations. Semin Hematol 2000;37:348–357.
13. Murphy KM, Levis M, Hafez MJ, et al. Detection of FLT3 internal tandem duplication and D835 mutations by a multiplex polymerase chain reaction and capillary electrophoresis assay. J Mol Diagn 2003;5:96–102.
14. Gale RE. Evaluation of clonality in myeloid stem-cell disorders. Semin Hematol 1999;36:361–372.
15. Arstila TP, Casrouge A, Baron V, et al. Diversity of human alpha beta T-cell receptors. Science 2000;288:1135.
16. Macintyre EA, Delabesse E. Molecular approaches to the diagnosis and evaluation of lymphoid malignancies. Semin Hematol 1999;36:373–389.
17. Butler JE. Immunoglobulin gene organization and the mechanism of repertoire development. Scand J Immunol 1997;45:455–462.
18. Beishuizen A, Verhoeven MA, Mol EJ, et al. Detection of immunoglobulin kappa light-chain gene rearrangement patterns by Southern blot analysis. Leukemia 1994;8:2228–2236.
19. Langerak AW, Szczepanski T, Van Der BM, et al. Heteroduplex PCR analysis of rearranged T-cell receptor genes for clonality assessment in suspect T-cell proliferations. Leukemia 1997;11:2192–2199.
20. Plasilova M, Risitano A, Maciejewski JP. Application of the molecular analysis of the T-cell receptor repertoire in the study of immune-mediated hematologic disease. Hematol J 2003;8:173–181.
21. Brown KE. Molecular diagnosis of viral disease in hematology patients. Semin Hematol 1999;36:352–360.
22. Precursor B-cell and T-cell neoplasms. In Jaffe ES, Harris NL, Stein H, et al., eds. World Health Organization Classification of Tumours. Pathology and Genetics of Tumours of Haematopoietic and Lymphoid Tissues. Lyon: IARC Press; 2001:109–117.
23. Mature B-cell neoplasms. In Jaffe ES, Harris NL, Stein H, et al, eds. World Health Organization Classification of Tumours. Pathology and Genetics of Tumours of Haematopoietic and Lymphoid Tissue. Lyon: IARC Press; 2001:119–187.
24. Jebbink J, Bai X, Rogers BB, et al. Development of real-time PCR assays for the quantitative detection of Epstein-Barr virus and cytomegalovirus, comparison of TaqMan probes, and molecular beacons. J Mol Diagn 2003;5:15–20.
25. Li H, Dummer JS, Estes WR, et al. Measurement of human cytomegalovirus loads by quantitative real-time PCR for monitoring clinical intervention in transplant recipients. J Clin Microbiol 2003;41:187–191.
26. Brouha PC, Ildstad ST. Mixed allogeneic chimerism. Past, present, and prospects for the future. Transplantation 2001;72:S36–S42.
27. Kreyenberg H, Holle W, Mohrle S, et al. Quantitative analysis of chimerism after allogeneic stem cell transplantation by PCR amplification of microsatellite markers and capillary electrophoresis with fluorescence detection: the Tuebingen experience. Leukemia 2003;17:237–240.

28. Leclair B, Fregeau CJ, Aye MT, et al. DNA typing for bone marrow engraftment follow-up after allogeneic transplant: a comparative study of current technologies. Bone Marrow Transplant 1995; 16:43–55.
29. Monaco AP. Chimerism in organ transplantation: conflicting experiments and clinical observations. Transplantation 2003;75:13S–16S.
30. Fernandez-Aviles F, Urbano-Ispizua A, Aymerich M, et al. Serial quantification of lymphoid and myeloid mixed chimerism using multiplex PCR amplification of short tandem repeat-markers predicts graft rejection and relapse, respectively, after allogeneic transplantation of CD34+ selected cells from peripheral blood. Leukemia 2003;17:613–620.
31. Nuckols JD, Rasheed BK, McGlennen RC, et al. Evaluation of an automated technique for assessment of marrow engraftment after allogeneic bone marrow transplantation using a commercially available kit. Am J Clin Pathol 2000;113:135–140.
32. Alizadeh M, Bernard M, Danic B, et al. Quantitative assessment of hematopoietic chimerism after bone marrow transplantation by real-time quantitative polymerase chain reaction. Blood 2002;99: 4618–4625.
33. Klein J, Sato A. The HLA system. First of two parts. N Engl J Med 2000;343:702–709.
34. Klein J, Sato A. The HLA system. Second of two parts. N Engl J Med 2000;343:782–786.
35. Cao K, Chopek M, Fernandez-Vina MA. High- and intermediate-resolution DNA typing systems for class I HLA-A, B, C genes by hybridization with sequence-specific oligonucleotide probes (SSOP). Rev Immunogenet 1999;1:177–208.
36. Tiu R, Gondek L, O'Keefe C, et al. Clonality of the stem cell compartment during evolution of myelodysplastic syndromes and other bone marrow failure syndromes. Leukemia 2007;21: 1648–1657.

30

Interpretation of Functional Genomics

Adrian Wiestner and Louis M. Staudt

The paradigm of "nature or nurture" juxtaposes genetically determined traits to the formative environment. When we consider gene expression in a given cell or organism, these apparent opposites converge. Genes required for cell lineage determination and genes required for cellular responses to environmental conditions are equally transcribed into RNA. Not all genes, however, are expressed in all cells at all times. Thus, the "transcriptome," the genes that are expressed in a given cell at a given time, is only a fraction of the genome. The transcriptome integrates cell lineage, cellular functions, activity of regulatory or oncogenic pathways, and response to external factors. In hematologic malignancies, the quantitative analysis of the transcriptome has revolutionized disease classification and has provided unprecedented prognostic information. DNA microarrays have been particularly successful for analyzing expression of thousands of genes in parallel (1). Here the focus is on this novel, powerful technology: we briefly review technical principles and conceptual aspects of data analysis and discuss select clinical applications of this method.

GENE EXPRESSION PROFILING ON DNA MICROARRAYS

DNA microarrays consist of solid supports onto which probes have been attached that detect the presence of a specific mRNA. Each array consists of thousands of such probes, and each probe will specifically hybridize to one distinct mRNA. To measure gene expression, mRNA is extracted from the sample of interest and labeled with a fluorescent dye. The labeled mRNA is then placed onto the array where pairing between mRNA strands and their complementary probes takes place. After this hybridization step unbound mRNAs are washed off, and the level of gene expression in the specimen can be determined by quantifying the fluorescent signal bound to a given probe. The method is highly quantitative and accurately detects changes in gene expression over 1000-fold range.

One microarray technology commonly used employs oligonucleotide probes that are synthesized directly on the solid support. These oligonucleotide arrays contain sequence specific oligonucleotide probes to detect a distinct mRNA and corresponding oligonucleotides that contain a mismatch to control for nonspecific binding. Samples are labeled with a fluorescent dye and hybridized to the array, which yields an absolute measure of mRNA abundance. Affymetrix GeneChip arrays are common commercially available oligonucleotide arrays that, depending on the specific array type, can quantify the expression of approximately 47,000 transcripts (Human Genome U133 Plus 2.0, Affymetrix, Santa Clara, CA).

Custom-made spotted microarrays are also in wide use. These arrays often contain cDNA sequences of several hundred base pairs that have been amplified by polymerase chain reaction (PCR) and are then robotically spotted onto the solid support. The template for these arrays is commonly a cDNA library derived from the tissue of interest with or without the addition of selected named genes. Alternatively, presynthesized oligonucleotides complementary to an mRNA can be spotted. Spotted DNA microarrays typically use two fluorescent channels; one channel is dedicated to the sample of interest while the second channel is used to analyze a comparator sample. The comparator mRNA can be derived from normal cells, a pool of cell lines, or a relevant control cell type. The comparator mRNA serves as a control for the performance of the hybridization as a whole and for the quality of the array probes. One example of a custom-spotted DNA microarray is the "Lymphochip," which was developed to study B-cell malignancies (2). This array contains roughly 15,000 cDNA spots representing about 12,000 genes that have been selected to represent different stages of B-cell development and different B-cell malignancies.

GENE EXPRESSION SIGNATURES IN MOLECULAR DIAGNOSIS, OUTCOME PREDICTION, AND TARGETED CANCER THERAPY

Microarray experiments typically yield several thousand data points per sample. The amount of data generated in such studies can easily overwhelm researcher and statistician alike and makes "by the eye" analysis of the data virtually impossible. A number of analytical techniques aid in the interpretation of microarray data (3–6). In a so-called unsupervised analysis, statistical methods are used to visualize patterns of shared gene expression and to identify distinct groups of samples. This approach is independent of external data. "Supervised" approaches instead rely on statistical tests to relate gene expression characteristics to known biologic or clinical characteristics.

Unsupervised Analysis: Pattern Discovery by Hierarchical Clustering

One commonly used unsupervised strategy is called hierarchical clustering (3). This analysis identifies genes that share a similar expression pattern across all samples. For example, hierarchical clustering will group genes together that are highly expressed in one group of samples and expressed at low levels in a second group. Genes that are involved in the same cellular function are often coordinately expressed and thus form a distinct "gene expression signature" of a particular biologic process (7). Gene expression signatures capture biologic characteristics including cell type, differentiation state, cellular functions, and activity of signaling pathways and thereby provide a framework in which the complexity of microarray data can be related to the biology of the study samples. Hierarchical clustering is a valuable tool to discover such patterns of coordinately expressed genes. The strength of this analysis is the focus on distinct biologic functions, represented by sets of genes contributing to the same process rather than isolated genes. For example, to proliferate, a cell simultaneously expresses a set of hundreds of genes involved in cell cycle progression, DNA replication, and metabolism, which upon hierarchical clustering can be visualized as a proliferation signature. Gene expression studies often use a single array per sample. The apparent lack of replicates is sometimes felt to make such data inferior. However, signature-based analysis strategies intrinsically are based on numerous replicates, which are more valuable biologically as opposed to technical replicates.

Hierarchical clustering can not only identify genes with coordinate expression across samples but can also group samples that share a common pattern of gene expression. The result of hierarchical clustering of samples is highly dependent on the set of genes chosen. The hierarchical clustering algorithm may be dominated by a few genes with a high degree of variability between samples, such as immunoglobulin genes in B-cell malignancies. A large set of coordinately expressed genes may have an overriding influence on the results of hierarchical clustering. For example, hundreds of genes may be differentially regulated in cells that differ in proliferation rate, and these proliferation signature genes may dominate hierarchical clustering and obscure other interesting biological differences between the samples. Therefore, it may be beneficial to narrow the list of genes considered in hierarchical clustering. With these caveats, hierarchical clustering can identify heterogeneity among tumor samples that may be very important clinically (2,8,9). Thus, hierarchical clustering is an especially useful tool for "question-driven" as opposed to "hypothesis-driven" analysis of a data set and can uncover unexpected associations.

Gene expression signatures that are experimentally defined and verified are increasingly catalogued and made available for statistical analysis (5,7,10). Signature-based analysis algorithms can provide molecular classifications of cancer types, establish prognoses, identify cancer subtypes with sensitivity to specific pharmacologic interventions, establish optimal drug combinations, and facilitate the discovery of novel pathway inhibitors. Strategies that have proven particularly effective are gene set enrichment analysis (GSEA) and the connectivity map. GSEA provides a statistical measure of the probability that a set of genes contains a predefined functional signature (6). This method can test whether gene expression difference expressed between two tumor types are due to, for example, differential activity of the NF-kB signaling pathway; similarly, the effect of a drug can be related to a distinct signaling pathway. To link these characteristic of cancer and drug, the connectivity map was developed (5). In essence, the gene expression profile is used to match tumor biology with the mechanism of action of a pharmaceutical agent. Guided by such methods, gene expression profiling is likely to transform drug development and ultimately clinical cancer therapy.

SUPERVISED ANALYSIS: BUILDING MOLECULAR PREDICTORS OF DIAGNOSIS, PROGNOSIS, AND TREATMENT RESPONSE

"Supervised" analytical methods use biologic or clinical data to search for gene expression differences that are diagnostically or prognostically most informative. To derive a molecular predictor of survival one can, for instance, use the Cox proportional hazard method to identify gene expression characteristics associated with a distinct outcome. This initial step may yield several hundred genes depending on the sample size and significance cutoffs chosen. To further organize data, hierarchical clustering can be used to identify specific gene expression signatures that reflect those biologic processes that impact on survival. The pattern of gene expression signatures represented by a molecular outcome predictor and the optimal number of genes vary between different diseases and analytical techniques. In a large study of diffuse large B-cell lymphoma (DLBCL), 17 genes representing several signatures related to differentiation, tumor proliferation, and tumor host interactions were combined to form the best prognostic score (11). In chronic lymphocytic leukemia (CLL), in contrast, a single gene, ZAP-70, was the most differentially expressed gene between biologic and prognostically distinct subtypes of the disease (12).

CHALLENGES OF GENE EXPRESSION PROFILING

Not surprisingly, a method that yields quantitative data concerning many thousands of genes in hundreds of samples poses statistical obstacles. We will focus briefly on three aspects; a recent review provides a more detailed discussion (13).

Data Reproducibility: The Value of Training and Validation Sets

The extremely large amount of data derived from gene expression studies increases the likelihood of finding chance associations between clinical variables and gene expression, increasing the likelihood that a model derived in one data set may not be reproducible in an independent data set. One approach against such overfitting problems is to randomly assign the cases in a study to two independent sets. The "training set" is used to derive the model, while the "validation set" is used to test the general applicability of the model. Because this method requires a large number of samples, a modification of this approach, termed "leave one out cross-validation" is often used. In this method, the model is derived from all samples within the study except one, and the model can then be applied to categorize the independent sample. The sample left out is rotated until all samples have served as independent validation samples. Overall, the leave one out cross-validation is less rigorous than the use of independent training and validation sets.

Multiple Testing Corrections: The Concept of False Discoveries

To analyze gene expression data, the traditional probability testing has to be corrected for the innumerable tests that can be performed on such large datasets. Because the p value is designed to test a distinct hypothesis, a correction for multiple testing is necessary to avoid numerous false positive calls. The false discovery rate (FDR) predicts the likely number of false positive discoveries within a nominally significant set of variables. The FDR is computed as the number of expected chance findings at a given p value divided by the number of observations at this significance cutoff.

Real and Apparent Discrepancies Between Different Gene Expression Studies

A quality control study sponsored by the Food and Drug Administration involving different laboratories and different array platforms found excellent reproducibility of microarray measurements. While establishing, in principle, the robustness of the method, apparent and real discrepancies between reported studies can have many reasons, including faulty annotation of probes, lack of specificity of spotted array features, technical differences in hybridization and signal detection, and different analysis strategies that seemingly yield discrepant gene lists (14). The use of different platforms may result in gene lists that only partially overlap but nevertheless capture the same biologic characteristics. Because a gene expression signature that identifies a distinct diagnostic entity or cellular process may be composed of several hundred genes, not all of which are equally represented and equally well measured on different platforms. Therefore, the rank order of these genes can substantially differ between two studies. Comparison of the entire set of differentially expressed genes, not only the top ranked genes, may be required in order to detect commonality (15). With the increasing standardization of technical platforms and more robust analysis algorithms, the reproducibility of microarray studies may already have surpassed the reproducibility of immunohistochemical or flow cytometric methods.

CLINICAL APPLICATION OF GENE EXPRESSION PROFILING

Gene expression profiling is in rapid transition from a research test to clinical application. Because of ready tissue availability, most clinical gene expression studies to date have been performed in malignancies. Table 30.1 summarizes select informative studies, and several recent reviews provide more detailed discussions (16–19); the majority of these studies are retrospective, often based on archival material, and large scale prospective studies have been initiated only recently.

Obtaining Gene Expression Profiling for Individual Patients

Gene expression profiling has generally been undertaken in large studies, often incorporating hundreds of patients, offering the possibility to view a specific sample in the context of the whole study and to assign a patient accurately to prognostic groups with a well-defined survival probability. The interpretation of a single patient's gene expression profile obtained outside of such a study and possibly obtained on a different experimental platform is a challenge, but the problem likely will be solved as algorithms for molecular diagnoses improve. Of importance, the molecular predictor of survival following treatment with a novel therapeutic agent may well be different from the survival predictor developed in retrospective studies. In addition, the interpretation of gene expression data is highly dependent on the clinical annotation of the study samples. For these reasons, patients should be enrolled in well-designed, prospective clinical trials that incorporate gene expression profiling into the trial design.

Select Prospective Clinical Trials Incorporating Gene Expression Profiling

Diffuse large B-cell non-hodgkin's lymphoma: randomized phase III study of rituximab, cyclophosphamide, adriamycin, vincristine, and prednisone (R-CHOP) compared with dose-adjusted etoposide, adriamycin, vincristine, cyclophosphamide, prednisone, and rituximab (EPOCH-R) http://www.clinicaltrials.gov/ct/show/NCT00118209?order=100

Mantle cell lymphoma: phase II study of bortezomib in combination with dose-adjusted EPOCH-R http://www.clinicaltrials.gov/ct/show/NCT00131976?order=1

T-cell large granular lymphocytic leukemia: phase II study of cyclosporine treatment http://www.clinicaltrials.gov/ct/show/NCT00363779?order=14

Chronic lymphocytic leukemia/small lymphocytic lymphoma: phase II study of lenalidomide in previously treated patients http://www.clinicaltrials.gov/ct/show/NCT00465127?order=36

Acute lymphoblastic leukemia: decitabine for relapsed, refractory disease http://www.clinicaltrials.gov/ct/show/NCT00349596?order=39

Multiple myeloma: total therapy III for newly diagnosed myeloma http://www.clinicaltrials.gov/ct/show/NCT00081939?order=9

Additional trials can be found at www.clinicaltrials.gov.

TABLE 30.1. *Select Gene Expression Profiling Studies in Hematologic Malignancies*

Diagnosis	Major Findings and Conclusions	Reference
ALL, AML	Proof or principle study that monitoring gene expression can be used to classify tumor types. In this study, an unsupervised analysis of gene expression profiles could accurately differentiate AML and ALL.	(4)
B-ALL	Identified distinct GESs for each of the cytogenetically defined prognostic subgroups of B-ALL in 360 pediatric cases and derived a molecular predictor that accurately classified patients into subgroups. Identified a novel subset of B-ALL not characterized by a diagnostic cytogenetic abnormality.	(20)
T-ALL	Showed that aberrant expression of key transcription factors is a central pathogenetic mechanism in 59 cases of T-ALL. Correlated GESs associated with overexpression of HOX11, TAL1, and LYL1 to distinct stages of T-cell differentiation and identified prognostic subgroups within T-ALL.	(21)
B-ALL	Tested leukemic cells from 173 children for drug sensitivity in vitro and derived a gene expression based score of drug resistance that predicted outcome in two independent cohorts.	(22)
AML	Within a cohort of 285 patients defined 16 subgroups of AML based on gene expression signatures. Differences were driven in large part by known chromosomal lesions, mutations, and oncogene expression, but novel subtypes with normal karyotypes were also identified. Gene expression identified a unique high-risk subgroup with very high relapse risk and a 5-year survival of 18%.	(23)
AML	Derived a gene expression outcome predictor in AML that provided improved prognostic information compared with known prognostic factors and that was equally predictive in patients with normal karyotypes as in patients with distinct cytogenetic abnormalities.	(24)
BL	Distinguished BL from DLBCL based on high expression of c-myc regulated genes and decreased expression of MHC class I and NF-kB target genes. Patients with the molecular signature of BL had a better survival when treated with intense chemotherapy regimens.	(25)
BL	Developed a gene expression based molecular diagnosis of BL that reliably identified BL. In addition, there was a group of lymphomas with intermediate signatures. Survival was better for BL than DLBCL.	(26)
CLL	Showed that CLL subtypes subdivided by immunoglobulin genotype have a common characteristic gene expression signature. Gene expression profiles related CLL B cells more to normal memory B cells than to naïve, germinal center derived, or CD5+ B cells.	(27)
CLL	Provided evidence that CLL can be viewed as a single disease characterized by a common GES. However, the two CLL subtypes, defined by immunoglobulin genotype, differentially expressed several hundred genes between subtypes, including ZAP-70.	(28)
CLL	Confirmed ZAP-70 as the most differentially expressed gene between subtypes defined by Ig-genotype in 107 patients and derived tests for its use as a prognostic marker in CLL.	(12)
CLL	Identified an in vivo fludarabine-mediated gene expression signature in CLL cells of patients undergoing the first treatment cycle and showed that the fludarabine induced gene expression signature is a p53 driven response.	(29)

TABLE 30.1. *Select Gene Expression Profiling Studies in Hematologic (continued)*

Diagnosis	Major Findings and Conclusions	Reference
DLBCL	Identified two molecularly and clinically distinct diseases within DLBCL that differentially express genes associated with different stages of B-cell differentiation. One subgroup termed Germinal Center B-cell like DLBC (GCB DLBCL) had a favorable 5-year survival and expressed genes characteristic of germinal centre B cells, while the second subgroup termed "Activated B-cell like DLBCL (ABC DLBCL)" expressed genes typically induced during activation of B cells.	(2)
DLBCL	Used supervised algorithm to define a molecular outcome predictor for 58 patients undergoing CHOP chemotherapy and identified two groups with 5-year survival rates of 70% versus 12%. Differences between microarray platforms hampered identification of DLBCL subgroups identified by Alizadeh et al (2).	(30)
DLBCL	Reproduced earlier finding of distinct subgroups in 240 patients with DLBCL and demonstrated that these subgroups have distinct oncogenic events. An outcome predictor that integrates 17 genes and confers prognostic information independent of IPI-scores with overall 5-year survival rates of 73% in the best quartile versus 15% in the lowest quartile could be derived.	(11)
DLBCL	Described a diagnostic algorithm for the classification of cancers by gene expression based on Bayesian statistics. GCB DLBCL and ABC DLBCL subgroups were identified in a set of 274 patients analyzed on the Lymphochip and in 58 independent patients profiled on Affymetrix arrays by Shipp et al (30).	(15)
FL	Derived a molecular predictor of survival based on two gene expression signatures that divided patients into 4 quartiles with median survival of 3.9, 10.8, 11.1, and 13.6 years. These signatures represent gene expression in nontumor-derived stroma and immune cells.	(31)
MCL	Described a molecular diagnosis of MCL and defined a MCL subset lacking Cyclin D1 expression. Derived a molecular measurement of tumor proliferation based on gene expression that identified quartiles of patients with a median survival ranging from 0.8, 6.7 years. Described MCL as a disease of cell cycle dysregulation with several cooperating pathogenic events.	(32)
MM	Used a supervised analysis in 532 newly diagnosed patients, identified 70 genes that were linked to early death. Five-year projected survival was 78% for the low-risk group and 28% for the high-risk. The high risk score was present in 13% of patients at diagnosis but in 76% at relapse. A subset of 17 was enough to accurately capture the prognostic information.	(33)
MM	In a set of 414 newly diagnosed patients, unsupervised analysis identifies gene expression signatures that delineate 7 MM subtypes characterized by distinct genetic lesions and variable clinical characteristics. Low-risk disease (4 subtypes) has a projected 4-year survival of 79% compared with high-risk disease (3 subtypes) with 51%.	(9)
PMBL	Identified PMBL as a molecularly distinct subgroup of DLBCL with a favorable prognosis and defined a molecular diagnosis of PMBL based on the expression of 46 genes. Provided evidence of a relationship between PMBL and Hodgkin lymphoma.	(34)
PMBL	Defined PMBL as a distinct subtype of DLBCL characterized by low expression of components of the B-cell receptor signaling pathway and expression of genes also expressed in Reed-Sternberg cells of Hodgkin lymphoma.	(35)

ALL, acute lymphocytic leukemia; AML, acute myelogenous leukemia; B-ALL, acute B-cell lymphoblastic leukemia; BL, Burkitt's lymphoma; CHOP, cyclophosphamide, adriamycin, vincristine, and prednisone; CLL, chronic lymphocytic leukemia; DLBCL, diffuse large B-cell lymphoma; FL, follicular lymphoma; GES: gene expression signature; Ig: immunoglobulin gene; IPI, international prognostic index; MCL, mantle cell lymphoma; MHC, major histocompatibility complex; MM, multiple myeloma; PMBL, primary mediastinal B-cell lymphoma; T-ALL, acute T-cell lymphoblastic leukemia.

OUTLOOK

In the near future, one may expect the routine use of DNA microarrays in the clinical laboratory. While it is possible to translate some of the insights gained from gene expression profiling into tests such as immunohistochemistry or flow cytometry, the number of genes necessary for the best molecular classification is rapidly expanding, making these other diagnostic techniques perhaps temporary measures. Such conventional methods are semiquantitative, while gene expression profiling is highly quantitative, capable of making precise molecular diagnoses and yielding important prognostic information. Besides providing an unprecedented amount of data, the use of arrays in the clinical laboratory could simplify and standardize diagnostic testing on a single technical platform that yields information currently obtained only from several different techniques. In addition, microarrays provide a digital fingerprint of a specimen that can be analyzed by computer-based diagnostic algorithms and easily stored. Such data will not only accelerate the transition to a molecular diagnosis of cancer but will also lead to more effective treatment through individualized cancer therapy.

REFERENCES

1. Staudt LM. Molecular diagnosis of the hematologic cancers. N Engl J Med 2003;348:1777–1785.
2. Alizadeh AA, Eisen MB, Davis RE, et al. Distinct types of diffuse large B-cell lymphoma identified by gene expression profiling. Nature 2000;403:503–511.
3. Eisen MB, Spellman PT, Brown PO, et al. Cluster analysis and display of genome-wide expression patterns. Proc Natl Acad Sci U S A 1998;95:14863–14868.
4. Golub TR, Slonim DK, Tamayo P, et al. Molecular classification of cancer: class discovery and class prediction by gene expression monitoring. Science 1999;286:531–537.
5. Lamb J, Crawford ED, Peck D, et al. The Connectivity Map: using gene-expression signatures to connect small molecules, genes, and disease. Science 2006;313:1929–1935.
6. Subramanian A, Tamayo P, Mootha VK, et al. Gene set enrichment analysis: a knowledge-based approach for interpreting genome-wide expression profiles. Proc Natl Acad Sci U S A 2005;102: 15545–15550.
7. Shaffer AL, Wright G, Yang L, et al. A library of gene expression signatures to illuminate normal and pathological lymphoid biology. Immunol Rev 2006;210:67–85.
8. Valk PJ, Delwel R, Lowenberg B. Gene expression profiling in acute myeloid leukemia. Curr Opin Hematol 2005;12:76–81.
9. Zhan F, Huang Y, Colla S, et al. The molecular classification of multiple myeloma. Blood 2006;108:2020–2028.
10. Nevins JR, Potti A. Mining gene expression profiles: expression signatures as cancer phenotypes. Nat Rev Genet 2007;8:601–609.
11. Rosenwald A, Wright G, Chan WC, et al. The use of molecular profiling to predict survival after chemotherapy for diffuse large-B-cell lymphoma. N Engl J Med 2002;346:1937–1947.
12. Wiestner A, Rosenwald A, Barry TS, et al. ZAP-70 expression identifies a chronic lymphocytic leukemia subtype with unmutated immunoglobulin genes, inferior clinical outcome, and distinct gene expression profile. Blood 2003;101:4944–4951.
13. Tinker AV, Boussioutas A, Bowtell DD. The challenges of gene expression microarrays for the study of human cancer. Cancer Cell 2006;9:333–339.
14. Sotiriou C, Piccart MJ. Taking gene-expression profiling to the clinic: when will molecular signatures become relevant to patient care? Nat Rev Cancer 2007;7:545–553.
15. Wright G, Tan B, Rosenwald A, et al. A gene expression-based method to diagnose clinically distinct subgroups of diffuse large B-cell lymphoma. Proc Natl Acad Sci U S A 2003;100:9991–9996.
16. Bullinger L. Gene expression profiling in acute myeloid leukemia. Haematologica 2006;91: 733–738.
17. Rizzatti EG, Wiestner A. Underlying mechanisms of hematologic malignancies revealed by gene expression profiling. Drug Discov Today Dis Mech 2006;3:507–514.
18. Wiestner A, Staudt LM. Towards molecular diagnosis and targeted therapy of lymphoid malignancies. Semin Hematol 2003;40:296–307.

19. Zhan F, Barlogie B, Shaughnessy J Jr. Toward the identification of distinct molecular and clinical entities of multiple myeloma using global gene expression profiling. Semin Hematol 2003;40: 308–320.
20. Yeoh E-J, Ross ME, Shurtleff SA, et al. Classification, subtype discovery, and prediction of outcome in pediatric acute lymphblastic leukemia by gene expression profiling. Cancer Cell 2002;1: 133–143.
21. Ferrando AA, Neuberg DS, Staunton J, et al. Gene expression signatures define novel oncogenic pathways in T-cell acute lymphoblastic leukemia. Cancer Cell 2002;1:75–87.
22. Holleman A, Cheok MH, den Boer ML, et al. Gene-expression patterns in drug-resistant acute lymphoblastic leukemia cells and response to treatment. N Engl J Med 2004;351:533–542.
23. Valk PJ, Verhaak RG, Beijen MA, et al. Prognostically useful gene-expression profiles in acute myeloid leukemia. N Engl J Med 2004;350:1617–1628.
24. Bullinger L, Dohner K, Bair E, et al. Use of gene-expression profiling to identify prognostic subclasses in adult acute myeloid leukemia. N Engl J Med 2004;350:1605–1616.
25. Dave SS, Fu K, Wright GW, et al. Molecular diagnosis of Burkitt's lymphoma. N Engl J Med 2006;354:2431–2442.
26. Hummel M, Bentink S, Berger H, et al. A biologic definition of Burkitt's lymphoma from transcriptional and genomic profiling. N Engl J Med 2006;354:2419–2430.
27. Klein U, Tu Y, Stolovitzky GA, et al. Gene expression profiling of B-cell chronic lymphocytic leukemia reveals a homogeneous phenotype related to memory B cells. J Exp Med 2001;194: 1625–1638.
28. Rosenwald A, Alizadeh AA, Widhopf G, et al. Relation of gene expression phenotype to immunoglobulin mutation genotype in B-cell chronic lymphocytic leukemia. J Exp Med 2001;194: 1639–1647.
29. Rosenwald A, Chuang EY, Davis RE, et al. Fludarabine treatment of patients with chronic lymphocytic leukemia induces a p53-dependent gene expression response. Blood 2004;104:1428–1434.
30. Shipp MA, Ross KN, Tamayo P, et al. Diffuse large B-cell lymphoma outcome prediction by gene-expression profiling and supervised machine learning. Nat Med 2002;8:68–74.
31. Dave SS, Wright G, Tan B, et al. Prediction of survival in follicular lymphoma based on molecular features of tumor-infiltrating immune cells. N Engl J Med 2004;351:2159–2169.
32. Rosenwald A, Wright G, Wiestner A, et al. The proliferation gene expression signature is a quantitative integrator of oncogenic events that predicts survival in mantle cell lymphoma. Cancer Cell 2003;3:185–197.
33. Shaughnessy JD Jr., Zhan F, Burington BE, et al. A validated gene expression model of high-risk multiple myeloma is defined by deregulated expression of genes mapping to chromosome 1. Blood 2007;109:2276–2284.
34. Rosenwald A, Wright G, Leroy K, et al. Molecular diagnosis of primary mediastinal B-cell lymphoma identifies a clinically favorable subgroup of diffuse large B-cell lymphoma related to Hodgkin lymphoma. J Exp Med 2003;198:851–862.
35. Savage KJ, Monti S, Kutok JL, et al. The molecular signature of mediastinal large B-cell lymphoma differs from that of other diffuse large B-cell lymphomas and shares features with classical Hodgkin lymphoma. Blood 2003;102:3871–3879.

Appendix
Cytokines Approved for Clinical Use

Pierre Noel

ERYTHROPOIETIN (EPOIETIN ALFA, PROCRIT™, EPOGEN™)

Epoietin alfa (EPO) Indications

- Anemia of chronic renal failure patients (Dialysis [+] or dialysis [−]).
- Anemia in zidovudine-treated human immunodeficiency virus (HIV)-infected patients.
- Anemia in patients undergoing chemotherapy.
- Reduction of allogeneic blood transfusions in surgical patients.

In adult patients with chronic renal failure (CRF), doses of 50 to 100 U/kg 3 times weekly are required to maintain a hematocrit in the mid- to high 30s. The intravenous (IV) route of administration is recommended in dialysis patients; the IV or subcutaneous (SC) administration routes can be utilized in patients with CRF not undergoing hemodialysis. Patients with CRF treated with EPO experienced an increased risk of serious cardiovascular disease when treated to target higher hemoglobin levels. The dose of EPO should be individualized to achieve and maintain hemoglobin levels between 10 and 12 g/dL and should be reduced in patients who respond rapidly (>1 g/dL increase in hemoglobin over a period of 2 weeks) to minimize the risk of serious cardiovascular events. In zidovudine-treated adult patients with HIV with a serum erythropoietin of <500 mU/ml who are receiving a dose of zidovudine <4200 mg/week, the recommended starting dose is 100 U/kg as an IV or SC injection 3 times a week for 8 weeks. The dose of EPO should be titrated to avoid transfusions and not to exceed a hemoglobin of 12 g/dL. Patients with endogenous erythropoietin levels >500 mU/ml are unlikely to respond to EPO. In adult anemic cancer patients undergoing chemotherapy, the initial recommended dose of EPO is 150 U/kg SC three times a week or 40,000 U subcutaneously (SC) weekly. Therapy should not be initiated if the hemoglobin is >10 g/dL. Patients with serum erythropoietin levels >200 mU/mL are unlikely to respond to EPO. In some recent clinical studies erythropoiesis stimulating agents (ESA) shortened overall survival and/or increased the risk of tumor progression or recurrence in patients with breast, nonsmall cell lung, head and neck, lymphoid, and cervical cancers; because of these findings, EPO use is not recommended in patients receiving myelosuppressive therapy when the anticipated outcome is cure. In adult surgical patients, the reduction of allogeneic transfusion can be achieved with an EPO dose of 300 IU/kg/day for 10 days prior to surgery, on the day of surgery, and for 4 days after surgery. An alternate dose schedule is 600 U/kg SC in once-a-week doses starting 3 weeks prior to surgery plus a fourth dose on the day of surgery. All patients should receive iron supplementation. The preoperative hemoglobin should be between 10 and 13 g/dL. In surgical patients not receiving prophylactic anticoagulation, EPO increased the rate of deep venous thrombosis. Deep venous thrombosis prophylaxis should be considered in this setting.

Prior to and during treatment with EPO, the patient's iron stores should be evaluated. Most patients require iron supplementation during therapy with EPO. Blood pressure may rise during treatment of anemia with EPO; hypertension should be controlled before initiation of therapy. The hemoglobin levels need to be monitored regularly while patients are being treated with EPO.

Allergic reactions and antibody mediated pure red cell aplasia have been associated with the use of EPO. EPO contains albumin; it carries a very small risk of transmission of viral diseases.

DARBEPOIETIN ALFA (ARANESP™)

Darbepoietin alfa differs from recombinant human EPO by having sialylated carbohydrate content increasing the molecular weight, prolonging its half-life and increasing its biologic in vivo activity.

Darbepoietin alfa is indicated for the treatment of anemia with chronic renal failure and the treatment of anemia associated with nonmyeloid malignancies because of chemotherapy. In adult patients with anemia associated with renal failure, the recommended starting dose is 0.45 mcg/kg administered intravenously (IV) or SC once per week. Alternatively, in patients not undergoing hemodialysis an initial dose of 0.75 μg/kg may be administered SC once every 2 weeks.

Darbepoietin alfa has been associated with an increased risk of cardiovascular events in patients with chronic renal failure. The risk of cardiovascular events is higher in patients who have target hemoglobin of 14 g/dL compared with patients who have target hemoglobin of 10 g/dL. The dose should be titrated to achieve and maintain target hemoglobin of 10 to 12 g/dL. In patients with nonmyeloid cancer receiving chemotherapy the recommended doses of darbepoietin alfa are 2.25 μ/kg SC weekly or 500 mcg SC every 3 weeks. Therapy should not be initiated at hemoglobin levels >10 g/dL. The goal of darbepoietin alfa treatment in the cancer setting is to avoid transfusions.

Blood pressure may rise during treatment of anemia with darbepoietin alfa; hypertension should be controlled before initiation of therapy.

Seizures and serious cardiovascular events have been reported in patients who had a rapid rate of increase in hemoglobin; the dose of darbepoietin alfa should be reduced if the hemoglobin increase exceeds 1.0g/dL in any 2-week period.

Clinical studies in cancer patients treated with erythropoiesis stimulating agents reported shortened overall survival and/or increase in the risk of tumor progression in patients with breast, nonsmall cell lung, head and neck, lymphoid and cervical cancer; because of these findings, darbepoietin alfa use is not recommended in patients receiving myelosuppressive therapy when the anticipated outcome is cure.

Darbepoietin alfa is supplied in two formulations: one containing polysorbate 80 and another containing albumin. Albumin is associated with a small risk of transmitting viral diseases.

METHOXY POLYETHYLENE GLYCOL-EPOETIN BETA (MICERA™)

Methoxy polyethylene glycol-epoetin beta is a continuous erythropoietin receptor activator (C.E.R.A) that can be administered monthly. It has an extended half-life of 130 hours and a low clearance as well as unique receptor-binding properties.

Methoxy polyethylene glycol-epoetin beta is indicated in the treatment of anemia associated with chronic renal disease. The recommended starting dose in patients not currently treated with an erythropoiesis stimulating agent is 0.6 μg/kg once every 2 weeks IV or SC.

The warnings and precautions that apply to all erythropoiesis stimulating agents also apply to methoxy polyethylene glycol-epoetin beta (pure red cell aplasia, cardiovascular events, hypertension, effect on tumor growth).

GRANULOCYTE COLONY-STIMULATING FACTOR (G-CSF, FILGRASTIM, NEUPOGEN™)

Filgrastim regulates the production of neutrophils within the bone marrow and also impacts on their function.

Granulocyte Colony-Stimulating Factor Indications

- Nonmyeloid malignancies undergoing myelosuppressive chemotherapy with an expected risk of severe neutropenia and fever.
- Acute myeloid leukemia, following induction or consolidation therapy.
- Nonmyeloid malignancies undergoing myeloablative chemotherapy followed by marrow transplantation.
- Mobilization of peripheral blood hematopoietic cells.
- Severe chronic neutropenia.

Granulocyte colony stimulating factor (G-CSF) can be administered SC or IV; the usual recommended dose is 5 μg/kg per day.

Patients treated with G-CSF have experienced allergic-type reactions, severe sickle-cell crises, bone pain, splenomegaly, and splenic rupture. G-CSF has the potential of stimulating the proliferation of myeloid leukemic cells.

PEGYLATED GRANULOCYTE COLONY-STIMULATING FACTOR (PEGFILGRATIM, NEULASTA™)

Pegfilgrastim is produced by covalently conjugating a 20-kd polyethylene glycol molecule to the N-terminus of filgrastim. The pegfilgrastim molecule is larger than the threshold for renal clearance, prolonging its half-life in circulation.

Pelfilgrastim is indicated to decrease the incidence of febrile neutropenia in patients with non-myeloid malignancies receiving myelosuppressive chemotherapy associated with a clinically significant incidence of febrile neutropenia. The adult recommended dose is 6 mg SC administered once per chemotherapy cycle.

Splenic rupture, adult respiratory distress syndrome, allergic reactions, severe sickle-cell crises, and proliferation of myeloid leukemic cells have been described in patients treated with filgrastim, which is the parent compound of pegfilgrastim.

GRANULOCYTE-MACROPHAGE COLONY-STIMULATING FACTOR (GM-CSF, SARGRAMOSTIM, LEUKINE™)

Sargramostim induces a dose-dependant increase in neutrophils and, to a lesser extent, monocytes and eosinophils. When GM-CSF is discontinued, the leukocyte counts decrease to pretreatment levels over 3 to 5 days.

Granulocyte-Macrophage Colony Stimulating Factor Indications

- Following induction chemotherapy in patients with acute myeloid leukemia over the age of 55.
- Mobilization of peripheral blood hematopoietic progenitor cells.
- Myeloid reconstitution following autologous bone marrow transplantation for non-Hodgkin's lymphoma, Hodgkin's lymphoma, and acute lymphoblastic leukemia.
- Myeloid reconstitution after allogeneic marrow transplantation.
- Allogeneic and autologous bone marrow transplantation engraftment failure or engraftment delay.

GM-CSF can be administered SC or IV. The usual daily recommended dose is 250 μg/m^2.

The use of GM-CSF is potentially associated with fluid retention, capillary leak syndrome, pleural and pericardial effusions, sequestration of granulocytes in the pulmonary circulation, supraventricular arrhythmias, as well as renal and hepatic dysfunction. GM-CSF has the potential to stimulate the proliferation of myeloid leukemic cells.

INTERLEUKIN-11 (OPRELVEKIN, NEUMEGA™)

Oprelvekin is a thrombopoietic growth factor that stimulates the proliferation of megakaryocytic progenitors and induces megakaryocyte maturation; it also promotes the integrity of gastrointestinal mucosal epithelial cells.

Oprelvekin stimulates platelet production in a dose-dependent manner with peak platelet counts 14 to 21 days following its administration.

Oprelvekin is indicated for the prevention of severe thrombocytopenia in patients with nonmyeloid malignancies undergoing myelosuppressive chemotherapy. Oprelvekin is not recommended for use following myeloablative chemotherapy.

The usual recommended dosage is 50 μg/kg given once a day SC. The use of Oprelvekin has been associated with allergic or hypersensitivity reactions, including anaphylaxis, papilledema, fluid retention, edema, arrhythmias, pleural effusions, and electrolyte imbalances.

ROMIPLOSTIM (NPLATE™)

Romiplostim is a thrombopoietin receptor agonist indicated for the treatment of thrombocytopenia in patients with chronic immune idiopathic thrombocytopenia who have had an inadequate response to corticosteroids, immunoglobulins, or splenectomy.

The recommended initial dose is 1 μg/kg once a week SC followed by weekly dose adjustments based on response.

It is recommended to use the lowest dose of Romiplostim to achieve and maintain a platelet count >50,000/ μL as necessary to reduce the risk of bleeding.

Romiplostim is associated with an increased risk of marrow fibrosis secondary to reticulin fiber deposition.

Index

Page numbers in italic denote figures; those followed by *t* denote tables